PHOTO GUIDE OF
NURSING SKILLS

PHOTO GUIDE OF
NURSING SKILLS

Sandra F. Smith, RN, MS, ABD
National Nursing Review

Donna J. Duell, RN, MS, ABD
Cabrillo College

Barbara C. Martin, RN, MS, CS
University of Tulsa

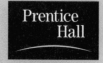

Prentice
Hall

Upper Saddle River, New Jersey 07458

Library of Congress Cataloging-in-Publication Data

Smith, Sandra Fucci.
    Photo guide of nursing skills / Sandra F. Smith, Donna
J. Duell, Barbara C. Martin.
        p.   cm.
    Includes bibliographical references and index.
    ISBN 0-8385-8174-9
    1. Nursing—Atlases.   2. Nursing assessment—
Atlases.   3. Physical diagnosis—Atlases.   I. Duell,
Donna, 1938–   II. Martin, Barbara, M.S.   III. Title.
    [DNLM: 1. Nursing Process—Atlases.   2. Nursing
Care—methods—Atlases. WY 17 S659p 2001]
RT48.S64 2001
610.73'022'2—dc21

                                                        2001021434

Publisher: Julie Alexander
Executive Editor: Maura Connor
Acquisitions Editor: Nancy Anselment
Development Editor: Sue Bredensteiner
Editorial Assistant: Mary Ellen Ruitenberg
Marketing Manager: Nicole Benson
**Director of Manufacturing
 and Production:** Bruce Johnson
Managing Editor: Patrick Walsh
Production Editor: North Market Street Graphics
Production Liaison: Cathy O'Connell
Manufacturing Manager: Ilene Sanford
Photographer: Ron May Photography
Interior Art: Janet Bollow and Stephen Chapot
Creative Director: Maria Guglielmo
Cover Design: Joe Sengotta
Interior Design: Wanda España
Composition: North Market Street Graphics
Printing and Binding: Banta, Menasha

Pearson Education LTD.
Pearson Education Australia PTY, Limited
Pearson Education Singapore, Pte. Ltd.
Pearson Education North Asia Ltd.
Pearson Education Canada, Ltd.
Pearson Educaciòn de Mexico, S.A. de C.V.
Pearson Education—Japan
Pearson Education Malaysia, Pte. Ltd.
Pearson Education, Upper Saddle River, New Jersey

Notice: Care has been taken to confirm the accuracy of information presented in this book. The authors, editors, and the publisher, however, cannot accept any responsibility for errors or omissions or for consequences from application of the information in this book and make no warranty, express or implied, with respect to its contents.

The authors and publisher have exerted every effort to ensure that drug selections and dosages set forth in this text are in accord with current recommendations and practice at time of publication. However, in view of ongoing research, changes in government regulations, and the constant flow of information relating to drug therapy and drug reactions, the reader is urged to check the package inserts of all drugs for any change in indications of dosage and for added warnings and precautions. This is particularly important when the recommended agent is a new and/or infrequently employed drug.

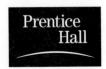

10 9 8 7 6 5 4 3 2
ISBN 0-8385-8174-9

CONTENTS

UNIT V.   SKIN AND TISSUE INTEGRITY   247

CHAPTER 10.   HEAT AND COLD   249

CHAPTER 11.   WOUND CARE AND DRESSINGS   271

UNIT VI. MOBILITY

CHAPTER 12. BODY MECHANICS AND POSITIONING

CHAPTER 13. EXERCISE AND AMBULATION

CHAPTER 22. BOWEL ELIMINATION

UNIT XI. OXYGENATION AND CIRCULATION

CHAPTER 23. RESPIRATORY SKILLS

PREFACE

Photo Guide of Nursing Skills has been designed to present nursing skills in a unique format: step-by-step photographs of essential skills that student nurses learn as part of their professional education. Mastery of this content is critical, since much of the time that nurses spend with clients is devoted to skill performance. There is no easier way to learn and master a skill than to visualize it as a step-by-step sequential process. This format enables the student to see, rather than just read about, each skill.

The authors have separated the skills into units containing chapters that progress from basic to intermediate level of difficulty. Each chapter includes introductory material providing the theoretical foundation necessary to understand the skill components; step-by-step photos and/or line drawings depicting each skill; clinical notes and safety alerts—additional information necessary for skill mastery; and Beyond the Skill material as an adjunct to the skill itself.

Key features include:

- More than 1300 full-color photos and line drawings, with minimal accompanying text, illustrate over 300 step-by-step procedures. This book, including essential basic to intermediate level skills, will serve as a useful supplement to any textbook that addresses fundamental concepts of nursing.

- Text material that includes quick-reference clinical content, safety alerts, charts and tables, and Beyond the Skill adjunct material to supplement the individual steps for each skill.

- A Critical Thinking Focus section at the end of each unit. Exercises focus on nursing competencies to assist learners in integrating knowledge, judgment, and skill. A section on unexpected outcomes and alternative nursing actions assists students in analyzing outcomes and contributes to rational problem solving and decision making. A self-check evaluation section is included at the end of each chapter.

- Clear, logical, and straightforward page layout and presentation of material. This allows the student to learn the steps of skill performance with minimal reliance on the text copy.

Photo Guide of Nursing Skills is a heavily illustrated, full-color presentation of necessary basic and intermediate skills for students enrolled in all types of nursing programs. This book provides a useful supplement to any text that focuses on basic nursing concepts, and will especially assist those individuals who learn most efficiently through visual cues rather than by verbal means.

The three authors, after completing the fifth edition of *Clinical Nursing Skills,* realized that a different type of skills textbook would fill a gap at the fundamental level of nursing education. As a result of many long hours of discussion, they elected to present essential skills in an illustrated format with a step-by-step approach for students who learn more easily through visualization. Thus, the creation of this photo guide.

The authors wish to thank all those who helped and contributed to this textbook, including Ron May, the photographer; Karen Hoxeng, the project concept director; the various editors and proofreaders; the indexer; and the reviewers of the text.

TEXT FEATURES/PEDAGOGY

Anyone preparing for a career in nursing, or providing health care at home, will benefit from this full-color visual presentation of all basic and intermediate nursing procedures. The unique and easy-to-follow format divides each procedure into logical steps, complete with appropriate illustrations, descriptions, and rationales. A strong emphasis on *critical thinking throughout the text*

helps students "think outside the box" by identifying a variety of unexpected patient responses and applying the appropriate nursing action.

As the title *Photo Guide to Nursing Skills* implies, this book provides an illustrated "how to" of basic and intermediate nursing skills. The clean design and efficient use of photos and illustrations enables students to see, rather than read about each skill.

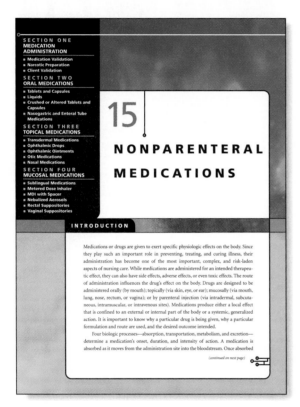

Every **chapter** opens with a summary of the preparation and completion protocols to orient the student and provide a review tool.

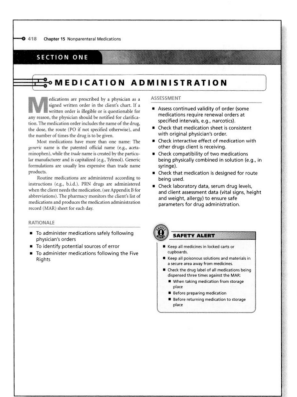

Each **section** opens with a list of specific rationales and assessment bullets to reinforce the content presented.

Each skill is presented with an equipment list and follows an easy step-by-step format with a color photo or line art illustration. There are over 1300 full-color illustrations and photos in the text.

Glove Icons remind the student that gloves are needed starting at the appropriate step

Clinical Notes highlight important information about clinical practice and patient care

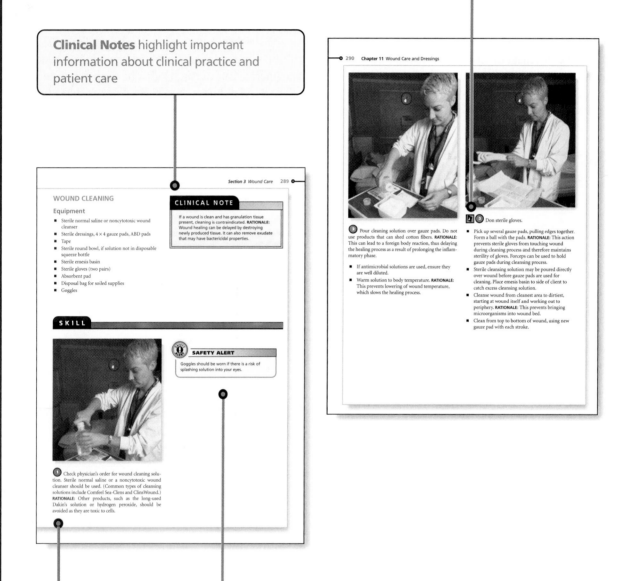

WOUND CLEANING

Equipment

- Sterile normal saline or noncytotoxic wound cleanser
- Sterile dressings, 4 × 4 gauze pads, ABD pads
- Tape
- Sterile round bowl, if solution not in disposable squeeze bottle
- Sterile emesis basin
- Sterile gloves (two pairs)
- Absorbent pad
- Disposal bag for soiled supplies
- Goggles

CLINICAL NOTE

If a wound is clean and has granulation tissue present, cleaning is contraindicated. **RATIONALE:** Wound healing can be delayed by destroying newly produced tissue. It can also remove exudate that may have bactericidal properties.

SKILL

SAFETY ALERT

Goggles should be worn if there is a risk of splashing solution into your eyes.

① Check physician's order for wound cleaning solution. Sterile normal saline or a noncytotoxic wound cleanser should be used. (Common types of cleansing solutions include Comfeel Sea-Clens and ClinsWound.) **RATIONALE:** Other products, such as the long-used Dakin's solution or hydrogen peroxide, should be avoided as they are toxic to cells.

② Pour cleaning solution over gauze pads. Do not use products that can shed cotton fibers. **RATIONALE:** This can lead to a foreign body reaction, thus delaying the healing process as a result of prolonging the inflammatory phase.

- If antimicrobial solutions are used, ensure they are well diluted.
- Warm solution to body temperature. **RATIONALE:** This prevents lowering of wound temperature, which slows the healing process.

③ Don sterile gloves.

- Pick up several gauze pads, pulling edges together. Form a ball with the pads. **RATIONALE:** This action prevents sterile gloves from touching wound during cleaning process and therefore maintains sterility of gloves. Forceps can be used to hold gauze pads during cleansing process.
- Sterile cleansing solution may be poured directly over wound before gauze pads are used for cleaning. Place emesis basin to side of client to catch excess cleansing solution.
- Cleanse wound from cleanest area to dirtiest, starting at wound itself and working out to periphery. **RATIONALE:** This prevents bringing microorganisms into wound bed.
- Clean from top to bottom of wound, using new gauze pad with each stroke.

Rationales for each step are presented in bold type to help students identify and connect the *why* behind the *how*

Safety Alerts emphasize necessary precautions and warnings to ensure optimum patient care

Beyond the Skill focus on skills that the student should be aware of but may not use in initial clinical practice

BEYOND THE SKILL

ALTERNATE METHODS FOR BLOOD PRESSURE

By Palpation
1. Palpate brachial artery while inflating cuff to 30 mm Hg above level at which radial artery pulsations are no longer felt.
2. Slowly release pressure, noting first palpated beat. **RATIONALE:** First palpated beat is systolic pressure and should be same point at which last pulsation was felt when inflating cuff.
3. Remove cuff and note palpated systolic pressure.

By Electronic Robotic Unit
Follow steps 1 to 5 for taking a blood pressure.
6. Inflate cuff (while palpating radial artery) to level 30 mm Hg above level at which radial pulsations are no longer felt. Note reading on manometer. **RATIONALE:** This procedure assures that cuff is inflated to pressure exceeding client's systolic pressure.
7. Deflate cuff and wait 60 sec to clear venous congestion (often, steps 6 and 7 are not done in clinical practice).
8. Inflate cuff to level 30 mm Hg above palpated systolic pressure.
9. Deflate cuff gradually at constant rate by opening valve on pump (2 mm Hg/sec). Systolic and diastolic readings will register digitally on readout panel. **RATIONALE:** Slower or faster deflation may yield false readings.

By Continuous-Monitoring Device
1. Attach cuff to air hose by firmly pushing valve from cuff into air hose and twisting to secure fit.
2. Wrap cuff securely around extremity (usually arm).
3. Position extremity at level of heart. **RATIONALE:** Allows for accurate reading; if arm is below heart level, reading will be higher than normal.
4. Turn power switch ON. Set arterial pressure alarm limits by pushing *alarm* button to ON and both HIGH and LOW parameters by depressing *alarm* button until parameters read out on digital display. **RATIONALE:** Alarm parameters provide safety factor by alerting nurse when reading exceeds parameters.
5. Press *start* button for approximately 4 sec. **RATIONALE:** Activates printer for readout of blood pressure, including systolic, diastolic, mean arterial pressure, and heart rate.
6. Press *start* button again to begin timed blood pressure reading.

BEYOND THE SKILL

Drainage Pouches for Wounds

Pouches or drainage bags are used for the following purposes:
1. Collecting drainage, particularly if it is excessive
2. Measuring drainage
3. Protecting skin from drainage
4. Containing drainage
5. Containing microorganisms to decrease their spread to other areas
6. Decreasing frequency of dressing changes

Care for clients with drainage bags includes the following:
1. Don clean gloves.
2. Remove dressings and place in disposal bag.
3. Measure drainage from pouches, as ordered.
4. Remove clean gloves and don sterile gloves.
5. Clean drain site with sterile cleansing solution and cotton applicator sticks or forceps and cotton balls. Use new applicator sticks or cotton balls for each site.
6. Apply sterile dressings as ordered. Drainage pouches may be left open for assessment.

Charting is reinforced at the end of every section to provide students with information on what is important to document

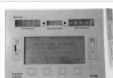

Set temperature control at 98.6°F (37°C). Lower temperature 2 to 3°F every 15 min until 90°F is reached (or set temperature according to physician's order or hospital policy). Keep blanket on at set temperature until client's body temperature is close to normal. Gradually increase blanket temperature over 6 hrs or turn machine off and monitor client's temperature. **RATIONALE:** Determines client's ability to maintain body temperature without use of cooling blanket.

- Remove cooling blanket when client's temperature is stabilized.

SAFETY ALERT

Maintain safety measures for clients on hypothermia blankets by using these guidelines:

- Monitor client's body temperature every 15 min. (This is automatically recorded when rectal temperature probe is used.)
- Check automatic temperature control for accuracy every 4 hrs by taking client's temperature with external thermometer. Use appropriate type of thermometer (oral, rectal, axillary) based on client's condition.
- Monitor all vital signs every 30 min during hypothermia treatment. Monitor every 2 hrs for 24 hrs after treatment is discontinued.
- Monitor with ECG if client has cardiac condition.
- Observe client closely for signs of shivering (ECG muscle tremor artifact, visible facial muscle twitching, hyperventilation, verbalized sensations). If shivering occurs, obtain order for IV medications (usually chlorpromazine). **RATIONALE:** Shivering increases heat production by thermogenesis.
- Observe obese clients for fluid balance alterations.
- Check physician's orders for and apply thigh-high support stockings, because stockings prevent venous stasis.
- Monitor client's skin condition and bony prominences every 2 hrs. **RATIONALE:** Client is at risk for altered tissue integrity when skin temperature is low and skin is moist.
- Observe client for signs of edema, particularly dependent edema. **RATIONALE:** Edema can be caused by increased cellular permeability, acidotic shock due to shivering, fluid imbalance, or hypothermia.

CHARTING

- Client's vital signs, particularly temperature
- Untoward effects of treatment and actions taken
- Settings on cooling blanket
- Condition of skin

Each chapter concludes with a **Self-Check Evaluation.** This well-designed review tool helps students cement their knowledge base by reviewing the material in three different ways through:

■ Matching Terms
■ Multiple Choice Questions
■ Critical Thinking Application

Answers found at the back of the text reinforce the learning process.

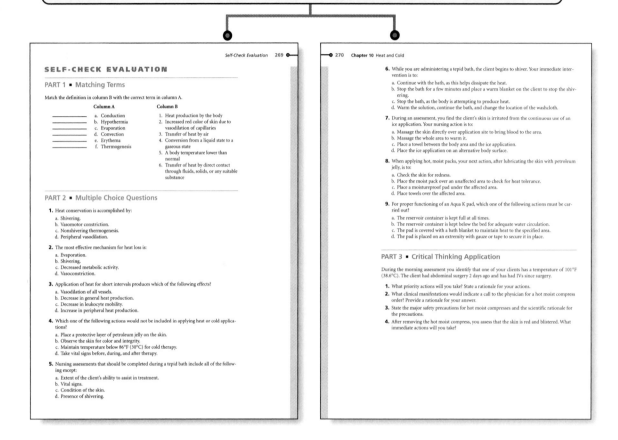

SELF-CHECK EVALUATION

PART 1 ■ Matching Terms

Match the definition in column B with the correct term in column A.

Column A	Column B
a. Conduction	1. Heat production by the body
b. Hypothermia	2. Increased red color of skin due to vasodilation of capillaries
c. Evaporation	3. Transfer of heat by air
d. Convection	4. Conversion from a liquid state to a gaseous state
e. Erythema	5. A body temperature lower than normal
f. Thermogenesis	6. Transfer of heat by direct contact through fluids, solids, or any suitable substance

PART 2 ■ Multiple Choice Questions

1. Heat conservation is accomplished by:
  a. Shivering.
  b. Vasomotor constriction.
  c. Nonshivering thermogenesis.
  d. Peripheral vasodilation.

2. The most effective mechanism for heat loss is:
  a. Evaporation.
  b. Shivering.
  c. Decreased metabolic activity.
  d. Vasoconstriction.

3. Application of heat for short intervals produces which of the following effects?
  a. Vasodilation of all vessels.
  b. Decrease in general heat production.
  c. Decrease in leukocyte mobility.
  d. Increase in peripheral heat production.

4. Which one of the following actions would not be included in applying heat or cold applications?
  a. Place a protective layer of petroleum jelly on the skin.
  b. Observe the skin for color and integrity.
  c. Maintain temperature below 86°F (30°C) for cold therapy.
  d. Take vital signs before, during, and after therapy.

5. Nursing assessments that should be completed during a tepid bath include all of the following except:
  a. Extent of the client's ability to assist in treatment.
  b. Vital signs.
  c. Condition of the skin.
  d. Presence of shivering.

6. While you are administering a tepid bath, the client begins to shiver. Your immediate intervention is to:
  a. Continue with the bath, as this helps dissipate the heat.
  b. Stop the bath for a few minutes and place a warm blanket on the client to stop the shivering.
  c. Stop the bath, as the body is attempting to produce heat.
  d. Warm the solution, continue the bath, and change the location of the washcloth.

7. During an assessment, you find the client's skin is irritated from the continuous use of an ice application. Your nursing action is to:
  a. Massage the skin directly over application site to bring blood to the area.
  b. Massage the whole area to warm it.
  c. Place a towel between the body area and the ice application.
  d. Place the ice application on an alternative body surface.

8. When applying hot, moist packs, your next action, after lubricating the skin with petroleum jelly, is to:
  a. Check the skin for redness.
  b. Place the moist pack over an unaffected area to check for heat tolerance.
  c. Place a moistureproof pad under the affected area.
  d. Place towels over the affected area.

9. For proper functioning of an Aqua K pad, which one of the following actions must be carried out?
  a. The reservoir container is kept full at all times.
  b. The reservoir container is kept below the bed for adequate water circulation.
  c. The pad is covered with a bath blanket to maintain heat to the specified area.
  d. The pad is placed on an extremity with gauze or tape to secure it in place.

PART 3 ■ Critical Thinking Application

During the morning assessment you identify that one of your clients has a temperature of 101°F (38.6°C). The client had abdominal surgery 2 days ago and has had IVs since surgery.

1. What priority actions will you take? State a rationale for your actions.
2. What clinical manifestations would indicate a call to the physician for a hot moist compress order? Provide a rationale for your answer.
3. State the major safety precautions for hot moist compresses and the scientific rationale for the precautions.
4. After removing the hot moist compress, you assess that the skin is red and blistered. What immediate actions will you take?

A **Glossary** of important terms, **Bibliography**, and **Appendices** essential to abbreviations, conversions, and medication administration are found in the back of the text as well.

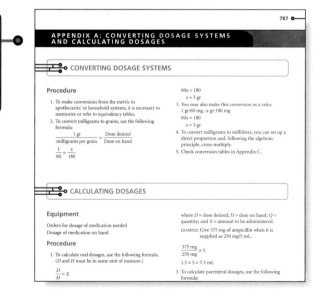

APPENDIX A: CONVERTING DOSAGE SYSTEMS AND CALCULATING DOSAGES

CONVERTING DOSAGE SYSTEMS

Procedure

1. To make conversions from the metric to apothecaries' or household systems, it is necessary to memorize or refer to equivalency tables.
2. To convert milligrams to grains, use the following formula:

$$\frac{1\ gr}{\text{milligrams per grain}} = \frac{\text{Dose desired}}{\text{Dose on hand}}$$

$$\frac{1}{60} = \frac{x}{180}$$

$$60x = 180$$
$$x = 3\ gr$$

3. You may also make this conversion as a ratio:
  1 gr:60 mg :x gr:180 mg
$$60x = 180$$
$$x = 3\ gr$$
4. To convert milligrams to milliliters, you can set up a direct proportion and, following the algebraic principle, cross-multiply.
5. Check conversion tables in Appendix C.

CALCULATING DOSAGES

Equipment

Orders for dosage of medication needed
Dosage of medication on hand

Procedure

1. To calculate oral dosages, use the following formula. (D and H must be in same unit of measure.)

$$\frac{D}{H} = X$$

where D = dose desired; H = dose on hand; Q = quantity; and X = amount to be administered.

EXAMPLE: Give 375 mg of ampicillin when it is supplied as 250 mg/5 mL.

$$\frac{375\ mg}{250\ mg} \times 5$$

$$1.5 \times 5 = 7.5\ mL$$

3. To calculate parenteral dosages, use the following formula:

PHOTO GUIDE OF NURSING SKILLS

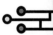

1

LEGAL AND ETHICAL PRACTICE

INTRODUCTION

As you enter the profession of nursing, you will have many wonderful and rewarding experiences. You will need to know about legal and ethical issues in order to provide safe client care. Knowledge of legal and ethical principles and policies will protect clients, families, and health care workers from untoward outcomes.

Clients' rights may conflict with the nursing function; therefore, you should be familiar with the key elements of these rights. Rights include consent, confidentiality, and involuntary commitment. Clients' rights may be modified by the client's mental or physical condition. Clients' rights may be moral or legal or both; a legal right can be enforced in a court of law. Within a health care system, all clients retain their basic constitutional rights, such as freedom of expression, equal protection, due process of law, and freedom from cruel and unusual punishment, as well as the other constitutional protections.

Legal issues and regulations play a dominant role in nursing practice. The law provides a framework for establishing nursing actions in the care of clients. Laws determine and set boundaries that maintain a standard of nursing practice. A thorough grounding in legal and ethical protocols, the issue of clients' rights, and nursing standards as defined by government and the American Nurses Association (ANA) will allow you to achieve and be rewarded by the highest level of legal and ethical practice.

LEGAL AND ETHICAL PROTOCOLS

Understanding the client's rights and the Nurse Practice Act in the state in which you practice will make you aware of potential consequences of nursing actions. As a nurse, you will be held *accountable* and *responsible* for your actions. To be *accountable* means that you are answerable for all your activities surrounding client care. Accountability can be observed and measured by a variety of factors. Nursing actions are evaluated against a set of standards, frequently referred to as *standards of performance.* Nurses must be competent because they are judged according to predetermined factors. To be *responsible* means that the nurse is conscientious and honest in all professional activities. A good example of responsibility is not betraying confidential information concerning clients in the hospital. Client information belongs only in the nursing unit and must not be discussed in the cafeteria or hallways. Nurses must respect clients' rights and abide by the Patient's Bill of Rights.

AMERICAN NURSES ASSOCIATION CODE FOR NURSES

All nurses must function within the nurses' code of ethics. The code of ethics is a set of formal guidelines governing professional action. The code of ethics assists the nurse in problem solving where judgment is required. The ANA Code for Nurses is the most common document outlining nurses' professional actions and responsibilities. In addition to the ANA Code for Nurses, other professional nursing organizations have written codes of ethics that their members must uphold. Nurses who violate these codes will be subject to review and possible disciplinary action.

American Nurses Association Code for Nurses

1. The nurse provides services with respect for human dignity and the uniqueness of the client, unrestricted by considerations of social or economic status, personal attributes, or the nature of the health problems.

2. The nurse safeguards the client's right to privacy by judiciously protecting information of a confidential nature.

3. The nurse acts to safeguard the client and the public when health care and safety are affected by the incompetent, unethical, or illegal actions of any person.

4. The nurse assumes responsibility and accountability for individual nursing judgments and actions.

5. The nurse maintains competence in nursing.

6. The nurse exercises informed judgment and uses individual competence and qualifications as criteria in seeking consultation, accepting responsibilities, and delegating nursing activities to others.

7. The nurse participates in activities that contribute to the ongoing development of the profession's body of knowledge.

8. The nurse participates in the profession's efforts to implement and improve nursing standards.

9. The nurse participates in the profession's efforts to establish and maintain conditions of employment conducive to high-quality nursing care.

10. The nurse participates in the profession's effort to protect the public from misinformation and misrepresentation and to maintain the integrity of nursing.

11. The nurse collaborates with members of the health professions and other citizens in promoting community and national efforts to meet the health needs of the public.

Source: American Nurses Association, *Code for Nurses with Interpretive Statements.* Washington, DC: American Nurses Association, 1985.

CLIENTS' RIGHTS

State and federal regulations governing health care facilities mandate that certain rights be afforded clients receiving health care. All but 10 states have some provision for the rights of clients. Hospitals must have established policies discussing client rights and how staff members are to adhere to them. It is the nurse's responsibility to know what the document states in each facility and how the information is provided to the client.

The Client's Bill of Rights document sets forth clients' right to considerate and respectful care, the right to obtain current information regarding their health status from the physician, the right to receive the necessary information required to give informed consent, the right to refuse treatment, and the right to expect reasonable continuity of care. These are just a few examples of statements included in the document. The Client's Bill of Rights is clearly displayed in each facility where clients receive treatment. Nurses must be familiar with these rights and uphold and abide by them.

ADVANCE DIRECTIVES

The Patient Self-Determination Act (PSDA) of 1990 is federal law that applies to all health care institutions receiving Medicaid funds. This act does not apply to federal facilities such as Veterans Administration hospitals that do not receive Medicare or Medicaid funds. The act requires that all individuals receiving medical care must be given written information about their rights under state law to make decisions about medical care, including the right to accept or refuse medical or surgical treatment. Individuals must also be given information about their rights to formulate advance directives.

Advance directives allow the clients to participate in choosing their health care providers (nurses and physicians), decide who has access to their medical records, specify the type of medical treatment they desire, consent to or refuse treatments, and choose the agent who will make health care decisions if they are unable to do so. Advance directives are written and signed before health care becomes necessary. They must be signed and witnessed, and copies must be kept on file in the physician's office and the hospital. The witness should not be a hospital employee, relative, or heir to the client's estate.

The PSDA describes and defines advance directives such as the living will and the durable power of attorney for health care. The major difference between a living will and a durable power of attorney for health care is that the durable power of attorney is more flexible. A living will is used if the client's condition is terminal or if the client is in a permanently unconscious state. The durable power of attorney addresses all types of health care decisions, including life-sustaining treatments.

LIVING WILL

This type of advance directive indicates the client's wishes regarding prolonging life using life support measures, refusing or stopping medical interventions, or making decisions about his or her medical care when he or she is diagnosed as having a terminal or permanent unconscious condition. It does not apply to any other health care decision. Living wills are executed while the client is competent and able to make sound decisions. As conditions change, a living will needs to be evaluated for relevance. Because states differ in their acceptance of living wills as legal documents, you must be familiar with what is acceptable in the state in which you practice nursing.

DURABLE POWER OF ATTORNEY FOR HEALTH CARE

This legal document must be prepared and signed while the client is competent. The document gives power to make health care decisions to a designated individual in the event the client is unable to make competent decisions. The designated person is obligated to follow the directives outlined in the document. The document gives the designated person specific decisions or the authority to make any and all health care decisions the client would make if able. Decisions regarding withdrawing or using life support, organ donation, or consent to treatment or procedures are included in the directives. As long as the client is competent, no one may make treatment decisions for the client.

According to the American Nurses Association, nurses must play a primary role in implementation of the law. The formation of advance directives is an important decision and will inevitably involve nurses, who spend more time with clients and their families than other health care workers. The nurse is one of several health care professionals who have the responsibility for ensuring that the advance care directives initiated by the client are current and are reflective of the client's choices. Each nurse should know the laws of the state in which she or he is practicing pertaining to advance directives. It is imperative that nurses assist the client and family in making end-of-life care decisions before it is necessary.

CONSENT TO RECEIVE HEALTH SERVICES

Consent is the client's approval to have his or her body touched by specific individuals, such as doctors, nurses, and laboratory technicians. *Informed consent* refers to the process of informing the client prior to obtaining consent regarding treatment such as tests and surgery, and must be understood by the client in terms of the intended outcome and the potential harmful results. The client may rescind a prior consent verbally or in writing.

A consent form may only be signed by a mentally competent adult. Court-authorized persons may give consent for mentally incompetent adults. In an emergency situation where the client is in immediate danger of serious harm or death, a consent form may not be required.

The nurse's liability in terms of consent is to ensure that the client is fully informed before being asked to sign the consent form. The client must be provided with information regarding any potential harmful effects of the treatment. In most cases, this is the responsibility of the physician. If this is not done, it may result in the nurse being held personally liable. The nurse must also respect the right of the mentally competent adult client to refuse health care; however, a life-threatening situation may alter the client's right to refuse treatment.

PATIENT RIGHT TO KNOW ACT

Though not yet enacted, this act will encourage health care providers to exercise their best medical, ethical, and moral judgment in advising clients. It will prohibit health maintenance organizations from interfering with communication between provider and client. This act will also permit clients access to all information relevant to decisions concerning their health care. The act would guarantee that if clients are treated in an emergency room, the health plan is prohibited from arbitrarily refusing to pay for covered emergency benefits.

LEGAL ASPECTS

The Nurse Practice Act defines professional nursing and distinguishes between those actions that the nurse can practice independently and those actions that require a physician's order before completion. Each state has the authority to regulate and administrate health care professionals. Although the provisions of Nurse Practice Acts are quite similar from state to state, it is imperative that the nurse know the specific licensing requirements and the grounds for license revocation defined by the state in which the nurse works.

Legal and ethical standards for nurses are complicated by many federal and state statutes and the continually changing interpretation of them by the courts. Nurses are faced with the possibility of legal action based on negligence, malpractice, invasion of privacy, and other grounds.

THE NURSE PRACTICE ACT

The Nurse Practice Act is a series of statutes enacted by a state to regulate the practice of nursing in that state. The Nurse Practice Act defines the scope of practice, education, licensure, and grounds for disciplinary actions. Nurse Practice Acts are quite similar throughout the United States, but the professional nurse is held legally responsible only for the specific requirements for licensure and regulations of practice defined by the state in which she or he works.

The responsibilities of the professional nurse involve a level of performance for a defined range of health care services, including assessment, implementation, and evaluation of nursing action, as well as teaching and related services such as counseling. Skills and functions that professional nurses perform in daily practice include:

- Provide direct and indirect client care services
- Perform and deliver basic health care services
- Implement testing and prevention procedures
- Observe signs and symptoms of illness
- Administer treatments per physician's order
- Observe treatment reactions and responses
- Administer medications per physician's order
- Observe medication responses and any side effects
- Observe general physical and mental conditions of individual clients
- Document nursing care
- Supervise allied nursing personnel
- Coordinate members of the health care team

NURSE LICENSURE

The authorization to practice nursing is defined legally as the right to practice nursing by an individual who holds an active license issued by the state in which she or he intends to work. The licensing process is administered by the Board of Registered Nursing (BRN). This board may also grant endorsement or reciprocity to an applicant who holds a current license in another state. The applicant for RN licensure must have attended an accredited school of nursing, be a qualified nursing professional or paraprofessional, or have met specific prerequisites if licensed in a foreign country.

STANDARDS OF CLINICAL NURSING PRACTICE

The Standards of Clinical Nursing Practice consist of two components, Standards of Care and Standards of Professional Performance. These standards were first published in 1973 by the American Nurses Association and have

---

American Nurses Association Standards of Care

I. Assessment: The nurse collects patient health data.

II. Diagnosis: The nurse analyzes the assessment data in determining diagnoses.

III. Outcome Identification: The nurse identifies expected outcomes individualized to the patient.

IV. Planning: The nurse develops a plan of care that prescribes interventions to attain expected outcomes.

V. Implementation: The nurse implements the interventions identified in the plan of care.

VI. Evaluation: The nurse evaluates the patient's progress toward attainment of outcomes.

Source: American Nurses Association, *Standards of Clinical Nursing Practice* (2nd ed.). Washington, DC: American Nurses Association, 1998.

been revised in 1991 and updated in 1998. The Standards of Care describe the specific function and activities of nurses and provide criteria for evaluating the quality and effectiveness of nursing care. Six defined standards encompass the use of the nursing process in the delivery of client care. The standards are authoritative descriptions of the responsibility and accountability of the professional nurse. These standards apply to nursing practice in any setting.

The Standards of Professional Performance describe a competent level of behavior in the professional role. These behaviors relate to quality of care, performance appraisals, education, collegiality, ethics, collaboration, research, and resource allocation.

Standards for specialty roles, such as those in critical care and oncology, elaborate on appropriate expectations for the various professional role standards (ANA Standard of Clinical Nursing Practice, 1991).

American Nurses Association Standards of Professional Performance

   I. Quality of Care: The nurse systematically evaluates the quality and effectiveness of nursing practice.

  II. Performance Appraisal: The nurse evaluates one's own nursing practice in relation to professional practice standards and relevant statutes and regulations.

 III. Education: The nurse acquires and maintains current knowledge and competence in nursing practice.

  IV. Collegiality: The nurse interacts with, and contributes to the professional development of, peers and other health care providers as colleagues.

   V. Ethics: The nurse's decisions and actions on behalf of patients are determined in an ethical manner.

  VI. Collaboration: The nurse collaborates with the patient, family, and other health care providers in providing patient care.

 VII. Research: The nurse uses research findings in practice.

VIII. Resource Utilization: The nurse considers factors related to safety, effectiveness, and cost in planning and delivering patient care.

Source: American Nurses Association, *Standards of Clinical Nursing Practice* (2nd ed.). Washington, DC: American Nurses Association, 1998.

LIABILITY AND LEGAL ISSUES

Each state defines and regulates the grounds for professional misconduct. Even though many states have similar standards, the practicing nurse must know how her or his state defines professional misconduct. The penalties for professional misconduct include probation, censure and reprimand, suspension of license, or revocation of license. The state's Board of Registered Nursing (BRN) has the authority to impose any of these penalties for professional misconduct. Any one of the following actions would be considered professional misconduct.

- Obtaining an RN license through misrepresentation or fraudulent methods
- Giving false information on application for license
- Practicing in a grossly negligent or incompetent manner
- Practicing when one's ability to practice is severely impaired
- Being habitually drunk or dependent on drugs
- Furnishing controlled substances to oneself or to another person
- Impersonating another certified or licensed practitioner or allowing another person to use one's license for the purpose of nursing
- Being convicted of or committing an act constituting a crime under federal or state law
- Refusing to provide health care services on the grounds of race, color, creed, or national origin
- Permitting or aiding an unlicensed person to perform activities requiring a license
- Practicing nursing while one's license is suspended
- Practicing medicine without a license
- Procuring, aiding, or offering to assist at a criminal abortion
- Representing oneself to the public as a nurse-practitioner without being certified by the BRN as a nurse-practitioner (in some states)

LEGAL ISSUES AND DRUG ADMINISTRATION

One of the major roles the nurse performs each day is the administration of medications. Failure to give the correct medication or improper handling of drugs may result in serious problems for the nurse due to strict federal and state statutes relating to drugs. The Comprehensive Drug Abuse Prevention Act of 1970 provides the fundamental federal regulations for compounding, selling, and dispensing narcotics, stimulants, depressants, and other controlled items. Each state has a similar set of regulations.

Guidelines for Drug Administration

- Nurses must not administer a specific drug unless allowed to do so by the particular state's Nurse Practice Act.

- Nurses must not administer any drug without a specific physician's order.

- Nurses are to take every safety precaution in whatever they are doing.

- Nurses are to be certain that their employer's policy allows them to administer a specific drug.

- Nurses must not administer a controlled substance if the physician's order is outdated.

- A drug may not lawfully be administered unless all the preceding items are in effect.

- Nurses are not permitted to fill prescriptions and in most states cannot write prescriptions.

- General rules for drug dispensing:
  1. Never leave prepared medicines unattended.
  2. Always report errors immediately.
  3. Send labeled bottles that are unintelligible back to the pharmacist for relabeling.
  4. Store internal and external medicines separately if possible.

Noncompliance with federal or state drug regulations can result in liability. Violation of the state drug regulations or licensing laws is grounds for the Board of Registered Nursing to initiate disciplinary action.

NEGLIGENCE AND MALPRACTICE

The doctrine of negligence rests on the duty of every person to exercise due care in his or her conduct toward others in situations where injury may result. For liability to be found, there must be a duty of care on the part of the nurse and a causal relationship between damage or harm to the client as well as an act or omission to act by the nurse.

Gross negligence is the intentional failure to perform a duty in reckless disregard of the consequences affecting the client. It is viewed as a gross lack of care to such a level as to be considered willful and wanton.

Criminal negligence also consists of a duty on the part of the nurse and an act that is the proximate cause of the injury or death of a client. This type of negligence is usually defined by statute and as such is punishable as a crime (see Table 1-1). The act being punished would be flagrant and reckless disregard of the safety of others and/or a willful disregard for the injury liable to follow so as to convert the act into a crime when it results in personal injury or death. One is not negligent unless one fails to exercise the degree of reasonable care that would be exercised by a person of ordinary prudence under all the existing circumstances in view of probable danger of injury.

Malpractice is any professional misconduct that is an unreasonable lack of skill or fidelity in professional duties. In a more specific sense it means bad, wrong, or injurious treatment of a client resulting in injury, unnecessary suffering, or death to a client proceeding from ignorance; carelessness; lack of professional skill; disregard of established rules, protocols, principles, or procedures; neglect; or malicious or criminal intent.

It is the nurse's legal duty to provide competent, reasonable care to clients. To ensure that this occurs, the nurse must know the standard of care, develop consistent patterns of practice that meet the standard, and reflect her or his actions in accurate and complete documentation. Legal action against nurses has been increasing over the past decade. Nursing actions that constitute a breach of a standard of care and that can lead to injury of a client include such actions as not inserting a Foley catheter correctly, not taking appropriate steps to decrease a client's temperature, not reporting unusual or worsening condition of the client to his or her physician, and not preventing falls. All of these situations can lead to malpractice suits.

Legal doctrine holds that an employer may also be liable for negligent acts of employees in the course and scope of employment. Physicians, hospitals, clinics, and other employers may be held liable for negligent acts of their employees. This doctrine does not support acts of gross negligence or acts that are outside the scope of employment.

TABLE 1-1	ACTIONS COVERED BY CIVIL VERSUS CRIMINAL LAW
Civil Law	**Criminal Law**
Contract	Assault
Unintentional tort	Battery
Intentional tort	Murder
Negligence	Manslaughter

CRITICAL THINKING FOCUS

SECTIONS ONE, TWO, AND THREE ▪ Legal and Ethical Practice

Potential Problems

- Students are overheard discussing clients in the cafeteria.

- The American Nurses Association Code for Nurses cannot be found in the hospital setting to use as a reference.

- The Client's Bill of Rights is not displayed in an accessible area in the hospital.

- A seriously ill client is admitted to the hospital without advance directives.

- There is concern that someone is impersonating an RN.

- You determine that a nurse is not practicing within the guidelines of the Nurse Practice Act.

Possible Outcomes

- Remind students of their responsibility and accountability to maintain confidentiality.
- Discuss students' role in maintaining confidentiality of clients' records and information.

- Seek help from the facility's librarian in obtaining a copy for each nursing unit.
- Write directly to the ANA to request a copy.
- Locate a copy in one of the many textbooks that reproduce the code.

- Discuss the issue with the nursing executive and ask for the document to be placed in the lobby or hallway where it can be viewed by all clients and visitors.

- Ask the client's spouse or children to assist the client in obtaining the written document.
- Ensure that the signed document is placed on the chart and the physician has a copy.
- Remember, hospital staff members do not act as witnesses to this document.

- Notify the nurse executive of your concern.
- Notify the Board of Registered Nursing.

- Document your findings.
- Talk directly to the person and ask for clarification of her or his actions.
- If the practice is outside the scope of the Nurse Practice Act, notify the nurse manager.

SELF-CHECK EVALUATION

PART 1 ▪ Matching Terms

Match the definition from column B that best describes each term in column A.

Column A

_____ a. Accountable
_____ b. Responsible
_____ c. Nurses' code of ethics
_____ d. Clients' Bill of Rights
_____ e. Living will
_____ f. Durable power of
attorney for health care

Column B

1. States client's rights regarding medical care or treatment
2. Answerable for client care activities
3. Indicates client's wishes regarding prolonging life
4. Conscientious in all professional activities
5. Formal guidelines governing professional action
6. Gives power to a designated individual for health care issues if client unable to make decisions

PART 2 ▪ Multiple Choice Questions

1. The set of formal guidelines for governing RNs' professional action is called:

a. Patient's Bill of Rights.
b. Nurses' code of ethics.
c. Professional responsibility.
d. ANA Standards of Nursing Practice.

2. Standards of nursing practice are best defined as:

a. Authorization statements describing the nurse's accountability and responsibility.
b. Standards that ensure that nursing procedures are the same in all states.
c. Guidelines for ethical practice.
d. Statements that identify the nurse's role in providing care.

3. Advance directives are best described as:

a. Consent forms for medical care by physicians and nurses.
b. Clients' rights for informed consent while hospitalized.
c. Statements giving the right to determine health care decisions to the next of kin in emergency situations.
d. Documents that allow the client to make legal decisions regarding future health care.

4. Gross negligence is best described as:

a. Not providing total care to clients during hospitalization.
b. Lack of care to such a level as to be considered willful or wanton.
c. Flagrant and reckless disregard for the safety of others.
d. Professional misconduct that is an unreasonable lack of skill in professional duties.

5. Which one of the following best describes the grounds for professional misconduct?

a. Practicing in a clinic before receiving your state board examination results.
b. Assisting a nursing student to learn the technique for starting an IV.
c. Drinking alcoholic beverages prior to coming to work on the night shift.
d. Allowing a seriously ill client to sign out of the hospital against medical advice (AMA).

6. Which one of the following terms best illustrates civil law?

    a. Assault and battery.

    b. Manslaughter.

    c. Negligence.

    d. Homicide.

7. Which one of the following statements about consent is true?

    a. A statement of informed consent is signed at the time of hospital admission.

    b. A consent form must be signed before emergency surgery can be performed for a life-threatening event.

    c. Confidential information regarding communicable diseases cannot be released without consent of the client.

    d. A client may verbally rescind a prior consent.

PART 3 ▪ Critical Thinking Application

As you are admitting a client to the nursing unit, he tells you this is his first hospitalization. He is 68 years old with the diagnosis of terminal cancer of the pancreas. He was just diagnosed two days ago.

1. What documents would be most appropriate for this client to sign?

2. Provide the intent of each document you identified.

3. What is the nurse's role in this activity?

2

DOCUMENTATION AND CARE PLANNING

INTRODUCTION

Documentation encompasses all methods of relaying client information to appropriate health care workers. Nursing documentation communicates assessment data to all other members of the health care team who are coordinating the treatment regime. Nursing documentation is a critical component of the client's medical record. It is used to help obtain reimbursement from insurance companies and Medicare. Inadequate or inappropriate nursing documentation has led to very large revenue losses in many institutions. What you document and how you document play a major role in reimbursement for client care services. Medicare and insurance companies rely on daily documentation of the client's ongoing need for care when they review the client's records for reimbursement. They evaluate the appropriate billing of supplies and equipment by reading nursing notes and other documentation forms describing the client's care. If a treatment or use of special equipment is not noted in the nursing documentation, reimbursement is denied. The old adage, "If it isn't charted, it didn't happen," is still alive and well. Most of the insurance companies, and Medicare, look for

(continued on next page)

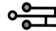

nursing documentation that supports nursing diagnoses, appropriate client teaching, and discharge planning.

Client care plans are an integral part of providing nursing care. Without them, quality and consistency of client care may not be obtained. Client care plans provide a means of communication among nurses and other health care providers. The care plan should serve as a focal point for client care assignments and reporting. Used together, documentation and care planning assist the health care team in its efforts to provide care of the highest scope and quality.

SECTION ONE

DOCUMENTATION

Documentation includes client charting using a variety of methods, client care plans or critical pathways, medication records, flowcharts and graphics, and unusual occurrence reports. Each document represents specific information about the client and his or her progress during hospitalization, clinic visits, or home care visits. State law and Medicare's conditions of participation determine what must be charted. For example, the Minimum Data Set (MDS) is a standardized assessment tool that must be completed for each client in a long-term care facility. The American Nurses Association, the Joint Commission on Accreditation of Healthcare Organizations (JCAHO), and the Health Care Financing Administration (HCFA) require that documentation include initial and ongoing assessments, variations from the assessment, client teaching, response to therapy, and other relevant data regarding the client's condition or statements. JCAHO standards include information about establishing policies regarding the frequency and documentation of client assessment. Agencies and facilities also develop policies and procedures regarding specifics relative to the documentation systems in place in the agency.

Documentation communicates nursing assessments, interventions, and evaluation outcomes to all members of the health care team. It is the most important activity a nurse performs in the care of clients. Nurses' charting is scrutinized by medical records personnel in the facility, certifying agencies, licensing organizations, quality improve-

ment committees, and Medicare and insurance companies. If a client were to take legal action through the court system, judges and attorneys would have access to all documentation.

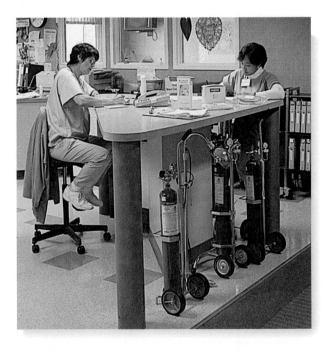

● **FIGURE 2-1** *Charting is completed immediately following client care.*

CLINICAL NOTE

MALPRACTICE CONCERNS

Malpractice concerns can be diminished if you provide the best care you can, maintaining the standards of clinical practice, working within the Nurse Practice Act, and following facility policies and practices. After completing client care, ensure that you precisely chart your observations, interventions, and communications; this is the best deterrent to later legal problems. The following inaccurate or incomplete charting entries are those that are usually scrutinized in malpractice suits.

- Timely vital signs entries
- Medications given
- Client responses
- Discharge teaching
- Changes in a client's condition

Source: *Mastering Documentation,* 2nd ed. Springhouse, PA: Springhouse Corporation, 1999, pp. 325–342.

CHARTING GUIDELINES FOR POTENTIAL LEGAL PROBLEMS

These guidelines will assist you in charting proactively and will protect both you and the employer from potential litigation. Keep in mind that you never alter a medical record except as indicated in the guidelines. Never erase, obliterate, or deface a medical record. Do not try to improve charting or entries after the fact. Charting requires good judgement based on proper assessment, specific nursing interventions, and the client's plan of care.

- Use the nursing process in your documentation.
- Use specific assessment parameters, not global assessments ("IV running well").
- State objective facts, not assumptions.
- Place a direct quote from a client or family member in quotation marks.
- Be professional in your charting; do not make interpretations.
- Chart significant events and client responses.
- Chart potentially serious situations; include observations and who you reported the findings to, and whether actions were taken based on the communication.

- Do not use words such as *mistake* or *accident;* write specifically what incident occurred and what actions were taken.
- Do not use tentative or vague statements such as *appears* or *apparently.*
- Use correct language and medical terms. Do not use slang, pat phrases, or abbreviations that are not generally accepted.
- Use correct grammar and spelling.
- Do not chart for someone else.
- Do not chart ahead of time. Chart after the care is complete, but do not wait until the end of the shift.
- Do not alter a medical record. Draw a single line through an incorrect entry and initial and date the error.
- Write in late entries when you think about them; do not try to go back into earlier charting and insert the information. Label the information as "late entry" and put the time it actually happened in the entry.
- Countersign care given by assistive staff only if the facility allows you to countersign, and then do so only after you review the entry and are familiar with the care provided to the client.

THE CHARTING PROCESS

The format of the chart varies from facility to facility. Most important is the content included in each of the documents. The notes should describe the assessment that is completed at the beginning of the shift. This information provides a baseline for changes in the client's condition that may occur later. If there are no changes, this fact should be entered as the final note. Some facilities require that all parts of the assessment be documented, others only that abnormalities be documented.

As the shift progresses, certain aspects of the client's condition and actions need to be documented. These may include changes in assessment findings, changes in vital signs, changes in the client's mental or emotional status, reactions to any unscheduled or PRN medications, the client's response to teaching, or untoward effects of treatments.

CHARTING AND THE NURSING PROCESS

The nursing process provides the framework for decision making throughout all phases of nursing care. It is important to relate the nursing process to charting because, for experienced nurses, the process may become only a mental exercise. The nurse thinks through the situation, makes decisions, takes action, and observes the results. Unless the entire process is recorded on the client care plan and documented in the chart, the next nurse who encounters a similar situation with the same client is deprived of important and potentially valuable background data. For students, this will also become a familiar routine with practice in charting. To master the art of documentation, it is necessary to practice charting with each skill performed in the skills laboratory. For beginning students, charting should be checked by the instructor before the information is entered into the client's chart. Remember, this is a legal document and under scrutiny by many individuals.

DOCUMENTATION SYSTEMS

There are five recognized methods or systems of charting used in health care facilities. Each facility selects the system that meets its individual needs and also meets legal and regulatory requirements. The five systems include source-oriented charting (narrative), problem-oriented medical records (POMR), focus charting, problem-intervention-evaluation (PIE), and charting by exception (CBE).

COMMON CHARTING FORMATS

- Narrative charting
- Problem-oriented medical records
- Focus charting
- PIE charting
- Charting by exception

Source-Oriented Charting

This system, commonly referred to as *narrative charting,* is the most common form of charting used in acute, long-term, ambulatory, and home care settings. The term *source-oriented* refers to information that is organized and presented according to its source. For example, there are separate sections for doctors' progress notes, nurses' notes, and respiratory therapy notes. In this system, nursing units may use different types of documentation forms: a medical floor may use nurses' notes without flowsheets, and critical care units may make extensive use of flowsheets. There is no consistency within the system.

Regardless of the type of nurses' notes or documents used, at the beginning of the shift the nurse performs a physical assessment on each client to determine the client's current status. This information is usually the first entry in narrative charting. When changes occur, the time is noted next to the appropriate system and the change is documented. If no changes occur during the shift, no other charting of this type may be necessary. Flowsheets are commonly used in conjunction with this system. Special sheets such as neurologic monitoring sheets and diabetic sheets are used as necessary. Flowsheets eliminate the need to write excessive notes and avoid duplication of information; flowsheets do not negate the need for narrative descriptions, however.

Narrative charting is based on chronology rather than systems. Information is charted in chronological order, regardless of the subject of the note. Hospitals usually have maximum time requirements for this type of note, with common parameters being every 2 or 3 hrs. Although there may be requirements for frequency of charting, there is usually no requirement for charting content. This leads to the primary deficiency of narrative charting; it is very easy to chart without specifying why the client is in the hospital or the client's overall condition.

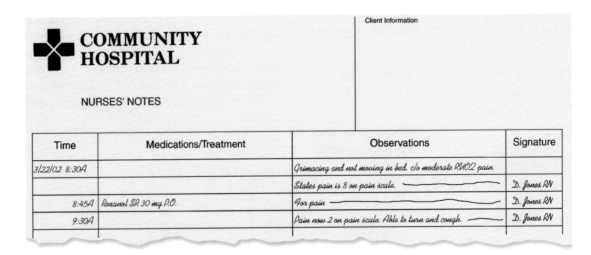

● **FIGURE 2-2** *Nurses' notes.*

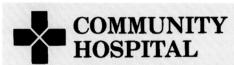

COMMUNITY HOSPITAL

ICU NEURO/SPINAL FLOW CHART

Date: 3/22/02		Time:	8 am		
		Right: size	4 mm		
		Reaction	s		
Pupils		Left: Size	4 mm		
		Reaction	s		
		Visual Acuity	c		
Mental Status					
C O M A	Eyes Open	Spontaneously			
		To Speech			
		To Pain	+		
		Never			
S C A L E	Verbal Response	Clear			
		Confused			
		Inappropriate	+		
		Incomprehensible			
		None			
M O V E M E N T	Arms	Normal Power			
		Weakness	+		
		Flexion			
		Extension			
		No Response			
	Legs	Normal Power			
		Weakness	+		
		Flexion			
		Extension			
		No Response			
Reflexes		Gag/Cough	0		
		Corneal	+		
		Babinski R/L	+ / +		
		Oculocephalic	0		
Respiratory		Pattern	Reg.		
		Rate	28		
Seizures		Type	0		
		Duration			
Fluid Drainage from Ears or			0		
		Nose	0		

Signature _____ D. Jones RN _____

● **FIGURE 2-3** *Neurologic flow sheet.*

Rules for Charting Narrative Notes

Care providers can help ensure accurate records by adopting these specific but easy rules in the care environment.

1. Use black ink, not felt pen or pencil. Black ink microfilms best.

2. Correct errors by drawing a line through the error, writing the words *mistaken entry* (ME) above it, and then initialing the error. The error must be readable. Ink eradication, erasures, or use of occlusive materials is not acceptable. The word *error* is no longer advised because juries tend to associate the word *error* with an actual nursing care mistake.

3. Sign each entry with your first initial, last name, and status; for example, SN for student nurse, LVN for licensed vocational nurse, or RN for registered nurse. Script, not printing, is used for the signature. Each signature should appear at the right margin of the nurses' notes.

4. Notes should appear on each succeeding line. Lines should not be omitted in the nurses' notes. Draw a horizontal line to fill up a partial line. Continuous charting is done for each entry unless a time change occurs. You do not need a new line for each new idea or statement.

5. Entries should be concise. Complete sentences are not required. Start each entry with a capital letter, and end the entry with a period even if the entry is a single word or phrase.

6. The date is entered in the data column on the first line of every page of nurses' notes and whenever the date changes.

7. The time is entered in the time column whenever a new time entry occurs. Do not put time changes in the text of the nurses' notes. If only one time is entered for block charting, enter the last time you were with the client.

8. Chart objective facts, not your interpretations: for example, chart "Ate 100%," not "Good appetite." If the client complains, place the complaint in quotation marks to indicate that it is his or her statement: for example, " 'c/o chest pain radiating down left arm.' "

9. Objective data is to be charted as well. In addition to the statement offered by the client, the nurse should chart her or his observations: "Skin cold and clammy. Diaphoretic. Vital signs stable."

10. Refusal of medications and treatments must be documented. Place a circle around the time the medication or treatment is to be given in the appropriate areas of the chart. Enter an explanation as to the reason the medication was not given into the nurses' notes.

11. Sign each entry before the chart is replaced in the chart rack. An entry is not to be left unsigned. If all the charting is completed for the shift at one time, place a single signature at the end of the charting.

12. Accuracy is important. Describe behaviors rather than feelings. This allows other health team members to determine the client's actual problems.

TABLE 2-1	NARRATIVE CHARTING	

Advantages	Disadvantages
■ Portrays a complete picture of the client over an extended period of time.	■ Lacks systematic structure, leading to difficulty determining data relationships.
■ Can be used in conjunction with flowsheets and other documentation systems.	■ Time-consuming.
■ Quick method of charting chronological data.	■ Frequently lacks information on client care outcomes.
■ Familiar method of charting.	■ Difficult to monitor data for quality assurance.
■ Easy to use.	■ Relevant information found in several areas in chart.
	■ Difficult to track problems.
■ Is flexible and can be used in all types of clinical settings.	■ Charts can be long and contain repetitive information.

13. Chart only those abbreviations and symbols approved by the facility. Information can be misinterpreted or misleading when unfamiliar abbreviations are used.

14. Spell correctly, using proper terminology and grammar.

15. Write legibly. If your writing is not legible, then print.

16. Only chart what you have personally done or observed. An exception to this rule is when you are responsible for charting for nonprofessional personnel.

17. Do not use the word *client* in the chart. The chart belongs to that client.

18. Do not double-chart. If something appears on a flowsheet, it does not need to appear on the nurses' narrative record unless there is an alteration from normal.

19. Do not squeeze information into a space because you forgot to chart it earlier. Add the information on the first available line. Write in the time the event occurred, not the time you entered the information.

20. The following information should be charted: (1) physicians' visits; (2) times the client leaves and returns to the unit, mode of transportation, and destination; (3) medications (chart immediately after given), including dosage, route of administration (if parenteral, where given), whether pain was relieved (if pain medication), and side effects; and (4) treatments (chart immediately after given).

A new form of narrative charting, assessment-intervention-response (AIR), has been introduced that presents a more efficient and effective method of organizing and simplifying this type of charting. In the assessment (A) section of the chart, the nurse summarizes data and impressions of problems found via assessment. The

---

THE AIR FORMAT

A Respirations 30 and labored. Rales bilateral in the bases.

I Deep breathing and coughing, incentive spirometer with Mucomyst. Up in chair.

R Respiration 24, decreased intensity of rales but still present.

---

intervention (I) section is for summaries about interventions based on assessment findings. The summary may include a condensed nursing care plan or plans for additional monitoring. The response (R) section focuses on the client's response to nursing interventions. Each assessment and intervention is labeled so that other nurses can chart pertinent responses. With appropriate flowsheets and the AIR method of narrative charting, client care is more clearly and concisely documented.

Problem-Oriented Medical Records

The problem-oriented medical records (POMR) documentation system is the second major type of charting system and is used in acute, long-term, and home health care settings. This system differs from source-oriented narrative charting not only in format but in philosophy. POMR focuses on the client's status rather than on the source of the information, such as the department or member of the health care team originating the information. Only one set of progress notes is used, and all personnel caring for the client record their data on the same set.

In its purest form, a POMR system consists of five distinct parts: (1) the initial baseline data obtained from

COMMUNITY HOSPITAL

NURSING ASSESSMENT DATA BASE

Date	Time	Room #	Admit ambulatory ___ guerney ___ by: W/C ✓ ambulance ___
3/22/02	4 pm	110A	

T.P.R.	B/P RT	B/P LT	Height	Weight
99⁸-110-24	160/90	164/94	5'6"	200#

Instructed in use of:

Yes	No	
✓		Telephone
✓		Bed-Controls
✓		Lights
✓		Nurse call System
✓		Visiting hours

Articles at bedside (describe item)

	Item	Description
✓	Ring	Yellow Metal
	Watch	
✓	Money (amt.)	$10.50
✓	Eyeglasses	
	Hearing Aid	

	Contact Lenses	
	Dentures: Upper	✓
	Lower	✓
	Other	

Reason for No: ___ Other ___

Tests completed on admission

	Lab Work	
✓	UA	
✓	X-ray	Chest
	Other	

Above information obtained by: KMend, RN

Previous illness	Meds taken @ home on routine basis	Meds taken today state time	Meds brought to hospital
Diabetes	Lasix 40 mg P.O.		None
✓ Hypertension	Digoxin 0.25 mg P.O.		
✓ Heart Disease			
Lung Disease			
Other			

Disposition of Meds: Home / Pharmacy

Allergies:

✓	FOOD	Shellfish, Citrus fruit
✓	DRUGS	ASA, Codeine
	None Known	

● **FIGURE 2-4** *POMR database record.*

all departments involved in the client care, (2) a problem list, (3) a plan of care for each problem, (4) progress notes, and (5) a discharge summary. The database is made up of information from and about the client that is used to develop the problem list. Because the POMR system is systematic and well defined, the database consists of specific types of data, including the chief complaint, personal and family medical history, allergies and reactions, medications taken at home, physical assessment, mental and emotional assessment, and lifestyle.

The categories of POMR closely approximate the steps in the nursing process. The database and problem list equate to assessment; the initial plan equates to planning; the progress notes discuss interventions; and the discharge summary is an evaluation. After the database is completed and the problem list is initiated, the client care plan is formulated.

The POMR system uses the subjective, objective, assessment, plan (SOAP) or subjective, objective, assessment, plan, implementation, evaluation (SOAPIE) charting format to document client information. A separate SOAP or SOAPIE note must be written in the progress notes for each identified problem. Problems are not combined into one entry. It is not always necessary to include

COMMUNITY HOSPITAL

NURSING PROBLEM LIST

Date Problem Began	Prob. #	Problem	Date Resolved	Date Recurred
3/22/02	1	Altered Urinary Elimination R/t incontinence.		
3/22/02	2	Unilateral Neglect R/t right-sided weakness.		
3/22/02	3	Altered Nutrition: Less than Body Requirement R/t aversion to eating and difficulty swallowing.		
3/22/02	4	Impaired Skin Integrity R/t emaciation.		

● **FIGURE 2-5** *POMR problem list.*

SOAPIE CHARTING FORMAT

Subjective: Client's symptoms and own description of problem.

Objective: Clinical findings; include observations and factual data (for instance, intake and output, vital signs, drainage, presence of rash).

Assessment: Your conclusions about the problem based on subjective and objective data. Nursing diagnoses may be written here.

Plan: What you decide to do about the problem.

Implementation: Your nursing interventions.

Evaluation: How the implementation worked.

CLINICAL NOTE

SOAP AND SOAPIE CHARTING

Problem 1

Fluid volume, excess. Related to poor compliance to medication administration.

S "My rings are tight and my shoes don't fit."

O Fingers are edematous. 3+ pitting edema of both ankles.

A Due to fluid overload as a result of refusing diuretics.

P Elevate feet. Explain necessity for diuretics. Administer drug, obtain order for IM med if nec. Observe dietary intake of Na^+ to determine if compliant to diet.

I Client education completed regarding use of Lasix.

E Could state signs and symptoms of low potassium.

Problem 2

Ineffective airway clearance, related to pain.

S "I'm having difficulty bringing up mucus."

O Lungs sound congested, rales present bilaterally in lower bases.

A Unable to breathe and cough due to high abdominal incision.

P Elevate HOB 45 degrees. Enc. coughing and deep breathing. Medicate for pain q3h. Splint inc. when coughing.

I Expectorating large amounts of clear mucus.

E (Evaluation is not always included in this charting.)

the implementation (I) or evaluation (E) portions of the note; however, the SOAP parts should always be included even if the client does not supply subjective statements.

The discharge summary includes both a summary of the client's hospitalization and documentation of client teaching. The SOAPIE notes are used as the charting format, and a summary should be written for each remaining problem on the problem list. Problems that have been resolved during hospitalization are noted with the date they occurred.

✚ COMMUNITY HOSPITAL

Client Information

PROGRESS NOTES

Date	Note progress of case, complications, change in diagnosis, condition on discharge
3/22/02	Mr. Rappaport was admitted to the restorative care unit on 3/15/00 with right-side weakness, difficulty swallowing,
	inability to perform ADL's, 10# weight loss, and coccyx area reddened with Stage 1 pressure ulcer. Laboratory values WNL,
	except for a urinary tract infection 1 week prior to admission which has been resolved with P.O. Gantrisin (Problem #1)
	Continues to exhibit right-sided weakness. Unable to perform ADL's right handed (Problem #2) O.T. working on alternative
	ways to become independent in ADL's. Instructions given to client to swallow on left side. Weight loss has stabilized, dietitian
	working with client to determine food preferences. Hi-protein, hi-calorie liquids between meals started 4/10/00. (Problem #3)
	Skin care with transparent dressings continues. Area remains unchanged. (Problem #4) Plan is to begin preparation for
	discharge. Instructions on dietary needs and skin care given to wife and daughter. O.T. will continue at home to work on
	ADL's. ———————————————————————————— D. Jones RN

● **FIGURE 2-6** *POMR discharge summary.*

Other Problem-Based Methods

The problem identification, intervention, evaluation (PIE) charting format is a newer, condensed version of the problem-oriented charting system. The PIE charting format is well suited for acute care areas where the client's condition changes quickly. The PIE system organizes information according to the client's problems and integrates the client's plan of care into progress notes that simplify the documentation process. This type of charting uses the nursing process and nursing diagnosis while incorporating the plan of care into the nurses' progress notes.

The PIE system does not use the traditional nursing care plan. Client problems, teaching needs, and discharge planning needs are identified during the initial client assessment [the problem (P) element of the PIE format]. Based on the assessment, nursing diagnoses are identified and numbered on a problem list. Interventions (the I in the PIE format) that are carried out are documented for each specific nursing diagnosis. Each shift performs an evaluation (the E in the PIE format) of the client's response to the intervention and its impact on problem resolution.

PIE DOCUMENTATION

P#1: Pain r/t postoperative incisional drainage tube placement.

P: Instruct in use of PCA and positioning for comfort.

I: Instruction given on how to use PCA pump. Positioned on unoperative side with pillows to back and between knees.

E: Using PCA appropriately, pain tolerable, identified as 3 on pain scale. Positioning has assisted in decreasing pain and allowed client to rest comfortably for longer periods of time.

Because of the many changes necessary when implementing POMR, hospitals often use only part of it or are changing to it in stages; therefore it is common to find situations in which parts of several systems are in use. For example, SOAP nursing notes may be used, with the remainder of the chart being source-oriented, or physicians may use the problem list and SOAP progress notes while the nurses use systems charting.

TABLE 2-2	PROBLEM-ORIENTED CHARTING

Advantages	Disadvantages
■ Focuses on client problem.	■ Difficult to obtain agreement on what should be included in record.
■ Implements problem-solving approach.	■ Physicians vary in their acceptance of all disciplines using same list.
■ Retrieving information about each problem is easy.	■ Duplication of information necessary on several forms.
■ Problem resolution is clearly documented.	
■ Problem list assists in identifying priority needs of client.	■ Need for constant updating of problem list and determining person responsible.
■ May be used effectively in acute or long-term care settings.	■ Format is frequently not used in pure form, making it difficult to use effectively.
■ Documentation format is consistent.	■ Not efficient because each problem requires a separate POMR entry.
	■ Incorporates use of care planning, which is the responsibility of the RN; therefore it is difficult to use LVNs in documentation system.
■ Effectively uses nursing process in documentation.	
■ Readily used in conjunction with standard nursing care plan.	
■ Integrated documentation system promotes collaboration among all health care providers.	
■ PIE charting uses flowsheet, which decreases documentation time and redundancy.	

Focus Charting

Focus charting is a documentation system used in acute and long-term care, and is consistent with JCAHO requirements for documenting client responses and outcomes. A focus charting system begins with a client assessment followed by formulation of client-centered topics of concern and concise documentation of client status. The term *focus* is used instead of the word *problem*. Using the term *focus* eliminates the negative connotations of *problem*. Each client concern, or focus, is usually written as a nursing diagnosis. In some instances, client behavior, change in health status, or a significant event such as hemorrhage, and signs and symptoms may also be the focus of the plan.

FOCUS CHARTING

D Client found grimacing, hands clenched, and body rigid. Verbalized pain at 9 on pain scale.

A Administered 15 mg MS IV push. Called physician to request PCA for client.

R Pain moderately relieved after 35 min. Able to understand instructions in use of PCA.

Focus charting is similar to SOAP charting except for the use of the term *focus* instead of *problem*. The data-action-response (DAR) format is used on the progress notes. Data (D) includes the information that supports the focus, action (A) is the nursing intervention used to treat the problem, and response (R) is how the client responds to the intervention and the outcome.

Charting by Exception

The charting by exception (CBE) format is used in both acute and long-term care facilities. This type of charting requires documentation of only significant or abnormal findings. CBE utilizes a nursing database, a problem-oriented plan of care, nursing diagnoses, protocols and standards of practice, flowsheets, and SOAP progress notes. CBE has a nursing focus and promotes continuity of care through the tracking of client data from admission to discharge. Initial and ongoing health assessments are documented only as exceptions. Normal findings are preprinted on forms and used as guidelines for each body system. These guidelines use standards that provide a normal assessment to chart against. If the client is within normal limits on the physical assessment, *WNL* can be documented or checked off on a checklist. This form of charting is just the opposite of the other types of formats, in which both normal and abnormal assessment findings are recorded.

Both a nursing and physician order flowsheet are used to document the physical assessments and implementation of physician and nursing orders. The forms contain the teaching record and discharge notes as well. Nurses chart only when the client does not meet the predetermined standard or norm; therefore, when narrative charting is found in the chart, other nurses know that something unusual has occurred.

TABLE 2-3	FOCUS CHARTING	
Advantages		**Disadvantages**
■ Uses a data-action-response format that is easy to follow.		■ Can require multiple flowsheets and checklists.
■ DAR charting provides clues that help direct documentation in a process-oriented way.		
■ Is flexible and adaptable for most clinical settings.		
■ Is based on nursing process.		
■ It is easy to find information about specific client problems.		
■ Nurses can document problems that do not appear on the problem list.		

TABLE 2-4	CHARTING BY EXCEPTION

Advantages	Disadvantages
■ Documenting only significant data saves time.	■ It is time-consuming to prepare clear guidelines and standards of care.
■ It decreases multiple data entries and thus the amount of documentation needed.	■ It is not conducive to interdisciplinary charting.
■ It eliminates redundant charting, and identifies abnormal data.	■ Guidelines must be understood and used by all nursing staff members for this format to be effective.
■ Flowsheets can be kept at the bedside, which promotes immediate and complete charting.	■ There are still some legal reimbursement issues related to CBE. "If it isn't charted, it wasn't done" is still a prevailing attitude in some legal situations.
■ It has a nursing focus and promotes continuity of client care.	
■ It provides tracking of clients from admission through discharge.	

Computer-Assisted Charting

Computerized charting systems have several advantages over other methods of charting. The first is improved legibility. Computerized charting also decreases recording time and costs, results in fewer errors, and promotes communication among health care team members. Computerized medical records establish a database for each client that allows client information to be accessible during subsequent admissions. This type of charting system also increases the database for client care, education, research, and quality improvement. Chart reviews and coding are much easier with computerized charting systems, and that increases the accuracy of client billing data, facilitating accurate reimbursement.

Computerized charting is very useful in home health care. Nurses can document client care while still in the field. Accuracy of documentation is increased because client care can be documented right after it is provided. Client information can be transmitted to various agencies as well as directly to the physician's office.

Computer-assisted charting can be accomplished at a nurses' station or at the bedside. When the equipment is available, practically all necessary documentation can be done at the bedside. This includes vital signs, admission assessment, nursing assessment, intake and output records, client education records, and client care plans. Once the information is entered into the computer, it can be disseminated to different reports without the nurse's intervention. Some of the documentation systems offer packages, such as customized flowsheets for each nursing unit in the hospital, and individualized critical pathways for each service area in the facility. Laboratory results, respiratory therapy notes, and client care documentation are fully integrated into the electronic chart. Management reports can also be generated through this type of system. Shift reports, client acuity, and client care plan variance can be generated in some systems.

Computer systems record, store, and retrieve many pieces of data about the client that must be communicated throughout the hospital for the client to receive optimal care. For example, when a client is admitted and the physician enters orders into the computer, many things happen automatically. The dietary department is notified of diet needs, the pharmacy is notified of medications and IVs that are ordered, the laboratory is notified of required tests. It is no longer necessary for the nurse to make out and deliver requests to all these departments and then arrange for delivery or pickup of the desired items.

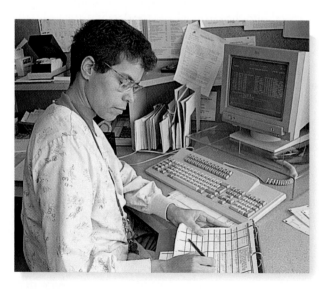

● **FIGURE 2-7** *In computer-assisted charting, entry data becomes part of the permanent record.*

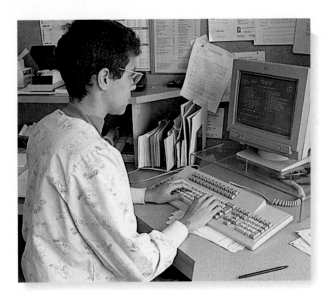

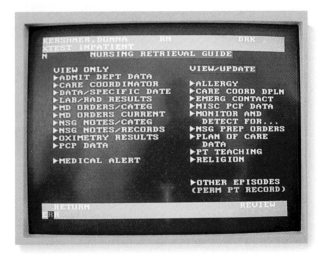

● **FIGURE 2-10** *Nurses choose a specific category of data from the screen.*

● **FIGURE 2-8** *Client data is entered into a computer at the nurses' station.*

Each nursing unit has several computer terminals, and there may be terminals at the bedside as well. Before the terminal is accessed, the sign-on code must be entered. Each person accessing information must have his or her own sign-on code. This prevents unauthorized people from accessing confidential information. After sending the code by pressing a SEND button, the nurse can select the section of the record needed. The light pen is pointed at the data category, and after the button on the pen is pressed, the selection comes up on the screen. The most common category selections are nurses' notes, physicians' orders, laboratory or x-ray reports, and client care plans.

Hospitals usually have programs that contain special matrices of nursing retrieval guide(s). Once the retrieval guide appears on the screen, the nurse can choose the specific category of data needed. Much of the routine ordering and care a nurse gives can be charted rapidly and completely in a matter of seconds using this system.

When the nurse has completed the charting, the information is displayed. At this time the nurse can make additions, corrections, or deletions. If the data displayed is correct, the nurse enters the data and it becomes a permanent part of the computer record for that client, and a hard copy is printed out to be put in the chart.

At the time the client is discharged, the nursing discharge summary is completed. This shows not only the client's physical condition, but also the status of client teaching and follow-up plans. Again, it is simply punched or tapped into the terminal and the data is displayed. This information and the client instruction sheet generated by the computer are sent home with the client.

In addition to making the charting of client care and communication between departments much simpler and less time-consuming, the computer provides reference material for common nursing problems. For example, a matrix may show the signs and symptoms associated with diabetes mellitus. If the nurse is unsure of the signs and symptoms of the different forms of the disease, she or he can easily find them in the computer, and if needed, the information may be printed out and put in the chart. In this way the nurse can be quickly updated about the client's condition and thereby provide optimal care.

As in many professions, the use of the computer in nursing and medicine has become more common and its possible uses are rapidly expanding. In the very near future, automated speech recognition will allow nurses to document data into the computer by just speaking.

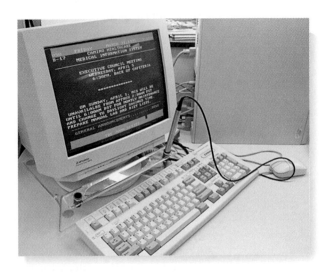

● **FIGURE 2-9** *A light pen is used to record information into a computer terminal.*

```
CCU    -9065              - EL CAMINO HOSPITAL -

01/04/02      12:50 PM

                NURSING DATA        **PRINT**    3


BED 404B
MATSON, EDWARD

                    01/04/02
09:30AM  RESPIRATORY ASSESSMENT. . . . LUNG
SOUNDS: CLEAR BILAT POST--DENIES
SHORTNESS OF BREATH ON ROOM AIR. (LCC )
09:30AM  MUSCULOSKELETAL ASSSESSMENT. . . .
CIRCULATION: PEDAL PULSE PRESENT
BILATERAL. . . . CIRCULATION: --1+ PEDAL
EDEMA BILATERALLY. (LCC )
09:30AM  CARDIOVASCULAR ASSESSMENT --NO
SALINE LOCK. (LCC )
09:30AM  ABDOMINAL ASSESSMENT. . . .
ABDOMEN: SOFT. . . . BOWEL SOUNDS: PRESENT
        (LCC )
```

● **FIGURE 2-11** *Example of nurses' notes documented in computer.*

```
CCU 9061      EL CAMINO HOSPITAL
01/04/02 12:49 PM   QAZ$$P    PAGE 001        MEDICAL CARE PLAN
BRAUN, SALLY                      F 65  CC13  SERV   MED
ADM: 01/01/02   MURPHY, PAUL MD            07:00 AM 01/04/02
CARE COORINDATOR: JANE DAYTON, RN
======================================================================
ADVANCE DIRECTIVE: N              ACCOM CODE:  **/STD ACCOM-CRIT CARE
DIAGNOSIS:

  DIVERTICULITIS OF COLON 56211
  CLINICAL PATH: EMERGENT COLORECTAL SURGERY
  01-03-02: PERFORATED CECUM; FECAL PERITONITIS; ILEOCOLECTOMY

VITAL SIGNS:

  01/03  VITAL SIGNS, T-P-R/BP, Q2H, (CCAC)

DIET AND FLUID BALANCE:

  01/03  DIET: NPO-EXC-ICE, (CCAC)
  01/03  IV LINE-START D5/.45% NACL, 1000ML W, KCL 20MEQ, CONT TIL DC'D,
         125ML/HR (31/125GTT) *CONT TIL DC'D*, <01/03/99-..>, (CCAC)
  01/03  CONNECT NG TUBE, SUCTION LOW CONTINUOUS, (CCAC)
  01/03  IRRIGATE/INSTILL, NG TUBE, WITH NORM SALINE, 20ML, Q4H, OR PRN,
         <01/03/99-..>, (CCAC)
  01/03  RECORD I 7 O, (CCAC)
  01/03  FOLEY CATH TO GRAVITY DRAINAGE, (CCAC)
  01/04    #2 197 IV LINE- D5/.45% NACL, 1000ML W, KCL 20MEQ, 125ML/HR
         (31/125GTT) *CONT TIL DC'D*, SCHED FOR APPROX 01:10 AM

HYGIENE/ACTIVITY/SAFETY:

  01/03  ACTIVITY, AMBULATE WITH ASSIST, (CCAC)
  01/03  POSTIONING: ELEVATE HD OF BED 30DEG, (CCAC)
  01/04  ACTIVITY, UP IN CHAIR-WITH ASSISTANCE--WHEN EXTUBATED, (CCAC)
OTHER CATEGORIES INCLUDED ARE:


MISCELLANEOUS ORDERS
ALLERGIES
SCHEDULED MEDICATIONS
UNSCHEDULED AND PRN MEDICATIONS
RESPIRATORY THERAPY ORDERS
OTHER DEPARTMENTS
BASIC CARE NEEDS
UNIVERSAL DATA
```

● **FIGURE 2-12** *Client care plan.*

Also, handwriting recognition programs are being tested and will soon be available. This will allow nurses to write rather than type information into a book-sized computer. The reward and the result of learning to use a computer is more efficient nursing care as well as much less time spent on paperwork.

MINIMIZING LEGAL RISKS OF COMPUTERIZED CHARTING

The American Nurses Association, the American Medical Record Association, and the Canadian Nurses Association offer guidelines and strategies for computer safety in charting.

- Your personal password or computer signature should not be given to anyone—neither another nurse on the unit, a float nurse, nor a physician. The hospital issues a short-term password with access to certain records for infrequent users.

- Do not leave a computer terminal unattended after you have logged on. (Most computers do have a timing device that shuts down a terminal when it has not been used for a certain amount of time.)

- Computer entries are part of the client's permanent record and, as such, cannot be deleted. It is possible, however, to correct an error before the material has been stored. If the entry has already been moved to storage, handle the error by marking the entry "mistaken entry," add correct information, and date and initial the entry.

- Once information about a client is stored, it is difficult to delete accidentally. Do check that stored records have backup files. This is an important safety check. If you inadvertently delete a part of the permanent record (this is difficult to do, since the computer always asks if you are sure), type an explanation into the computer file with the date, the time, and your initials. Submit an explanation in writing to your supervisor.

- Do not leave computer information about a client displayed on a monitor where others have access to it. Also, do not leave printed files unattended. Keep a log that accounts for every copy of a computerized file that you have generated from the system.

- A positive diagnosis of human immunodeficiency virus (HIV) or hepatitis B virus (HBV) is part of the client's confidential record. Disclosure of this information to unauthorized people may have legal implications. If a diagnosis is entered like any other diagnosis, take steps to follow your hospital's confidentiality procedures. Check your state's special protocols for treatment of a client's HBV or HIV status.

TABLE 2-5	COMPUTER-ASSISTED CHARTING
Advantages	**Disadvantages**
■ It allows quick communication between departments.	■ Computer systems are expensive to purchase and update.
■ Information can be accessed quickly.	■ Downtime can create problems of not receiving information or information not being charted on time.
■ Confidentiality of records is maintained.	■ Charting time may be increased if the number of terminals is insufficient.
■ Bedside computers increase accuracy and speed of documentation.	■ Nurses rely on computers and don't question information when it may be wrong.
■ Nursing information systems improve documentation and meet JCAHO standards.	
■ Client outcomes can be tracked.	
■ Speed and completeness of reimbursement are increased through accurate documentation.	
■ Information is legible.	

CARE PLANNING

According to guidelines established by the Joint Commission on Accreditation of Healthcare Organizations (JCAHO), the client or family must be involved in the development of the care plan and it must be interdisciplinary. Critical or clinical pathways are becoming more popular because of the interdisciplinary requirement of JCAHO. Client care plans provide a vital communication link among nurses. The care plan is the focal point for client care assignments and reporting between shifts.

TYPES OF CARE PLANS

Client care plans consist of two types: an individualized care plan, completely written by the nurse and/or other health team member for each specific client, and a standard client care plan. Nursing departments tend to use the standard care plan due to the time constraints of writing an individualized care plan. Standard care plans are usually written for the most frequent admission diagnoses for the hospital.

The standard care plan, based on the facility's standards of nursing practice, contains guidelines that outline the usual problems or needs that occur with a specific diagnosis. It contains a list of the usual nursing actions or interventions and the standard, or usual, expected outcomes for each problem.

INDIVIDUALIZING CARE PLANS

All clients must have an individualized plan of care even though the standard care plan is used as the base. To individualize the care plan, space is usually provided at the end of the preprinted form to allow the nurse to identify unusual problems or needs. Standard care plans are individualized by activating only those problems that pertain to a particular client. Nurses add other problems at the bottom of the form to further individualize the care plan.

All care plans, whether individualized or standard, include client needs or problems, nursing diagnoses, expected outcomes or goals, nursing interventions, and time frames for when goals should be attained.

● **FIGURE 2-13** *Individualized client care plan.*

		CLIENT CARE PLAN			Client Information

✚ COMMUNITY HOSPITAL

Discharge Criteria
1) Lungs clear to auscultation.
2) Voiding qs and continent of urine.
3) Verbalizes an understanding of discharge instructions and medications.
4)

Admitting Diagnosis

Relevant Info:

Date	Problem/Need	Expected Outcome/Goal	CP	DL	Nursing Interventions	Update / DC	Initial
3/22/02	① 1. Ineffective Breathing Pattern related to pain.	Absence of respiratory complications.	q2h x24h then q4h x48h then q8h q3-4 h	POD 3 3/25 3 pm	1a. Encourage turning, coughing and deep breathing exercises (TCDB) q2h. b. Teach client to splint incision when coughing. c. Instruct in use of breathing device, if ordered. d. Place in semi-Fowler's position. e. Assess need for pain med. f. Medicate for pain 1/2hr. before TCDB. g. Auscultate breath sounds.		
	2. Altered Urinary Elimination related to incontinence.	Continent of urine. Absence of urinary tract infection (UTI).	q4h	cath. out	2a. Check urinary output for signs and symptoms of UTI, i.e. color, odor, consistency. b. Provide catheter care according to protocol. c. Force fluids to 2500mL. d. Give cranberry juice, 240mL q shift.		
3/22/02	③ 3. Knowledge Deficit related to administration of discharge meds.	Verbalizes understanding of discharge meds, including listing signs and symptoms of side effects.	q24h	prior to disch	3a. Instruct in action of Maxaquin b. Review side effects with client and/or family. c. Have client state signs and symptoms of side effects prior to discharge. d. Provide Take Home Medication pamphlet.		
	4. Impaired Skin Integrity related to prolonged immobility.	Skin clean and intact.	q4h q2h	prior to disch	4a. Provide skin care. Use lotion. b. Turn side to side. c. Keep linens dry and wrinkle free.		

*You may use approved abbreviations from the facility when writing care plans.

● FIGURE 2-14 *Preprinted standardized client care plan using nursing diagnosis format.*

TABLE 2-6	STANDARD AND COMPUTERIZED CARE PLANS	
	Standard	**Computerized**
Advantages	■ Standards of care are established for diagnoses, which provides effective care for each client. ■ Continuity of care is established. ■ All nurses provide the same level of care. ■ Documentation time is decreased. ■ Documentation is accurate.	■ Preparation time for writing individualized care plans is decreased. ■ Care plans are written by clinical experts in the field.
Disadvantages	■ The nursing staff will not individualize the standard care plan for each client.	■ Nurses must carefully determine the relevance and appropriateness of the care plan for each individual client.

CRITICAL PATHS
OR CLINICAL PATHWAYS

This type of documentation is used primarily with managed care delivery systems. In this system, traditional nursing care plans do not exist. A critical path or clinical pathway is a standardized multidisciplinary plan of care developed for clients with common or prevalent conditions. It is a tool developed collaboratively by all health team members to facilitate achievement of client outcomes in a predictable and established time frame. The clinical pathways are used on each shift to direct and

Use Ortho Admit Orders	Day 1 Admit/ to OR in 24–36 hrs. Date _____	Day 2 Post Operative Day (POD) 1
Assessment **A** *If mechanical fall with no medical hx of problems, then surgery immediately. If hx of medical problems eval. suggested.*	• Adm. assessment, q 8 hr. ✓ Basic assessment, CMS, Drsg HV, I&O, IV, skin assess, B/S, flatus. **q 4 hr. Post-op** ✓ VS, O₂ protocol. SpO₂ reading (see graphic)	• q 8 hr. ✓ Basic assessment, CMS, HV Drsg, I&O, SpO₂, VS, IV site, skin assess. sign. • BID ✓ Homan sign. Oxygen protocol.
Physical Activity **P** • Ambulate BID if able.	• Bedrest, move in bed with assistance. • Pre admit activity level:	• OOB chair. • Commode with help. • Transfer & gait training.
Treatment **T** *Hip Precautions for hemiarthroplasty only*	• Incentive Spirometry (IS), TCDB, TED/Sequential Compression Device (SCD). • Foley cath. insert	• TED/SCD, I.S., TCDB. • Foley cath. remains if needed. • *Hip Precaution for hemiathroplasty only*
Medications IV, PO, IM, SQ, etc. **M**	• Ancef pre operative. • Ancef 8 hr. × 24 hr. (after Surgery). Antiemetic PRN, Anticoagulant.	• Stool softener • Iron supp. BID (hold if GI upset). • Anticoagulant.
IV Fluids/Blood Products **I**	• Transfuse blood if needed. • IV at 75–100cc till tol. P.O. then switch to IVL.	• IV at TKO or IVL.
Nutrition **N**	• Advance diet as tolerated.	• Diet as tolerated.
Comfort/Pain **C**	• PCA or other pain medication as ordered by Surgeon or Anesthesia.	• PCA or other pain medication as ordered by Surgeon or Anesthesia.
Education **E**	• Pre & Post op. Patient Clinical pathway, TED/SCD, Analgesia method. • Discharge plan reinforced.	• Reinforce Post op. & Clinical pathway, TED/SCD, Analgesia method.

ALL DISCIPLINES SIGN & INITIAL EACH DAY. IF OUTCOME NOT MET, LIST AS A PROBLEM.

11-7	11-7
11-7	11-7
7-3	7-3
7-3	7-3
7-3	7-3
3-11	3-11
3-11	3-11
3-11	3-11

● **FIGURE 2-15** *Clinical pathway for operative hip.*

monitor client care. The plan indicates the actions and interventions to be achieved at designated times in order to meet the criteria for reimbursable length of stay. For example, a client with a total hip replacement has a critical path that states time frames for being out of bed, gait training, and ambulation listed under the physical activity section of the form. On the second postoperative day, the client should move from bed to chair with assistance. Nursing diagnoses are not always incorporated into the critical path. Documentation of nursing activities completed in response to the critical path varies according to facility policies and guidelines. Some facilities initial each day's completed tasks on the critical path document, whereas others use flowcharts and narrative charting.

If the client does not achieve the expected outcome in the specified time, a *variance* occurs, and an individual plan of care is developed that may then incorporate nursing diagnoses. For example, if a client is unable to ambu-

NORMAL ASSESSMENT FINDINGS	ADMITTING ASSESSMENT	
	CODE	Abnormal Findings
Neurological Assessment Alert and Oriented to person, place, time Behavior appropriate to situation and memory is intact Extremities with symmetry of strength No numbness or paresthesia; face symmetrical Verbalization clear and understandable		
Cardiovascular Assessment Regular rhythm, rate 60–100/min, BP stable No peripheral edema No dizziness, chest pain or pressure		
Respiratory Assessment Regular rate 10–20/min Breath sounds clear and unlabored No sputum or sputum clear, white, or pale yellow		
Gastrointestinal Assessment Abdomen soft, non-distended with bowel sounds BM's within at least 3 days prior Light to dark brown, formed stool No emesis or diarrhea		
Nutrition Assessment See Nutrition Risk Eval. for adm. only Taking average of 75% diet over last 3 days. Tolerating food and fluid. No difficulty chewing or swallowing or mouth pain.		
Genitourinary Assessment Urine clear to yellow. No signs current infect., drainage, trauma, bleeding, retention.		
Musculoskeletal/Mobility Assessment No redness, swelling or deformity Normal ROM of extremities		
Integumentary Assessment Skin color within patient's normal, Afebrile. Skin dry and intact with no rashes, lesions or ecchymosis.		
Intravenous Assessment (all sites) Site without signs or symptoms of redness, swelling or pain Dressing dry and intact Cath is intact when discontinued		Document on MAR
Pain Management Assessment Pain free (obtain order if needed)		Chart *response* to med on MAR or Pain Flowsheet
Surgical Site Assessment Incision edges approximated if visible No evidence of inflammation or purulent drainage Suture, staples, steri-strips, dressings dry & intact if applicable		
Knowledge and Education Assessment Demonstrate readiness and willingness, capability and resource to learn about condition and self care Understands diagnosis and treatment plan States understanding of verbal or written instructions		
Discharge Planning See Disch. Planning Risk Assess. for adm. only Able to manage ADL's without difficulty, or has adequate support system in place Able to return to previous living situation.		
Psychosocial Assessment Appropriate behavior for condition and age range Cooperative with no signs of distress, or depression, manageable anxiety		
Tubes/Equipment—(if present) CT to underwater seal at 20 cm suction drains serosanguineous fluid, no air leak. NG in place draining greenish-brown fluid, irrigates well if ordered. Foley cath drains clear yellow urine. Hemovac/JP in place, compressed, draining serosanguineous		Carry name of tube, suction, and location to Assessment Record
If referrals made, order in computer and record on top RAND. Computer ord: Social Services (SS) Social Services Update (SSUP) Dietitian referral and Nutrition Score (DIETSCR)		

The left side of the form contains:

Chief Complaint: _____

History of Present Illness: _____

Previous Hospitalizations/Chronic Illness: _____

Current Medications:
☐ None ☐ Sent home ☐ Pharmacy

Name	Dose	Freq.	Last Dose

Risk Evaluation: Falls/Skin
☐ Disoriented or Confused
☐ History of Fall
☐ Neurological disorder
☐ Patient is 70+
☐ Physically impaired
☐ Restlessness or Agitation
☐ Urgency and/or Incontinent
☐ Syncope and/or dizziness
☐ Receiving hypnotics, laxatives/ diuretics
☐ Visual impairment

Additional Risk for Skin
☐ Venous stasis
☐ Edema
☐ Poor Nutrition
☐ Diabetes
☐ Thyroid condition
☐ Steroid dependency
☐ If admitted with pressure ulcer automatic skin risk assessment

☐ No risk identified ☐ Risk Identified ≥ 3 items checked
☐ Initiate pt. prone to falls std. ☐ Initiate Skin Risk Assessment

Nutrition Risk Evaluation: (Total checkboxes to obtain score)
Poor appetite one week prior to admission . . . .(2) ☐
Unintentional weight loss of more than 10 lbs. . . . . . .(2) ☐
Difficulty swallowing . . . .(1) ☐
Major surgery in the past month . . . .(1) ☐
Enter "DietScr" if Score = 3 or more   SCORE _____

Social or Cultural Variables: Circle Y (yes) or N (no)
Alcohol: Y N How much: _____
Smoking: Y How long: _____ How much: _____
      N ☐ Quit/When: _____
Recreational Drugs: Y N What: _____
Language: ☐ English ☐ Other _____
Cultural or spiritual factors or preferences that may contribute to patient's response to illness and treatment: Y N
Identify problems on the Multidisciplinary Problem Record

Information for Admission Database obtained from:
☐ Patient ☐ Other _____

PLAN OF CARE: _____
☐ Unit Standard of Care
☐ Clinical Pathway for _____
Discharge Plan _____ Estimated DC date _____
Patient stated long-term goal: _____

Additional Standards Implemented:
☐ Neuro Patient   ☐ Orthopedic Patient
☐ Cardiac Patient   ☐ Pre- and Post-op Patient
☐ Respiratory Patient   ☐ Prone to Falls
☐ Other _____   ☐ Potential for Skin Breakdown
_____ R.N. _____ Date

● **FIGURE 2-16** *Admitting assessment data collection sheet.*

late by day three, a nursing diagnosis can be used to individualize the client's variance from the critical pathway expectations. An individualized care plan is initiated, and charting continues on the variance until it is resolved. The individualized section of the care path is usually found on the back of the form. In the sample clinical pathway for operative hip, the form used to chart the variance is termed the Multidisciplinary Problem Record. The problem is identified and listed as Problem 1. In the space provided for the problem, a nursing diagnosis is used or a client problem is listed. Interventions are developed and an evaluation section is added. All other documentation continues on the care path.

In addition to the pathway and multidisciplinary problem record, clinical pathways may also include an admitting assessment and a nursing history. An ongoing admission database, including a discharge plan, risk assessment, and multidisciplinary team conference, is included as part of the total package for the pathway.

CRITICAL THINKING FOCUS

SECTION ONE ▪ Documentation

Potential Problems

- Nursing intervention is not entered into chart within appropriate time frame.

- Information is charted on wrong client's chart.

- A nurse asks you to chart on a client's chart a treatment that she has completed.

- A physician asks you for your password to the computer so he can enter his orders.

Possible Outcomes

- Make entry at the next line of document. Label entry *late entry*.

- Draw line through entry, write date, and sign your name.
- Write the words *mistaken entry* (ME) above line.

- Explain to the nurse that you cannot chart something you have not done yourself. If she says it is OK because you observed her, refuse to chart entry and notify your instructor or nurse manager.

- Explain to the physician that each individual must use his or her own password.
- Ask him if he needs assistance to retrieve his own password or if he needs to obtain one.

SECTION TWO ▪ Care Planning

Potential Problems

- Client is placed on critical pathway after surgery, but is not able to meet criteria (perform activities as scheduled).

- Plan of care established on standard care plan being used for client is not accurate.

Possible Outcomes

- Individual plan of care must be initiated.

- Individualize those areas where care plan is not appropriate for client.
- Update care plan to include current information.

SELF-CHECK EVALUATION

PART 1 ▪ Matching Terms

Select the definition from column B that most accurately describes the charting format in column A. Not all definitions will be used.

Column A

a. Charting by exception
b. Narrative charting
c. Problem-oriented medical records
d. Focus charting

Column B

1. Format contains a database, problem list, and progress notes.
2. Differences from the initial assessment are documented.
3. Charting focuses on client's status.
4. Flowsheets are part of documentation format.
5. All charting is done on progress notes.
6. Chronological charting is used.
7. Frequency of charting input is stated in hospital policy.
8. DAR format is used for charting.

PART 2 ▪ Multiple Choice Questions

1. Charting is one of the nurse's most important functions. Which of the following is the most important purpose of charting?

a. To communicate to other members of the client's health care team.
b. To evaluate the staff's performance.
c. To provide information for a nursing audit.
d. To enable physicians to monitor nursing care.

2. Which of the following items would you always include in a client's chart?

1. Initial assessment at beginning of shift.
2. Abnormalities noted during assessment.
3. Changes in client's condition.
4. General verbatim comments.
5. Client's response to teaching.
   (a) All of the above.
   (b) All but 4.
   (c) All but 4 and 5.
   (d) 2, 3, and 5.

3. Which of the following statements is the best explanation of a source-oriented system of charting?

a. This system is based on problems, and the information is charted in chronological order.
b. It is a common and efficient way of organizing client information according to the source of information.
c. This system focuses on the client's status rather than on the source.
d. Systematic and well-defined, this method consists of five distinct parts.

4. A well-organized POMR system includes progress notes that have a specific format called SOAP. This acronym translates as:

    a. Subjective, objective, assessment, plan.

    b. Summary, objective documentation, assessment, promoting care.

    c. Symptoms, observations, assessment, plan.

    d. Subjective, objective, assessment, priority problems.

5. A major advantage of a computer-based documentation system is:

    a. All health care staff members can chart in the nursing notes.

    b. The system provides reference material for common nursing problems.

    c. Nurses do not need to check physicians' orders as they are transferred to the appropriate department for implementation.

    d. Information is readily available with minimal delays.

6. Charting by exception (CBE) is best described as a system of charting that:

    a. Does not encompass the use of nursing diagnosis.

    b. Necessitates a complete nursing assessment at the beginning and end of each shift.

    c. Requires a data entry every 2 hrs in the nursing notes.

    d. Only addresses client changes when the predetermined norm is not met.

7. Which one of the following statements is *true* regarding minimizing the legal risks of charting?

    a. The password you use to enter the computer is not given to a physician to assist him or her with data entry.

    b. Computer entries are deleted when they are no longer relevant to client care.

    c. The nurse must be extremely careful when entering data into the computer, as it is very easy to delete information.

    d. It is important that records have backup files as a safety factor.

PART 3 ▪ Critical Thinking Application

Complete the nurses' notes in narrative format from the following clinical situation: Jane Bowman, a 24-year-old woman, was admitted to the surgical unit following an appendectomy. She is now 8 hrs postop and complaining of incisional pain when you come on duty at 11:00 P.M. After report, you administer meperidine (Demerol) 50 mg and promethazine (Phenergan) 25 mg IM in the left ventrogluteal area. When making nursing rounds at 1:00 A.M., you observe the client sleeping. At 3:00 A.M. she is awake and you check her dressing. It is in place, dry, and without drainage. The client is able to turn side to side without assistance. Her vital signs are stable, and she is able to turn, cough, and deep breathe effectively. There is an unproductive cough with the deep breathing and coughing.

NURSES' NOTES

Time	Medications/Treatment	Observations	Signature

3

MEDICAL ASEPSIS

INTRODUCTION

Clients may enter the health care facility with an infection or may develop an infection while in the facility. Clients in health care settings are at risk for acquired infections, termed *nosocomial infections*. These infections occur because hospitals harbor many different types of microorganisms, some of which are resistant to antibiotics. Clients come into contact with many different health care workers over the course of a day and are subjected to any number of invasive procedures. The longer the client's hospital stay, the greater his or her risk of developing an infection. Infection control principles help prevent the spread of infection or disease by maintaining medical asepsis and standard precautions in the delivery of client care.

Handwashing is the single most important act that prevents the spread of infection. Contact transmission by contaminated hands—of either health care workers or clients themselves—is the most common form of contamination from microorganisms. It is estimated that 50 percent of nosocomial infections can be eliminated or reduced by handwashing.

(continued on next page)

The use of clean gloves by health care workers when providing specified nursing care procedures will reduce the likelihood of the spread of microorganisms. Latex and vinyl are the two most common materials used in gloves. Latex-free gloves are available and should be provided for medical personnel allergic to latex. Latex gloves are commonly used for procedures requiring fine motor skills and procedures that take a lengthy period of time to complete. Vinyl gloves can be used for other client care, such as handling specimens, emptying bedpans, or providing personal hygienic care. Vinyl gloves are less expensive; however, they provide less protection than latex gloves. Even if gloves are used to provide client care, handwashing is done before and after gloves are used.

PREPARATION PROTOCOL: FOR MEDICAL ASEPSIS

Complete the following steps before each skill.

1. Determine if nonantimicrobial (usual) or antiseptic cleansing agents are required for client care.
2. Determine if orange sticks or antiseptic-impregnated scrub brushes are necessary.
3. Check if usual 30-sec hand wash is sufficient.
4. Identify need for gloves for client care.
5. Identify most appropriate type of gloves for client care when needed.

COMPLETION PROTOCOL: FOR MEDICAL ASEPSIS

Make sure the following steps have been completed.

1. Remove gloves, if used, and place in appropriate container.
2. Wash hands for 30 sec following client care.
3. Dry hands thoroughly using paper towels.

SECTION ONE

HANDWASHING

Handwashing is done before and after all client contact. This includes the handling of all equipment, preparation of medications, and documenting in the chart. In medical asepsis, handwashing is most effective if adequate friction is used during the hand scrub, all surfaces of the hands and wrists are cleaned thoroughly, and sufficient time is used for the procedure. Thirty seconds is the recommended time for handwashing when medical asepsis is required. Surgical asepsis requires a much greater length of time to complete, and the area to be cleansed includes the hands, wrists, and arms up to the elbow.

It is important to use a soap dispenser and paper toweling rather than bar soap and cloth toweling to decrease microorganisms on the hands. This will assist in preventing the spread of infection to the clients, other health care workers, and yourself.

RATIONALE

- To decrease number of bacteria on the hands
- To prevent spread of microorganisms from health care worker or environment to client
- To prevent spread of microorganisms between clients

ASSESSMENT

- Assess type of handwashing procedure that needs to be completed—medical or surgical asepsis.
- Determine type of soap to be used— nonantimicrobial or antiseptic cleansing agents.
- Determine length of time for handwashing.

CLINICAL NOTE

PRINCIPLES OF HANDWASHING

- Wash hands thoroughly at the beginning of the shift before providing client care.
- Wash hands for 30 sec before and after providing client care.
- Wash hands before and after preparing medications.
- Wash hands after handling soiled linen, equipment, or supplies.
- Wash hands between contact with different clients.
- Wash hands after removing gloves.
- Wash hands after you have sneezed or coughed.
- Wash hands before and after eating.
- Wash hands just before leaving the nursing unit.

SAFETY ALERT

To help prevent the spread of infection, nurses must wash their hands for 30 sec before and after each direct contact with a client or each use of client care items.

HANDWASHING

Equipment

- Nonantimicrobial soap following 1997 Healthcare Infection Control Practices Advisory Committee (HICPAC) recommendations
- Orangewood stick for cleaning nails, if available

- Running warm water
- Paper towels
- Trash basket

SKILL

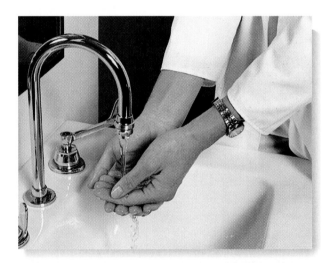

① Ensure that paper towel is hanging down from dispenser.

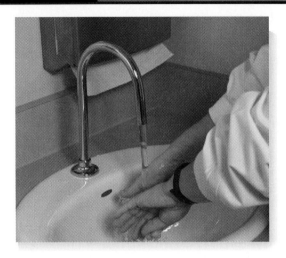

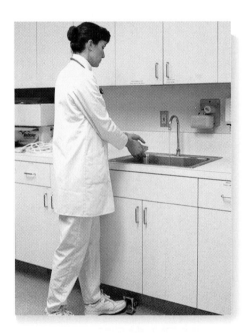

② Stand in front of but away from sink. **RATIONALE:** Uniform should not touch sink to avoid contamination.

- Turn on water using foot pedal or faucet so that flow is adequate, but not splashing.

③ Wet hands under running water. **RATIONALE:** Wetting hands facilitates distribution of soap over entire skin surface.

- Adjust temperature to warm. **RATIONALE:** Cold does not facilitate sudsing and cleaning; hot is damaging to skin.

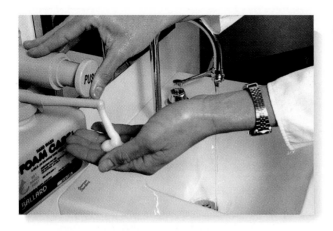

4 Place small amount (one or two teaspoons) of liquid soap on hands. Soap should come from a dispenser, not bar soap. **RATIONALE:** This prevents spread of microorganisms.

CLINICAL NOTE

Clean under your fingernails with an orangewood stick. This should be done at the start of every day and if your hands are heavily contaminated.

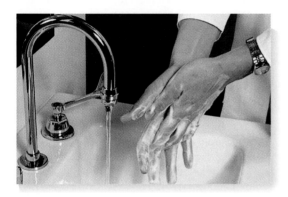

5 Rub vigorously, using a firm, circular motion, while keeping fingers pointed down lower than wrists. Start with each finger, then between fingers, then palm and back of hand. Wash hands for at least 30 sec.

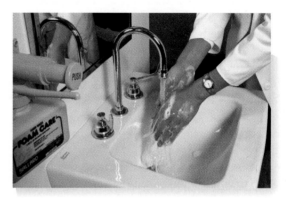

6 Rinse hands under running water, keeping fingers pointed downward. **RATIONALE:** This position prevents contamination of arms.

- Resoap hands, rewash, and rerinse if heavily contaminated.

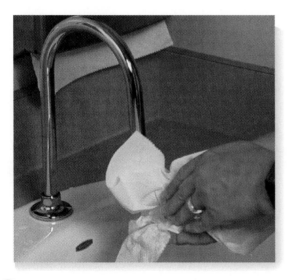

7 Dry hands thoroughly with a paper towel. **RATIONALE:** Moist hands tend to gather more microorganisms from the environment.

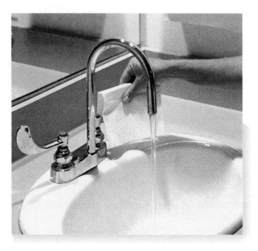

8 Turn off water faucet with dry paper towel if not using foot pedal. Restart procedure at step 3 if hands touch sink anytime between steps 3 and 8.

SECTION TWO

DONNING AND REMOVING GLOVES

The Centers for Disease Control and Prevention (CDC) guidelines for glove use should be readily available in the nursing unit. Using gloves will protect health care workers from acquiring microorganisms on their hands. Gloves will also prevent the transmission of organisms to clients and other health care workers. Hands are washed and dried thoroughly before and after gloving. Clean, nonsterile gloves should be worn when touching blood, body fluids, secretions, excretions, and contaminated items. Gloves are put on just before touching mucous membranes and nonintact skin. Remove gloves immediately if torn or excessively soiled, and after use. Gloves should be discarded immediately and not reused. Hands must be washed before touching uncontaminated items and environmental surfaces or giving care to another client.

Washing hands thoroughly after using latex gloves may assist in the prevention of future latex allergies. Using vinyl gloves instead of latex to provide routine client care will help prevent allergies and be less costly. It is also important to determine if gloves are actually needed for each client care activity. In many cases, gloves are unnecessary and place the nurse at risk of developing an allergy if she or he wears them unnecessarily. For those nurses with latex allergies, latex-free gloves must be provided.

CLINICAL NOTE

GLOVE SELECTION

■ Use examination gloves for procedures involving contact with mucous membranes, unless otherwise indicated, and for client care or procedures that do not require use of sterile gloves.

■ Use sterile gloves for procedures involving contact with normally sterile areas of the body.

■ Change gloves between clients.

■ Do not wash, disinfect, or reuse surgical or examination gloves.

■ Use general-purpose utility gloves (rubber household gloves) for housekeeping tasks that involve potential blood contact and for instrument cleaning and decontamination procedures.

RATIONALE

■ To prevent spread of microorganisms from health care worker or environment to client

■ To prevent spread of microorganisms from client to health care worker

■ To prevent spread of microorganisms between clients

ASSESSMENT

■ Determine most appropriate glove for client care.

■ Assess client for potential latex allergies.

■ Assess nurses for potential latex allergies.

■ Assess need for latex-free equipment for client care.

SAFETY ALERT

Latex allergy or hypersensitivity can be life-threatening, so know the primary symptoms.

■ Contact dermatitis

■ Type IV hypersensitivity with symptoms of localized swelling, redness, itching, and hives

■ Type I hypersensitivity, potentially dangerous, with symptoms of bronchospasm, generalized edema, difficulty breathing, cardiac arrest, and other major systemic symptoms

DONNING AND REMOVING GLOVES

Equipment

- Clean gloves
- Trash receptacle

SKILL

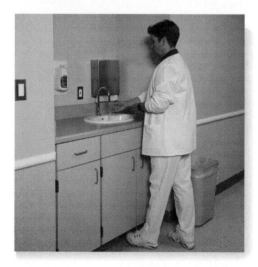

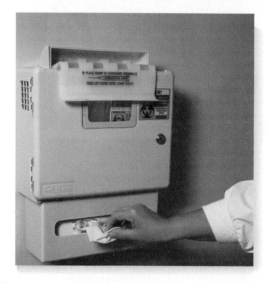

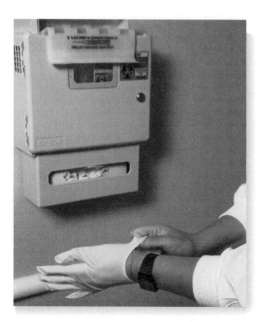

1 Wash your hands.

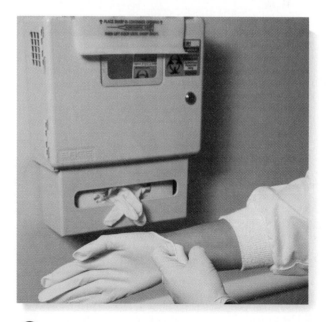

2 Remove glove from dispenser.

3 Hold glove at wrist edge and slip fingers into openings. Pull glove up to wrist.

4 Place gloved hand under wrist edge of second glove and slip fingers into opening.

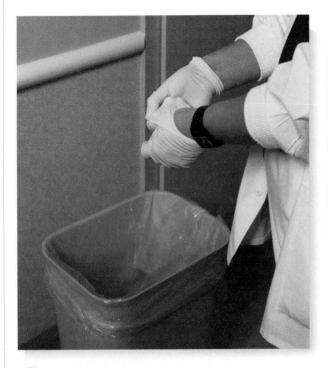

5 Remove glove by pulling off. Touch only outside of glove at cuff, so that glove turns inside out.

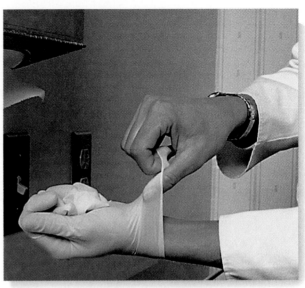

6 Place rolled-up glove in palm of second hand. Remove second glove by slipping one finger under glove edge and pulling down and off so that glove turns inside out. Both gloves are removed as a unit.

SAFETY ALERT

Ungloved hands should not touch anything that is moist coming from a body surface. The moisture coming from a body surface should be considered potentially contaminated.

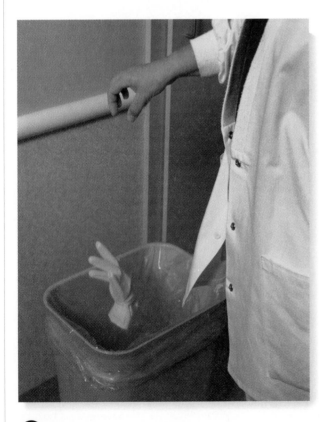

7 Dispose of gloves in proper container, not at bedside. Wash your hands.

CHARTING

- Infection control measures used
- Clean gloves used for procedure
- Use of latex-free gloves

CRITICAL THINKING FOCUS

SECTIONS ONE AND TWO ▪ Medical Asepsis

Unexpected Outcomes

- Infection occurs in client.

- Allergic reaction occurs in client.

- Nurse develops allergic reaction to latex.

Alternative Nursing Actions

- Assess mode of transmission of microorganism.
- Check that gloving technique is appropriate.
- Review handwashing technique.
- Attend in-service education program on infection control procedures.

- Notify physician.
- Health care providers change to latex-free gloves.
- Change all latex equipment to latex-free equipment.

- Notify nurse manager of allergy.
- Ensure adequate supply of latex-free gloves and equipment on unit.
- Use only latex-free gloves when providing client care.

SELF-CHECK EVALUATION

PART 1 ▪ Matching Terms

Select the description from column B that best describes the term in column A. Not all descriptions will be used.

Column A

_____ a. Medical asepsis
_____ b. Surgical asepsis
_____ c. Latex gloves
_____ d. Vinyl gloves

Column B

1. Maintaining equipment free from micro-organisms
2. Using nonantibacterial soap for handwashing
3. Using germicidal soap for handwashing
4. Used during client care activities requiring fine motor skills
5. Used during routine client care activities
6. Used for clients or health care workers who are allergic to latex

PART 2 ▪ Multiple Choice Questions

1. Nosocomial infections are best described as infections that are:

a. Life-threatening.
b. Acquired in the hospital.
c. Caused by gram-negative organisms.
d. Easily killed by using nonantibacterial soaps.

2. In medical asepsis, the spread of microorganisms is prevented by the use of _____ and _____ asepsis.

a. Clean, surgical.
b. Medical, surgical.
c. Sterile, clean.
d. Prevention, medical.

3. Which one of the following statements regarding use of gloves is *true?*

a. Gloves should be changed between clients only if soiled with body fluids.
b. Health care workers with cuts on their hands should wear double gloves the entire shift.
c. Gloves should be worn when there is potential for contact with blood and body fluids.
d. Gloves should be worn when taking vital signs on all clients.

4. Handwashing should take _____ seconds and is completed by keeping the fingers pointed _____.

a. 30, upward.
b. 30, downward.
c. 60, upward.
d. 60, downward.

5. The most effective method of preventing the transmission of infection is:

a. Wearing a mask if the organism is airborne.
b. Wearing gloves when giving client care.
c. Wearing a gown when giving client care.
d. Good handwashing.

6. In which situation are gloves *not* necessary?

a. When in contact with urine.
b. When suctioning clients.
c. When changing an ostomy pouch.
d. When delivering a food tray to an AIDS client.

PART 3 ▪ Critical Thinking Application

You are assigned to care for the following three clients:

▪ James Dunn, a 26-year-old male, admitted with a gunshot wound to the abdomen. He has just returned from the OR after an exploratory laparotomy and has a temporary colostomy. His abdominal dressing is moist and has a moderate amount of serosanguineous drainage present. He requires the use of a urinal and assistance with turning and moving.

▪ Cynthia Maloney, a 65-year-old female, two days postop thoracotomy with lower right lobe resection for cancer. Her dressing is dry and intact. Her IV is infusing slowly but doesn't appear to be infiltrated. She needs assistance going to the bathroom and with ambulation.

■ Paul Barnes, a 78-year-old male, admitted this morning for possible prostatic cancer. He has been having laboratory tests and is scheduled for surgery later today. He has BRPs until his preop medication is given.

1. Indicate when medical asepsis principles are carried out with client care for each of the three clients. Be specific with your response.

2. For each client, indicate when gloves should be worn and the specific type of gloves needed.

3. Is there a need for surgical asepsis to be used with any of the clients? If so, identify client(s) requiring surgical asepsis. Provide a rationale for your answer.

4

INFECTION CONTROL

INTRODUCTION

Infection control involves monitoring the client, the environment, and health care workers to prevent the spread of infection. Immediate procedures are instituted when infection is present. These procedures involve the handling of linen, food trays, equipment, and supplies used in client care.

Barriers to Infection

An individual's ability to resist infection is determined by the state of the body's immune system and by the person's general health. Factors that contribute to susceptibility to infection include altered nutritional status, stress, fatigue, disease, drugs, metabolic functions, and age. Clients with severe underlying diseases are most likely to develop nosocomial infections. The body is protected against infection by immunities, by the inflammatory process, and by anatomic barriers that include the skin and mucous membranes.

The anatomic barrier is unable to protect the body against infection when the integrity of the skin or mucous membrane is broken. In this case, both resident and transient flora or bacteria have a direct route to the internal tissue of the body. To pre-

(continued on next page)

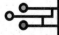

vent the spread of infection, the body's internal defense mechanisms mobilize and begin clearing and repairing the damaged site.

The second way disease or infection is prevented is through immunity, antitoxins, and vaccines. Natural immunity is inherited. Acquired immunity occurs after an individual has been exposed to a disease or infection or has been vaccinated.

The third way the body resists infection is through the inflammatory process. Inflammation activates various systems in the body (plasma, clotting, kinin). Blood flow to the inflamed area is increased, and, in many cases, there is drainage of inflammatory debris to the external environment.

Conditions Predisposing to Infection

Certain conditions and invasive techniques predispose clients to infection because the integrity of the skin is broken or the illness itself establishes a climate favorable for the infectious process to occur. Among the most common are surgical wounds, changes in the body's immune system, and alterations in the respiratory tract or genitourinary tract. Implants such as heart valves, prosthetic grafts, or vascular grafts can lead to nosocomial septicemia. The extensive use of IV therapy in clients has increased infections dramatically.

Nosocomial Infections

These infections are acquired while the client is hospitalized and were not present or incubating at the time of hospital admission. Nosocomial infections result in a high morbidity and are estimated to cause or contribute to 80,000 deaths annually in the United States. Many of these infections are caused by pathogens transmitted from one client to another by health care workers. Nosocomial infections are usually caused by poor handwashing techniques or no handwashing between clients. It has been estimated that compliance with proper handwashing techniques by health care workers is as low as 30 to 50 percent. Compliance with handwashing procedures is higher among nurses than among physicians and other health care personnel; however, it is still very low. It was identified in a study of 2800 opportunities for handwashing that there was only a 48 percent compliance with handwashing practices. Before high-risk procedures, in intensive care units, and in areas where highly susceptible clients were, there was even less compliance with handwashing procedures. In other studies, not only was handwashing omitted, but when it was done, the hands were washed for an average of only 8.5 to 9.5 sec. It is obvious that a major responsibility of nurses is to prevent nosocomial infections from occurring in the hospitalized client. Therefore, handwashing is the most important intervention practiced in nursing and must be completed following strict policies and procedures.

Three major organisms are responsible for a very large percentage of nosocomial infections: *Clostridium difficile,* methicillin-resistant *Staphylococcus aureus,* and vancomycin-resistant enterococcus. *C. difficile* is a gram-positive, spore-forming bacterium with significant nosocomial potential. It is often resistant to anti-microbial therapy, due to its protective spore, and is therefore able to proliferate relatively unimpeded in the hospital setting. It is inherent in the colon and works as a pathogen by releasing toxins into the lumen of the bowel. The toxins cause destruction at the site. The destruction of this large area can produce profound sepsis. Because so many hospitalized clients require antibiotic therapy, the bacterium is very prevalent. This nosocomial infection is also a problem because *C. difficile* is relatively resistant to cleaning and handwashing agents. It is therefore spread by health care workers and by contact with equipment that has not been properly disinfected.

Methicillin-resistant *S. aureus* (MRSA) is very commonly found in hospitals and long-term care facilities. Unfortunately, this organism has become increasingly resistant to methicillin and other synthetic penicillins. Vancomycin, the drug of choice to treat

MRSA more recently, is also losing its effectiveness as a treatment for *S. aureus*. Health care workers easily transmit MRSA to clients because it frequently colonizes skin. The colonization is seldom recognized and thus transmission of the organism to other clients is easily accomplished. It usually occurs when invasive procedures such as IV therapy, respiratory therapy treatments, and surgical procedures are part of the client's hospitalization.

Vancomycin-resistant enterococcus (VRE) is a gram-positive bacterium that is part of the normal flora of the gastrointestinal tract. It is capable of producing significant infections in certain situations. It is the second most frequent cause of nosocomial infections. VRE was formerly treated with ampicillin or vancomycin in combination with gentamicin, but clients with VRE are frequently resistant to all other antimicrobial therapies. This leaves these clients with bacterial infections for which there is no pharmaceutical treatment. In April 2000, the Food and Drug Administration (FDA) approved a new super antibiotic called Zyvox, the first entirely new type of antibiotic in 35 years. This drug is now reserved to fight infections that are resistant to other antibiotics. It is the drug of choice for VRE and MRSA.

PREPARATION PROTOCOL: FOR INFECTION CONTROL

Complete the following steps before each skill.

1. Check client's plan of care and physician's orders.
2. Determine specific type of isolation precautions that need to be implemented.
3. Gather all necessary equipment.
4. Wash hands.
5. Don appropriate isolation attire.
6. Take all equipment, linens, and supplies into room.
7. Identify client.

COMPLETION PROTOCOL: FOR INFECTION CONTROL

Make sure the following steps have been completed.

1. Ensure client is comfortable and his or her care has been completed.
2. Place linen in linen hamper.
3. Place garbage in red isolation bag.
4. Place reusable items in red isolation bag and label with contents.
5. When bag is one-half to three-fourths full, close bag and place near door for transport to "dirty" utility room.
6. Place new bag in containers as needed.
7. Take isolation attire off and place in appropriate red bag.
8. Wash hands inside room.
9. Wash hands outside room at nearest sink.

STANDARD PRECAUTIONS

The Centers for Disease Control and Prevention (CDC) instituted guidelines using a two-tier system in 1996. *The First Tier, Standard Precautions,* is used for the care of all clients in hospitals. Standard precautions apply to blood, all body fluids, secretions, and excretions, whether or not they contain visible blood; nonintact skin; and mucous membranes. These precautions are designed to reduce the risk of transmission of both recognized and unrecognized sources of infection in hospitals.

The *Second Tier, Transmission-Based Precautions,* covers three sets of precautions based on the routes of transmission. These categories are designed to be used with clients documented or suspected to be infected or colonized with highly transmissible or epidemiologically important pathogens for which additional precautions must be used to interrupt transmission to others in the hospital. The three types of transmission-based precautions include airborne precautions, droplet precautions, and contact precautions.

Airborne precautions reduce the risk of airborne transmission of infectious agents, such as rubeola, varicella, and *Mycobacterium tuberculosis.* The small-particle droplet residue can stay suspended in the air for long periods of time. Because the droplets can be dispersed widely by air currents, they may be inhaled by a susceptible host within the same room or even over longer distances.

Droplet precautions are used to prevent the trans-mission of diseases such as meningitis, pneumonia, scarlet fever, diphtheria, rubella, and pertussis. Droplets are generated by the client primarily during coughing, sneezing, and talking. Droplets are also spread during suctioning and bronchoscopy procedures. Transmission occurs when the droplets containing the microorganisms generated from the infected person are propelled a short distance through the air and deposited on the host's mucous membranes (conjunctiva, nasal mucosa, or mouth). These droplets do not remain suspended in the air; therefore special ventilation or air handling in the room is not required.

Contact precautions are used for clients known or suspected to have serious illnesses easily transmitted by direct contact, such as herpes simplex, staphylococcal infections, hepatitis A, respiratory syncytial virus, and wound or skin infections. Contact transmission is the most frequent mode of transmission of nosocomial infection in the hospital. Contact transmission is divided into two subgroups: direct contact and indirect contact transmission.

- Direct contact transmission involves a direct body surface-to-surface contact and physical transfer of microorganisms between a susceptible client and an infected or colonized person. This can occur during direct client care activities such as bathing, turning, or providing other hygienic care. Direct contact transmission can also occur between two clients.

- Indirect contact transmission involves client contact with contaminated instruments, needles, or dressings. Contaminated hands of health care workers may transmit microorganisms through this route.

All three types of precautions may be used at one time when multiple routes of transmission are suspected in a client. These precautions are always used in conjunction with Standard Precautions.

Health care providers should follow these guidelines when caring for clients.

- Wash hands thoroughly after removing gloves and before and after all client contact.

- Wear gloves when there is direct contact with blood, body fluids, secretions, excretions, or contaminated items. This includes neonate before first bath. Wash as soon as possible if unanticipated contact with these body substances occurs.

- Protect clothing with gowns or plastic aprons if there is possibility of being splashed or directly contacting contaminated material.

- Wear masks, goggles, or face shield to avoid being splashed; this includes during suctioning, irrigation, and deliveries.

- Do not break or recap needles; discard them intact into puncture-resistant containers.

- Place all contaminated articles and trash in leakproof bags. Check hospital policy regarding double-bagging.

- Clean spills quickly with a 1:10 solution of bleach or according to facility policy, or with Environmental Protection Agency (EPA)-approved germicide if spill occurs in an HIV/AIDS client's room.

- Place clients at risk for contaminating the environment in private rooms with separate bathroom facilities, or with other clients with same infectious organism.

- Transport infected clients using appropriate barriers (i.e., mask and gown).

TABLE 4-1	HICPAC* RECOMMENDATIONS FOR TRANSMISSION-BASED PRECAUTIONS		
	Contact	**Droplet**	**Airborne**
Purpose	Prevent transmission of known or suspected infected or colonized microorganisms by direct hand or skin-to-skin contact that occurs when providing direct client care. Conditions in which contact precautions are required: diphtheria, herpes simplex, scabies, staphylococcus infection, hepatitis A, and respiratory syncytial virus wound or skin infection.	Prevent transmission of large-particle droplets, larger than 5 μm (i.e., diphtheria, pertussis, streptococcal pharyngitis, pneumonia, scarlet fever, meningitis, rubella).	Prevent transmission of small-particle residue of 5 μm or smaller droplets (i.e., measles, varicella, tuberculosis).
Client placement	■ Private room. ■ Can be placed in room of client with same microorganism.	■ Private room. ■ Can be placed in room of client with same diagnosis.	■ Private room. ■ Can be placed in room of client with same diagnosis. ■ Monitor negative air pressure. ■ Keep door closed. ■ Keep client in room.
Respiratory protection	■ Mask not necessary.	■ Use mask when working within 3 ft of client.	■ Respiratory protective equipment. ■ Do not enter room of clients with rubeola or varicella if susceptible to these infections.
Gloves and gown	■ Wear gloves when entering room. ■ Change gloves after contact with infective material, such as wound drainage or fecal material. ■ Wash hands immediately after removing gloves. ■ Wear gown when working with clients with diarrhea, ostomies, or wound drainage not contained in dressing. ■ Wear gown if contact with client or environment will occur.	■ Follow standard precautions.	■ Follow standard precautions.
Client transport	■ Transport only if essential. ■ Ensure precautions are maintained to minimize risk of transmission.	■ Transport only if essential. ■ Place mask on client when outside room.	■ Transport only if essential. ■ Place mask on client when outside room.
Client care items	■ Client care items and environmental surfaces are cleaned daily. ■ Dedicate equipment to single client use (i.e., stethoscope, thermometer).		

*Hospital Infection Control Practices Advisory Committee.

Adapted from Department of Health and Human Services: CDC, *Federal Register,* "Recommendations for Isolation Precautions in Hospitals," updated February 18, 1997.

RATIONALE

- To prevent the transmission of microorganisms from nurse to client, client to nurse, client to client, or to other health care workers
- To prevent compromised clients from acquiring nosocomial infections

ASSESSMENT

- Assess extent of isolation attire required by client's condition.
- Assess equipment and supplies needed before entering isolation room.
- Determine type of isolation room necessary for client.
- Determine type of transmission precautions that need to be implemented.

STANDARD PRECAUTIONS (TIER ONE)

Equipment

- Nonantimicrobial soap
- Paper towels
- Clean gloves
- Mask or respiratory device
- Face shield, if needed
- Gown
- Sharps container

SAFETY ALERT

- Standard Precautions are designed to be used for all clients in the hospital.
- Standard Precautions reduce the risk of microorganism transmission from health care worker to client, client to client, and health care worker to health care worker.
- These precautions apply in the following situations:
  - Contact with blood
  - Contact with body fluids, excretions, and secretions (except for sweat)
  - Contact with nonintact skin
  - Contact with mucous membranes

SKILL

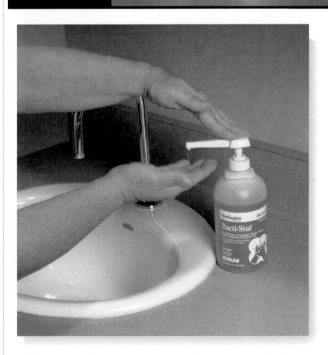

1 Wash hands after contact with blood, body fluids, secretions, excretions, or contaminated objects, whether gloves are worn or not. **RATIONALE:** Donning gloves with unclean hands can transfer microorganisms outside of gloves.

- Wash hands using nonantimicrobial soap for routine handwashing.
- Wash hands using antimicrobial agent or antiseptic agent for control of specific outbreaks of infection.
- Wash hands immediately after removing gloves.
- Protect hands by applying skin protectants or using alcohol-based hand rinses and gels containing emollients if soap and water causes dermatitis.

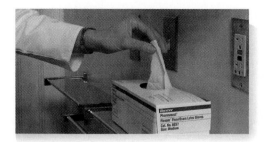

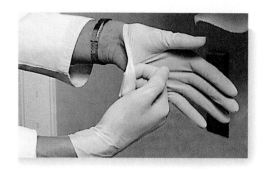

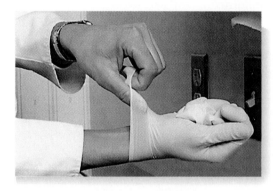

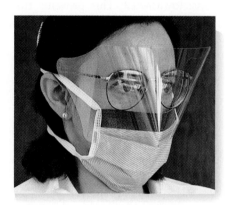

2 Wear gloves when touching blood, body fluids, secretions, excretions, or contaminated items. Clean gloves are used in most cases. If there is risk of transmitting microorganisms, sterile gloves should be worn.

3 Change gloves after contact with infectious material that may have high concentrations of microorganisms (fecal material and wound drainage).

4 Remove gloves immediately after client care and before touching noncontaminated surfaces or objects. **RATIONALE:** This reduces risk of transmission of microorganisms in environment or to other clients.

- Wash hands immediately after removing gloves.

5 Wear mask, goggles, or face shield if there is potential for splashes or sprays of blood, body fluids, secretions, or excretions. **RATIONALE:** These devices prevent microorganisms from splashing into eyes or mucous membranes.

BEYOND THE SKILL

Waterless Antiseptic Agents

Waterless antiseptic agents should be placed at client's bedside to facilitate hand hygiene.

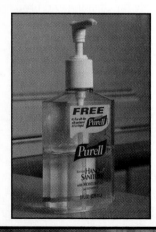

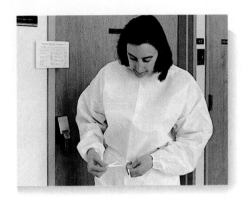

6 Wear clean, nonsterile gown if there is potential for splashes or sprays of blood, body fluids, secretions, or excretions. **RATIONALE:** This prevents transfer of microorganisms to you, or potentially to other clients.

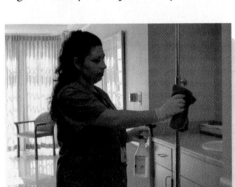

8 Handle client care equipment that is soiled with blood, body fluids, secretions, or excretions carefully to prevent transfer of microorganisms to others and to environment.

- Place single-use equipment in appropriate receptacle for disposal.
- Clean, if appropriate, and place reusable equipment in appropriate area for return to central supply for cleaning and processing.

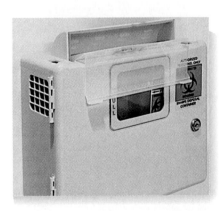

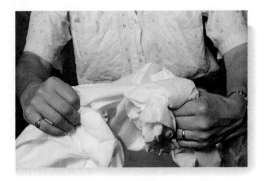

7 Remove soiled gown by turning it inside out and placing it in appropriate receptacle. **RATIONALE:** This prevents transfer of microorganisms from client to nurse's uniform.

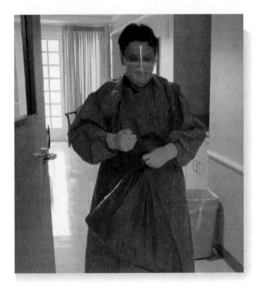

9 Dispose of linen that is soiled with blood, bloody fluids, secretions, or excretions by placing in biohazard bag. Send bag to laundry for cleaning. **RATIONALE:** Microorganism transmission risk is negligible if linen is handled, transported, and laundered appropriately.

10 Prevent injuries from sharps or needles by placing them in puncture-resistant container. Do not recap, bend, or break needles. **RATIONALE:** These actions can cause accidental needle sticks.

 SAFETY ALERT

Many health care facilities are prohibiting the use of acrylic nails due to the spread of infections and fungus to immune-compromised clients.

SAFETY ALERT

No special precautions are needed for dishes, glasses, cups, or eating utensils. Hot water and detergents are sufficient to decontaminate these items.

TRANSMISSION-BASED PRECAUTIONS (TIER TWO)

Equipment

- HEPA or N95 respirator mask
- Mask
- Clean gloves
- Gown

Preparation

CLINICAL NOTE

Negative-pressure ventilation pulls air away from hallways and exhausts it out of the room to areas away from air intake vents. Six to 12 air exchanges each hour are required to provide microbial dilution within the room. Ultraviolet irradiation lamps can be used to supplement ventilation systems when the risk of tuberculosis transmission is high.

STANDARD PRECAUTIONS
For all patient care

PROCEDURE	🖐	🧤	🧍	😷	🥼
Talking to patient					
Adjusting IV fluid rate or non-invasive equipment					
Examining patient *without* touching blood, body fluids, mucous membranes	X				
Examining patient *including* contact with blood, body fluids, mucous membranes	X	X			
Drawing blood	X	X			
Inserting venous access	X	X			
Suctioning	X	X	Use gown, mask, eyewear if bloody body fluid splattering is likely		
Inserting body or face catheters	X	X	Use gown, mask, eyewear if bloody body fluid splattering is likely		
Handling soiled waste, linen, other materials	X	X	Use gown, mask, eyewear only if waste or linen are extensively contaminated and splattering is likely		
Intubation	X	X	X	X	X
Inserting arterial access	X	X	X	X	X
Endoscopy	X	X	X	X	X
Operative and other procedures which produce extensive splattering of blood or body fluids.	X	X	X	X	X

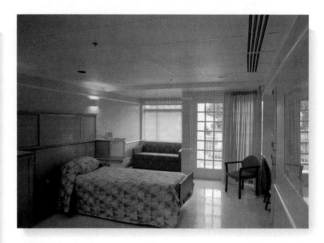

2 Place client in private room with directional air flow, negative-pressure ventilation system with minimum of 6 to 12 air exchanges per hour. If private room is not available, client can be placed in room with another client infected with same microorganism. **RATIONALE:** Cross contamination will not occur if same organism is involved.

 Follow Standard Precautions (Tier One) skill.

SKILL

Airborne Precautions

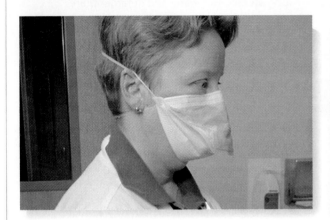

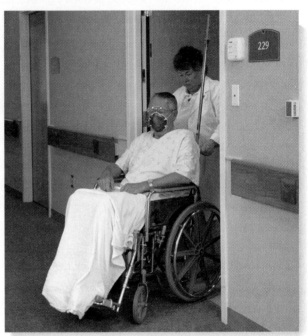

 1 Use respiratory N95 or HEPA filter respirator when entering room of a client who is suspected or known to have primary *M. tuberculosis.*

- Remove mask and place in plastic bag until next use. It can be left in anteroom or in designated area on nursing unit.

SAFETY ALERT

Each health care worker must be fitted for a *particulate respirator* to ensure that the mask fits properly over the nose and mouth. Masks are stored in zippered plastic bags when not in use. Masks can be used repeatedly and are worn until it becomes difficult to breathe through them. This indicates the mask is clogged. Health care workers who are susceptible to *M. tuberculosis,* rubeola, or varicella should not enter rooms where clients are known or suspected to have these infections.

2 Place surgical mask on client if he needs to be transported outside room. Taking client out of room should be done only if absolutely necessary. **RATIONALE:** There is a risk of transmission to other clients and health care workers, particularly if client is coughing or sneezing.

TABLE 4-2	POTENTIAL PATHOGENS THAT WARRANT TRANSMISSION-BASED PRECAUTIONS
Type of Precautions	**Potential Pathogen Examples**
Airborne	Tuberculosis, measles, varicella
Droplet	Diphtheria; mycoplasma pneumonia; pertussis; mumps; rubella; or streptococcal pharyngitis, scarlet fever, or pneumonia in children or infants
Contact	Gastroenteritis; *C. difficile; Escherichia coli;* shigella; hepatitis A; herpes simplex virus; pediculosis; scabies

Droplet Precautions

Contact Precautions

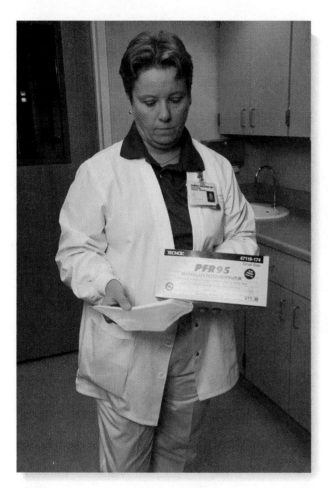

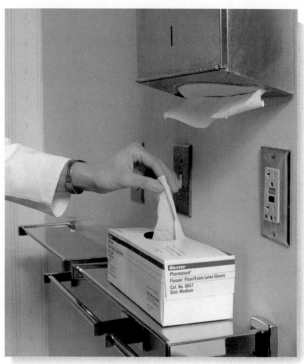

 ① Wear mask if working within 3 ft of client. As in airborne precautions, place surgical mask on client if transportation outside room is necessary.

① Wear clean gloves when touching blood, body fluids, secretions, excretions, or contaminated items.

- Change gloves after each contact with infectious material.
- Remove gloves before leaving client's room.
- Wash hands using antimicrobial agent immediately after removing gloves. Do not touch anything in room after handwashing.
- After exiting room, wash hands at nearest sink.

SAFETY ALERT

Masks must be changed every 30 min or if they become damp. **RATIONALE:** Effectiveness is greatly reduced after 30 min or when masks are moist.

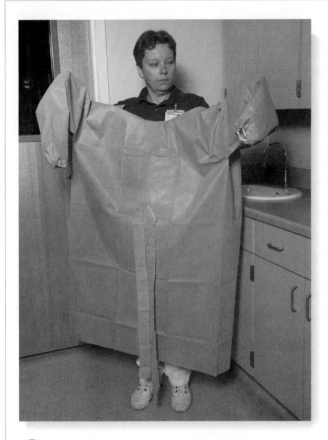

2 Wear gown when entering room if there is possibility of contact with contaminated surfaces or items, or if client is incontinent or has diarrhea, colostomy, or wound drainage not contained by dressing.

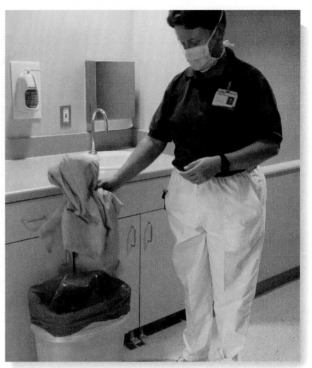

3 Remove gown in room, fold gown inside out as it is being removed, and dispose of gown in appropriate receptacle.

- Wash hands, remove mask and dispose of it in appropriate receptacle.

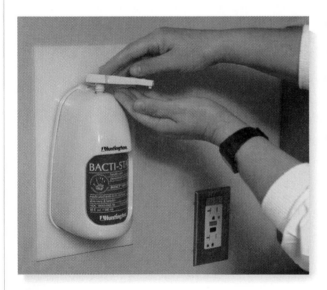

4 Wash hands in room and immediately after leaving room at nearest sink.

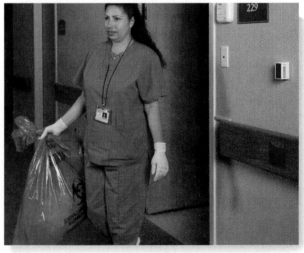

5 Dispose of one-use equipment in biohazard bag and place in receptacle in "dirty" utility room.

- Leave reusable equipment in room until client is discharged or no longer needs equipment.

CHARTING

- Standard precautions maintained
- Client's response to care
- Specimen sent to laboratory if appropriate

SECTION TWO

ISOLATION PRACTICES

Isolation practices relate to techniques used to prevent the spread of infection to other health care workers, clients, or the nurse. The techniques include proper handwashing, cleaning of reusable equipment, donning and removing isolation attire, and proper disposal of soiled linen and equipment. Single-bag techniques can be used if the disposable bag is sturdy and impervious to microorganisms and if contaminated articles can be placed in the bag without contaminating it. Double-bagging must be done if the outside of the bag is contaminated, if the bag can be penetrated, or if the contaminated material is heavy and could break.

The nurse must know the correct precautions to take to prevent transmission of the specific microorganism. These precautions must be followed with each client contact in order for isolation practices to be effective. Means of preventing the transfer of pathogens from one person to another are sometimes referred to as *barriers.* The most commonly used barriers include the gowns, masks, and gloves worn by health care providers. Private rooms, the use of waterproof disposal bags for linen and trash, and bagging of contaminated equipment also fall into the category of barriers against the spread of infection.

Private rooms are preferred for all clients with infections. The private room will prevent direct or indirect contact transmission. When possible, the room should include handwashing and toilet facilities and an anteroom to reduce the risk for transmission of microorganisms. The use of a directional air flow, negative-pressure ventilation system is particularly helpful to prevent the spread of airborne organisms.

RATIONALE

- To prevent spread of microorganisms between clients and/or health care workers
- To prevent immunosuppressed clients from acquiring nosocomial infections
- To dispose of equipment, linens, and garbage using appropriate methods

ASSESSMENT

- Determine appropriate isolation attire required for client's condition.
- Determine appropriate method of disposing of equipment, linen, and garbage.
- Determine appropriate method of donning isolation attire.
- Determine appropriate method of taking off isolation attire when exiting client's room.

PROTECTIVE ATTIRE

Equipment

- Disposable gloves
- Gown
- Mask
- Protective eyewear

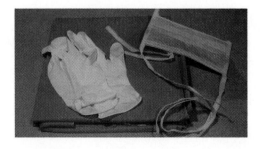

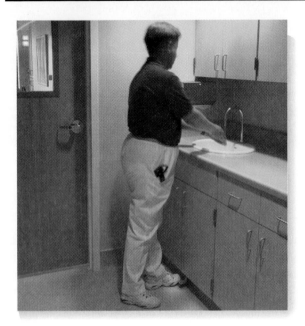

1 Wash and dry hands thoroughly.

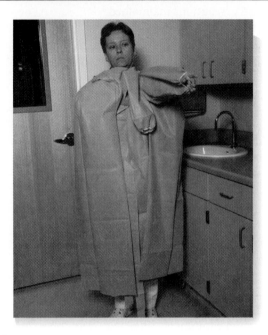

2 Put on gown by placing one arm at a time through sleeves.

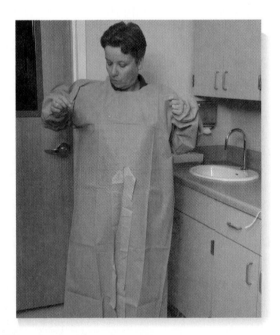

3 After both arms are placed in sleeves, wrap gown around body so it covers clothing completely. **RATIONALE:** Gowns are worn when it is likely that nurses' clothing will come in contact with blood, body fluids, secretions, or excretions.

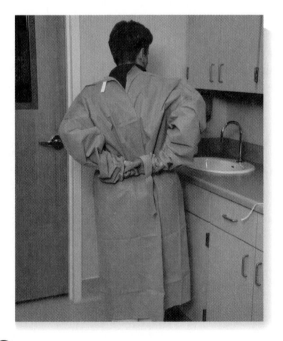

4 Bring waist ties from back to front of gown and tie (or, as shown, tie in back, according to hospital procedure).

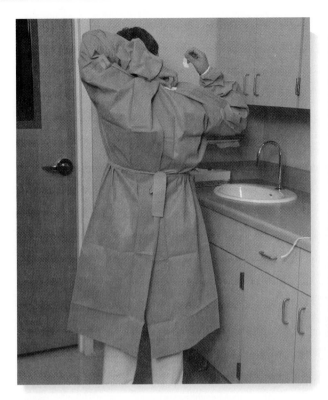

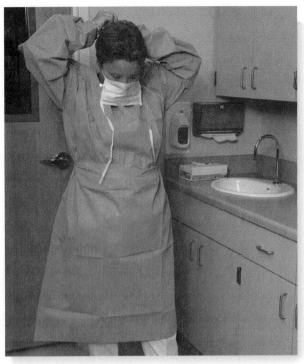

5 Tie gown at neck or adhere Velcro strap to gown. (In some hospitals, gown must be tied at neck before tying waist ties; check hospital procedure.)

6 Don mask. **RATIONALE:** Masks are worn when there is anticipated contact with respiratory droplet secretions, client has persistent cough and does not cover mouth, or suction will be performed.

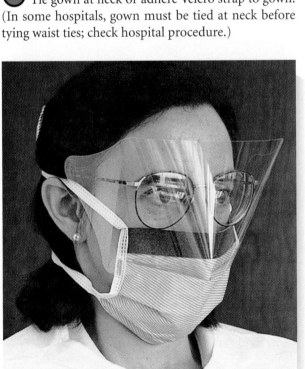

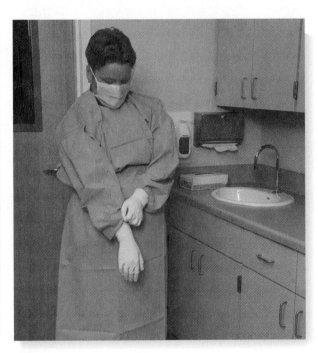

7 Don protective eyewear, such as face shield, if appropriate for client care. **RATIONALE:** Face shields will protect the nurse from splashing of blood or body fluids while caring for clients.

8 Don disposable gloves. **RATIONALE:** Gloves will prevent contamination of hands when there is contact with blood, body fluids, secretions, or excretions.

EXIT A CLIENT'S ROOM

Equipment

- Linen hamper
- Garbage bag

SKILL

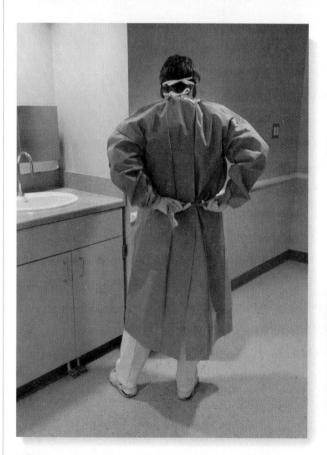

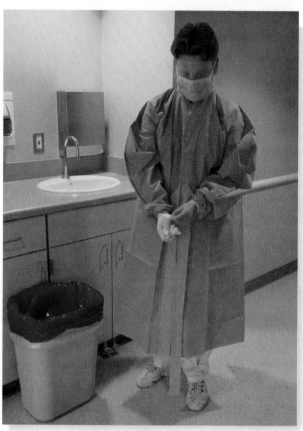

1 Remove gown by first untying string at waist (or in back, as shown in photo). **RATIONALE:** Any surface below waist level is considered contaminated; therefore strings at waist are untied before gloves are removed.

2 Remove first glove by pulling it off so glove turns inside out. Place rolled-up glove in palm of second hand.

- Remove second glove by slipping one finger under glove edge and pulling down and off so that glove turns inside out.

- Dispose of both gloves in garbage bag.

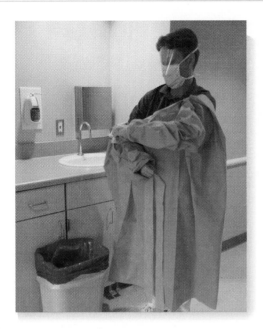

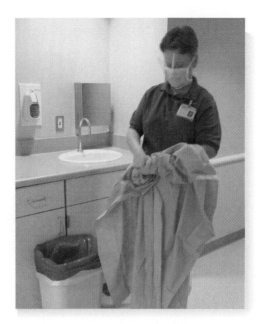

3 Untie gown at neck. **RATIONALE:** Back of neck is considered clean, and tie should not be touched with contaminated gloves.

■ Take off gown by pulling down from shoulders first and then pulling arms out of gown.

4 Turn gown inside out as you pull it off. **RATIONALE:** Inside of gown is not considered contaminated, and therefore, if it accidentally touches your uniform, uniform will not be contaminated.

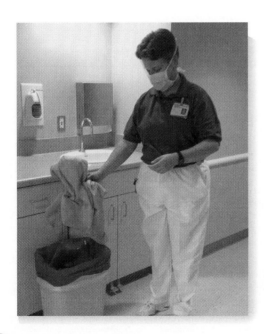

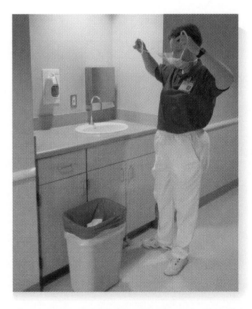

5 Dispose of gown in linen hamper; if disposable, place in garbage bag. **RATIONALE:** Gowns are only worn once to prevent contamination.

6 Remove protective eyewear, if worn. Remove mask and place in receptacle.

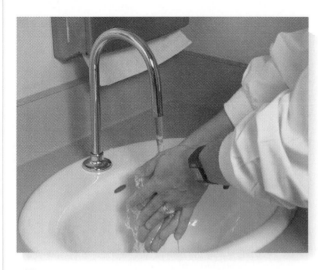

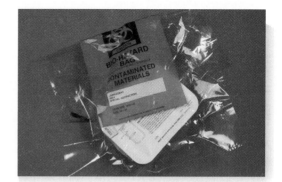

8 Dispose of all soiled equipment or contaminated material in appropriate receptacle.

- Deposit linen in appropriate linen hamper.
- Send specimens to laboratory.
- Wash hands again.

7 Wash hands in room. After exiting room, wash hands at nearest sink.

ISOLATION ITEM DISPOSAL

Equipment

- Large red isolation bags
- Specimen container

- Plastic bag with biohazard label
- Laundry bag
- Puncture-resistant container for sharps and needles
- Gloves
- Antimicrobial agent or antiseptic agent

SKILL

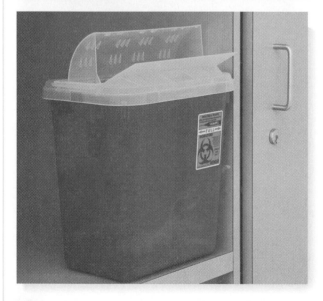

1 Place all sharps, needles, or sharp objects in puncture-resistant container immediately after use. When container is full, take to "dirty" utility room and place in appropriate receptacle.

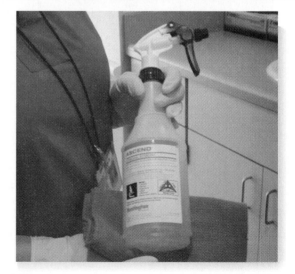

2 Clean all reusable large equipment thoroughly with antimicrobial or antiseptic agent if required by hospital policy.

- Place note on equipment, "from isolation room."
- Set equipment near door.

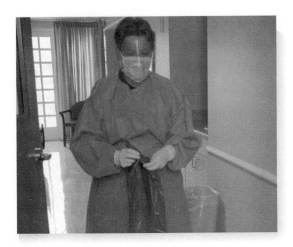

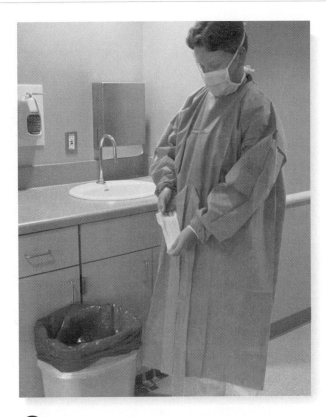

3 Place reusable small equipment, such as procedure trays, in red bag after thoroughly cleaning instruments or equipment.

- Label bag with name of equipment and set near door. **RATIONALE:** Appropriate separation of equipment and labeling alerts central supply staff that equipment is contaminated and special handling needs to be carried out.

- Replace all bags (linen, garbage bags) in appropriate containers in room before removing isolation attire.

4 Remove isolation attire and place in appropriate receptacle.

- Wash hands thoroughly.

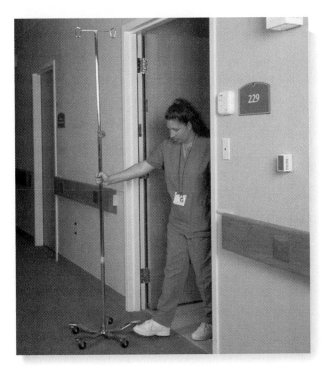

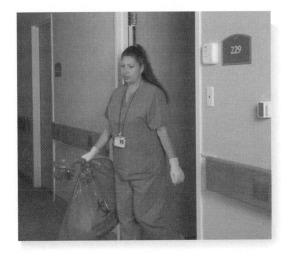

5 Take equipment to "dirty" utility room for return to CSR for cleaning after leaving isolation room.

6 Dispose of all garbage in red plastic bags. Double-bag if appropriate (see "Double-Bag Equipment and Linen" skill).

- Take bags to appropriate receptacle in "dirty" utility room or dispose of bags directly in trash bin after leaving isolation room. **RATIONALE:** All garbage from isolation room is considered contaminated.

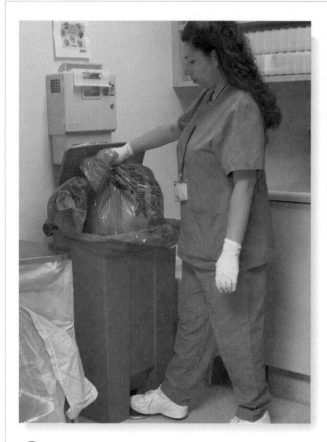

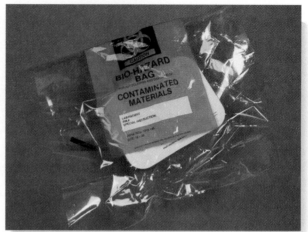

8 Send specimen from isolation client to laboratory.

■ Mark specimen container with client's name, type of specimen, and the word *isolation* before entering isolation room.

■ Collect specimen, and place container in clean plastic biohazard bag outside room. **RATIONALE:** Use clear bags so that laboratory personnel can see specimen easily.

7 Take all red biohazard bags to specified area for disposal.

CLINICAL NOTE

GUIDELINES FOR DISPOSING OF CONTAMINATED EQUIPMENT

■ **Disposable glass:** Place in isolation bag separate from burnable trash and direct to appropriate hospital area for disposal.

■ **Glass equipment:** Bag separately from metal equipment and return to CSR.

■ **Metal equipment:** Bag all equipment together, label, and return to CSR.

■ **Rubber and plastic items:** Bag items separately and return to CSR for gas sterilization.

■ **Dishes:** Require no special precautions unless contaminated with infected material; then bag, label, and return to kitchen.

■ **Plastic or paper dishes:** Dispose of these items in burnable trash.

■ **Soiled linens:** Place in laundry bag, and send to separate area of laundry room for special care. If possible, place linens in hot-water–soluble

bag. This method is safer for handling, as bag may be placed directly into washing machine. (Double-bagging is usually required because these bags are easily punctured or torn. They also dissolve when wet.)

■ **Food and liquids:** Dispose of these items by putting them in the toilet—flush thoroughly.

■ **Needles and syringes:** Do not recap needles; place in puncture-resistant container.

■ **Sphygmomanometer and stethoscope:** Require no special precautions unless they are contaminated. If contaminated, disinfect using the appropriate cleaning protocol based on the infective agent.

■ **Thermometers:** Dispose of electronic probe cover with burnable trash. If probe or machine is contaminated, clean with appropriate disinfectant for infective agent. If reusable glass thermometers are used, disinfect with appropriate solution.

BEYOND THE SKILL

CLEANING WASHABLE ARTICLES

Equipment

- Article to be cleaned
- Antiseptic solution or antimicrobial soap (according to hospital policy)

- Clean gloves
- Paper towels

Procedure

1. Wash your hands and don clean gloves.
2. Rinse article under cold running water. **RATIONALE:** Cold water removes organic material. Hot water coagulates protein of organic material (pus, blood) and makes it adhere to surface.
3. Wash with antiseptic solution or hot soapy water using friction. Use brush to clean between grooves, if necessary.
4. Rinse well with hot water.
5. Dry thoroughly.
6. Place in red bag, label, and set near door.
7. Remove gloves and wash hands.

DOUBLE-BAG EQUIPMENT AND LINEN

Equipment

- Two disposable red sturdy isolation bags
- Items to be removed from room
- Gloves

SAFETY ALERT

If the outside of the bag is contaminated, if the bag could be easily penetrated, or if contaminated material in the bag is heavy and could break the bag, double-bagging should be used for safety.

SKILL

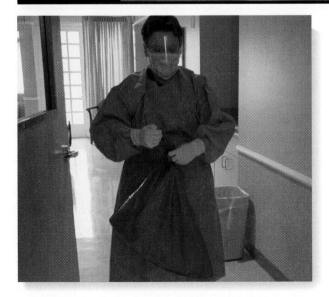

1 Before leaving room, prepare disposable items for removal.

- Close isolation bag when it is one-half to three-fourths full.
- Close bag inside isolation room.

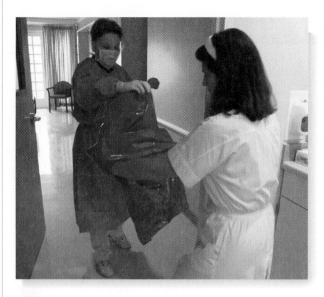

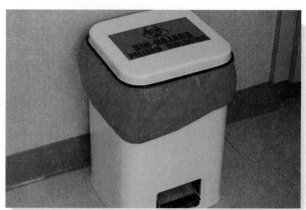

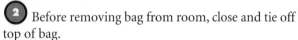 Set up new bags for continued use inside room. Bags are usually red with the word *biohazard* printed on the outside.

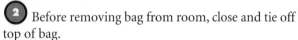 Before removing bag from room, close and tie off top of bag.

- Place bag from inside room into a bag held open by a second health care worker outside room.
- Place bag into second bag without contaminating outside of bag.
- Secure top of bag by tying knot in top of bag.
- Take bag to designated area where biohazard material is collected, usually "dirty" utility room.

CHARTING

- Type of isolation protocol being practiced
- Client's reactions to sensory deprivation
- Specimens sent to laboratory
- Unusual findings relative to isolation

CRITICAL THINKING FOCUS

SECTION ONE ▪ Standard Precautions

Unexpected Outcomes

- Contaminated material or body fluid comes in contact with your skin or mucous membranes.

Alternative Nursing Actions

- Report incident, and complete unusual occurrence report (very important for follow-up legal and medical implications).
- Follow hospital guidelines for postexposure prophylaxis.
- HIV exposure should be immediately reported, as most hospitals offer AZT preventive therapy. This therapy should be administered within 1 hr and not more than 24 hrs after exposure.
- Obtain AIDS antibody test in ensuing months.
- Continue to monitor own health status and carry out specific activities to build immune system.
- Do not smoke or drink excessively.
- Eat well-balanced meals with reduced fat intake.
- Take vitamin supplements designed to boost immune system (zinc, vitamin C, beta-carotene, vitamin A, coenzyme Q10). Check with nutritionist or holistic physician for complete protocol.
- Exercise frequently.
- Obtain adequate sleep and rest.
- Learn and practice stress reduction activities (stress is known to lessen effectiveness of immune system).

SECTION TWO ▪ Isolation Practices

Unexpected Outcomes

- Outbreak of infection occurs in isolation environment.

Alternative Nursing Actions

- Identify cause of outbreak, and contact infection control practitioner for consultation.
- Examine handwashing and infection control practices among staff.
- Attend in-service education program on isolation techniques to increase your awareness of appropriate procedures.

SELF-CHECK EVALUATION

PART 1 ▪ Matching

Match the definition from column B with the correct term from column A.

Column A

_____ a. Contamination
_____ b. Antimicrobial
_____ c. Asepsis
_____ d. Antibody
_____ e. Disinfectant
_____ f. Barrier

Column B

1. Absence of disease-producing microorganisms
2. Technique that reduces the risk of cross contamination
3. Introduction of disease or infectious material into a normally sterile object
4. Agent that prevents the development or pathogenic action of microbes
5. Protein substance developed by the body to fight disease organisms
6. Chemical agent used to destroy or reduce microorganisms on inanimate surfaces

PART 2 ▪ Multiple Choice Questions

1. When removing an isolation gown, you should:

   a. Untie neck strings, remove gloves, untie waist strings.
   b. Untie waist strings, remove gloves, untie neck strip.
   c. Remove gloves, untie waist strings, wash hands.
   d. Remove gloves, untie neck strings, wash hands.

2. To pull the isolation gown down over your arms, you should:

   a. Grasp the outside of the gown through the sleeve at the shoulder and pull it down.
   b. Pull the sleeve wristlet until it comes off the arm.
   c. Grasp the inside of the gown and the neck and pull the gown inside-out as you take it off.
   d. Grasp the neck strings and pull them down until the gown is over the hands.

3. The most effective method of preventing the transmission of infection is:

   a. Wearing a mask if the organism is airborne.
   b. Wearing gloves when giving client care.
   c. Wearing a gown when giving client care.
   d. Good handwashing.

4. Disposal precautions are followed for:

   a. Isolation equipment.
   b. Syringes and needles.
   c. Thermometers.
   d. Plastic items.

5. In which situation are gloves *not* necessary?

   a. When in contact with urine.
   b. When suctioning clients.
   c. When changing an ostomy pouch.
   d. When delivering a food tray to an AIDS client.

6. Which of the following is *not* considered a protective barrier?

    a. Protective eyewear.
    b. Gloves.
    c. Ace bandage.
    d. Mask.

PART 3 ▪ Critical Thinking Application

You are assigned to care for two clients. One client has just returned from surgery for an abdominal resection. The second client is hospitalized with an acute case of tuberculosis.

1. Is this assignment appropriate considering the two diagnoses? Provide a rationale for the answer.

2. What special precautions will you take when providing care for these two clients?

3. CDC guidelines are specific for clients with tuberculosis. Identify the differences in providing care for this client versus other clients requiring barrier nursing.

4. You are assigned to take both clients' vital signs, complete a focus assessment, and provide hygienic care. You need to monitor IVs and complete a dressing change for the client with the abdominal resection, and complete client teaching for the client with tuberculosis. Develop a time management plan and a rationale for the time frames and activities.

5. Describe the procedure for leaving the tuberculosis client's room. Provide a rationale.

UNIT

III

Personal Care and Safety

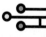

5

SAFE CLIENT ENVIRONMENT

INTRODUCTION

As a nurse, one of your primary responsibilities is to ensure that your clients feel that they are in a safe and comfortable health care environment.

From a holistic viewpoint, the term *environment* can generally be defined as the total of all conditions and influences, both external and internal, that affect the life and development of an organism. As human beings, we are constantly exposed to changing physical, biologic, and social conditions. To survive, we continually assess our relationship to our changing surroundings. We learn how to make adjustments that help us control and improve our environment. This complex process is called *adaptation*. Adaptation includes psychologic and physiologic adjustments. People in most situations are able to control or adapt to their immediate surroundings. Each of us adjusts to our immediate environment in a way that is unique to us. When the environment changes suddenly—for instance, when we are hospitalized—we may not be able to adapt independently to our immediate surroundings safely and comfortably. It is at this point that assistance must be provided.

(continued on next page)

Even though nurses are not responsible for the proper function of electrical systems in a facility, they need to be alert for potential problems. It is, however, the responsibility of nurses to identify the placement of *red switches* in case of power outages. Electrical power is provided only to those switches when power is lost. Most agencies do not allow clients to bring in their own electrical devices. In some facilities they are allowed to bring in battery-operated devices, but not rechargers.

Health and safety issues are always of paramount importance to ensure the client's safety is maintained throughout hospitalization. Nurses must be aware of the health and safety policies and procedures of the facility. All staff must follow these policies and procedures to ensure the client's safety. Fire and disaster drills need to be done routinely, and nurses must be tested on the procedures and must frequently review the protocols to be followed.

Latex allergies have become more prevalent in both clients and health care staff over the past several years. It is estimated that 8 percent to 17 percent of health care workers are allergic to latex. The Americans with Disabilities Act (ADA) requires employers to make reasonable accommodations for employees, unless it would cause an undue hardship for the employer. Reasonable accommodations include, among other things, providing latex-free gloves and equipment. Clients who have latex allergies must be identified to ensure that latex-free equipment is used in caring for them. Asking about latex allergy should be as common as asking about medication allergies. If the allergy is severe, the client may need to be placed in a private room that has been cleaned thoroughly to remove latex powder residue.

When clients require the use of restraints—drug or physical—JCAHO Guidelines for Restraints must be followed. The client's plan of care must address the use of restraints and indicate appropriate safety measures. Most of the regulatory bodies that govern health care facilities have very specific guidelines that need to be followed. If the guidelines are violated, fines can be imposed and nurses may be held liable for their actions.

PREPARATION PROTOCOL: FOR SAFE CLIENT ENVIRONMENT

Complete the following steps before each skill.

1. Familiarize yourself with specific safety protocols before caring for client.
2. Gather appropriate equipment for client care.
3. Introduce yourself to client and explain nursing care you will be giving or safety protocols that will be carried out.
4. Obtain appropriate safety equipment and protective devices.

COMPLETION PROTOCOL: FOR SAFE CLIENT ENVIRONMENT

Make sure the following steps have been completed.

1. Remove safety equipment and protective devices; clean and store according to facility policy.
2. Ensure client is left in a secure and comfortable position.
3. Ensure all restraints are appropriately applied before leaving room.
4. Notify appropriate personnel if potential or actual safety violation has occurred.
5. Complete an Unusual Occurrence Report if safety violation has occurred with client.

CLIENT ENVIRONMENT

Providing a safe environment involves a number of people, including the client, visitors, and health care providers. Providing protection from hazardous situations and education concerning safety precautions is one of your most important responsibilities as a nurse.

Clients who are moved from their usual environment into one that is often frightening and unfamiliar may act in ways that are very different from their usual behavior. A threatening situation can interfere with the individual's adaptation to the immediate surroundings. A safe environment includes the design of the room, color scheme, decor, furniture, lighting, ventilation, noise control, and safety measures that prevent mechanical injuries. Not only the room itself, but also the health care facility's fire, disaster, and hazardous material protocols, promote a safe client environment.

RATIONALE

- To promote calm, therapeutic environment to assist client in resuming a healthy state
- To maintain good ventilation to prevent spread of microorganisms through system
- To provide client privacy during procedures and when client requests privacy
- To provide protection for client while in health care facility
- To provide safety devices for clients who require support
- To inform client about fire and disaster protocols

ASSESSMENT

- Assess client's ability to comprehend instructions about how to use potentially dangerous equipment.
- Evaluate client's ability to make judgments relative to safety issues.
- Assess need for specific precautions to promote safe environment.

PROVIDE A COMFORTABLE ENVIRONMENT

Equipment

- Adjustable hospital bed
- Overhead lighting above bed
- Electrical bed control panel easily accessible by client
- Side rails

- Adjustable over-bed table
- Nightstand
- Chair with firm back and arm rests, made of material that can be cleaned

SKILL

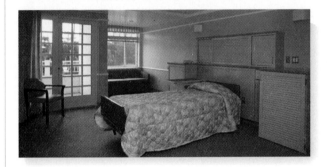

1 Arrange furnishings in a manner that is physically safe, comfortable, and aesthetically appealing for client.

- Clean furnishings at a time of day that coordinates with client's needs and activities. **RATIONALE:** Ambience of room and sense of order and cleanliness contribute to client's sense of well-being.

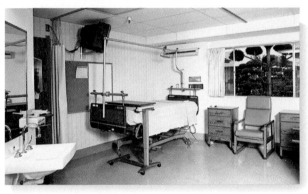

2 Ensure equipment is functioning appropriately.

 SAFETY ALERT

Bed height must be adjustable from LOW to HIGH position. **RATIONALE:** LOW position is used for client safety when client is not receiving nursing care. HIGH position is used during client care to protect health care worker's back.

Head and foot of bed can be elevated by electrical motors or manual cranks. Ensure cranks are returned under bed when not in use. **RATIONALE:** To prevent staff from injury as a result of hitting cranks while approaching bed.

Electrical controls must be fully functioning (controls are on foot or side of bed or on side rails).

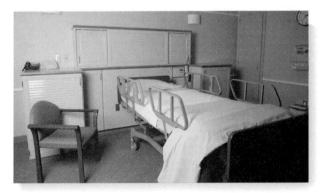

3 Provide chair with firm back and arm support for client comfort, and with material that is washable plastic or vinyl.

- Cover chair to ensure client is not sitting directly on chair material. **RATIONALE:** To promote client comfort and prevent contamination.

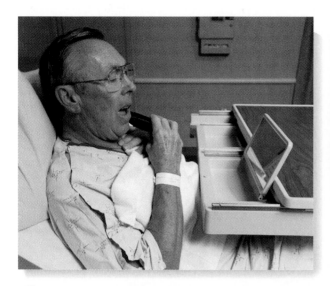

4 Ensure over-bed table is adjusted to correct height for client needs and safety.

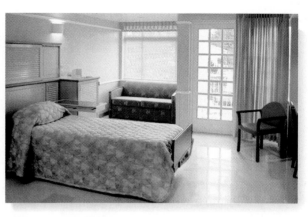

5 Ensure adequate ventilation; room air should contain adequate moisture; be free of irritating pollutants, odors, or noxious fumes; and be at a comfortable temperature.

■ A room with directional airflow negative-pressure ventilation may be needed for some clients.

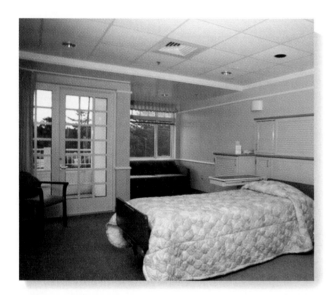

6 Provide adequate natural and artificial light. **RATIONALE:** Natural light is used to decrease feelings of isolation and encourages clients to continue their normal daily routine. It also helps wounds heal. Natural or artificial light is essential to preserve sight, for safety, and for accurate assessments and nursing care.

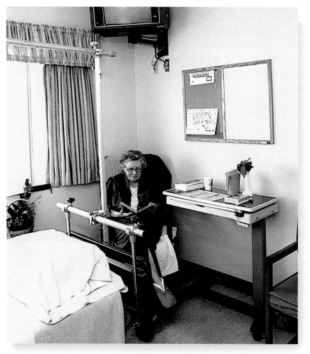

7 Provide adequate space for client's personal effects. **RATIONALE:** This allows client some control over part of their hospitalization.

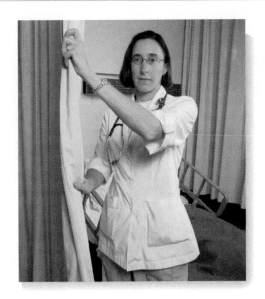

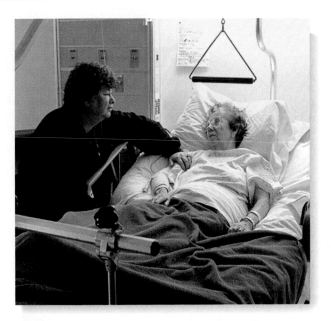

8 Provide privacy for client. **RATIONALE:** To prevent fear of exposure and loss of identity.

- Draw curtains before performing procedures.
- Close door to allow client time to rest and to keep noise level down.

9 Instruct client and family about environment and safety measures to ensure client's safety and comfort.

PREVENT MECHANICAL INJURIES

Equipment

- Side rails, hand rails
- Alarm system

- Restraints
- Locks for movable equipment such as beds, wheelchairs, and gurneys

SKILL

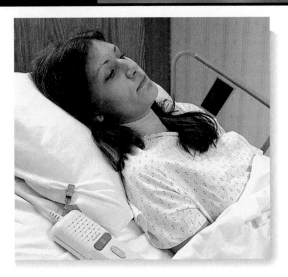

1 Orient new clients to surroundings, including use of call light.

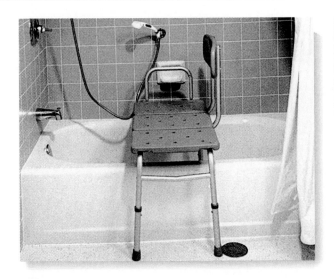

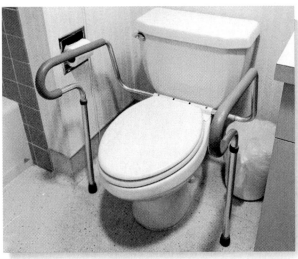

2 Instruct ambulatory clients in use of shower controls and shower chair.

3 Ensure that rails are placed over toilet for clients with altered mobility.

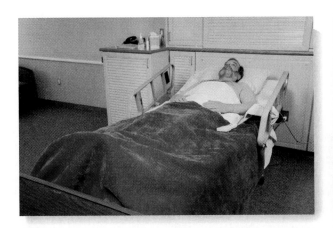

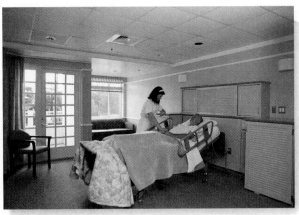

4 Place bed in LOW position when not providing direct client care.

5 Keep top side rails up for all clients.

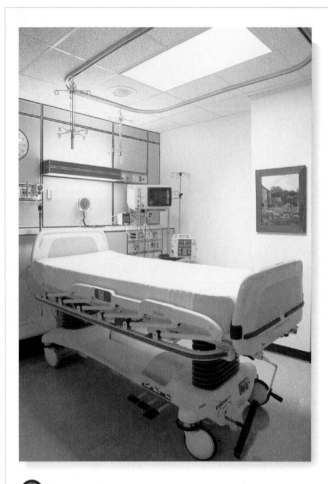

SAFETY ALERT

There is a tendency for clients who have multiple falls to repeat the type and location of the fall on successive falls, (e.g., use of commode). Studies have identified a variety of fall risk factors that have led to the development of a number of fall risk assessment tools. Clients at high risk for falls generally demonstrate more than one of the following:

- History of falls
- Advanced age
- Sensory or motor impairment
- Urgent need for elimination
- Postural blood pressure instability

6 Keep three-quarter side rails up for all heavily sedated, elderly, confused, and immediate postsurgical clients. When all side rails are up, it indicates need for checks every 15 min. **RATIONALE:** This is considered a form of restraint.

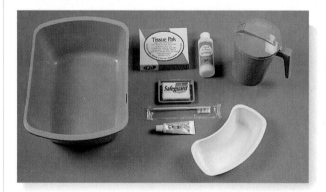

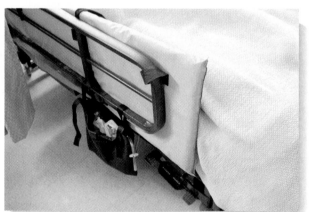

7 Place articles such as call light, cups, and water within client's reach.

8 Pad bed rails for clients with high risk for seizures.

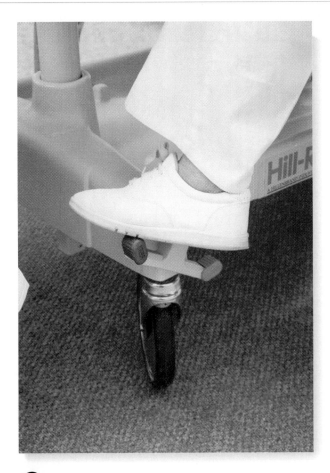

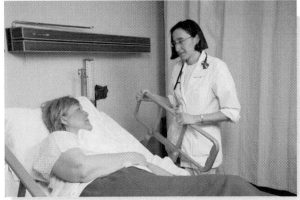

10 Tell clients who are weak, sedated, or in pain, or who have had surgery, to ask for assistance before getting out of bed.

SAFETY ALERT

Ensure floors are free of debris that might cause clients to slip and fall. Spilled liquids should be wiped up immediately. Encourage housekeepers to use signs for slippery areas. Check to see that client's unit and hallway are neat and free of hazardous obstacles, such as footstools, electrical cords, or shoes.

9 Remind agency personnel to lock beds, wheelchairs, and gurneys and to release locks only after client is secured for transport.

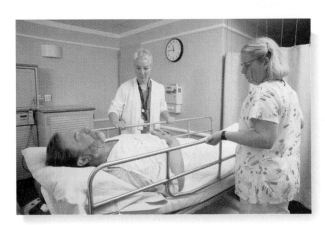

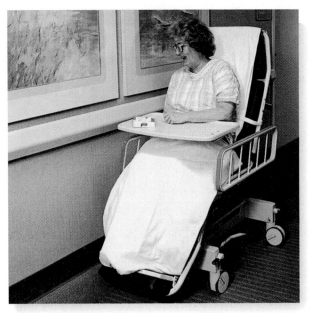

11 Use two staff members to transport client on gurney or wheelchair when nondetachable equipment, such as chest tube system or IV poles, must accompany client in transport.

12 Ensure side rails are up and client has a Posey in place when in geri-chair.

BEYOND THE SKILL

PREVENTING INJURIES FOR HIGH-RISK CLIENTS

- Attend to acute changes in client's behavior (e.g., hallucinations, abrupt disorientation, altered responses, or cognitive impairment). Monitor client frequently.
- Continuously orient the disoriented client.
- Assess and respond to fluid elimination needs every 1 hr.
- Employ bed, chair, and wander alarms.
- Assign aides or elicit assistance of sitters or family to monitor high-risk client; make certain these people inform you when they leave client's side.
- Relocate high-risk client to room near nurses' station.
- Utilize recliner chair for client safety.
- Keep intercom open between client's room and nurses' station.
- Secure physician's specific orders if restraints are deemed absolutely necessary.

PREVENT THERMAL/ELECTRICAL INJURIES

Equipment

- Fire extinguishers
- Covers for heat and cold application devices
- Electric cords and plugs in good repair

SKILL

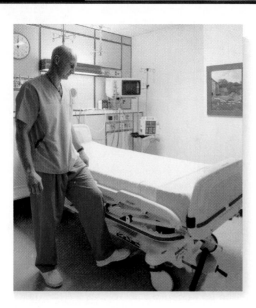

1 Make sure all electrical equipment is routinely checked and maintained. Report and do not use any apparatus that produces a shock, has broken plug or ground pin, or has frayed cord.

SAFETY ALERT

- Store all combustible materials securely to prevent spontaneous combustion.
- Make sure that all staff and employees participate in and understand fire safety measures, such as procedures for extinguishing fires and the plan for evacuating clients.
- Report and do not use any apparatus that produces a shock, has a broken plug or ground pin, or has a frayed cord.

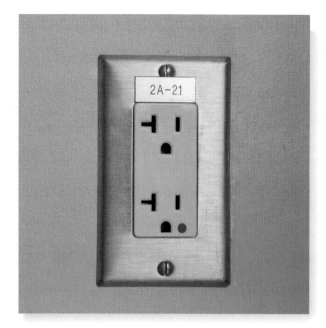

2 Use three-prong "hospital-grade" plugs for all equipment. The third, long prong is grounding device. If three-prong plug is not on clinical equipment, notify biomedical engineering department.

- When unplugging cord, pull by plug, not cord.
- Do not use extension cords.
- Unplug all electrical equipment before moving it.
- Do not use cords that are frayed; this can cause shock or fire.

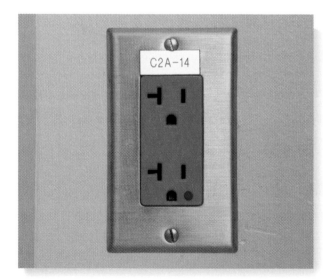

3 In case of power outage, emergency power is delivered to lights by red switch toggle. Power is usually available from these switches within 15 sec and is supplied from generator source in facility.

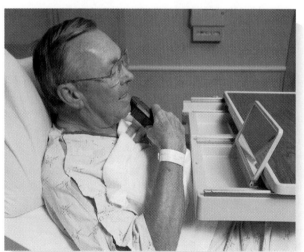

4 Have all electrical appliances brought to agency by clients (radios, electric razors, hair dryers, etc.) inspected by agency staff. These appliances must be battery powered. (Some facilities do not allow any electrical appliances from home, so check agency policy.)

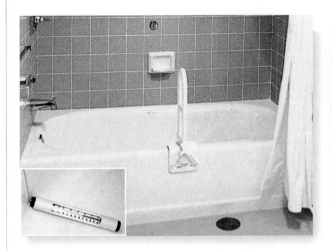

5 Make sure water in tub or shower is not more than 110°F (95°F for those with circulatory insufficiency).

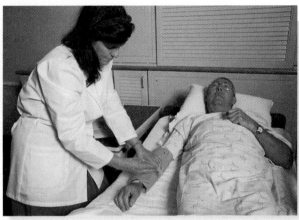

6 When heating pads, sitz bath, or hot compresses are used, check client frequently for redness. Maximum temperature should not exceed 105°F (95°F for those with circulatory insufficiency). **RATIONALE:** To prevent burning client.

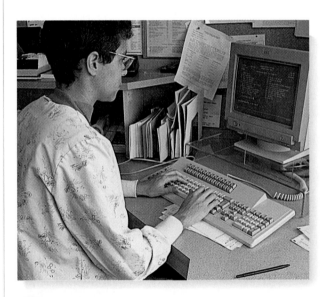

7 Do not stack liquids or other items on top of computer monitors or other electrical equipment.

CLINICAL NOTE

Hospitals do not allow smoking in their facilities. JCAHO standards require hospital smoking policies to be disseminated and enforced throughout hospital buildings. There may be designated smoking areas outside the building. Inform clients and visitors about hospital smoking regulations. Do not allow confused, sedated, or severely incapacitated clients to smoke without supervision. A physician may write orders for an exception to this policy for an individual client.

PREVENT LATEX ALLERGIES

Equipment

- Latex-free gloves
- Latex-free syringes
- Latex-free IV tubing and bags of solution
- Latex-free cart with supplies

SKILL

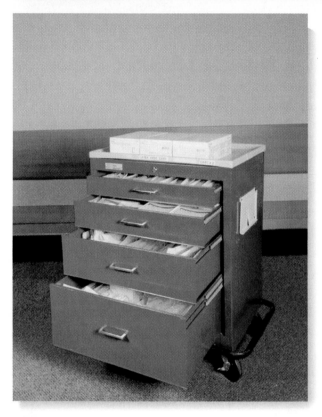

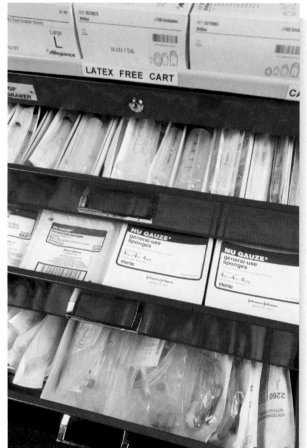

1 Obtain latex-free cart when client is identified as having latex allergy.

- Place cart just inside client's room.
- Ensure that anaphylaxis medication is on cart and available if signs of anaphylactic shock occur.

2 Check that cart is supplied with gauze pads, latex-free syringes, suction catheters, IV tubing, and latex-free gloves.

SAFETY ALERT

Clients with allergies to avocados, bananas, kiwifruit, or chestnuts may have latex cross-sensitivity. Signs of allergic reaction include facial swelling, rhinitis, eye symptoms, generalized urticaria, and respiratory distress shortly after exposure to latex. Anaphylaxis can occur in some clients.

CLINICAL NOTE

Nurses with latex allergies are required to have reasonable workplace accommodations. This includes latex-free gloves and equipment, and, if necessary, a change in assignment to decrease exposure to latex powder. This may require reassignment to a latex-free environment with a separate ventilation system.

- Incidents involving mechanical, chemical, or thermal trauma
- Client and/or family education provided regarding safety

- Safety devices used, including type of side rails in place
- Latex-free equipment cart in room
- Allergy symptoms present for clients with latex allergy

SECTION TWO

HEALTH, SAFETY, AND DISASTERS

Knowledge and awareness of fire and disaster procedures is a major part of all facility orientation programs and yearly in-service education updates. Students are required to go through an orientation program, as are all new employees.

Knowing how to react quickly during a fire or disaster may save the lives of clients, staff, and visitors. The agency also provides services for disaster victims from the community; therefore, nurses must be familiar with the disaster plan and follow it precisely.

Health care workers must follow radiation safety precautions for themselves as well as for the client and family if the client is receiving radiation therapy. The guidelines for safety precautions are an effort to keep radiation exposure as low as reasonably possible.

FIRE SAFETY

Equipment

- ABC fire extinguisher

SKILL

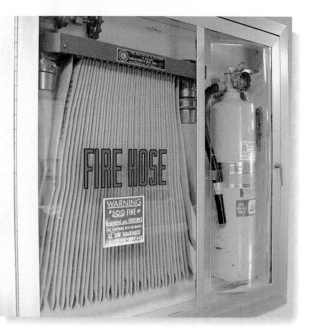

① Be familiar with location and use of fire extinguisher as well as agency policy and procedures regarding pulling of fire alarm pull boxes and evacuation of clients.

- Rescue anyone in danger and move him or her to a safe place.
- Pull fire alarm and call designated emergency number for facility.
- Secure burning area by closing all doors and windows.
- Attempt to put out fire with ABC extinguishers.
  —Pull plastic lock off extinguisher.
  —Aim extinguisher toward base of fire.
  —Squeeze handle.
  —Spray solution toward base of fire.
- Fire extinguishers should not be pointed directly at clients.

DISASTER PREPAREDNESS

Equipment

- Disaster plan in easy view of staff

SAFETY ALERT

Be familiar with emergency phone number used for disaster emergencies in each facility.

SKILL

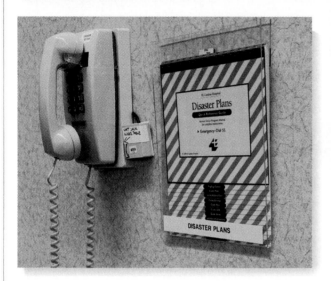

1 Be familiar with disaster plan and manual in the nursing unit. Perform mock disaster scenarios on routine basis. **RATIONALE:** To maintain skill level and knowledge of procedures if disaster occurs.

- After notification of disaster, agency paging system will use designated code to notify all personnel of disaster, e.g., "Attention, please— Code IV."
- Directions will be given for specific personnel to report to designated area of facility for assignment. Students have assigned responsibilities in each facility. Be sure to know what is expected of you in a disaster. If paging system is not available, personnel will receive information by telephone.
- Staff who are at home when disaster occurs are instructed to listen to local emergency broadcast system for directions regarding return to facility. Follow specific directions on how, when, and where to return to facility.
- During a disaster, many facilities allow staff to bring their children with them when they report back to the hospital.

CLINICAL NOTE

An ABC fire extinguisher is the most common type of extinguisher used. It contains graphite and can be used on any type of fire.

If fire is not extinguished, remove clients from area using one of three methods:

- Place blanket (or bedspread) on floor. Lower client onto blanket. Lift up head end of blanket and move client out of danger.
- Use two-person swing method: Place client in sitting position. Form "seat" by having two people clasp forearms and shoulders. Lift client into "seat" and carry out of danger.
- Carry client using back-strap carry method: Step in front of client. Place client's arms around your neck. Grasp client's wrists and hold tight against your chest. Pull client onto your back and carry to safety.

SAFETY ALERT

If a bomb threat is received:

- Listen to the caller and keep him or her talking.
- Listen for background noises, accents, language, etc.
- Ask the caller where the bomb is and whether it is timed to go off.
- Write down everything the caller says.
- Notify the security officer on duty. Do not use beepers or radio transmitters until the bomb threat is cleared. Use only the telephone. The security officer on duty will notify the administrator on call.
- If a bomb threat protocol is in place, it needs to be followed. Usually the administrator on call is designated to initiate the protocol.

RADIOACTIVE MATERIALS SAFETY

Equipment

- Protective shields for x-ray
- Film badge, if required
- Sign for client's door indicating radioactive material in use

SKILL

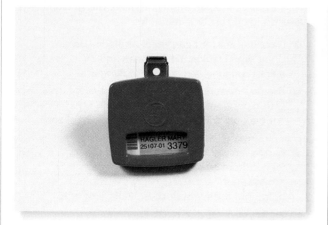

1 Wear film badge when client has radioactive material in place.

- Lead aprons and shields are used as protection, particularly if bedside x-rays are being taken.
- All individuals assisting with procedure must wear shield. This includes family members in client's room.
- Limit time at bedside; provide only essential nursing care when radioactive implants are used for client. If possible, limit time of exposure to 15 min per day for each caregiver. Limit visitors to 1 hr per visitor per day.

CLINICAL NOTE

GENERAL GUIDELINES FOR RADIATION PRECAUTIONS

Radioactive Implant

- Wear rubber gloves at all times when providing care.
- Wash gloves before removing and place in designated waste container.
- Wash hands with soap and water after removing gloves.
- Dispose of all bed linens in contaminated linen bag.
- Wrap all nondisposable items that have come in contact with client's blood, saliva, or gastric juices in plastic bag. Send to appropriate agency department for decontamination.
- Notify radiation safety officer if clothes or shoes become contaminated.

Systemic Radioactive Material

- Lab specimens are not to be taken without consent of radiation safety officer.
- Use disposable dietary tray.
- Handle all excreta and secretions with gloves.
- Have client flush twice after using toilet.
- Shielding is not required.
- No visitors without special instructions.
- Keep gloves, dressings, linens, and trash in contaminated container.

CHARTING

- Radioactive precautions in place
- Client's reaction to radiation therapy
- Incidents affecting client if fire or disaster occurs

SECTION THREE

RESTRAINTS

Restraints are classified as chemical or physical. According to the Health Care Financing Administration (HCFA) Acute Medical and Surgical Care Standards, a chemical restraint uses drugs in addition to or instead of the client's regular drug regimen to control extreme behavior during an emergency. Commonly used drugs are sedatives, psychotropics, and neuroleptics. Drugs must be addressed in the client's plan of care and medical record. A physical restraint by definition is any manual method or physical or mechanical device that restricts freedom of movement or normal access to the client's body, material, or equipment, and that is attached to or adjacent to the client's body such that the client cannot easily remove it. Holding a client in a manner that restricts his or her movements constitutes restraining a client.

In 1992 the Food and Drug Administration (FDA) issued a safety alert stating that at least 100 restraint-related deaths and injuries were occurring yearly, with many more likely going unreported. As a result of these findings, the FDA made a statement identifying the following points: clients' right to be free from restraint; health care facilities' obligation to develop written policies regarding restraint; proper staff documentation of the need for restraint; appropriate selection of restraining devices; better labeling by manufacturers of these devices; proper application of the devices; and frequent client monitoring.

Clients placed in restraints are more likely to suffer injury than clients who are not restrained. Even the use of side rails can be hazardous; clients have become entrapped between the mattress and side rails.

Since the FDA safety alert, consumer advocacy groups and government regulatory agencies have emphasized restraint-free care and recommended use of alternatives to restraints. Specific standards have been developed for clients in nursing homes and nonpsychiatric and psychiatric settings. Standards are outlined for each setting relative to the client population served in that setting. With the strict mandated procedures to ensure protection of clients' rights regarding physical restraint, nurses must be knowledgeable and follow these procedures. Nurses' conduct relative to the use of restraints is judged against the standard of practice. A nurse can be held liable if there is evidence that standards have been ignored or violated. If restraints must be used, a physician's order must be obtained. Documentation must be factual and include the client behavior that precipitated the use of restraints. All alternative interventions tried before restraints were applied must be documented.

RATIONALE

- To identify clients who need to be protected from injury
- To employ preventive measures before restraints are implemented
- To identify most appropriate type of restraint for client
- To apply restraints appropriately to prevent circulatory and range-of-motion complications

ASSESSMENT

- Assess client's behavior (confusion, agitation, or anxiety) to determine need for restraints.
- Assess client's risk factor for falls or injury.
- Assess need to implement nonrestraint measures of protection.
- Identify least restrictive and most appropriate type of restraint for client.
- Assess client every 15 min while in restraints.
- Assess client's emotional response to restraints.

TORSO/BELT RESTRAINT

Equipment

- Safety belt restraint

SKILL

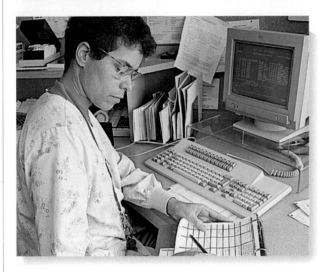

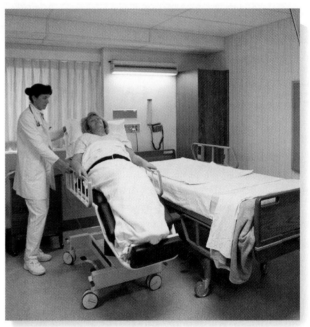

1 Check physician's order for type of restraint, justification or purpose, length of time to be used, and criteria for removal. **RATIONALE:** Restraints cannot be used on a PRN basis.

- Determine if all other alternatives to protect client have been exhausted before restraints are applied.
- Determine if client is a risk to self or others.
- Determine if client is a risk for falling or removing devices such as IVs or endotracheal tubes.

2 Obtain belt. Some belts have key-locked buckle to prevent slipping and to provide snug fit.

- Explain necessity for safety belt to client and family.
- Place belt over client's lower abdomen or hips.
- Slip waist belt through flat buckle, adjusting to client's size.
- If key-locked buckle is used, snap hinged plate shut by hooking plain end of key over crossbar and lifting upward.
- Attach side belts to bed frame or side of geri-chair (see photo).

SAFETY ALERT

Clients with restraints must be assessed and documentation must occur every 15 min. Document type of restraint, LOC, response, resolution, and effect. Restraints must be removed, skin and circulation assessed, and range of motion, fluids and nourishment, and toileting provided every 2 hrs.

Justification for continuation of restraints must be renewed at least once every 24 hrs by the physician's written order.

CLINICAL NOTE

If the physician is not available, and a restraint must be used to protect the client from injury, a registered nurse may initiate the restraint. The physician's verbal or written order must be obtained within 12 hrs.

WRIST RESTRAINT

Equipment

- Padded wrist restraints
- Padding material, if wrist restraints are not padded

SAFETY ALERT

Attaching the restraint to the movable portion of the bed frame (not side rails) will prevent pressure on the limb when the client's position in the bed is changed.

SKILL

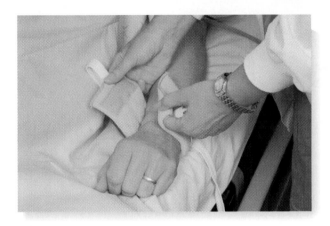

1 Apply padded portion of commercially prepared restraint around wrist or ankle.

- Pad bony prominences on wrist or ankle if nonpadded restraint is used.

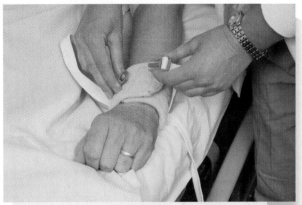

2 Secure restraint by pinching long pronged adapter and inserting into buckle end of restraint.

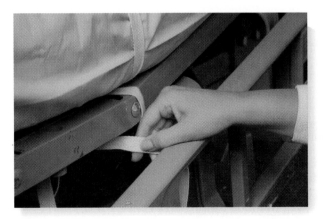

3 Using half-bow knot (quick-release knot), or square knot, if appropriate, attach other end of commercial restraint to movable portion of bed frame (not side rails).

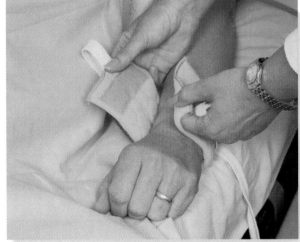

4 Release restraints and monitor every 2 hrs.

- Check limb circulation and skin condition.
- Provide range-of-motion exercises.
- Reposition client.
- Evaluate changes in client behavior.

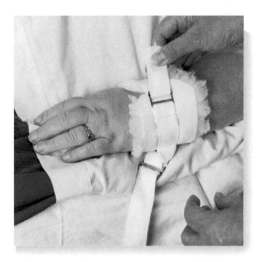

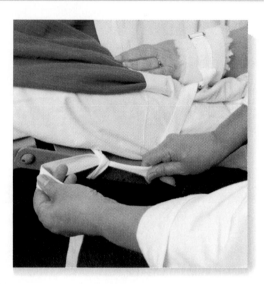

⑤ Alternate method: Apply padded wrist or ankle restraint.

⑥ Attach restraint to movable part of bed frame.

- Slide strap through slit in wrist area.
- Tighten strap securely. Ensure circulation is not impaired by keeping a two-fingerbreath space between restraint and client's wrist or ankle.

CLINICAL NOTE

Devices that serve multiple purposes, such as geri-chairs and side rails, constitute a restraint when they have the effect of restricting a client's movement and cannot be easily removed by the client. Tucking a sheet tightly so the client cannot move or placing a wheelchair-bound client so close to the wall that he or she cannot move constitutes client restraint.

VEST RESTRAINT

Equipment

- Appropriate size vest restraint

SKILL

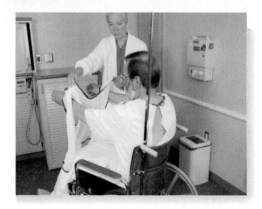

① Place vest Posey on client. Zipper-type vest is preferred. **RATIONALE:** Fastening Posey in back prevents client from strangulation on Posey if he or she slumps over in chair.

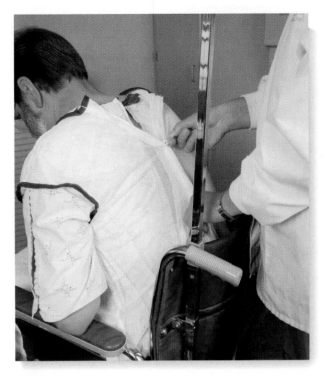

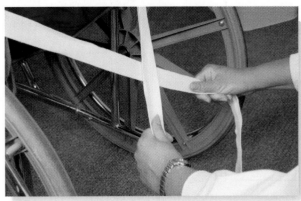

3 Pull vest tails under armrests and cross tails in back of chair. **RATIONALE:** Tying vest tails in back of chair prevents client from reaching them and untying vest.

2 Pull zipper up from bottom to top. Ensure there is adequate space between vest and client. **RATIONALE:** To prevent constriction from vest that is too tight.

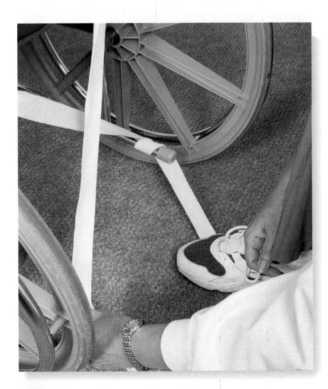

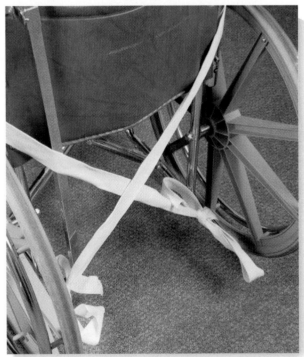

4 Wrap tails around immovable kickspur. **RATIONALE:** This will anchor tails and prevent client from slipping out of restraint.

5 Tie each tail to kickspur using half-bow knot. **RATIONALE:** This type of knot is used because it can be quickly released if necessary.

BEYOND THE SKILL

Tying a Half-Bow Knot

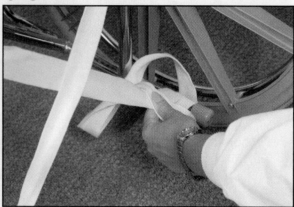

1. Place restraint tie around wheelchair kickspur. Bring free end up, around, under, and over attached end of tie and pull tight.

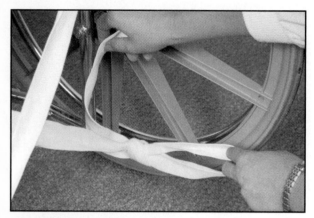

3. Tighten free end of tie and bow until knot is secure.

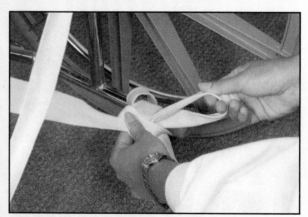

2. Take free end over and under attached end of tie, but this time make half-bow loop.

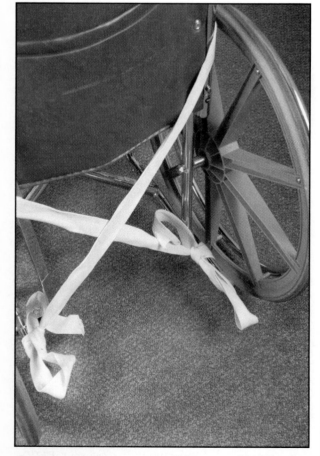

4. Ensure ties are secure on kickspur and half-bow knots are tight.

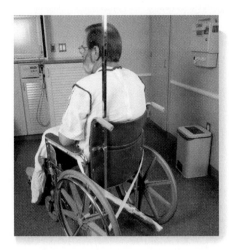

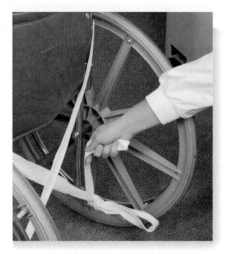

6 Check that vest Posey is not too tight and that client is comfortable.

7 To untie knot, pull end of tie and then loosen first crossover tie.

8 Alternate method: Place safety vest on client so that closed side of vest is in back and front side of vest crosses over chest. **RATIONALE:** This prevents choking if client slumps forward.

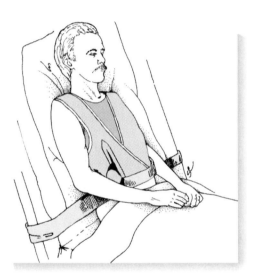

- Bring straps through slit in front of vest.
- Tie straps to movable part of bed frame or to kickspur on wheelchair. **RATIONALE:** Anchoring straps to movable part of bed allows restraint to move with bed if head of bed is moved up or down.

CLINICAL NOTE

Commercial thumbless mitts may be applied to clients whose hands must not reach IVs, Foley catheters, etc. Follow manufacturer's directions for applying and securing mitts. Remove mitts every 2 to 4 hrs, and wash and dry client's hands thoroughly. Provide range-of-motion exercises to hands. Reapply clean mitts.

CHARTING

- Specific behavior leading to use of restraints
- All alternative measures attempted before restraints applied
- Time and type of restraint applied

- Assessment of skin and circulation every 2 hrs
- Client's behavioral response to restraints
- Frequency of assessments and range-of-motion exercises

CRITICAL THINKING FOCUS

SECTION ONE ▪ Client Environment

Unexpected Outcomes

- Client, nurse, or visitor experiences accident or injury related to mechanical, chemical, or thermal trauma.

Alternative Nursing Actions

- Provide immediate first aid or care.
- Assess vital signs and notify physician.
- Report incident according to agency procedure. Unusual occurrence forms are used to protect injured individual, nurse, and agency.
- Review safety procedures to ensure safe environment.
- Report all malfunctioning equipment immediately to proper department.

SECTION TWO ▪ Health, Safety, and Disasters

Unexpected Outcomes

- Unfamiliarity with agency fire and disaster protocol results in poor performance.

- Radioactive implant becomes dislodged and falls out.

- Spillage of excreta from client undergoing systemic radioactive therapy occurs.

Alternative Nursing Actions

- Review protocols frequently to update knowledge base.
- Participate in fire and disaster drills to become familiar with protocols.

- Put on lead gloves, pick up implant with forceps, and place in lead-shielded container in client's room.
- Notify physician and agency radiation safety officer immediately.
- Never touch radioactive source directly.

- Cover spillage with absorbent material and notify radiation safety officer.

SECTION THREE ▪ Restraints

Unexpected Outcomes

- Skin abrasion, maceration, or rash occurs following application of restraints.

- Impaired circulation or edema occurs as evidenced by change in color, sensation, and movement, and blanching of nail beds.

Alternative Nursing Actions

- Reassess absolute need for restraint.
- Reassess application method.
- Increase padding of soft restraints before application.
- Keep restraints off as much as possible and have staff or family member stay with client.

- On observation of signs of neurovascular changes, immediately release restraints.
- Massage area gently to increase circulation.
- If extremity is edematous, elevate extremity above level of heart.

- Encourage range of motion.
- Request order for different type of restraint.

- Client unties restraints.

- Ensure restraints are tied securely to back of wheelchair or under bed frame.
- Reassess need for restraint.
- Exhaust alternative measures to restraints to promote safety.
- Anticipate and attend to client's needs.

- Client with history of falling develops acute cognitive changes.

- Alert all personnel that client is at high risk for fall.
- Review medication regimen (e.g., Demerol and psychoactive drugs can cause acute confusion).
- Assess for physiological causes (e.g., hypoxemia, infection, pain) and address alterations.
- Place bedside commode close to bed and remove obstacles; provide good lighting as well as night-light.
- Reduce environmental stimuli (e.g., television).
- Reorient client with each encounter.
- Move client for better surveillance.
- Employ monitoring alarm/device or engage family attendance.
- Request recliner chair.

SELF-CHECK EVALUATION

PART 1 ▪ Matching Terms

Match the definition in column B with the correct term in column A. Not all definitions will be used.

Column A

_____ a. Physical restraint
_____ b. Drug restraint
_____ c. Quick-release knot
_____ d. Kickspur
_____ e. Justification
_____ f. JCAHO

Column B

1. Joint Commission on Accreditation of Health Care Organizations
2. Manual or mechanical device used as a restraint
3. Half bow-knot
4. Square knot
5. Health Care Financing Administration
6. Restraint of client with medications in addition to usual drugs
7. Restraint of client with usual medications
8. Purpose of restraint
9. Post on underside of wheelchair

PART 2 ▪ Multiple Choice

1. Which of the following statements is true regarding wrist restraints?

 a. Restraints should be used on all elderly clients.
 b. Physician's orders are not required for soft restraints.
 c. When bony prominences are padded, circulatory impairment does not occur.
 d. Allow as much freedom as possible when restraints are applied.

2. Which of the following is an appropriate nursing action for preventing mechanical injuries?

 a. Listen to client's complaints.
 b. Always keep bed in LOW position between client care.
 c. Make sure floors are free of debris.
 d. Use restraints.

3. The first step in providing client safety during a fire is to:

 a. Pull the fire alarm.
 b. Turn off the oxygen source.
 c. Call the fire department.
 d. Remove the client from the area.

4. Orders for continuation or termination of restraint should be determined:

 a. Weekly.
 b. Daily.
 c. Every 8 hrs.
 d. When condition changes.

5. Which of the following nursing actions is inappropriate for a client using wrist restraints?

 a. Check limbs every 2 hrs for circulation.
 b. Change client's position every 2 hrs.
 c. Release restraints every shift.
 d. Put extremities through range of motion every 2 hrs.

6. The most restrictive form of restraint is:

 a. Humane belt.
 b. Torso vest.
 c. Wrist restraints.
 d. Chemical restraints.

7. Which of the following physical restraints does not need a physician's order or signed approval?

 a. Arm restraint post pacemaker implantation.
 b. Humane belt to remind client to call for assistance.
 c. Soft wrist restraints to prevent client from removing dressing.
 d. Hand mitts to prevent client from pulling Foley catheter.

8. Reasonable accommodations for nurses with latex allergies could include all of the following except:

 a. Providing latex-free gloves.
 b. Providing HEPA filter masks.
 c. Assignments in a latex-free environment.
 d. Providing latex-free IV equipment.

9. Which of the following types of equipment would not be considered necessary to promote a comfortable environment for the client?

    a. Adjustable over-bed table.

    b. Chair with a firm back and arm rests.

    c. Electrical bed control panel within client's reach.

    d. Television with remote control.

10. Which one of the following statements is most accurate about the use of side rails?

    a. There are no exceptions to having side rails up on clients.

    b. Three-quarter side rails are kept in the up position for all clients until assessment indicates otherwise.

    c. Top side rails are kept in the up position for all clients.

    d. Beds can be left in the high position as long as upper and lower side rails are in the up position.

11. Preventing electrical injuries is accomplished by all of the following actions except:

    a. Using extension cords on low-voltage equipment only.

    b. Unplugging cords before moving equipment.

    c. Pulling the plug, not the cord when unplugging a cord.

    d. Not using a frayed electrical cord.

12. Clients at risk for latex cross-sensitivity would most likely be allergic to:

    a. Bananas.

    b. Tomatoes.

    c. Shellfish.

    d. Peanuts.

13. If you receive a bomb threat, the most important action for you to take is:

    a. Keep the caller talking.

    b. Ask the caller to tell you about the bomb.

    c. Ask the caller what his or her name is.

    d. Determine why the bomb was placed in the area.

14. A film badge is worn when you are:

    a. Providing care for a client having a bedside chest x-ray.

    b. Assisting the x-ray technologist in holding a client when an x-ray is being taken.

    c. Caring for a client with radioactive implants.

    d. Working in a critical care unit where many x-rays are taken.

15. Before placing a restraint on a client, which one of the following activities must be carried out?

    a. Obtain permission from the client's family.

    b. Medicate the client with a neuroleptic medication.

    c. Obtain permission from the nursing administrator on call.

    d. Determine if all other alternatives to protect the client have been attempted.

PART 3 ▪ Critical Thinking Application

As you enter the room of 82-year-old Mrs. Lake, you find her with one leg over the side rail, making attempts to get out of bed unassisted. Mrs. Lake tells you she has to get to the bathroom and she needs to let her dog outside. She was admitted with a diagnosis of heart failure and was oriented on admission 2 days ago, but this change in behavior has been reported by nurses for the two previous shifts.

1. What assessment data will you gather before making a decision on an action to take?
2. Based on the information provided, list in priority the interventions you will carry out. Provide a rationale for your decision.
3. What is the protocol that must be followed before restraints can be applied?
4. If a physical restraint is indicated, what do you document? How often do you document findings, and how often do you check the client?

6

BATHING AND BEDMAKING

INTRODUCTION

Clients enter the hospital environment because of an accident or acute illness requiring immediate care, or because the physician has recommended diagnostic procedures or surgery. Hospitalization causes the client to alter everyday routines and activities of daily living. The ability to manage his or her own activities also may be disrupted as a result of illness or accident. The client may need nursing assistance even in the most basic actions, such as bathing and other personal care activities. Knowing when and how to intervene and performing skills such as bedmaking, bathing, and personal hygiene facilitate the client's process of adapting to the hospital's routine.

In addition to providing essential physical care, the nurse needs to take time to evaluate the client's ability to participate in his or her own care. It may be necessary to make modifications in the usual method of providing care to enable the client to have some independence. The time of day for bathing should be taken into consideration based on the client's needs, not just hospital protocol. This may be one of the few independent decisions he or she may be able to make. Nurses play a critical role in assisting clients to become self-sufficient after injury or hospitalization.

(continued on next page)

Bathing and bedmaking should not be considered just the task of giving a bed bath or making a bed. It is a time for client assessment, establishing a nurse-client relationship, and instituting client teaching. A total body assessment is accomplished during the bath. The client's overall physical condition is observed, as well as the presence of bruises, rashes, unusual signs, and injured areas. Mobility, self-care deficits, and personal habits are assessed while bathing clients.

The condition of the nails, hair, feet, and teeth is easily observed during the bath. Skin assessment is best accomplished during bathing. Maintaining skin integrity is an integral part of providing nursing care; being aware of the client's skin condition and alterations in skin integrity is a critical aspect of providing total client care. The skin is the first line of defense against microorganisms and infection entering the body. Increased perspiration interacts with bacteria on the skin to cause body odor, which can be offensive and promote bacterial growth. Regular bathing removes excess oil, perspiration, and bacteria from the skin surface. When injury or illness compromises the skin, the body becomes more susceptible to infection.

In addition to the bath, the client should be offered morning and evening care. Morning care consists of providing water and a washcloth to allow the client to wash his or her face and hands before breakfast. Oral hygiene should also be offered during this time. Assisting clients to the bathroom or offering a bedpan should be incorporated into this activity as well. Evening care is particularly important for clients on complete bed rest. Providing evening care prepares the client for a more restful sleep. Washing the client's face and hands, providing oral hygiene, and straightening out the bed to prevent wrinkles facilitates sleep and rest. Back care is also essential for bedridden clients to promote rest.

PREPARATION PROTOCOL: FOR BATHING AND BEDMAKING SKILLS

Complete the following steps before each skill.

1. Check client care plan for extent of assistance needed for bathing.
2. Gather equipment.
3. Check client's identaband.
4. Introduce yourself to the client and explain the nursing care you will be giving.
5. Provide privacy.
6. Wash your hands.
7. Don gloves as indicated.

COMPLETION PROTOCOL: FOR BATHING AND BEDMAKING

Make sure the following steps have been completed.

1. Discard bathwater, rinse and clean utensils, and replace in appropriate place.
2. Replace client care items in appropriate place.
3. Place linen in hamper.
4. Remove gloves (if used) and discard appropriately, then wash hands.
5. Return client to comfortable position.
6. Return equipment to appropriate location.
7. Wash your hands.
8. Document pertinent data and report as indicated.

Bedmaking

When the client is confined to bed even for a short time, comfort is essential in order to promote rest and sleep. Beds must be kept clean and free of debris and wrinkles, to prevent skin irritation and breakdown. The bed needs to be straightened frequently during the day to accomplish this. If the client is to remain in bed for an extended time, all care and daily routines are directed from the bed. It becomes the center of activity.

Special beds may be required for clients with specific needs. The client with altered skin integrity should be placed on an air-fluidized or static high-air-loss or static low-air-loss bed. In situations where specialized beds are required, follow the manufacturer's specific directions for making the bed. There are specific recommendations for each type of bed, which need to be carried out to provide the greatest benefit for the client.

SECTION ONE

BATHING

Routine bathing is an essential component of daily care. It is essential to the prevention of body odor, because perspiration interacts with bacteria to cause odor. Dead skin cells can lead to infection if impaired skin integrity occurs. Excessive bathing, on the other hand, can be dangerous to older clients. In the elderly, the skin may become dry and cracked, which can lead to infection.

Bathing promotes a feeling of self-worth by improving the person's appearance. Relaxation and improved circulation are added benefits that play a therapeutic role in care. Increased circulation results from the friction applied by the washcloth and helps maintain muscle tone as well as joint mobility. A warm or hot bath increases circulation through dilation of the vessels near the skin surface. This allows more blood flow and increased nutrition to the skin. Particularly for clients with burns, bathing is a therapeutic treatment that promotes healing.

Bathing is accomplished in a variety of ways, according to the client's needs, condition, and personal habits. Cultural differences must be considered when bathing clients. North Americans value personal cleanliness and often bathe at least once a day—some twice, depending on their activities. They find body odor very offensive, while in some cultures body odor is considered normal. In many cultures, bathing is done once a week.

The nurse also must be aware of cultural differences regarding issues of privacy, since it is often of great concern to clients. In some cultures, touching clients during the bathing process may be found offensive. In others, communal bathing is accepted. When preparing to bathe a client, consider the effect of cultural differences on the process, including the acceptability of a female nurse bathing an elderly male client or a male nurse bathing a female client.

RATIONALE

- To decrease possibility of infection by removing excessive debris, secretions, and perspiration from skin
- To prevent body odor
- To promote circulation
- To maintain muscle tone through active or passive movement during bathing
- To provide comfort for client
- To assess client's overall status, skin condition, level of mobility, and comfort

ASSESSMENT

- Assess client's need for bathing and other personal hygiene activities.
- Assess client's ability to perform his or her own care and determine how much assistance is required.
- Discuss client's preferences for the bathing procedure, bath, and personal articles.
- Assess client's skin.
- Assess client's cultural biases and habits associated with bathing.

BATH FOR AN ADULT CLIENT

Equipment

- Basin or sink with warm water (110° to 115°F [43° to 46°C])
- Soap and soap dish
- Personal articles (i.e., deodorant, powder, lotions)
- Laundry hamper
- Towels and washcloths (two or three of each)
- Gloves, if appropriate
- Bath blanket
- Clean pajamas or hospital gown
- Table for bathing equipment

SAFETY ALERT

Don clean gloves if there is a risk of exposure to body fluids when bathing a client. This will maintain Standard Precautions.

Preparation

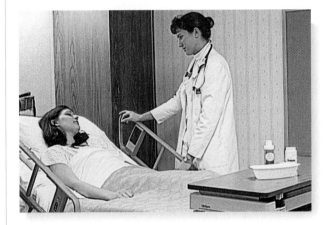

1 Provide a comfortable room environment (i.e., comfortable temperature, lighting).

- Talk with client about plan for bathing to meet personal care needs.
- Encourage client to bathe self. **RATIONALE:** To increase independence and promote exercise and a sense of self-worth.
- Explain any unfamiliar methods or procedures regarding bathing.

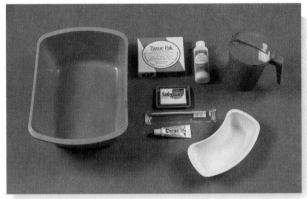

2 Collect necessary equipment, and place articles within reach on over-bed table.

- Ask client if he or she needs to void or defecate before starting the bath. **RATIONALE:** Warm water of the bath and movement can stimulate the client to void.
- Position the bed at a comfortable working height. Ensure privacy.

BEYOND THE SKILL

Making a Washcloth Mitt

1. Unfold washcloth. Place one corner of cloth in palm of your hand, just above fingers.

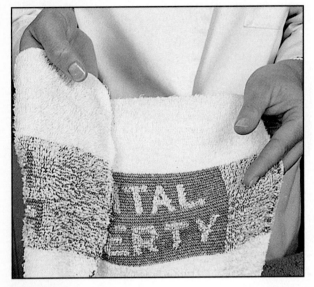

2. Wrap one edge of cloth around palm and fingers. Anchor cloth with thumb.

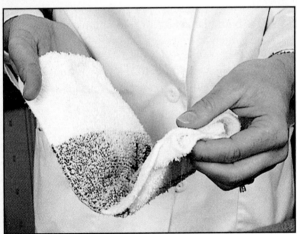

3. Bring far edge of cloth up and tuck under edge in palm of hand.

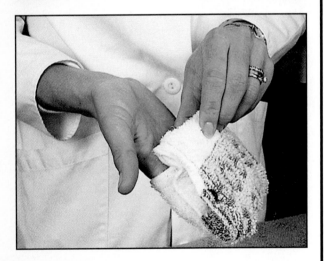

SKILL

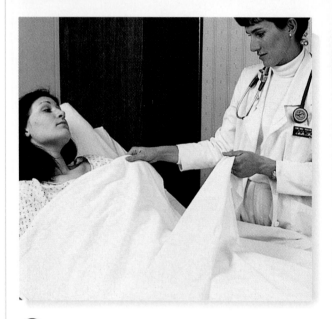

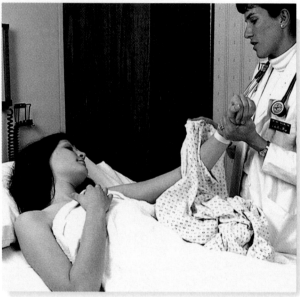

① Place bath blanket over client and over top linen. Loosen top linen at edges and foot of bed.

- Remove dirty top linen from under bath blanket, starting at client's shoulders and rolling linen down toward client's feet.
- Ask client to grasp and hold top edge of bath blanket to keep it in place while you pull linen to foot of bed.
- Place dirty linen in laundry hamper.

② Remove client's gown. Keep client covered with bath blanket.

- Place gown in laundry bag.
- Remove pillow if client can tolerate.
- Place towel under client's head.

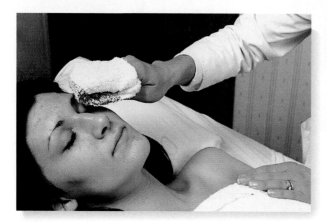

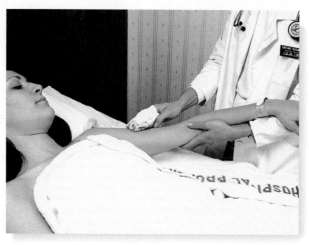

3 Make a mitt of the washcloth. Fold washcloth around your hand as illustrated previously. **RATIONALE:** This prevents the wet ends of the cloth from annoying the client.

- Bathe client's face. **RATIONALE:** Begin bath at cleanest area and work downward toward feet.
- Wash around client's eyes using clear water. With one edge of the face cloth, wipe from the inner canthus toward the outer canthus. **RATIONALE:** This prevents secretions from entering lacrimal duct. Using a different section of the washcloth, repeat procedure on other eye. Dry thoroughly.
- Wash, rinse, and dry client's forehead, cheeks, nose, and area around lips. Use soap with client's permission.
- Wash, rinse, and dry client's neck.
- Remove towel from under client's head.

4 Bathe client's upper body and extremities. Place towel under area to be bathed.

- Wash both arms by elevating client's arm and holding client's wrist. Use gentle strokes from the wrist toward the shoulder, including the axillary area. **RATIONALE:** Firm strokes from the distal to the proximal point will increase venous blood return.
- Wash, rinse, and dry client's axilla. Apply deodorant and powder if desired.

CLINICAL NOTE

During the bath, continually assess the client's skin and musculoskeletal system. Careful attention should be paid to verbal statements and nonverbal expressions. This data yields information about the client's overall condition.

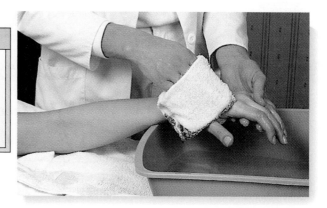

5 Wash client's hands by soaking them in the basin or with a washcloth.

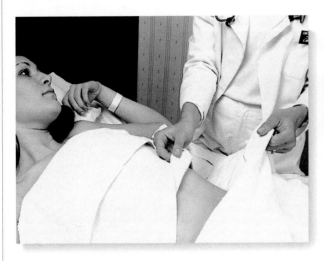

6 Keeping chest covered with the towel, wash, rinse, and thoroughly dry client's chest (especially under breasts, and apply powder or cornstarch if desired).

- Bathe client's abdomen. Using a towel over chest area and bath blanket, cover areas you are not bathing. Wash, rinse, and dry abdomen and umbilicus. Replace bath blanket over client's upper body and abdomen. **RATIONALE:** Replacing the bath blanket will provide for warmth and maintain privacy.

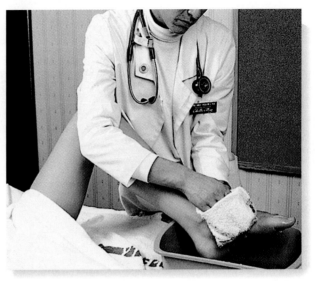

7 Bathe client's legs and feet. Place towel under leg to be bathed. Drape other leg, hip, and genital area with bath blanket.

- Carefully place bath basin on towel near client's foot.
- With one arm under the client's leg, grasp the client's foot and bend the knee. Place foot in basin of water.

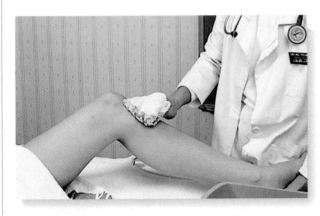

8 Bathe client's leg, moving from the ankle toward the hip. Rinse and dry client's leg.

- Wash client's foot with washcloth. Rinse and dry foot and area between toes thoroughly.
- Carefully move basin to other side of bed, and repeat procedure for client's other leg and foot.
- Change bathwater. Raise siderails when refilling basin. **RATIONALE:** This ensures client safety. Check water temperature before continuing with bath.

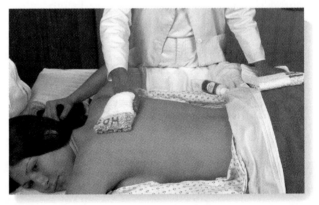

9 Help client turn to a lateral or prone position. Place towel under area to be bathed. Cover client with bath blanket.

- Wash, rinse, and dry client's back, moving from the shoulders to the buttocks.
- Provide back massage now or after completion of bath. (See "Back Care," p. 125–126.)

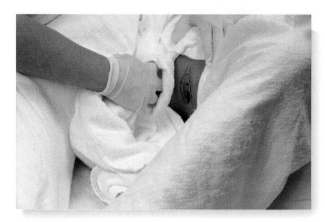
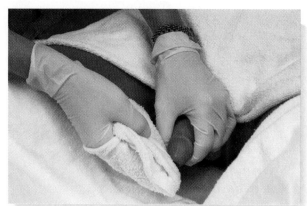

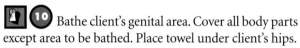 **10** Bathe client's genital area. Cover all body parts except area to be bathed. Place towel under client's hips.

- For a female client, clean from front to back. **RATIONALE:** This prevents contamination from the rectal area. Use a different section of the washcloth for each stroke. Wash, rinse, and dry thoroughly between all skin folds.

- For a male client: Carefully retract the foreskin on an uncircumcised penis. Wash, rinse, and dry gently and replace foreskin to its original position. Continue to wash, rinse, and dry penis, scrotum, and remaining skin folds.

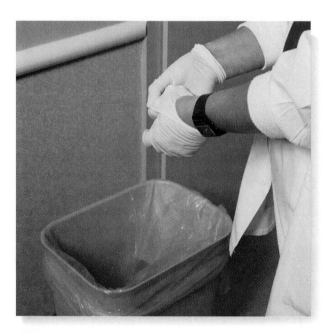

11 Remove gloves and place in receptacle.

- Assist client to dress in a clean hospital gown or pajamas.
- Clean and store bath equipment. Dispose of dirty linen.
- Proceed with any other personal hygiene activities as needed.
- Replace call light, lower bed, and place siderails in UP position before leaving client.

CLINICAL NOTE

TYPES OF BATHING

- **Complete bed bath:** The client, who is usually totally dependent, is bathed by the nurse due to physical or mental incapacity. The client is encouraged to complete as much of the bath as possible.
- **Partial bath:** Face, axillae, hands, back, and genital area are bathed. Partial bath may be completed by client or nurse.
- **Therapeutic bath:** This bath is used as part of a treatment regimen for specific conditions, such as skin disorders, burns, high body temperature, or muscular injuries. Medicinal substances, such as oatmeal, Aveeno, and cornstarch, may be included in the bathwater.
- **Shower:** This is preferred method of bathing if client is ambulatory or can be transported to use a shower chair.
- **Tub bath:** This is used by ambulatory clients as well as those who must be assisted by a device such as a Hoyer lift.
- **Cooling bath:** The client is placed in a tub of tepid water to reduce body temperature.

BEYOND THE SKILL

Morning and Evening Care

Morning Care

- Wash face and hands.
- Provide oral hygiene.
- Offer bedpan or assist to bathroom.

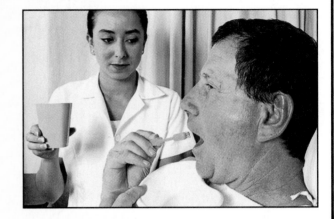

Evening Care

- Wash face and hands.
- Provide oral hygiene.
- Offer bedpan or assist to bathroom.
- Straighten linen; change as necessary.
- Remove elastic wraps, elastic hose, and binders and replace after providing hygienic care.

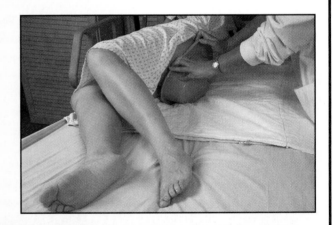

BACK CARE

Equipment

- Basin of warm water
- Washcloth
- Towel
- Soap
- Skin care lotion

SKILL

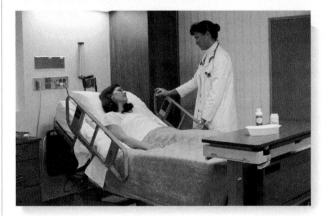

1 Explain purpose to client and ask if client wishes back care. **RATIONALE:** Back care promotes sleep, comfort, and relaxation for the client.

- Provide privacy.

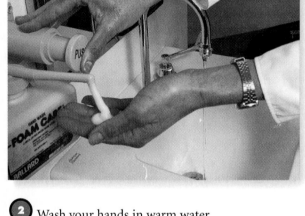

2 Wash your hands in warm water.

- Warm lotion bottle by running under warm water if necessary.

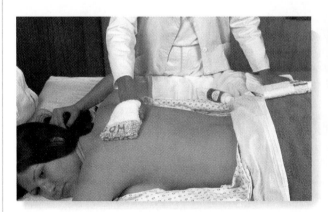

3 Place client in a comfortable position—in a lateral, or preferably, a prone position.

- Raise bed to comfortable height for working.
- Untie gown and pull linens down past client's waist level.
- Wash client's back with warm water and soap, if necessary. Dry thoroughly.

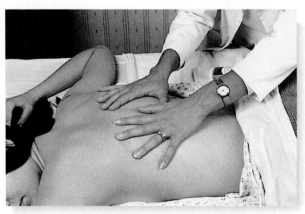

4 Place lotion on your hands. Once you have placed your hands on the client's back, keep them in constant skin contact until back care is complete. **RATIONALE:** This prevents "tickling" sensation.

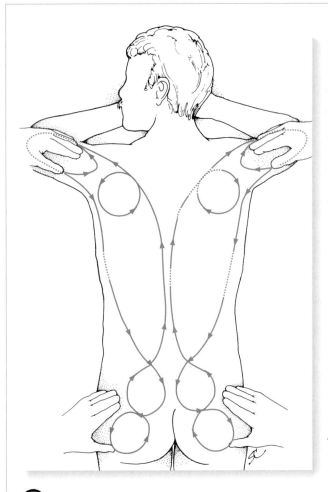

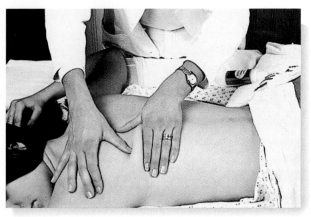

6 Use the kneading stroke, or petrissage, over the shoulders and along the back. Pick up the skin between the thumb and fingers as you move up the back. **RATIONALE:** Petrissage causes stimulation to the skin if done quickly and with firm pressure. This stroke should be done for 2 to 3 min.

- Assess the skin for color, turgor, and skin breakdown.

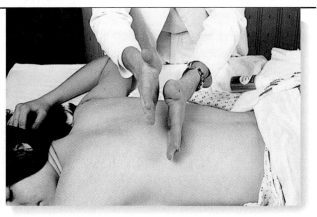

7 Use the tapotement stroke to stimulate circulation over the back. Lightly strike the back, using the fleshy sides of your hands, in a rhythmical movement up and down the back.

- This stroke should be used for only 1 to 2 min.
- Complete the massage with several long strokes over the entire back and buttocks.
- Tie the gown and reposition the client for comfort.
- Place the bed in LOW position with siderails in the UP position.
- Clean and store equipment. Place dirty linen in hamper.

5 Using your palms and fingers, slowly move in a circular motion along the side of the client's spine, across the scapular area, decreasing the pressure over the neck area, extending over the upper shoulders and then down the lateral aspects of the back using the effleurage stroke, applying firm and steady pressure. Decrease the pressure over the neck area.

- Move your hands down the center of the client's back to the sacral area.
- Massage with a figure-eight motion from the sacrum out over each buttock.
- Repeat the massage strokes for 3 to 4 min. **RATIONALE:** This stroke has a relaxing quality if done slowly and with light pressure.
- Rub lightly up and down the back a few strokes before lifting hands from client's back.

BEYOND THE SKILL

Alternate Methods for Bathing

Tub Bath

- Fill tub one-half full with 110° to 115°F (43° to 46°C) water.
- Cover all IVs, dressings, tubes, or catheters with plastic wrap to prevent from getting wet.
- Place towel or rubber mat in bathtub to prevent slipping.
- Place call light on chair or stool next to tub.

Shower

- Place shower chair in shower. Ensure rubber tips are in place on chair. **RATIONALE:** To prevent chair from slipping.
- Check water temperature.
- Bring client to shower.
- Assist client as needed with shower.

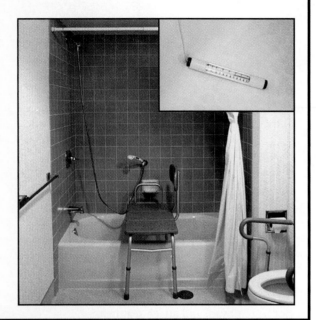

HYDRAULIC BATHTUB CHAIR

Equipment

- Towels and washcloths (two of each)
- Soap
- Clean gown, robe, and slippers

SKILL

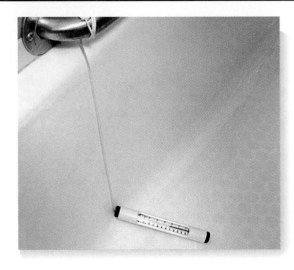

1 Fill tub with water and check temperature. **RATIONALE:** Temperatures over 105°F (41°C) can burn the client's skin, particularly in the older adult.

 SAFETY ALERT

Check that water temperature is not above 105°F (41°C) to prevent burning the client.

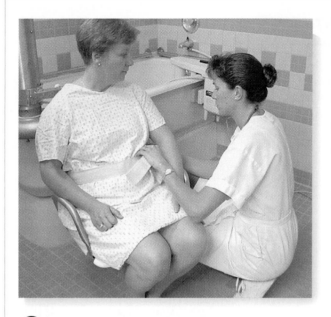

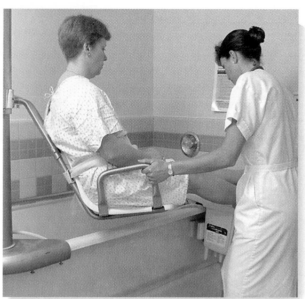

2 Release chair to lowest point beside tub, and place towel on floor under chair.

- Move client into bathtub chair, gown may or may not be removed, and attach seat belt.

3 Swing chair into position over tub.

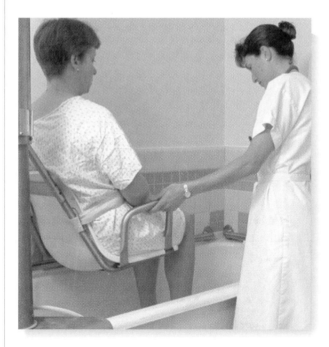

4 Direct client to move legs down, then lower chair into low position in tub filled with water.

- When client is finished bathing, reverse chair out of tub.
- Assist client to towel dry.
- Put clean gown, robe, and slippers on client and transport to room.

CHARTING

- Client's overall ability to participate in own care
- Type of bath given and by whom
- Condition of client's skin and any interventions provided for the skin (e.g., lotion)
- Client's educational needs regarding hygienic care
- Back care provided

SECTION TWO

BEDMAKING

The usual hospital bed is a standard twin-size bed in a frame that allows for different positions to facilitate care and comfort for the client. The height, head, and foot positions on most beds are electrically operated to assist both the client and the nursing staff. All hospital beds have siderails for client safety. There are several types of siderails, including one long siderail on each side of the bed or two half siderails on each side of the bed. If two siderails are on each side of the bed, one siderail is placed at the head of the bed and the second siderail is placed at the foot of the bed. When two half siderails are on one side of the bed, communication and bed position controls may be installed in the siderail at the head of the bed. The controls include a call light for the nurse, controls for the TV or radio, and controls for adjusting the bed height and the head and foot of the bed.

Bedmaking includes making an occupied, unoccupied, or surgical bed. Special beds may have their own specific methods and coverings. The manufacturer's directions should be followed to ensure the client has the full therapeutic effect from the bed.

RATIONALE

- To provide a clean, comfortable sleeping and resting environment for the client
- To eliminate irritants to the skin by providing wrinkle-free sheets
- To avoid client discomfort when making an occupied bed
- To properly dispose of bed linens to prevent cross contamination

ASSESSMENT

- Assess client's need for linen change.
- Determine if client's condition allows for linen change.
- Determine type and amount of linen necessary for a linen change.
- Check client's room for linen to ensure only necessary linen is brought into room.
- Assess client's ability and restrictions in turning during bedmaking.
- Assess client's ability to get out of bed during linen change.

CLINICAL NOTE

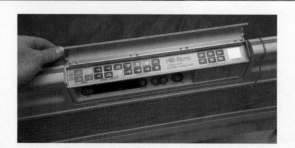

Some client beds, such as the Hill-Rom bed, have many features for client safety and comfort:

- Siderail lockouts
- Firm or soft mattresses
- Various position choices (e.g., Trendelenburg, chair position)
- Bed weights available

UNOCCUPIED BED

Equipment

- Chair or table
- Linen hamper
- Linen, in order of use: bath blanket, mattress pad, bottom sheet, drawsheet, incontinent pad as needed, top sheet, blanket, bedspread, pillowcase

Preparation

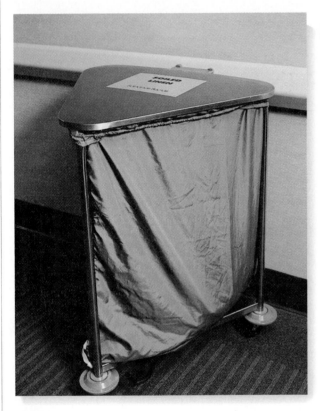

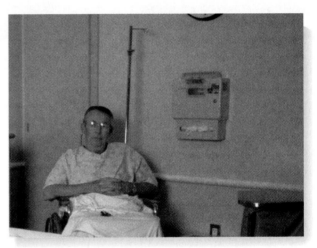

2 Assist client out of bed and into chair.

- Explain need for client to be out of bed during procedure.

1 Gather linen and hamper and bring into room.

SAFETY ALERT

Never place dirty linen on the floor, because doing so can cause cross contamination to occur.

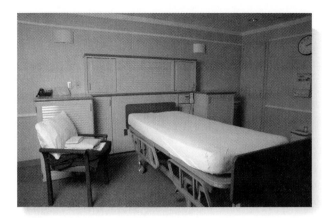

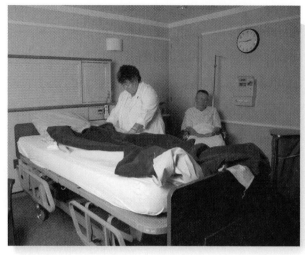

3 Wipe chair off before placing linen on chair.

- Place linen on chair.
- Remove call signal from linens.
- Adjust bed to a comfortable working height.
- Lower both siderails.

4 Loosen linen on all sides, including head and foot of bed.

SKILL

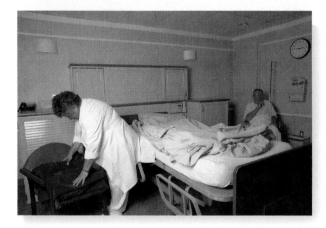

1 Remove spread and blanket. If they are to be reused, fold them and place on chair.

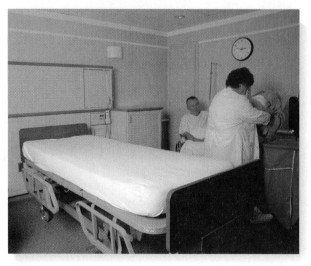

2 Remove top, draw, and bottom sheets and place in linen hamper. **RATIONALE:** Never place dirty linen on the floor as cross contamination occurs from this action.

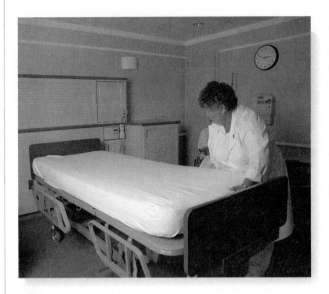

3 Push mattress to head of bed. Center mattress if necessary.

- If mattress pad is not changed, smooth out wrinkles and center pad on bed surface.

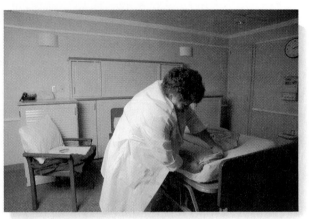

4 Place contour bottom sheet on mattress, make up one side of bed, then move to the other side of the bed and make it. **RATIONALE:** This step saves time and energy.

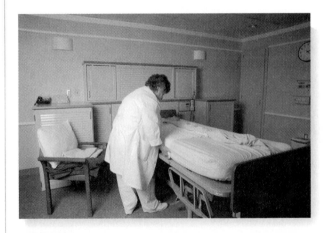

5 If the client needs a drawsheet, center drawsheet on bed and open to opposite side. Tuck drawsheet under mattress. Smooth out wrinkles.

- If a pull sheet is needed, fold drawsheet in half or quarters. Position sheet in middle of bed. **RATIONALE:** Pull sheets are used with heavy or difficult-to-move clients.

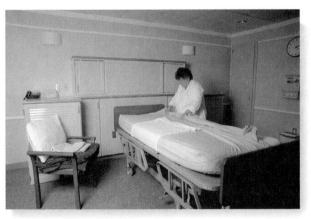

6 Move to other side of bed. Pull linen toward you and straighten out linen.

- Pull corners of the sheet over the top and bottom edges of the mattress.

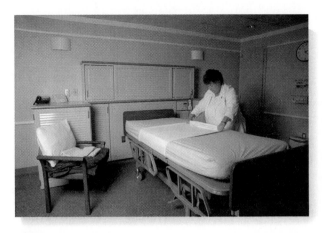

7 Tighten drawsheet (if used) and tuck under mattress. **RATIONALE:** To prevent wrinkles under client that could lead to pressure areas on back, buttocks, and heels.

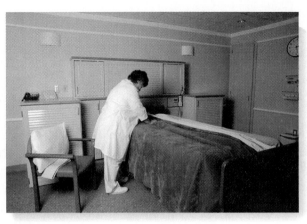

8 Place top sheet, blanket, and spread full length on top of bed.

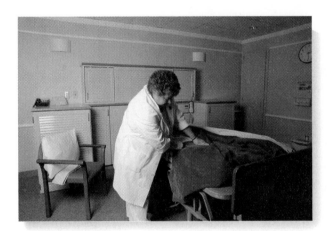

9 Tuck sheet, spread, and blanket well under foot of mattress, one side at a time.

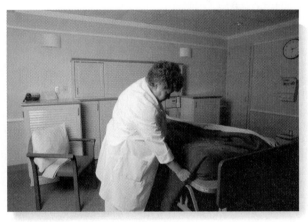

10 Miter corners at foot of bed, one side at a time.

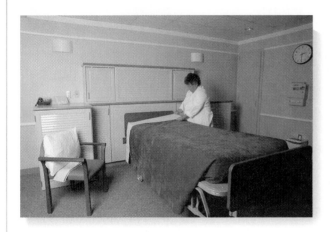

11 Pull edge of sheet over spread to form a cuff. **RATIONALE:** This prevents client's face from rubbing against the blanket.

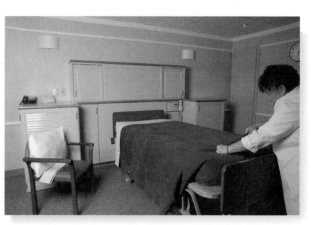

12 Make a small pleat at the foot of the bed. **RATIONALE:** To allow room for client's feet and decrease pressure on feet.

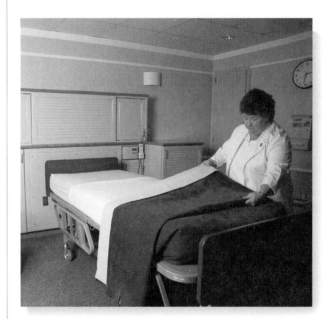

13 Fanfold linen to foot of bed. **RATIONALE:** To make it easier for the client to get into bed.

- Return bed to lowest position.
- Reattach call signal to linens.

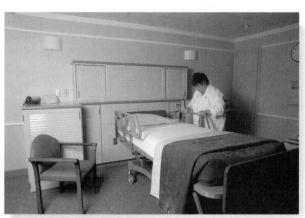

14 Place siderails in UP position.

- Dispose of soiled laundry.

FLAT BOTTOM SHEET

SKILL

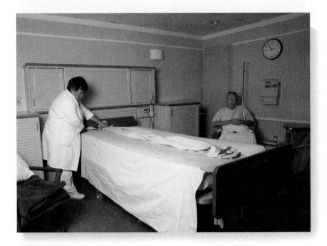

1 Complete step 1 in "Unoccupied Bed" skill.

- Place center fold of flat sheet in middle of mattress with end of sheet even with end of mattress at foot of bed.

- Unfold flat sheet and cover mattress.

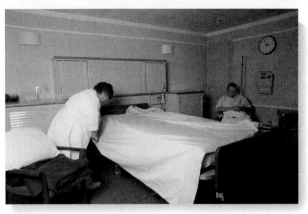

2 Tuck top of sheet under head of bed.

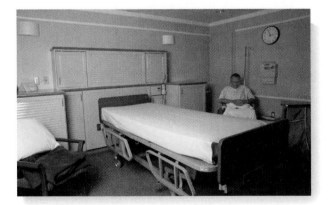

3 Miter corner of sheet at head of bed.

- Tuck remaining side of bottom sheet well under mattress.
- Move to other side of bed; miter corner at head of bed and tuck remaining sheet under mattress.

CLINICAL NOTE

PRINCIPLES OF MEDICAL ASEPSIS

- Keep linen hamper cover on at all times.
- Place dirty linen in hamper.
- Do not place dirty linen on floor.
- Discard all unused linen from client area.
- Do not transfer linen from one client room to another.
- Do not allow dirty linen to touch uniform.

BEYOND THE SKILL

Mitered Corner

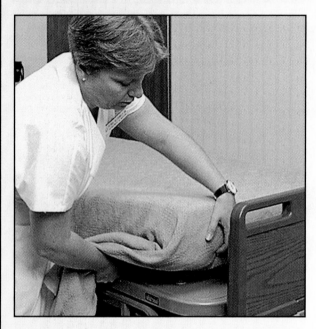

1. Tuck sheet and spread tightly under mattress.

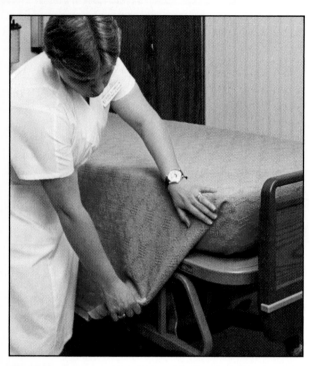

3. Place finger on sheet where it meets mattress and lower top of sheet over finger. **RATIONALE:** This action makes the mitered corner neat and tight.
   - Remove finger without disturbing folds, allowing bedding to hang freely.

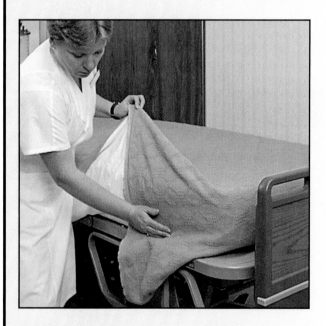

2. Grasp edge of sheet and spread with hand, and bring both onto mattress so that edge forms a right angle.
   - Tuck lower edge of sheet under mattress.

SURGICAL BED

SKILL

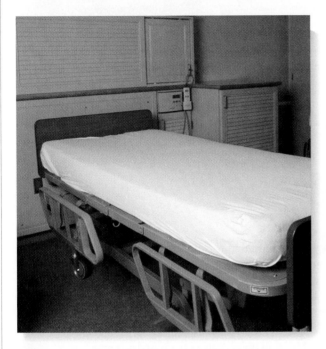

① Bring linen to room. Arrange chair and linen hamper in a convenient place for use. Wipe off chair before placing linen on it. Raise bed to highest position.

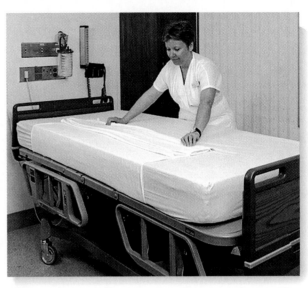

② Place bottom sheet on bed, using the same method as for making an unoccupied bed. Place a plastic or cloth drawsheet (or both) and absorbent pad on the bed if appropriate.

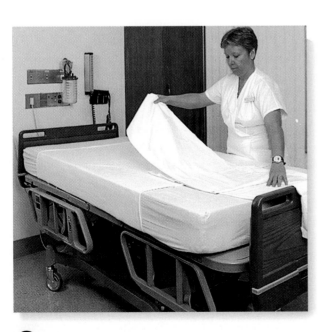

③ Place top sheet on bed.

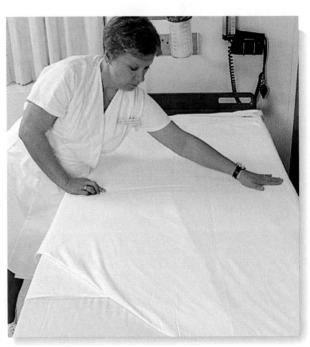

④ Fold bottom corner of sheet toward center of bed at opposite side. Repeat with top corner to form triangle.

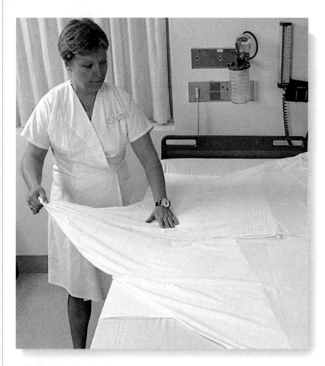

5 Pick up center point of triangle.

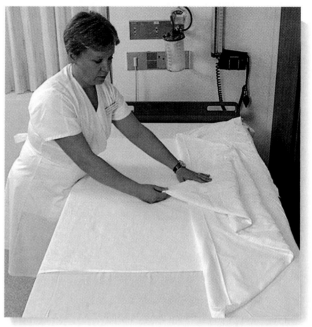

6 Fanfold linen to side of bed. **RATIONALE:** Folding linen at side of bed facilitates moving surgical clients into bed.

- Change pillowcase and leave on chair or at foot of bed.
- Move all objects away from bedside area.

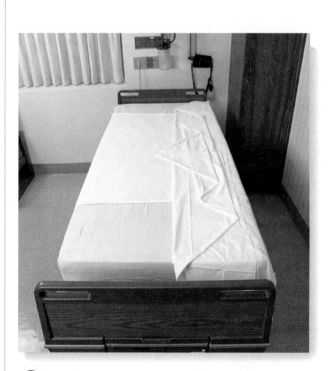

7 Leave bed in HIGH position to facilitate easy transfer of surgical client from gurney to bed. **RATIONALE:** This allows surgical gurney to be placed close to bed for client transfer.

PILLOWCASE CHANGE

Equipment

- Clean pillowcase

SKILL

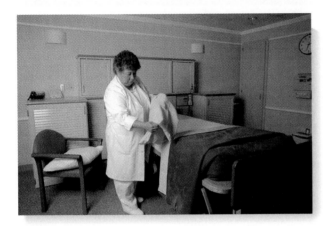

1 Pick up center of closed end of pillowcase.

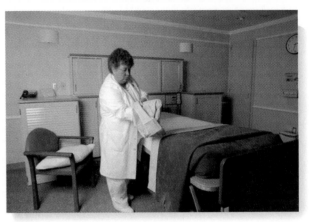

2 Continue to firmly grip end of pillowcase, then with your other hand gather pillowcase from open end and fold back (inside out) over closed end.

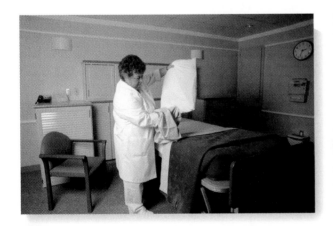

3 Pick up center of one end of pillow with the hand holding the gathered pillowcase. Pull pillowcase over pillow with other hand. Do not place pillow or case under arm or chin or in teeth. **RATIONALE:** Contamination occurs from using these methods.

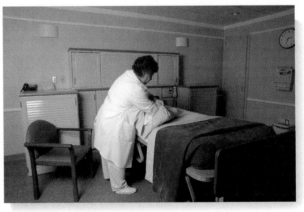

4 Adjust pillow corners in pillowcase by placing hand between case and pillow.

OCCUPIED BED

Equipment

- Chair or table
- Linen hamper

- Linen (in order of use): bath blanket, mattress pad, bottom sheet, plastic drawsheet as needed

SKILL

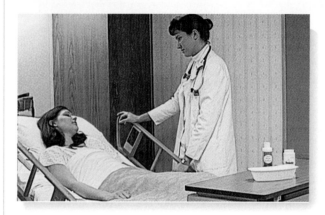

1 Talk with client and explain sequence of procedure. Arrange furniture and equipment (e.g., linen hamper and chair) for convenience of use.

- Wipe off chair or over-bed table before placing linen on it.
- Remove call signal from linen
- Pull curtain closed. **RATIONALE:** This provides privacy for the client.
- Help client into a supine position. Don gloves if bed linen is soiled with body fluids.

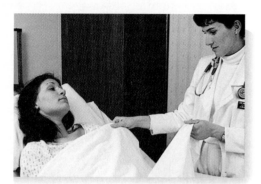

2 Adjust bed to comfortable working height and lower siderail on your side of bed. Make sure siderail on opposite side is in UP position. **RATIONALE:** This ensures client safety as client rolls to edge of bed.

- Loosen top linen. Remove spread, sheet, and blanket. At the same time, a bath blanket may be placed over the client. **RATIONALE:** Blanket keeps client warm during bed change.
- If blanket and spread are to be reused, fold them and place on chair. Place top sheet in linen hamper. Push mattress to head of bed. Center mattress if necessary.

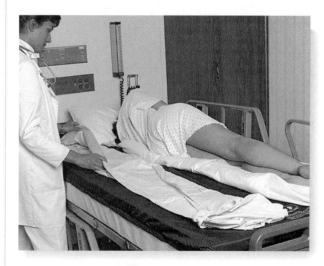

3 Assist client to side of bed; place in side-lying position facing away from you as near to the far siderail as possible.

- Loosen bottom linen on your side of bed.
- Push dirty linen under or as close as possible to the client.
- Smooth out wrinkles and recenter pad on bed surface if mattress pad is used. **RATIONALE:** Wrinkles may cause skin irritation.

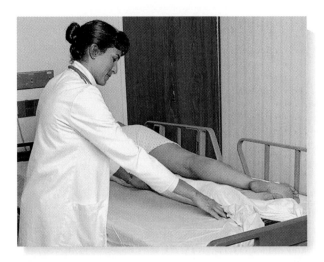

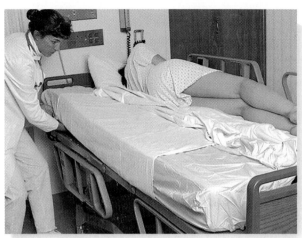

4 Unfold clean bottom sheet and cover mattress. Make sure clean bottom sheet is underneath any used linen. **RATIONALE:** This keeps clean linen uncontaminated.

- Place center fold of sheet in middle of mattress with end of sheet even with end of mattress.

5 Tuck top of sheet under head of bed, or position contour sheet around corner of mattress. Miter corner of bottom sheet at head of bed if not using contour sheet.

- Tuck remaining bottom sheet well under mattress from head to foot.
- Center plastic or cloth drawsheet on bed, if client requires a drawsheet, and fanfold half of the sheet under the client. Tuck side of sheet under mattress. Smooth out wrinkles.
- Fold cloth drawsheet in half or quarters if a pull sheet is needed. Position sheet in middle of bed. Fanfold half of pull sheet under client.
- Fanfold absorbent pad and center it on bed under client's buttocks. Place pad, absorbent side up and plastic side down, close to client.

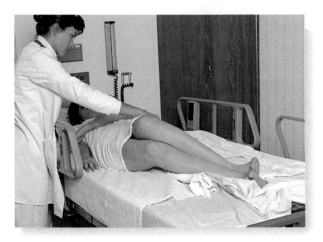

6 Help client roll over to other side of bed. Tell client why there is a hump of linen in the center of the bed. Make client comfortable.

- Raise siderail. Move to other side of bed. Lower siderail and loosen bottom sheet.

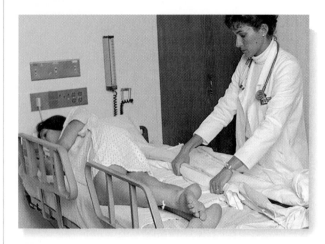

7 Move linen to other side of bed by gently pulling linen toward you. Pull dirty linen to side of bed and roll into a bundle at foot of bed or place linen in linen hamper. **RATIONALE:** This reduces the spread of microorganisms.

- Pull clean linen across mattress and straighten under client. Miter top corner of bottom sheet.
- Gather bottom sheet into your hand, lean away from bed, and pull linen downward at an angle. Tuck remaining bottom sheet well under the mattress. If a drawsheet is used, tighten and tuck it in the same way.

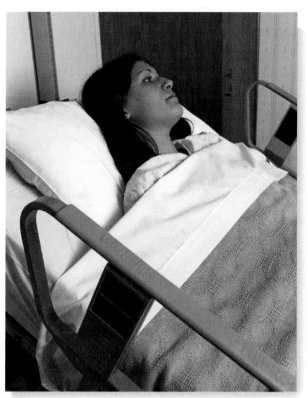

8 Help client into a supine position and adjust pillow. Place top sheet, blanket, and spread over client. Leave at least a 6-in. cuff at top of sheet at head of bed.

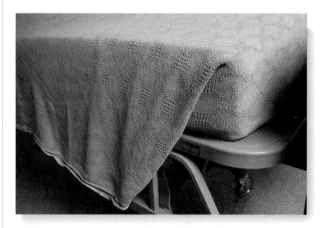

9 Miter corners at foot of bed. Pull up all layers of linen at client's toes. Make a small pleat. **RATIONALE:** This allows room for the client's feet and prevents sheets from rubbing on the client's toes.

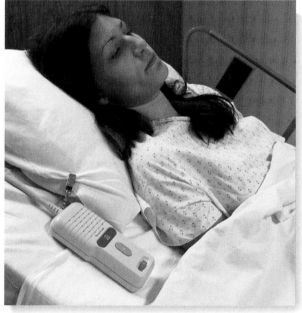

10 Return bed to lowest position. Position client for comfort. Reattach call signal to linens. Raise siderail. Dispose of soiled laundry. Wash your hands.

CHARTING

- Specific linen or equipment that causes discomfort for the client
- Special requirements for linen (e.g., certain detergents or elimination of starch)

- Use of pull sheets, incontinent pads, or specified ways to keep bed dry

CRITICAL THINKING FOCUS

SECTION ONE ▪ Bathing

Unexpected Outcomes

- Client is unwilling to have bed bath.

Alternate Nursing Actions

- Respect client's wishes.
- Offer to provide client with basin of water, washcloth, and towel to wash hands, face, and genitals.
- Provide back care if client allows.

- Client is too shy to allow nurse to provide bath.

- Determine if this is a cultural issue. Follow cultural beliefs and wishes.
- Determine if client prefers a different gender nurse or family member to give bath.
- Provide necessary assistance so client can do own bath.
- Have client wash hands, face, and genitals. Provide back care if client wishes.

- Client complains of dry, itchy skin following bath.

- Assess cause of itching.
- Apply lotion if not contraindicated.
- Change type of soap or avoid soap, depending on cause of dry skin.

SECTION TWO ▪ Bedmaking

Unexpected Outcomes

- Client refuses to have bed made.

Alternative Nursing Actions

- Assess reason for refusal. Client may be in pain or may not want to be disturbed.
- Offer to make the bed at a different time.
- Change only pillowcase and drawsheet, if client allows.
- Allow client to make this decision to promote client independence, if possible.

- Cross contamination occurs from improper linen disposal.

- Provide adequate linen hampers for nursing personnel.
- Provide in-service education program on infection control practices and require staff attendance.

- Client's skin becomes irritated from linen or begins to break down.

- Obtain hypoallergenic linen.
- Place special mattress under client.

SELF-CHECK EVALUATION

PART 1 ▪ Matching Terms

Match the definition in column B with the correct term in column A.

Column A	Column B
_____ a. Erythema	1. Movement in a regular course, as movement of blood through the heart and blood vessels
_____ b. Friction	
_____ c. Circulation	2. Folding top linen to foot or side of bed
_____ d. Effleurage	3. Alternate striking of fleshy part of hands on client's back as you move up and down the back
_____ e. Petrissage	
_____ f. Tapotement	4. Redness of skin associated with rashes, infection, and allergic reactions
_____ g. Fanfold	
	5. The act of rubbing
	6. Long stroking motions of the hands up and down the back
	7. Pinching the skin, subcutaneous tissue, and muscle as you move up and down the client's back

PART 2 ▪ Multiple Choice Questions

1. The appropriate temperature for bathing a client in a hydraulic bathtub chair is:

a. 100°F.
b. 105°F.
c. 110°F.
d. 115°F.

2. Which one of the following activities is *not* considered a part of evening care?

a. Provide mouth care.
b. Wash back.
c. Perform a complete linen change.
d. Replace binders or elastic hose.

3. The most accurate statement for providing morning care is:

a. It is provided for clients who will be discharged later in the morning.
b. It is only necessary for those clients who will be going to surgery later in the day.
c. It should be provided for bedridden clients.
d. It should be provided for clients who will not receive a bath until later in the morning.

4. The initial step in bathing a client on bed rest should be:

a. Removing the client's gown.
b. Removing the top linen.
c. Placing a bath blanket over the client.
d. Making a mitt with the washcloth.

5. The most appropriate sequence for bathing a client is:

a. Face, chest, abdomen, arms, legs, feet.
b. Eyes, forehead, cheeks, nose, lips.
c. Face, arms, axillae, abdomen, legs.
d. Arms, chest, abdomen, legs, back.

6. The main purpose for mitering the corners of the sheet is to:

    a. Secure the bottom sheet.

    b. Make the corners look neat.

    c. Keep bed linens tight.

    d. Follow nursing procedures.

7. An RN observes two team members placing the bed linens they have taken off a client's bed on the floor. The most appropriate intervention is to:

    a. Bring the staff members a clothes hamper and tell them to use it the next time.

    b. Explain the principles of medical asepsis to both team members.

    c. Tell them that this is unacceptable behavior and you will counsel both of them later.

    d. Do nothing because the linens are on their way to the laundry anyway.

8. All of the following scientific principles apply to bathing a client as a component of daily care *except*:

    a. Increased circulation results from the friction applied by the washcloth.

    b. It promotes a feeling of self-worth.

    c. Relaxation afforded by the bath plays a therapeutic role in the care of the client.

    d. It promotes venous constriction, which prevents pooling of blood in dependent areas.

PART III ▪ Critical Thinking Application

In reviewing the care plan and nurses' notes for Mr. Chavez, you note he has refused a bed bath the last two days. He is a third-day postoperative open-heart surgical client. When you enter the room you note a two-day growth of beard, and smell the client's breath and body odor.

1. Discuss your plan of action for Mr. Chavez's care.

2. Include psychosocial as well as physiological issues in your explanation.

7

PERSONAL HYGIENE

INTRODUCTION

Hygiene practices are considered primary care functions. These practices are basic to an individual's feeling of self-worth and independence. Basic hygiene functions include bathing, skin care, normal grooming functions, feeding, toileting, and dressing. Clients who are unable to perform these tasks are said to have a *self-care deficit*. Nurses focus on providing the necessary hygienic care while at the same time assisting the client to become more independent in these functions. Through their teaching role, nurses play a major and crucial role in assisting clients in returning to self-care independence.

Basic hygienic care is an integral part of the total treatment plan for a hospitalized client. Providing hygienic care gives the nurse an opportunity to complete assessment findings, particularly of the skin, mouth, hair, feet, and genitalia. This is also an excellent time for the nurse to communicate with the client and develop an interpersonal relationship. The client is provided basic care, in addition to the bath, which increases self-esteem and promotes cleanliness. Care of the skin, teeth, hair, and nails promotes good health by helping to protect the body from infection and disease. Proper nutrition is also required to promote the client's health and well-being.

(continued on next page)

The need to provide personal care depends on each client's physical state and the client's ability to care effectively for him- or herself. Before beginning hygienic care, first determine the extent of the client's involvement in completing the tasks. Establish a professional relationship with the client to prevent the client from feeling awkward that someone else has to assist or provide such personal care. This is an excellent time to determine the client's beliefs about hygienic care.

PREPARATION PROTOCOL: FOR PERSONAL HYGIENE

Complete the following steps before each skill.

1. Check client's plan of care for extent of assistance needed for personal hygiene tasks.
2. Gather equipment.
3. Check client's identaband.
4. Introduce yourself to the client and explain the nursing care you will be providing.
5. Provide privacy.
6. Wash your hands.
7. Don gloves as indicated.

COMPLETION PROTOCOL: FOR PERSONAL HYGIENE

Make sure the following steps have been completed.

1. Discard water, rinse and clean utensils, and replace equipment in appropriate area.
2. Place used linen in hamper.
3. Remove gloves (if used) and discard appropriately, then wash hands.
4. Return client to position of comfort.
5. Wash hands before leaving room.
6. Document pertinent data and report as indicated.

SECTION ONE

SKIN CARE

The skin is the first line of defense against microorganism invasion and infection. It is therefore critical that skin care be one of the most important components in providing personal hygienic care. The normal skin of healthy people has transient and resident microorganisms that are usually not harmful. However, during an illness increased perspiration causes body odor as it interacts with the bacteria residing on the skin. This promotes bacterial growth as well as being offensive. When injury or illness compromises the skin, the body becomes more susceptible to infection. Regular bathing routines remove the offending bacteria and promote healthy skin. In addition to bathing (see Chapter 6), the skin must be protected from breakdown. Applying skin lotions may not be enough to protect the skin. Special mattresses and beds may be needed for clients at high risk for skin breakdown.

The skin is the largest organ of the body and serves five major functions. (1) It protects the underlying tissue from injury and the intrusion of microorganisms. (2) It regulates body temperature through the processes of evaporation, radiation, and conduction. (3) It secretes sebum, an oily substance that has a bactericidal action as well as softening and lubricating effects on the skin and hair. (4) It produces and absorbs vitamin D (along with ultraviolet rays), which activates the precursor present in the skin. (5) It transmits pain, touch, and pressure sensations through nerve receptors.

Sweat glands found on the body surfaces are classified as apocrine glands or eccrine glands. The apocrine glands do not play a role in thermoregulation; that role is the primary function of the eccrine glands. The secretions from the apocrine glands are usually odorless unless there is decomposition or bacteria present on the skin, which causes the skin to emit an unpleasant odor known as body odor. The eccrine glands produce sweat that is used to cool the body through the process of evaporation. These glands are found on the palms of the hands, soles of the feet, and forehead. The sweat produced by these glands is composed of electrolytes, glucose, urea, and lactate. This is one of the reasons electrolyte imbalance is a major concern in clients with excessive perspiration.

RATIONALE

- To prevent skin breakdown for clients at risk or on bed rest
- To promote feelings of self-esteem by decreasing or preventing skin problems
- To prevent infections by maintaining intact skin
- To provide comfort for client
- To maintain skin cleanliness and prevent body odor

ASSESSMENT

- Assess overall condition of client's skin.
- Observe for changes in texture, color, and warmth.
- Observe for circulatory disturbances, i.e., dry, flaky skin, discoloration of the skin, signs of petechiae, or ulcers.
- Assess for signs of edema.
- Assess for presence of body odor.

MONITOR SKIN CONDITION

Equipment

- Artificial light for observation if natural light is insufficient
- Bath blanket, if appropriate
- Gown
- Clean gloves, if indicated

SKILL

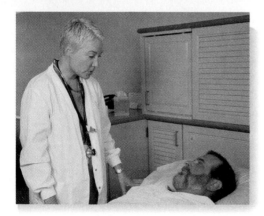

1 Explain monitoring process to client.

- Provide privacy for client; wash your hands.
- Remove linens and gown if necessary.

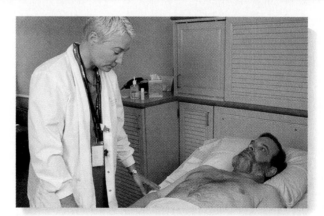

2 Compare color of client's skin with normal range of color within the individual's race. Observe for pallor (white color), flushing (red color), jaundice (yellow color), ashiness (gray color), or cyanosis (blue color).

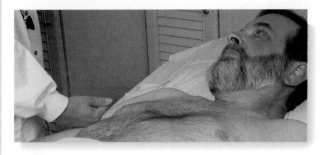

3 Place back of your fingers or hand on client's skin to check temperature. Consider temperature of room and of your hand. **RATIONALE:** The back of the hand is more sensitive to changes in temperature than the palm.

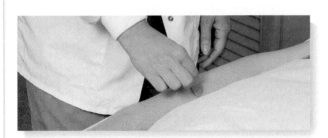

4 Gently pick up a small section of skin with your thumb and finger. Observe for ease of movement and speed of return to original position to check for skin turgor. **RATIONALE:** Degree of hydration is reflected in skin turgor or elasticity of skin.

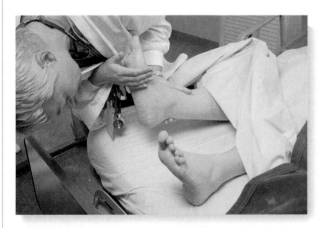

6 Observe for areas of broken skin (lesions) or ulcers. If present, wear gloves. Check if lesions are present over entire body or if they are localized.

- When checking skin temperature and texture, note client's response to heat, cold, gentle touch, and pressure.
- Correlate abnormalities in skin color with changes in skin temperature. **RATIONALE:** Skin temperature reflects blood circulation in the dermis.
- Observe for areas of excessive dryness, moisture, wrinkling, or flaking, and general texture of skin.
- Observe amount of oil, moisture, and dirt on skin surface. **RATIONALE:** Degree of moisture or dryness indicates disease states or hydration status.
- Note presence of strong body odors or odors in skin folds.

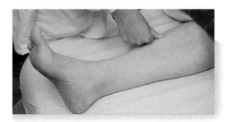

5 Press your finger firmly against client's skin for several seconds (especially in ankle area).

- After removing your finger, observe for lasting impression or indentation. **RATIONALE:** This identifies degree of edema based on level of indentation (1+ to 5+ indicates edema of 1 to 5 cm).

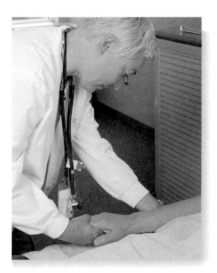

7 Check for skin discoloration (e.g., ecchymosis, petechiae, purpura, erythema, or altered pigmentation). **RATIONALE:** These signs are indications of generalized disease states, such as leukemia, vitamin deficiency, or hemophilia.

PREVENT SKIN BREAKDOWN

Equipment

- Skin lotion
- Pressure-relieving mattress, if needed
- Clean gloves, if open lesions present

SKILL

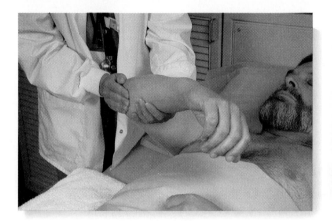

1 Observe client's most vulnerable body surfaces for ischemia, hyperemia, or broken areas.

- Keep skin clean and dry. Prevent soap, urine, feces, or excessive moisture from irritating skin.
- Protect healthy skin from drainage secretions.

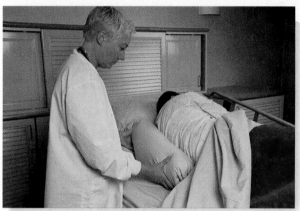

2 Change client's body position at least once every 2 hrs to rotate weight-bearing areas.

- Observe all vulnerable areas at this time.
- Keep linens clean, dry, and wrinkle free.
- Place client on special mattress or bed if indicated. (See page 143.)

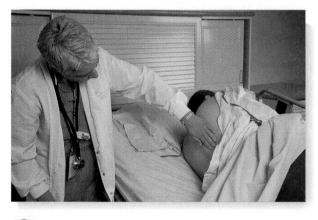

3 Massage client's skin and pressure-prone areas, if skin is not reddened. **RATIONALE:** Massage increases risk of breakdown in clients with reddened areas over bony prominences.

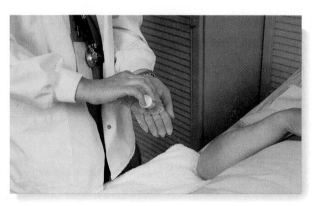

4 Lubricate dry, unbroken skin to prevent breakdown.

- Apply lotion to bedridden clients' sacrum, elbows, and heels several times during the day.

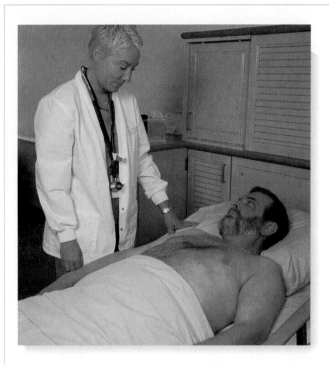

5 Teach client self-care principles.

- Encourage active exercises or range-of-motion exercises.
- Encourage client to eat a well-balanced diet with protein-rich foods and adequate fluids.
- Teach client and family how to prevent pressure areas and pressure ulcer formation.

TABLE 7-1	THERAPEUTIC BEDS	
Type of Bed	**Bed Features and Benefits**	**Client Recommendations**
Static low-air-loss Flexicair (MC3) KinAir Mediscus SMI 3000	Segmented cushions minimize shear and friction Automatic pressure adjustment Quick adjustment for CPR Built-in scale Bed-exit alarm Extended safety sides U-shaped cushions provide relief for head, sacral area, and heels	Clients at high risk for skin breakdown Clients with pulmonary problems— reduces risk of airborne contamination Clients with external fixators or heavy casts, or who are obese
Air-fluidized or static high-air-loss Clinitron (illustrated) Skytron Fluid Air SMI 5000	Fluidlike movement places minimum pressure on bony prominences Drying effect of beads prevents skin breakdown Offers softer surface than any other bed	Severe skin disorders Pressure ulcers Burns Generalized massive edema Poor wound healing Geriatric or orthopedic clients
Active low-air-loss EFICA-CC (illustrated) Biodyne Restcue Pulmonair 40	Built-in scale CPR deflation control Automatic pressure adjustment Gently pulsates or rotates side to side Protects skin integrity Promotes removal of pulmonary secretions Stimulates capillary blood flow	Massive edema Congestive heart failure Sepsis Critical care clients Pneumonia or other pulmonary problems with compromised skin integrity

BEYOND THE SKILL

Therapeutic Mattresses and Beds

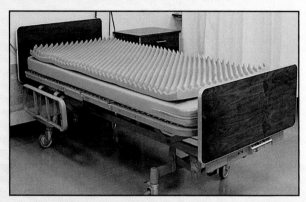

1. Eggcrate pressure mattresses circulate air and help to prevent skin breakdown.

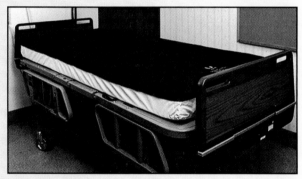

2. Gel nonpressure mattresses help to preserve skin integrity.

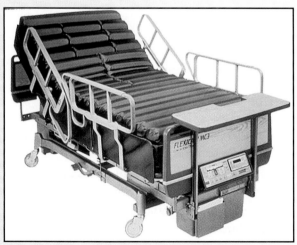

3. Static low-air-loss beds with segmented cushions help to minimize shear and friction. The Flexicair MC3 (illustrated courtesy of Hill-Rom) features automatic pressure adjustment. Other brands include KinAir, Mediscus, and SMI 3000.

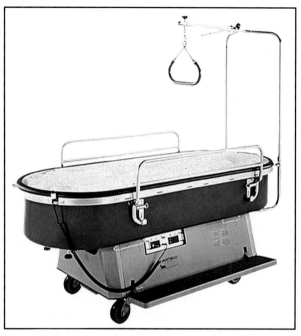

4. Air-fluidized or static high-air-loss beds provide fluidlike movement with minimum pressure on body prominences. The Clinitron (illustrated courtesy of Hill-Rom) offers a drying effect of beads that help prevent skin breakdown. Other brands include Skytron, Fluid Air, and SMI 5000.

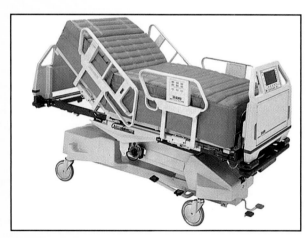

5. Active low-air-loss beds gently pulsate or rotate from side to side. The EFICA-CC (illustrated courtesy of Hill-Rom) offers automatic pressure adjustment. Other brands include Biodyne, Restcue, and Pulmonair 40.

CHARTING

- Client's skin condition: odor, temperature, turgor, sensation, cleanliness, integrity
- Client's mobility
- Turning frequency and client positioning
- Type of care given (e.g., massage, lotion)

- Client's complaints about skin or pressure ulcer
- Type of lesion, location, shape, color
- Alterations in sensation in skin lesion area
- Use of specialized mattress or bed

SECTION TWO

ORAL CARE

The condition of the oral cavity has a direct influence on an individual's overall state of health. Dental diseases require a host (the tooth and gum), an agent (plaque), and an environment (the presence of saliva and food). When plaque comes in contact with bacterial enzymes, carbohydrates, and acids, cavitation begins as the enamel of the tooth is decalcified. As long as food and plaque remain in the oral cavity, the possibility of dental decay increases.

It is important to maintain dental health in the hospitalized client. Maintaining dental hygiene begins with a good oral hygiene evaluation. Maintenance consists of brushing teeth or dentures, flossing, and using antiplaque mouthwash, if permitted.

RATIONALE

- To allow nurse to assess client's oral health status, knowledge, and routine for oral care
- To remove unpleasant tastes and odors from the oral cavity
- To provide comfort for client
- To remove plaque and bacteria-producing agents from oral cavity
- To provide client teaching on oral hygiene, if appropriate

ASSESSMENT

- Assess condition of client's oral cavity, teeth, gums, and mouth.
- Observe for color, lesions, tenderness, inflammation, intactness of teeth, and degree of moisture or dryness of oral cavity.
- Observe tongue.
- Evaluate the condition of gums and teeth.
- Assess for presence of dentures or bridges.
- Assess client's knowledge of oral hygiene techniques.

ORAL EVALUATION

Equipment

- Clean gloves
- Tongue blade (optional)
- Penlight

SKILL

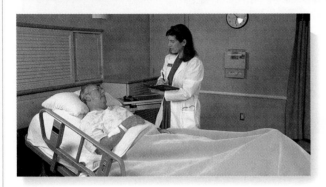

1 Place client in a Fowler's position, if possible. Assess client's physical condition. Consider diagnoses, treatments, fluid status, drugs, diet, and level of comfort or pain.

- Elicit any concerns, comments, or questions client may have about his or her oral health status.
- Determine last visit to dentist or dental hygienist. Elicit client's usual dental procedure or habits.

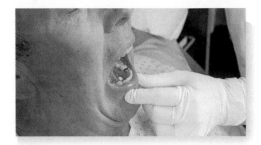

2 Inspect lips for fissures or unusual color. **RATIONALE:** Cheilitis is an inflammation of the lips. It frequently indicates a deficiency in vitamin B complex or can be caused by a bacterial infection.

- Inspect surface of mouth, especially buccal mucosa (it should be pink, smooth, and moist), for any abnormalities. **RATIONALE:** Alterations from normal may indicate presence of disease states such as measles, mumps, or Addison's disease.
- Examine condition of teeth and gums. Be alert to changes in gums. **RATIONALE:** Gingival hypertrophy, crevices between teeth and gums, pockets of debris, and bleeding with slight pressure are indicative of gingivitis.

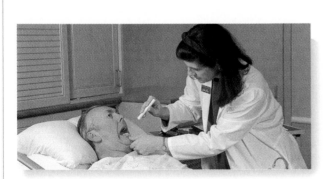

3 Examine tongue to determine abnormal findings and hydration status. Note any white patches, nodules, or ulcerations. **RATIONALE:** Deep fissures and dry mucous membranes are indicative of dehydration. Any lesion or ulcer persisting for more than 2 weeks should be assessed by the dentist.

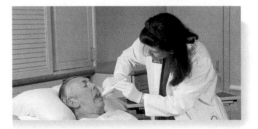

4 Determine oral hygiene needs based on assessment findings.

- Assess client's ability to care for self.
- Assess client's need for teaching. Consider educational level; physical, emotional, and mental state; previous experiences; and cultural differences.

BEYOND THE SKILL

Nurse-Client Teaching for Dental Health

Begin teaching the client about oral care during your initial assessment, if appropriate. Focus the teaching on oral health needs and care.

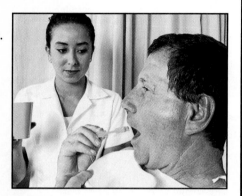

- Demonstrate and ask client to return demonstration of correct dental care techniques.
- Instruct in use of disclosure tablets or solution that temporarily stains dental plaque pink. This technique helps client see where plaque is left on teeth.
- After use of tablets or solution, instruct client to brush and floss until plaque is removed. All plaque may not be removed using this method.
- Encourage client to visit dentist when able.

ORAL HYGIENE

Equipment

- Toothbrush: small enough to reach back teeth; soft and rounded with nonfrayed rows of nylon bristles
- Dentifrice: client's choice, preferably one containing fluoride; special paste for dentures
- Cup of water
- Emesis basin or sink
- Dental floss: regular or fine, waxed or unwaxed, depending on client's needs
- Tissues or towel
- Mouthwash, if desired
- Clean gloves

SAFETY ALERT

Oral care following surgery or trauma to the face, oral cavity, or neck requires a specific physician's order. Oral hygiene is not done on a routine basis for these clients. Suctioning equipment is always present when oral hygiene is provided to these clients in order to prevent aspiration if the client is unable to handle secretions appropriately.

SKILL

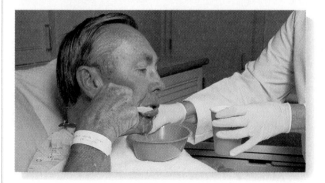

 Request that client open mouth wide and hold emesis basin under chin.

- Direct bristles of toothbrush toward gum line for all areas to be brushed. **RATIONALE:** This action removes food particles from gum line and stimulates gums.

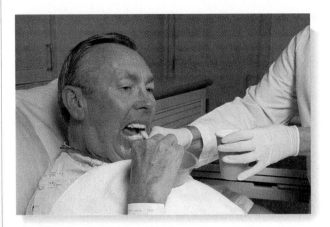

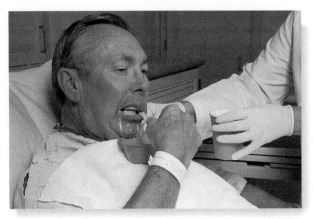

2 Keep brush positioned over only two or three teeth at a time. Use small rotating movements to cover outside surfaces of all teeth.

- Using brushing method just described, clean inner surfaces of all back teeth.
- To clean flat chewing surfaces, use a firm back-and-forth motion.

3 To clean inner surfaces of front teeth, use bristles on end of toothbrush and rotate brush back and forth across teeth.

- Lightly brush all areas of tongue. **RATIONALE:** This helps control breath odor.

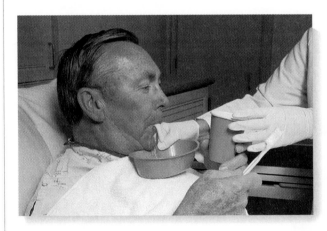

4 Rinse client's mouth thoroughly with water.

- Wipe off client's mouth and chin.
- Wash client's toothbrush, rinse and put it and the dentifrice away.

BEYOND THE SKILL

Flossing

Flossing is done as part of oral hygiene.

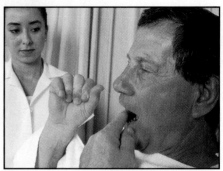

1. Floss thoroughly, using approximately 12 to 15 in of floss loosely wrapped around index fingers of both your hands.

2. Hold floss taut between your hands, and gently pull back and forth between each tooth.

3. Floss between each tooth by looping floss around each edge of the tooth and sliding floss down to the gum line. **RATIONALE:** This removes plaque that builds up between teeth.

4. Go as near gum line as possible without injury to gums. Pull floss back and forth gently, working back toward the biting surface of each tooth, until all teeth have been flossed. Use new section of floss for each tooth.

5. Floss each tooth several times until all particles of food are removed. **RATIONALE:** Gum disease and tooth decay can result if food particles remain on teeth and near gums.

6. Rinse client's mouth and wipe with towel.

DENTURE CARE

Equipment

- Denture toothbrush
- Denture cup
- Emesis basin
- Cleanser or effervescent tablets for dentures
- Clean gloves
- Mouthwash, if desired

SKILL

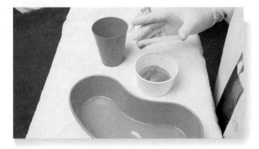

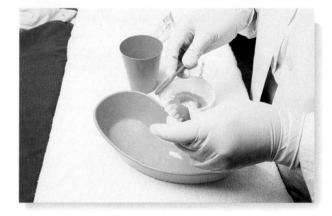

1 Help client remove dentures. If client is unable to do this, carefully place your finger on the edge of the upper denture. **RATIONALE:** This action breaks the seal at the roof of the mouth and allows the denture to slide out easily. The lower denture generally lifts out easily.

- If client is unable to clean own dentures, place them in an unbreakable container. Either wash dentures over an emesis basin or carry them to the sink.

2 Hold one denture in your hand. With other hand, use toothbrush or special denture brush and cleaning agent, such as a commercially prepared paste or solution, to brush denture. Use same brushing technique as with natural teeth.

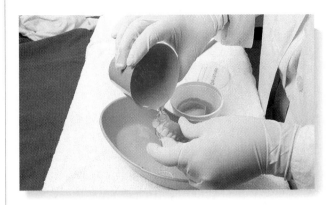

3 Rinse denture thoroughly in cold water.

- Clean second denture using same procedure as in step 2.
- Replace dentures in client's mouth after rinsing oral cavity with water or mouthwash.
- Place dentures in tight-fitting denture cup if client is not putting them in mouth immediately. Label denture cup with client's name and room number. Clean equipment and replace in appropriate area. Place denture cup in bedside stand or bathroom.

ORAL CARE FOR UNCONSCIOUS CLIENT

Equipment

- Mouth swabs, according to hospital policy
- Lubricant for lips
- Toothbrush
- Syringe (5 mL without needle) filled with water

- Yankauer suction catheter
- Emesis basin
- Padded tongue blade
- Clean gloves

SKILL

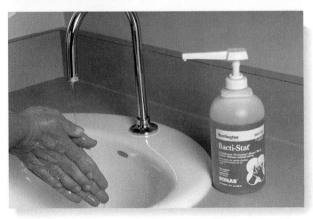

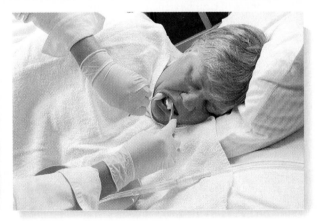

1 Wash hands before placing client in lateral, low-Fowler's or semi-Fowler's position. **RATIONALE:** To allow draining or suction of irrigation solution and toothpaste to prevent aspiration.

- Place suctioning equipment and emesis basin next to client for easy access.
- Put small amount of toothpaste on brush.
- Brush external surfaces of teeth in routine manner, using less water on brush.

2 Place padded tongue blade in client's mouth to hold mouth open and move cheeks and lips away from toothbrush. **RATIONALE:** This prevents client from closing down on toothbrush and accidentally biting your fingers if they are close to the client's teeth.

- Clean inner surfaces of teeth, using padded tongue blade to separate upper and lower sets of teeth. Brush teeth and tongue in usual manner.

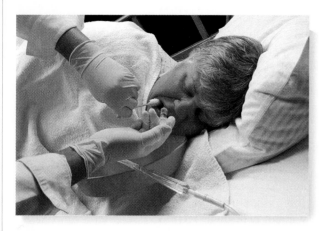

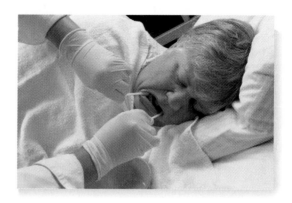

3 Rinse client's mouth carefully, using syringe to insert a small amount of water. No more than 5 mL of water should be inserted at one time. **RATIONALE:** To prevent aspiration.

4 Suction oral cavity with suction catheter to remove water and toothpaste.

- Wipe client's mouth with washcloth. Clean and replace equipment.
- Position client in a semi-Fowler's position for at least 30 min. **RATIONALE:** To prevent aspiration if water remains in mouth.

CHARTING

- Findings of oral evaluation: condition of gums, mucous membranes, mouth, and teeth
- Assessment of client's oral hygiene needs
- Oral care provided or observed
- Effectiveness of oral hygiene care on gums, mucous membranes, teeth

- Client's reaction and level of comfort
- Client teaching provided
- Client's participation in oral care

SECTION THREE

HAIR CARE

The appearance and condition of a client's hair may reflect his or her general physical and emotional status, individuality and feelings of worth, and ability to provide self-care. Hair is often neglected in clients who are very ill and require extensive nursing care actions. It is important that these clients receive appropriate interventions to maintain their hair in a nontangled, neat, clean manner.

Caring for the client's hair should be considered a regular function of hygiene care that is just as necessary as giving a bath. Regular assessment of the client's hair should be included in the client's overall assessment. This includes not just the hair, but beards and mustaches as well. Clients with long hair should have their hair braided to prevent the hair from becoming tangled or falling into an open wound.

RATIONALE

- To promote self-esteem
- To prevent irritation to the scalp and damage to the hair
- To maintain or improve the existing condition of the client's hair and scalp
- To prevent tangled hair during hospitalization

ASSESSMENT

- Assess client's hair care needs.
- Assess usual hair care routines, products, and appliances.
- Determine client's ability to care for own hair.
- Observe condition of hair and scalp.

HAIR CARE

Equipment

- Blunt-ended comb or pick
- Brush
- Towel
- Hair care products

SKILL

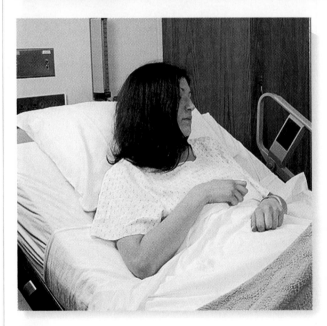

1 For routine hair care, determine client's hair care needs.

- Help client into a comfortable position to perform hair care.
- Collect and assemble equipment.
- Place towel over client's shoulders when combing and brushing hair.
- Brush or comb client's hair from scalp to ends, using gentle, even strokes.

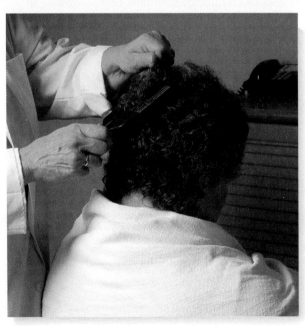

2 For tangled hair, hold hair above tangle to prevent discomfort.

- Using a wide-tooth comb, gently comb tangle, using short, gentle strokes. Work out tangle from ends of hair shafts toward scalp. Work on small amount of tangle at one time. **RATIONALE:** Working on large tangles results in broken ends and damaged hair shafts. *Note:* A small amount of white vinegar, conditioner, or alcohol can be used to make combing tangles easier.

BEYOND THE SKILL

Pediculosis

Equipment

- Isolation bags
- Treatment solution as ordered (i.e., gamma benzene hexachloride)
- Clean linen
- Fine-tooth comb; Disinfectant for comb
- Clean gloves

Skill

1. Examine hair using magnifying glass to detect head lice.
2. Remove and bag client's clothing and linens separately. Use isolation bags.
3. Apply solution ordered by physician (cream, lotion, or shampoo). Head lice requires treatment with miticide shampoo. Leave shampoo in place several minutes. **RATIONALE:** Prolonged use of shampoo can burn the scalp. (Body and pubic lice requires shower with soap followed by lotion application for 24 hrs).
4. Rinse hair thoroughly.
5. Comb through hair with fine-tooth comb.
6. Sterilize comb and brushes.
7. Examine hair closely for white nits on hair shafts. Repeat shampoo in 24 hrs as necessary.
8. Discuss cause, treatment, and preventive measures regarding lice infestation with client and family.

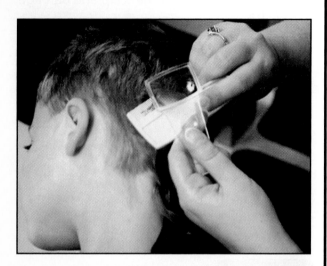

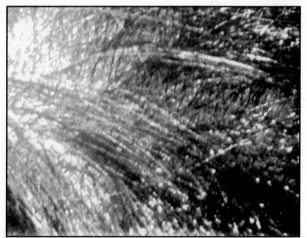

SAFETY ALERT

If you suspect a client may have an infestation of lice, ensure that good visual inspection is completed and proper treatment is carried out to prevent the spread of lice to other clients. This is most common in a pediatric setting; however, it can occur with adult clients as well.

CLINICAL NOTE

Due to the shorter lengths of hospital stays, shampooing clients' hair is seldom done in acute-care hospitals today. Dry shampoos can be used for clients on bed rest; however, they are not very effective for cleaning hair. The shampoo is easier and more effective if the client is able to go to the shower. If the client is unable to go to the shower, he or she can be placed on a gurney or in a wheelchair and taken to an area where there is a large sink.

BRAIDED HAIR

Equipment

- Comb or brush
- Barrette, ribbon, covered elastic band, or scrunchy

SKILL

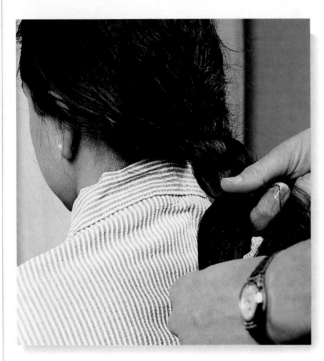

1 Position client in sitting position, if possible.

- Comb or brush hair. Remove tangles before braiding.
- Part hair into sections equal to number of desired braids.
- Divide each section into three equal strands.
- Begin braid so that base is not in a pressure area of the head.
- Weave the three strands, alternately placing right and left strands over middle one. Move strands smoothly from one hand to the other and keep strands in hands at all times. **RATIONALE:** The strands will release and the hair will unbraid if not kept in the hands at all times.
- Continue until ends of strands are reached. Fasten ends with barrette or covered elastic band. **RATIONALE:** Uncovered elastic bands will damage the hair shaft.

BEARDS AND MUSTACHES

Equipment

- Brush or comb
- Towel
- Mustache scissors

SKILL

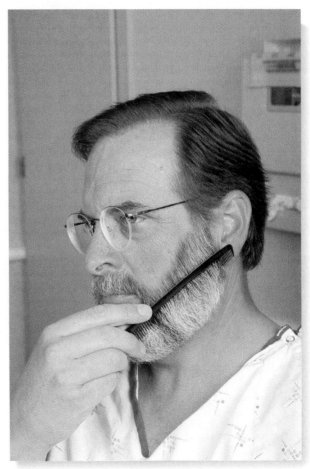

1 Determine extent of mustache or beard care needs.

- Help client to a comfortable position.
- Observe client's skin underneath beard or mustache.
- Comb or brush beard or mustache.
- Shampoo beard or mustache as needed.
- Assist client in trimming beard or mustache as needed.

SHAVING

Equipment

- Safety or electric razor
- Shaving cream (for straight razor or safety razor)
- Aftershave lotion (optional)
- Towels (two)
- Basin of warm water (for straight razor or safety razor)

Preparation

1 Raise client's bed into sitting position.

- Place towel over chest and under chin.
- Position mirror from over-bed table for client use.

CLINICAL NOTE

Before shaving a client, check if he has excessive bleeding tendencies due to pathologic conditions (hemophilia) or is taking anticoagulants or large doses of aspirin. In these cases, excessive bleeding can occur if the client is accidentally cut.

SAFETY ALERT

Don gloves if you are shaving client. **RATIONALE:** To protect yourself from potential blood as a result of an accidental nick.

Check hospital policy regarding the use of electric razors in the hospital. Some hospitals will allow only battery-operated razors.

SKILL

Straight or Safety Razor

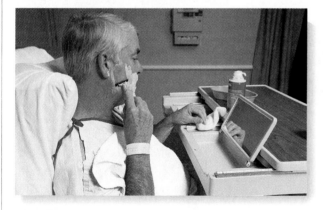

1 Moisten area to be shaved, then apply thick layer of shaving cream.

- Holding skin taut, use firm but small strokes in direction of hair growth and begin shaving from most lateral aspect of face and move toward center of face.
- Gently remove soap or lather with warm, damp towel. Inspect for areas missed.
- Apply aftershave lotion, if desired.
- Position client for comfort.
- Clean and dry razor and return razor and shaving lotion to bedside stand or bathroom.

Electric Razor

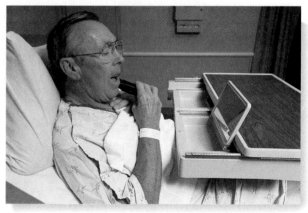

1 Start shaving from lateral aspect of face and move toward chin and upper lip area.

- Use rotating motion of razor as you move over each area of face.
- Apply aftershave lotion, if desired.
- Position client for comfort.
- Return razor to client's bedside stand or bathroom.

CHARTING

- Hair care assessment and needs
- Shampoo method, outcomes, problems encountered
- Client's tolerance for hair care

- Type of shave completed
- Unusual problems such as bleeding from shaving
- Outcome of pediculosis treatment

SECTION FOUR

FOOT CARE

The feet are especially susceptible to discomfort, trauma, and infection due to the amount of stress they must endure supporting an individual's weight when standing and walking. In addition, blood must travel the greatest distance from the heart to perfuse the lower extremities and feet. Therefore, problems with circulation may be related to problems with the feet. Several common foot problems seen in the hospitalized client include:

- **Incurvated or ingrown toenails:** Corners of the nail press into the skin, causing pain, ulceration, and infection.
- **Cracks and fissures between toes:** Often a result of very dry skin or athlete's foot.
- **Athlete's foot:** Fungal irritation that results in itching, burning, and dry skin.
- **Plantar warts:** Viral irritation that is deep, painful, and generally found on the sole of the foot.
- **Corns:** High calluses caused by pressure on toes, joints, or bony prominences.
- **Calluses:** Thickened epidermis over areas of skin caused by pressure.

Podiatrists must be called to the health care setting to do any type of foot care, except washing, for clients with diabetes or peripheral vascular disease. These clients are at high risk for infection, and if the skin is nicked during cutting of toenails or treatment of other foot conditions, the client's foot can easily become infected.

RATIONALE

- To determine extent of foot care needed
- To prevent infection and discomfort
- To determine need for podiatrist referral

ASSESSMENT

- Assess feet for clinical indications of peripheral vascular disease; warmth, color, capillary refill, discoloration, pulse, presence of edema, pain or discomfort when palpated.
- Assess feet for irritation, cracking, lesions, corns, calluses, deformities, and edema.
- Assess condition of toenails: color, contour, condition, length of nails.
- Assess cleanliness.

FOOT CARE

Equipment

- Basin of warm water
- Soap or emollient agent
- Washcloth
- Towels (two)

- Toenail clippers or scissors, according to facility policy
- Nail file
- Skin care lotion or lanolin
- Clean gloves as necessary

SKILL

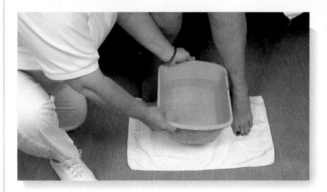

1 Gather equipment according to client's needs. Help client to edge of bed or into chair.

- Place towel on floor in front of client.
- Help client place feet in basin as needed. Add emollient agent to water, if desired.

Note: Check hospital policy regarding cutting nails. Some health care facilities allow only podiatrists to cut nails.

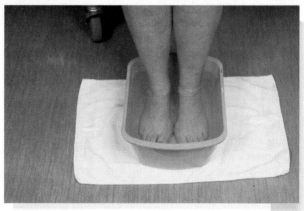

2 Soak feet for 10 min if client can tolerate.

- Use washcloth and soap to bathe feet as needed.
- Examine feet and nails while soaking and report unusual findings to physician.
- Obtain order for cutting nails or referring to podiatrist as needed.

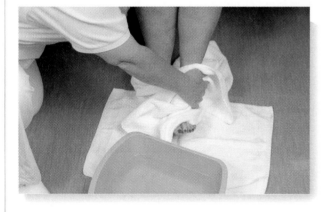

3 Dry each foot thoroughly with a second towel. Dry between each toe.

- Clean under nails using nail file as needed.
- Clip nails, if needed and allowed by facility policy. Cut toenails straight across with scissors or nail clipper. File rough edges with nail file. **RATIONALE:** Rounding off toenails may break skin or cause ingrown toenails.
- Apply lotion to feet, focusing on dry areas. Assist client into position of comfort.
- Return equipment to appropriate place.

CHARTING

- Findings from foot and nail assessment
- Identified foot and nail care needs
- Specific treatment provided

- Abnormalities observed and reported
- Referrals made, if appropriate

SECTION FIVE

PERINEAL AND GENITAL CARE

The perineum consists of the area between the thighs and from the anterior pelvis to the anus. This area contains organs and structures related to sexual function, reproduction, and elimination.

Hygienic care involves cleaning the perineum and genitalia to prevent bacterial growth, which can rapidly increase in this warm, dark, moist environment. Perineal care is provided as part of bathing activities, but it may also be required more frequently to prevent skin irritation, infection, discomfort, or odor. It is critical to provide frequent perineal care for clients who are incontinent. Urine or feces allowed to stay in contact with the skin for an extended period of time can lead to inflammation and then to excoriation of the area.

All clients are susceptible to perineal irritation or infection. Immobilized, incontinent, debilitated, comatose, or diabetic clients, or those with indwelling catheters, are at particularly high risk for perineal problems.

Providing perineal care can be a very sensitive issue. Clients often feel embarrassed; therefore, it is imperative that every precaution be taken to respect the client's privacy. The attitude of the nurse directly affects the client's response to this personal care activity.

RATIONALE

- To remove excessive secretions
- To decrease the growth of bacteria
- To promote healing after surgery and vaginal deliveries
- To prevent the spread of microorganisms in clients with indwelling catheters
- To promote client comfort and hygiene

ASSESSMENT

- Observe for signs of irritation, lesions, excoriations, or edema.
- Check for perineal itching or burning on urination.
- Assess for general comfort, comfort related to catheter placement, and catheter patency.

PERINEAL CARE FOR FEMALES

Equipment

- Bath blanket or sheet
- Towels (two)
- Protective pad
- Washcloth
- Clean gloves
- Wash basin
- Bedpan (optional)
- Soap or prescribed solution

SKILL

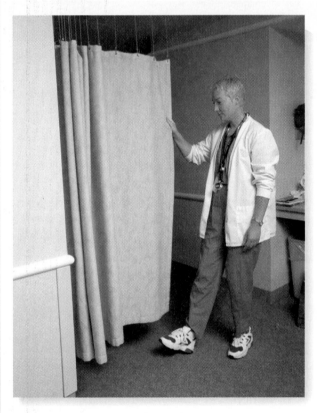

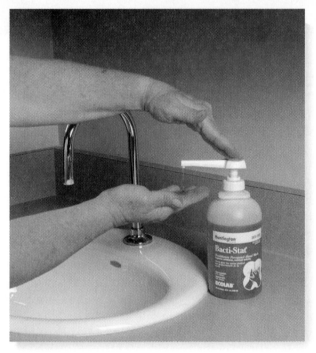

③ Wash hands and don gloves. **RATIONALE:** This prevents contamination of hands from body fluids or exudate.

① Complete Preparation Step 1 and 2 in "Bath for an Adult Client" skill, p. 118.

② Provide privacy for client by closing door and pulling curtain. **RATIONALE:** This provides privacy for client and lessens risk that someone will enter room while skill is being performed.

- Explain procedure to client.

- Pour warm water into basin.
- Place bed in HIGH position and lower siderail nearest you.
- Place protective pad on bed.
- Place client in dorsal recumbent position in bed. *Note:* Client can also be placed on the toilet, on a bedpan and positioned in a semi-Fowler's position in bed, or in a sitz bath for perineal care.

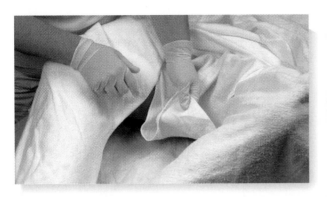

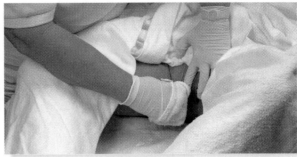

4 Drape client using bath blanket (see Chapter 21, p. ■■■, "Drape Client").

- Instruct client to bend knees and separate legs. **RATIONALE:** The perineal area can be cleansed more efficiently in this position.
- Lift corner of drape away from perineal area.
- Place washcloth into basin. Rub cloth with soap and wring out excess water. **RATIONALE:** This prevents the protective pad from getting excessively wet.

5 Fold washcloth into mitt or gather into palm of hand (see Chapter 6, p. 118, "Making a Washcloth Mitt").

- Separate labia with one hand to expose urethral and vaginal openings.
- Wash labia minora from front to back in a downward motion on one side.
- Change washcloth area and repeat cleansing stroke on opposite side. **RATIONALE:** This prevents cross contamination between areas.

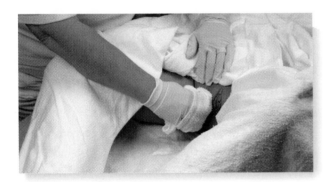

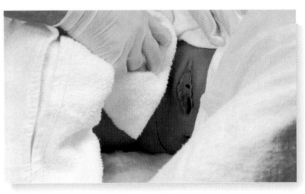

6 Place washcloth in water, resoap, wring dry, and gather into palm or hand or form a mitt using new section of washcloth to continue washing perineal area.

- Wash external labia (labia majora) and perineal area from front to back.

7 Change area of washcloth and cleanse opposite side of external labia and perineal area.

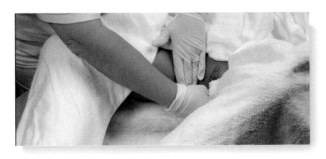

8 Change washcloth area and clean around anus.

- Thoroughly pat dry perineal and anal area. **RATIONALE:** To prevent moisture accumulation and potential fungus infections.

BEYOND THE SKILL

Alternative Method for Perineal Care

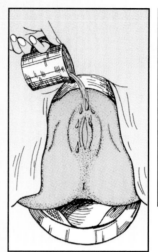
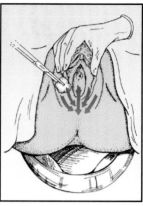

1. Place protective pad under client.
2. Place client in semi-Fowler's position on bedpan.
3. Have client bend knees and separate legs.
4. Pour warm water or prescribed solution over perineum while client is positioned on bedpan. **RATIONALE:** The perineum is more comfortably and effectively cleansed by this method. This method of perineal care is used frequently with clients who have had vaginal gynecological surgery or are in the postpartum period.
5. Wipe area from front to back using cotton balls or towel. Dry thoroughly.
6. Remove equipment, clean, and replace in appropriate area. Place protective pad in trash container.
7. Place client in position of comfort.

PERINEAL CARE FOR MALES

Equipment

- Bath blanket or sheet
- Towels (two or three)
- Protective pad
- Washcloth

- Wash basin
- Soap
- Clean gloves

SKILL

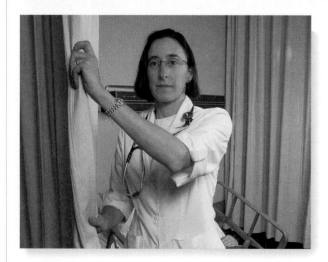

1 Provide privacy for client. Close curtain and door. **RATIONALE:** To prevent entry into room during procedure.

- Explain procedure to client. Gather equipment. Place protective pad under client.
- Place warm water in basin.

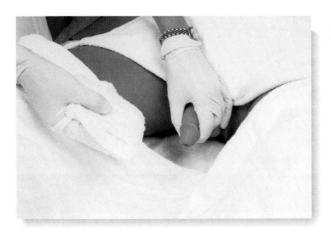

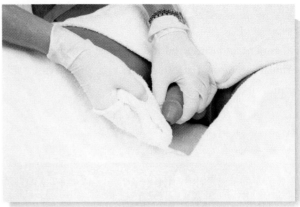

2 Cover client's legs with sheet or towel; cover abdomen with bath blanket or towel. Expose as little of genital area as possible. **RATIONALE:** This provides for client comfort and modesty.

- Place washcloth in basin. Apply soap to washcloth.
- Wring washcloth out to remove excess water. **RATIONALE:** This will prevent the protective pad from getting too wet.

3 Gently but securely hold shaft of penis in one hand.

- Starting at tip of penis, use circular motion with washcloth as you wash down toward shaft. *Note:* If the client has not been circumcised, retract his foreskin carefully to expose the glans of the penis. After cleansing the penis, replace the foreskin over the glans.
- Use new section of washcloth if washing over same area. **RATIONALE:** This prevents cross contamination.
- Rinse out washcloth and then rinse area thoroughly.

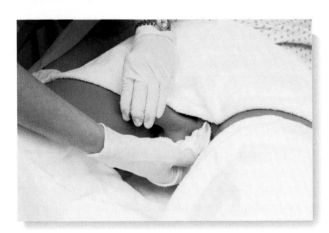

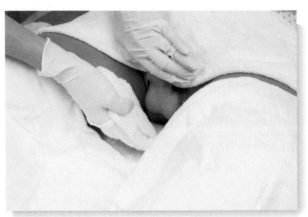

4 Wash around scrotum, using new section of the washcloth.

- Rinse out washcloth and then rinse area thoroughly.

5 Wash anal area last. **RATIONALE:** This prevents potential contamination from feces.

- Rinse out washcloth and then rinse area thoroughly.
- Dry all areas thoroughly. Clean and return basin to appropriate area. Discard linen in hamper.

- Assessment and care needs for perineal hygiene
- Perineal care provided and client's response to care
- Condition of perineum

CRITICAL THINKING FOCUS

SECTION ONE ▪ Skin Care

Unexpected Outcomes	**Alternative Nursing Actions**
▪ Skin is erythematous but remains intact.	▪ Monitor fluid and electrolyte balance and nutritional status.
	▪ Turn client at least every 2 hrs.
	▪ Obtain order for pressure-relieving mattress.
▪ Client cannot be positioned to avoid erythematous areas completely.	▪ Turn client at least every 2 hrs.
	▪ Do not turn on erythematous site.
	▪ Use protocol for Stage I ulcer treatment on affected area.
▪ Skin integrity is interrupted, even with skin care.	▪ Continue to use appropriate skin care products.
	▪ Use protocol for Stage II ulcer treatment on affected area.
	▪ Obtain order for air-fluidized bed.

SECTION TWO ▪ Oral Care

Unexpected Outcomes	**Alternative Nursing Actions**
▪ Even with increased oral hygiene, client still has halitosis.	▪ Use antiseptic mouthwash between oral hygiene care.
	▪ Notify physician; this could be a symptom of a systemic disease.
	▪ Evaluate client's nutritional intake; absent nutrients or imbalanced intake of fat, protein, or carbohydrates can result in bad breath.
	▪ Obtain a referral to a dentist; this could be a symptom of periodontal disease.
▪ Vigorous flossing results in bleeding and sore gums.	▪ Give client warm antiseptic mouthwash to relieve soreness.
	▪ Assess gums and obtain referral to dentist, if appropriate.
▪ Normal cleaning is not sufficient to remove debris and plaque in the unconscious client.	▪ Use toothbrush and dentifrice at least b.i.d. Keep suction nearby.

SECTION THREE ▪ Hair Care

Unexpected Outcomes	Alternative Nursing Actions
▪ Extreme matting, snarling, blood, or nonremovable substances appear in client's hair.	▪ If hair needs to be cut, check facility policy regarding hair cutting. Physician or family permission may be required. ▪ Rubbing alcohol applied to hair may remove blood or decrease matting and allow comb to go through hair.
▪ Client is cut during shaving with straight razor.	▪ Assess extent of cut. ▪ Place towel over area and apply pressure. ▪ If bleeding does not stop in a few minutes, or if cut is deep, notify physician. ▪ Complete an Unusual Occurrence Form.
▪ Shaving is difficult and painful for client.	▪ Place warm, moist towel over area to be shaved. ▪ Apply more shaving cream than usual. ▪ Ensure that razor is sharp. A new disposable razor may work better.
▪ Miticide is left on hair too long.	▪ Observe scalp frequently for signs of irritation after rinsing thoroughly. ▪ Notify physician for medication order. ▪ Do not repeat treatment until scalp is healed.

SECTION FOUR ▪ Foot Care

Unexpected Outcomes	Alternative Nursing Actions
▪ Client has excessively dry, scaly skin even after routine foot care.	▪ Apply alkali solutions as ordered, such as Epsom salts or bicarbonate of soda, to soften skin and remaining scales. ▪ Repeated soakings are usually necessary.
▪ Client's feet are excessively moist.	▪ Provide foot care b.i.d. ▪ Apply moisture-absorbing powder.
▪ Client has large calluses on feet.	▪ After soaking feet, obtain an order to rub a pumice stone or abrasive material on the callused area. Calluses are never cut from the skin due to possible scarring of the epidermis. ▪ For diabetic clients, obtain referral to a podiatrist.
▪ Client has mycotic nails.	▪ Obtain referral to podiatrist.

SECTION FIVE ▪ Perineal and Genital Care

Unexpected Outcomes	Alternative Nursing Actions
▪ Client has a foul odor even after perineal care.	▪ Obtain order for sitz bath. ▪ Request order for medicated solution. Pour solution over perineum. ▪ Discuss vaginal irrigation with physician.

- Discuss need for culture with physician. Medication may be indicated.

- Client develops urinary tract infection.

- Instruct client in proper technique for perineal care.
- Instruct female clients to cleanse from anterior to posterior aspects of perineum, using different sections of cloth for each wipe.
- Instruct male clients to cleanse from urethral opening down shaft of penis.

SELF-CHECK EVALUATION

PART 1 ▪ Matching Terms

Match the definition found in column B with correct term in column in A.

Column A	Column B
_____ a. Excoriation	1. Nonpathogenic normal body flora
_____ b. Mycotic	2. Presence of lice
_____ c. Calluses	3. Forerunner of dental caries and periodontal disease
_____ d. Plaque	4. Fungal infection
_____ e. Fungus	5. Abrasion of epidermis
_____ f. Epidermis	6. Outermost layer of the skin
_____ g. Pediculosis	7. Hypertrophy of horny layer of skin

PART 2 ▪ Multiple Choice Questions

1. Which one of the following actions is not considered a component of monitoring the skin condition of a client?
   a. Check for skin turgor.
   b. Observe color.
   c. Observe mentation.
   d. Check skin temperature.

2. Which one of the following skin colors indicates a potential problem is occurring with the client?
   a. Pink.
   b. Olive.
   c. Tan.
   d. Purplish.

3. Dental disease requires all of the following except:
   a. Plaque.
   b. Presence of fluoridated water.
   c. Presence of saliva and food in the oral cavity.
   d. A host; tooth and gum.

4. Client instruction for brushing the outside surface of the teeth should include:
   a. Brush for 2 to 3 min in each quadrant of the mouth.
   b. Brush one quadrant of the mouth using a horizontal brush stroke over the teeth.
   c. Use a small rotating movement over two or three teeth at a time.
   d. Use the bristles on the end of the toothbrush and rotate over surface of teeth.

5. The most important safety issue to remember when providing oral care to a comatose client is:

    a. Keep the client in a lateral position with head down.
    b. Use only toothettes or swabs for oral care.
    c. Keep a suction setup nearby.
    d. Do not rinse the client's mouth during oral care.

6. If a client has tangled hair, it is best to:

    a. Ask a relative to comb it during a visit.
    b. Comb the hair with a small-tooth comb to work out the tangles.
    c. Work the tangle out starting at the scalp and working down the shaft of the hair.
    d. Apply a small amount of vinegar or alcohol to the hair before combing.

7. Treatment for pediculosis usually consists of:

    a. Shampooing the hair twice a day with any shamoo for dry hair.
    b. Applying a prescription shampoo and leaving it in place for 12 hrs.
    c. Using a tar-based shampoo once a day for three days.
    d. Applying a miticide and leaving it in place for several minutes before rinsing.

8. It is important to prevent cross contamination of microorganisms while performing perineal and genital care for a female client. The most important action to prevent this is:

    a. Pour water directly over the perineum without touching the area with anything.
    b. Use a separate section of the washcloth for each stroke.
    c. Start the cleansing action at the lateral surface and move toward the labia.
    d. Use an antiseptic solution for the cleansing if there is any risk of cross contamination.

PART 3 ▪ Critical Thinking Application

You have been assigned to a 70-year-old man who was admitted yesterday for dehydration and poor nutrition leading to electrolye imbalance. He is unkempt and has severe body odor, and his teeth are in poor repair. He refused all personal care yesterday. At 8:00 this morning he also refused to allow you to do any personal hygienic care for him. He lives alone in a small apartment and states he cooks for himself.

1. How important is it that personal hygienic care be done for this client? State physiological and psychological implications for this client.

2. What action will you take to encourage him to accept nursing care?

3. Which two hygienic care activities are the most important for him at this time? Provide scientific data for your response.

8

ADMISSION AND ASSESSMENT

INTRODUCTION

The admission procedure can be a positive or negative experience for clients. If the procedure is impersonal, mechanized, or impolite, it can be a very negative experience; if handled with care and attention, it can be positive. The impressions formed by clients during the admission process strongly affect their attitude toward their total care. Because the admission procedure can be the client's initial introduction into the health care system, nurses should consider this process a key step in client care.

The process of admitting a client to a health care facility varies among institutions such as long-term care facilities, clinics, and hospitals. Regardless of the size or type of facility, however, the admission process is vitally important to providing safe, adequate care. Because the nurse-client relationship begins with admission, the nurse should have a thorough understanding of the standard admission procedure. If a client enters the hospital in an emergency situation, he or she may feel insecure or fearful because he or she has had little time to make plans concerning family, travel, finances, or employment. When a client enters the hospital for elective treatment or surgery, the nurse has a little more time to orient the client and prepare him or her for a hospital stay.

(continued on next page)

The first contact during the admission process is usually with the admitting receptionist, who assigns a hospital number and interviews the client. If the client cannot answer the questions required during this time, a relative is asked to supply the data. The information required includes insurance status, religious preference, family data, employment data, and advance directives. The client will also be asked to sign consent forms and send all valuables home with the relatives.

Prehospital laboratory procedures and x-rays should be done before admission for elective procedures. If not, the client should have them done immediately before being taken to his or her room or shortly after admission. Clients admitted under emergency situations will have their laboratory studies and x-rays completed in the emergency department or after they are admitted to the nursing unit.

In 1992, the Joint Commission on Accreditation of Healthcare Organizations (JCAHO) required every person admitted to the hospital to have an admission assessment completed or directed by a registered nurse within a specified time frame. The usual time frame is 1 to 2 hrs after admission.

Because clients may not be sure of their role while in the hospital, many hospitals have adopted versions of the American Hospital Association's Patient's Bill of Rights. This bill includes the following rights:

- To obtain information about one's illness or injury
- To refuse medication or treatment
- To participate in one's own care
- To know the rationale and risks of treatment
- To receive courteous care
- To ensure the client understands his/her rights.

Effective December 1991, The Patient Self-Determination Act was implemented. This act requires all Medicare and Medicaid recipient hospitals to provide clients with information regarding their rights to reject medical treatment and write advance directives. The admitting nurse should ensure that this is completed.

One of the first nursing interventions carried out while the client is being admitted, or shortly after the admission, is obtaining the client's health history and performing a physical assessment. This may be the first hospital experience for the client, and both of these activities must be done while maintaining privacy for the client. Curtains are closed, and health history questions should be asked quietly and in a professional manner, particularly when sensitive questions are asked.

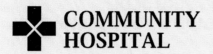

COMMUNITY HOSPITAL

LIST OF PATIENT RIGHTS IN CALIFORNIA

In accordance with section 70707 of the California Administrative Code, the hospital and medical staff have adopted the following list of patient rights. Each patient has the right to:

1. Exercise these rights without regard to sex or cultural, economic, educational, or religious background or the source of payment for his care.
2. Considerate and respectful care.
3. Knowledge of the name of the physician who has primary responsibility for coordinating his care and the names and professional relationships of other physicians who will see him.
4. Receive information from his physician about his illness, his course of treatment, and his prospects for recovery in terms that he can understand.
5. Receive as much information about any proposed treatment or procedure as he may need in order to give informed consent or to refuse this course of treatment. Except in emergencies, this information shall include a description of the procedure or treatment, the medically significant risks involved in this treatment, alternate course of treatment or nontreatment and the risks involved in each, and to know the name of the person who will carry out the procedure or treatment.
6. Participate actively in decisions regarding his medical care. To the extent permitted by law, this includes the right to refuse treatment.
7. Full consideration of privacy concerning his medical care program. Case discussion, consultation, examination, and treatment are confidential and should be conducted discreetly. The patient has the right to be advised as to the reason for the presence of any individual.
8. Confidential treatment of all communications and records pertaining to his care and his stay in the hospital. His written permission shall be obtained before his medical records can be made available to anyone not directly concerned with his care.
9. Reasonable responses to any reasonable requests he may make for service.
10. Leave the hospital even against the advice of his physicians.
11. Reasonable continuity of care and to know in advance the time and location of appointment as well as the physician providing the care.
12. Be advised if hospital/personal physician proposes to engage in or perform human experimentation affecting his care or treatment. The patient has the right to refuse to participate in such research projects.
13. Be informed by his physician or a delegate of his physician of his continuing health care requirements following his discharge from the hospital.
14. Examine and receive an explanation of his bill regardless of source of payment.
15. Know which hospital rules and policies apply to his conduct as a patient.
16. Have all patients' rights apply to the person who may have legal responsibility to make decisions regarding medical care on behalf of the patient.

● **FIGURE 8-1** *List of patient rights in California.*

PREPARATION PROTOCOL: FOR ADMISSION AND ASSESSMENT

Complete the following steps before each skill.

1. Check client's chart to determine that assigned room placement is appropriate.
2. Check physician's orders. Ensure physician is notified of client's admission and room number.
3. Gather equipment and necessary linens.
4. Wash hands. Don gloves if needed.
5. Introduce yourself to client and explain what you will be doing during each step.
6. Ensure client is in a comfortable environment.

COMPLETION PROTOCOL: FOR ADMISSION AND ASSESSMENT

Make sure the following steps have been completed.

1. Remove gloves, if used.
2. Place client in comfortable position.
3. Clean equipment and return to appropriate location.
4. Wash hands.
5. After initial assessment is completed, report unusual findings to physician.
6. Ensure that all laboratory and diagnostic tests have been ordered.
7. Ensure that all physician orders have been transcribed.
8. Notify pharmacy of medication orders.
9. Initiate client's plan of care—either care plan or clinical pathway.

SECTION ONE

ADMISSION OF CLIENT

The nurse assigned to care for the client should meet the client as he or she reaches the nursing unit. It is at this time that the nurse must begin to assess the client's needs and begin the plan of care. It is also at this time that the nurse establishes the nurse-client relationship.

When you meet a client, introduce yourself and any other personnel who will provide care, including the unit secretary. Explain your role and functions to the client. Your initial contact leaves a lasting impression, so try to present information in an uninterrupted, organized, and friendly manner. If other clients are in the room, introduce them to the new client.

RATIONALE

- To assist client to adapt to hospital environment with minimal distress
- To encourage client to participate in his or her own plan of care
- To provide client with an opportunity to verbalize his or her feelings about hospitalization
- To explain environment and usual procedures associated with hospital

ASSESSMENT

- Observe client's physical and emotional status at admission.
- Observe client's ability to adapt to environment of facility.
- Assess client's level of understanding of what is happening to him or her.
- Determine client's plan of care.

ADMISSION

Equipment

- Admission kit for personal hygiene
- Thermometer
- Blood pressure cuff and stethoscope
- Urine container, if UA not collected earlier
- Kardex card, client care plan, or clinical pathway
- Client's chart

SKILL

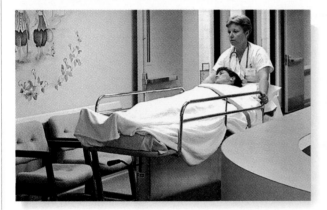

1 Client is admitted to nursing unit by gurney or wheelchair. If admitted by gurney, client is usually coming from emergency department and accompanied by a nurse.

- Introduce yourself to client and family as you take client to room.
- Introduce client and family to other staff members and clients in room.

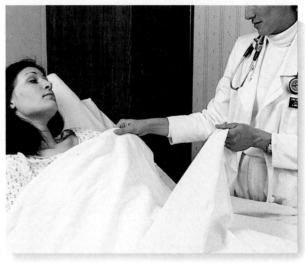

2 Place gown on client and assist him or her into bed. If appropriate, client can remain in a chair during initial orientation.

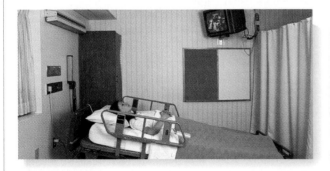

3 Explain equipment and hospital routines. Check that identaband information is correct and is placed on client's wrist. Place allergy band on wrist as needed.

- Determine if client needs additional information or has questions regarding hospitalization.

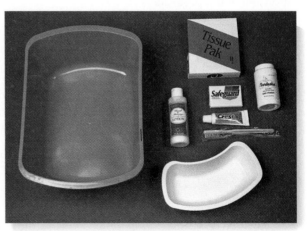

4 Place personal hygiene supplies in over-bed table drawer or nightstand.

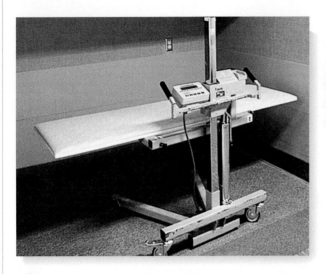

5 Obtain client's height and weight using bedside scale or standing scale.

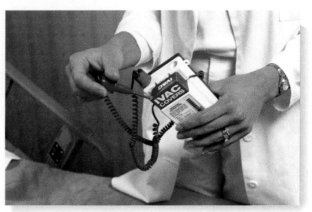

6 Take vital signs.

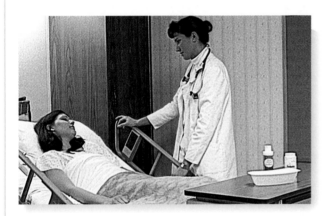

7 Obtain client's health history. **RATIONALE:** A complete health history provides total picture of client's condition and health problems.

CLINICAL NOTE

OBTAINING A NURSING HISTORY

- Past medical history or health problems, including those for which client was not hospitalized
- Signs and symptoms according to client's perceptions
- Assessment of health status (include lifestyle, habits)
- Diet and nutrition, hydration status, elimination, exercise, habits (i.e., smoking, drinking), sleep patterns, cognitive function
- Relationships and social support systems
- Values, beliefs, and religious or spiritual practices
- History of allergies, especially drugs and foods, and restrictions
- Medication history—use and allergies
- Risk factors for health—weight, smoking habit, age, general health, and so on
- Client's knowledge of illness (understanding of present illness) and expectations of care
- Risk analysis for discharge (ability to manage self-care at home)
- Special database for elderly client: level of independence, ability to complete activities of daily living (ADLs), toxic reactions or side effects of medications, history of recent loss of loved one, management of chronic conditions (arthritis, incontinence, etc.)

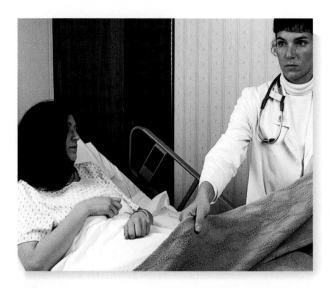

8 Complete bedside assessment. *Note:* A bedside assessment does not include a total physical assessment.

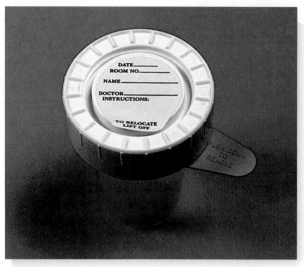

9 Obtain urine specimen, if not done earlier.

- Inform laboratory, ECG technician, and x-ray that client has been admitted. **RATIONALE:** Client needs to have admission laboratory specimens drawn, an ECG, and a chest film done for baseline data.

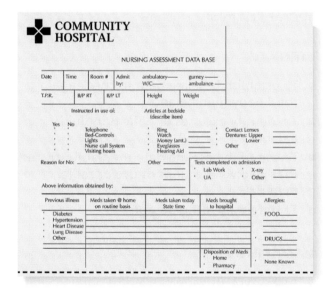

10 Document all findings on admission assessment data sheet.

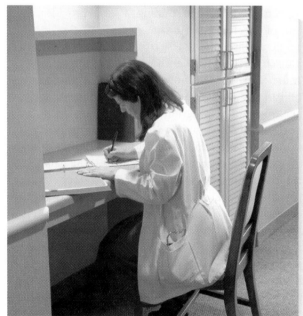

11 Begin client care plan or obtain appropriate clinical pathway and initiate plan of care.

- Notify physician that client has been admitted and obtain orders if not already on unit.

CHARTING

- Admission procedures
- Adaptation to hospital environment
- Admission assessment data including physical assessment, height, weight, and vital signs

- Laboratory specimens obtained
- Other diagnostic tests completed; ECG, chest x-ray

SECTION TWO

HEIGHT AND WEIGHT

In adult clients, the ratio of weight to height provides a general overview of health status. It is important to ask about the client's perception of his or her height and weight. This information provides a baseline for the usual finding versus the current finding. It also provides an indicator of the client's self-image.

Height and weight data is critical in the care of most hospitalized clients. A client's weight is necessary to determine appropriate amounts of anesthesia in some situations. Drug dosages are frequently calculated using the client's weight in kilograms. Some diagnostic studies require the client's weight in order to determine dosages of dye injection materials. Alteration in weight—either loss or gain—is a primary indicator of fluid balance, particularly in clients with cardiac or respiratory conditions. The nutritional status of clients, particularly long-term clients, can be evaluated using weight as a factor. It is important to remember that standardized weight and height charts should be used as guidelines only because each client is different.

There are several ways to measure height and weight, depending on the client's condition. The usual weight scale found in most hospitals has a built-in L-shaped height-measuring arm as well as the weight scale. A bedside scale is utilized for clients who are unable to stand. Many facilities also have a scale that allows wheelchair clients to be weighed in the chair. A movable bedside scale is most frequently used for daily weights. It is important to use the same scale and to weigh clients at the same time of the day, and with the same clothing on, especially if they have fluid balance problems.

RATIONALE

- To establish baseline data to check against total body fluid balance
- To identify excesses or deficits in fluid balance
- To establish baseline data for diagnostic tests that involve injections of dye or radioactive material
- To determine drug dosage

ASSESSMENT

- Assess type of scale needed to obtain client's height and weight.
- Determine need for daily weights.
- Evaluate necessity for weighing client at same time each day.

HEIGHT AND WEIGHT

Equipment

- Appropriate scale for client need
  - Portable bed scale
  - In-bed weight scale
- Balance beam scale
- Floor scale for wheelchair
- Paper towel (optional)

SKILL

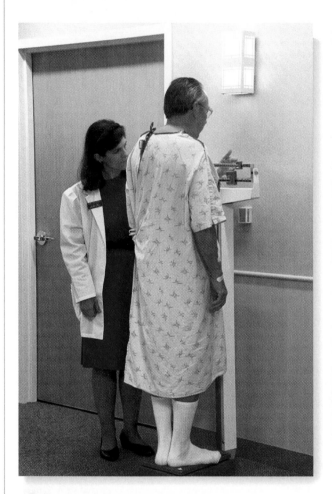

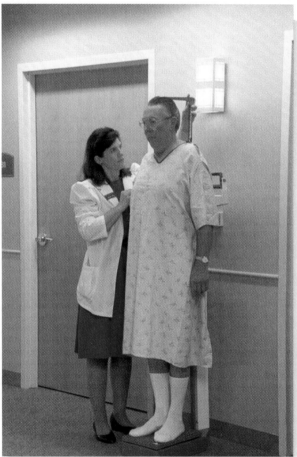

1 Transport client to scale.

- Balance scale before client steps on scale.
  RATIONALE: To ensure accuracy of weight reading.
- Place paper towel on scale or allow client to wear socks.
- Assist client to stand on scale.
- Move weights until weight bar is level or balanced.

2 Ask client to turn and place back of head toward balancing bar.

- Instruct client to stand erect. **RATIONALE:** To accurately measure height at top of head.
- Place L-shaped height bar on top of client's head.
- Document findings and return client to bed.
- Compare results with weight chart.

BEYOND THE SKILL

Alternate Methods for Weighing Clients

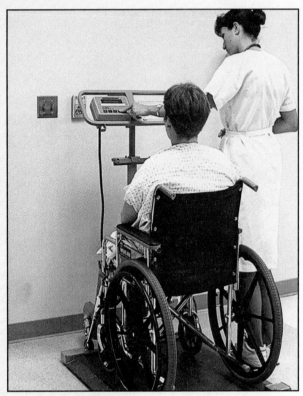

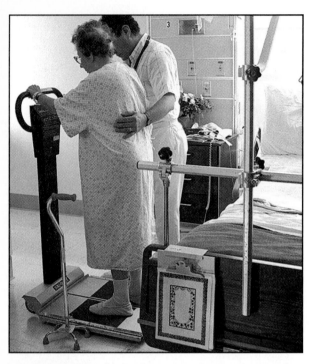

■ Wheelchair scales accommodate the needs of clients unable to stand to be weighed. A digital display panel reads the weight. Subtract the weight of the chair before recording the data.

■ Bedside portable scales are used most commonly in health care facilities for clients who can stand. On this particular scale, there is a digital readout.

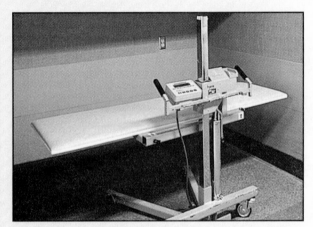

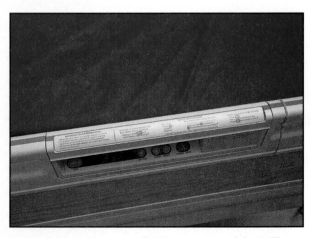

■ Bedside scales are used to weigh clients who are unable to stand. The scale is covered with a sheet, advanced to be placed snugly against the side of the client's bed, and positioned over the mattress. The client is then rolled and lifted onto the scale, and the weight is digitally recorded.

■ In-bed scales are available on many of the Hill-Rom beds. The client can be weighed at any time by just pressing a button on the panel at the end of the bed.

WOMEN Height Feet Inches	Small Frame Pounds	Medium Frame Pounds	Large Frame Pounds	MEN Height Feet Inches	Small Frame Pounds	Medium Frame Pounds	Large Frame Pounds
4 10	92–98	96–107	104–119	N/A	N/A	N/A	N/A
4 11	94–101	98–110	106–122	N/A	N/A	N/A	N/A
5 0	96–104	101–113	109–125	N/A	N/A	N/A	N/A
5 1	99–107	104–116	112–128	N/A	N/A	N/A	N/A
5 2	102–110	107–119	115–131	5 2	112–120	118–129	124–141
5 3	105–113	110–122	118–134	5 3	115–123	121–133	129–144
5 4	108–116	113–126	121–138	5 4	118–126	124–136	132–148
5 5	111–119	116–130	125–142	5 5	121–129	127–139	135–142
5 6	114–123	120–135	129–146	5 6	124–133	130–143	138–156
5 7	118–127	124–139	133–150	5 7	128–137	134–147	142–161
5 8	122–131	128–143	137–154	5 8	132–141	138–152	147–162
5 9	126–135	132–147	141–158	5 9	136–145	142–156	151–170
5 10	130–140	136–151	145–163	5 10	140–150	146–160	155–174
5 11	134–144	140–155	149–168	5 11	144–154	150–165	159–179
6 0	138–148	144–159	153–173	6 0	148–158	154–170	164–184
6 1	N/A	N/A	N/A	6 1	152–162	158–175	168–189
6 2	N/A	N/A	N/A	6 2	156–167	162–180	173–194
6 3	N/A	N/A	N/A	6 3	160–171	167–185	178–199
6 4	N/A	N/A	N/A	6 4	164–175	172–190	182–204

Source: Blue Cross/Blue Shield of Delaware, 1997; American Heart Association.

Height is in feet and inches, including shoes. **Weight** is in pounds, including indoor clothing. Assumption: Male indoor clothing with shoes weighed seven pounds. Female clothing with shoes weighed four pounds.

For girls between 18 and 25, subtract 1 pound for each year under 25.

CHARTING

- Height and weight (document on graphic sheet)
- Specific scale used for weight (place on chart or Kardex)
- Exact time of day client was weighed
- Clothing client was wearing when weighed

SECTION THREE

ADMISSION ASSESSMENT

The admission assessment includes two skills: obtaining the health history and performing a physical examination. When obtaining the health history, you should note such characteristics as hair, skin, posture, facial expression, and body language—in other words, the general appearance of the client. Use open-ended questions such as "tell me about . . ."; collect data about past health conditions, current problems, and present needs.

The information is obtained through objective (observed) and subjective (stated by the client) data collection.

Information obtained from the interview and the physical assessment constitutes the basis for identifying nursing diagnoses and establishing the individualized client plan of care. The nurse's role in assessing the client and obtaining a health history has expanded dramatically over the last 40 years. Today nurses must be adequately instructed to perform a total assessment, including the use of instruments—formerly the domain of physicians only. The skill of performing a physical assessment must be practiced repeatedly to acquire expertise.

The stethoscope is the primary instrument used for assessment. The diaphragm piece should be applied firmly to the skin. It enhances high-pitched sounds (breath sounds, normal heart sounds, bowel sounds). The bell piece should be placed very lightly to pick up low-pitched sounds, such as vascular sounds and abnormal heart sounds. If the bell is pressed firmly, it stretches the skin and acts as a diaphragm. Any movement of the tubing or chest piece by clothing or hands can cause extraneous noise that obliterates the sounds you want to hear.

An organized approach to the bedside physical examination is necessary so that important areas are not missed. Two methods of organization are the head-to-toe approach and the review-of-systems approach. A combination of the two approaches is often used and will be described in this chapter. Integration of the two methods increases the efficiency of the examination, thus saving time and also reducing client fatigue. For example, when examining the bedridden client, parts of the assessment can be combined to minimize the need for client repositioning. When the client is turned to the side for inspection of the skin of the buttocks and sacrum, the posterior lung fields can be assessed at the same time.

RATIONALE

- To gather objective and subjective data through examination and focused interview questions
- To identify relevant client problems
- To alert physician to any potential or developing problems
- To obtain baseline data so changes in client's condition can be identified throughout hospitalization

ASSESSMENT

- Assess all body systems in organized manner to prevent omission of critical information.
- Obtain complete health history that, in conjunction with assessment, provides data to determine client's nursing diagnosis and plan of care.
- Gather objective and subjective information during examination of each body system.
- Perform physical assessment using the four examination techniques correctly.

CLINICAL NOTE

HEALTH HISTORY
A complete health history includes the following elements:

- **Biographic information:** age, sex, educational level, marital status, living arrangements
- **Chief complaint:** condition that brought client to health care facility
- **Present health status or illness:** onset of problem; clinical manifestations, including severity of symptoms; pain characteristics if present
- **Health history:** general state of health, past illnesses, surgeries, hospitalizations, allergies, current medications, and general habits such as smoking
- **Family history:** age and health status of parents, siblings, and children; cause of death for immediate family members
- **Psychosocial factors, lifestyles:** cultural beliefs that influence health management; religious or spiritual beliefs
- **Nutrition:** dietary habits, preferences, or restrictions

EXAMINATION TECHNIQUES

Equipment

- Stethoscope

SKILL

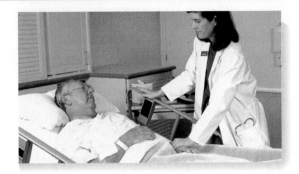

1 **Inspection:** Examine client's skin color and texture; check for lesions and hair distribution. Observe client while facing him or her in bed or chair.

- Look at overall body structure; observe gait and stance. Note all parts of body as examination proceeds. Inspection also evaluates verbal and behavioral responses and mental status.

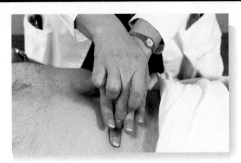

2 **Percussion:** Produces sound waves by using fingers as a hammer. Place interphalangeal joint of middle finger (place only this finger on skin surface) of nondominant hand on skin surface, and, using tip of middle finger of dominant hand, strike placed finger.

- Vibration is produced by impact of fingers striking against underlying tissue. Sound or tone of vibration is determined by body area or organ percussed. Normal lung areas produce resonant sound; liver sounds are dull; and flat sound is heard over muscle.

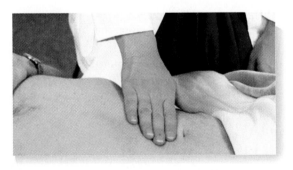

3 **Palpation:** Obtain information by using hands and fingers to palpate. Whether palpation is light or deep depends on area of abdomen being palpated.

- The palmar surface of fingers and finger pads is used to determine position, size, and consistency of organs, and presence of fluid accumulation or masses.
- The ulnar surface of the hand is used to distinguish vibration. Moisture and warmth of skin can also be determined during palpation.

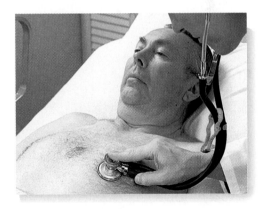

4 **Auscultation:** Place stethoscope on client's bare skin to listen for presence and characteristics of sound waves. Bell of stethoscope is used to detect low-pitched sounds; diaphragm detects high-pitched sounds.

- Note variations in intensity, pitch, duration, and quality of sounds.

ASSESSMENT

Equipment

- Stethoscope
- Penlight

SKILL

TABLE 8-1	ADMISSION ASSESSMENT

System	Objective Examination: Inspection, Auscultation, Palpation, and Percussion	Subjective Examination: Questions to Ask the Client
General appearance	<ul><li>Age-appropriate development</li><li>Interaction/cooperation with examiner</li><li>Grooming and hygiene</li><li>General nutritional appearance</li><li>Mood</li><li>Distress</li></ul>	<ul><li>How is your general health?</li><li>Have you had any significant health problems?</li><li>Why are you being seen today?</li></ul>
Neurological	<ul><li>Level of consciousness</li><li>Awareness of time, place, person, and situation</li><li>Verbal responses</li><li>Equality of movement and strength of extremities</li><li>Signs of discomfort or pain</li><li>Ability to follow commands</li><li>Long-term and short-term memory</li></ul>	Tell me<ul><li>Your name</li><li>Where you are</li><li>The date</li><li>Why you are here</li></ul>Assess client<ul><li>Use pain scale to rate pain</li><li>Have client describe and/or point to painful area</li><li>Ask about vision changes (blurring, etc.)</li><li>Ask about use of hearing aid</li></ul>
Integumentary (includes mucous membranes)	<ul><li>Temperature</li><li>Color</li><li>Moisture</li><li>Turgor</li><li>Lesions (include pressure ulcers)</li><li>Bruising</li><li>Oral mucous membranes (moisture, color, lesions)</li><li>Tongue (fissures, moisture, overgrowth)</li><li>Hair distribution</li><li>Nails</li><li>Dressings/wounds</li><li>Invasive insertion sites (IVs, tubes)</li></ul>	Do you have any<ul><li>Itching?</li><li>Burning?</li><li>Pain?</li><li>Drainage?</li><li>Lumps?</li><li>Rashes?</li></ul>

TABLE 8-1	ADMISSION ASSESSMENT

System	Objective Examination: Inspection, Auscultation, Palpation, and Percussion	Subjective Examination: Questions to Ask the Client
Cardiovascular	■ Pulse rate, rhythm, quality ■ Blood pressure ■ Neck vein distention ■ Heart sounds ■ Peripheral pulses ■ Capillary refill ■ Ankle edema ■ Activity tolerance ■ Leg discomfort with activity *Note:* Use approved rating scales for pain and edema	Do you have ■ Chest discomfort, pressure, or pain? ■ Palpitations? ■ Shortness of breath? ■ Dizziness or lightheadedness? Ask ■ When do symptoms occur? ■ How long has problem been occurring? ■ Location, duration, radiation ■ Does anything make it better/worse?
Respiratory	■ Breath sounds ■ Rate ■ Rhythm ■ Depth ■ Effort ■ Subcutaneous emphysema ■ Presence of supplemental oxygen ■ Assess correct use of incentive spirometer or coughing and deep breathing technique	■ Are you now, or do you ever feel, short of breath? ■ Do you have a cough? ■ Do you bring up any phlegm or sputum? ■ What is the amount, color, consistency, odor? ■ Are there any positions that are more/less comfortable for your breathing? ■ How many pillows do you use to sleep? ■ Smoking history
Gastrointestinal	■ Abdominal size, shape, contour ■ Skin appearance (veins, bruising) ■ Bowel sounds ■ Soft, firm, tender ■ Swallowing difficulty ■ Dentition ■ Nausea ■ Appearance of stool ■ Dressings ■ Drains and tubes (input, output, color, amount? ■ Colostomy or ileostomy site and output	■ How is your appetite? ■ Do you have any difficulty swallowing? ■ Do you ever choke? ■ Do you have any nausea? ■ What is your regular bowel movement pattern? Has there been a change? ■ Are you having any constipation or diarrhea? ■ What type of laxative do you use and how frequently? ■ Is there ever blood in your stool? ■ Have you vomited recently? ■ What was the color, consistency, amount) ■ Does your abdomen look like it usually does?

TABLE 8-1	ADMISSION ASSESSMENT (CONT'D)	

System	Objective Examination: Inspection, Auscultation, Palpation, and Percussion	Subjective Examination: Questions to Ask the Client
Gastrointestinal (con't.)	■ Incontinence of stool	■ Are you passing gas? ■ Recent weight gain/loss? ■ Are there any foods that you can't eat? Why?
Urinary	■ Urinary output amount ■ Clarity, color, odor, sediment ■ Bladder distention ■ Catheter site (meatus or urostomy) ■ Incontinence of urine	Do you ever have ■ Urgency, frequency, burning, hesitation? ■ Incomplete emptying? ■ Difficulty starting urine flow? ■ Blood in the urine? ■ Pain in lower abdomen (suprapubic area) or flanks? ■ How many times do you get up at night to urinate? ■ Do you ever have trouble getting to the bathroom in time?
Musculoskeletal	■ Limb range of motion, strength, and equality ■ Atrophy of any muscle mass ■ Posture (include significant scoliosis, kyphosis, or lordosis) ■ Transfer ability and gait stability ■ Ability to position and reposition self in bed ■ Correct use of mobility aids	Do you have ■ Joint stiffness? ■ Pain in any limb? ■ Cramps or spasms? ■ Problems getting out of chairs, up stairs, etc.? ■ Do you use a cane, walker, etc.?
Reproductive	Female ■ Menses regularity, duration, pain ■ Vaginal discharge ■ Breast exam (lumps, thickening, discharge, pain) ■ Frequency of Pap exams ■ Obstetrical history Male ■ Penile discharge ■ Impotence ■ Testicular exam ■ History of prostate problems	Female ■ Are your menses (periods) regular? ■ How long do they last? ■ Are they painful? ■ How many pads/tampons do you typically use? ■ Review sexual history (if appropriate) ■ Do you do breast self-exam? Male ■ Testicular pain ■ Do you do testicular self exam?

TABLE 8-2	GENERAL APPEARANCE ASSESSMENT	
System	**Objective Examination:** **Inspection, Auscultation, Palpation,** **and Percussion**	**Subjective Examination:** **Questions to Ask the Client**
General appearance	■ Age-appropriate development ■ Interaction/cooperation with examiner ■ Grooming and hygiene ■ General nutritional appearance ■ Mood ■ Distress	■ How is your general health? ■ Have you had any significant health problems? ■ Why are you being seen today?

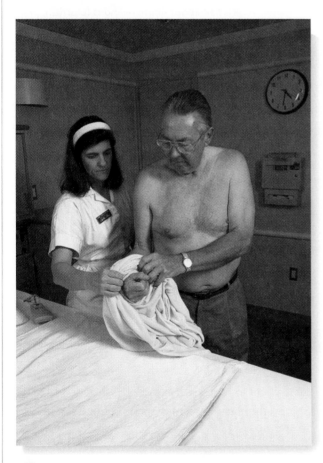

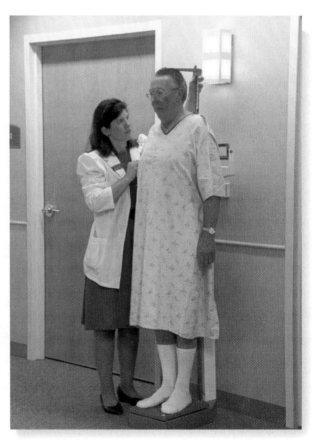

1 Assess client for general appearance as he or she is admitted to nursing unit.

2 Obtain vital signs.

■ Measure height and weight.

■ Age-appropriate development
■ Interaction and cooperation with examiner
■ Grooming and hygiene
■ General nutritional appearance
■ Mood
■ Distress

TABLE 8-3	NEUROLOGICAL ASSESSMENT	
System	**Objective Examination:** Inspection, Auscultation, Palpation, and Percussion	**Subjective Examination:** Questions to Ask the Client
Neurological	■ Level of consciousness ■ Awareness of time, place, person, and situation ■ Verbal responses ■ Equality of movement and strength of extremities ■ Signs of discomfort or pain ■ Ability to follow commands ■ Long-term and short-term memory	Tell me ■ Your name ■ Where you are ■ The date ■ Why you are here Assess client ■ Use pain scale to rate pain ■ Have client describe and/or point to painful area ■ Ask about vision changes (blurring, etc.) ■ Ask about use of hearing aid

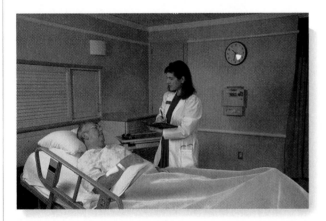

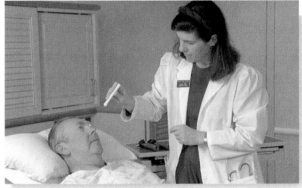

3 Assess level of consciousness: ask pertinent questions during physical assessment to gather subjective data from client.

■ Assess for motor response (decorticate or decerebrate posturing).

4 Darken room slightly to better observe pupillary reaction to light.

■ Have client look straight ahead.
■ Shine light in each eye, moving from side of head to eye.

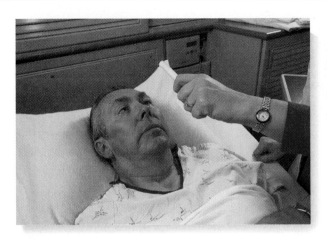

5 Observe each pupil for shape, equality of size, equality of reaction, and accommodation.

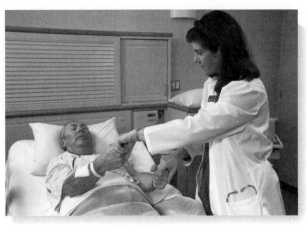

6 Assess hand grasp for strength and equality.

- This also allows assessment of ability to follow commands.

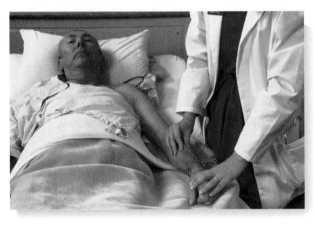

7 Assess skin turgor on forearm. Alternate site is over sternum. Skin with normal turgor should rapidly return to its original shape.

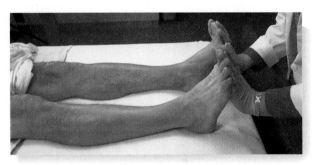

8 Assess bilateral plantarflexion as indicator of lower extremity strength.

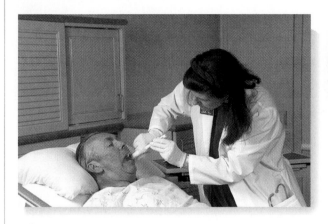

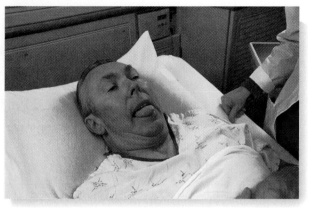

⑨ Inspect oral mucosa and dentition.

⑩ Inspect tongue for fissures, moisture, overgrowth, and symmetry.

TABLE 8-4	INTEGUMENTARY ASSESSMENT	
System	**Objective Examination:** **Inspection, Auscultation, Palpation,** **and Percussion**	**Subjective Examination:** **Questions to Ask the Client**
Integumentary (includes mucous membranes)	■ Temperature ■ Color ■ Moisture ■ Turgor ■ Lesions (include pressure ulcers) ■ Bruising ■ Oral mucous membranes (moisture, color, lesions) ■ Tongue (fissures, moisture, overgrowth) ■ Hair distribution ■ Nails ■ Dressings/wounds ■ Invasive insertion sites (IVs, tubes)	Do you have any ■ Itching? ■ Burning? ■ Pain? ■ Drainage? ■ Lumps? ■ Rashes?

TABLE 8-5	CARDIOVASCULAR ASSESSMENT	
System	**Objective Examination: Inspection, Auscultation, Palpation, and Percussion**	**Subjective Examination: Questions to Ask the Client**
Cardiovascular	■ Pulse rate, rhythm, quality ■ Blood pressure ■ Neck vein distention ■ Heart sounds ■ Peripheral pulses ■ Capillary refill ■ Ankle edema ■ Activity tolerance ■ Leg discomfort with activity	Do you have ■ Chest discomfort, pressure, or pain? ■ Palpitations? ■ Shortness of breath? ■ Dizziness or lightheadedness? Ask ■ When do symptoms occur? ■ How long has problem been occurring? ■ Location, duration, radiation ■ Does anything make it better/worse? *Note:* Use approved rating scales for pain and edema

CLINICAL NOTE

Use the diaphragm of the stethoscope for high-pitched sounds and the bell for lower-pitched sounds.

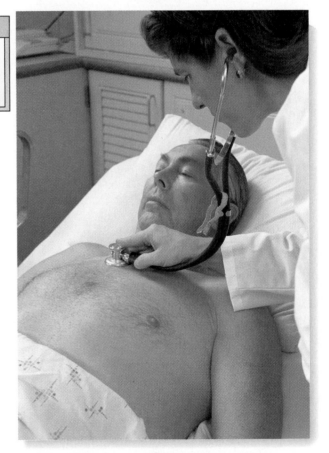

11 Auscultate heart sounds in organized manner.

■ Aortic sound (2nd intercostal space, right sternal border).

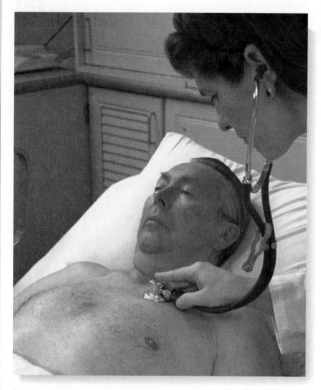

- Pulmonic sound (2nd intercostal space, left sternal border).

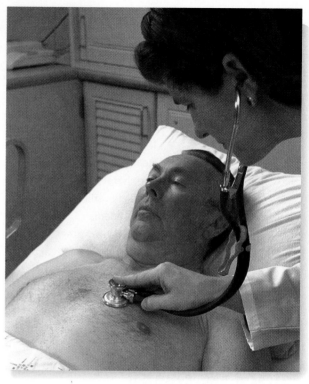

- Tricuspid sound (4th intercostal space, left sternal border)

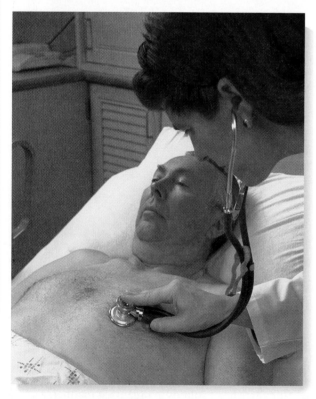

- Mitral sound (5th intercostal space, left midclavicular line).

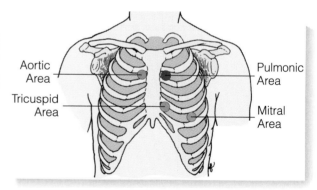

● **FIGURE 8-2** *Place stethoscope correctly to auscultate heart sounds.*

CLINICAL NOTE

Use an approved scale when palpating peripheral pulses for strength and equality, for example:

0	absent
1+	thready/weak
2+	normal
3+	bounding

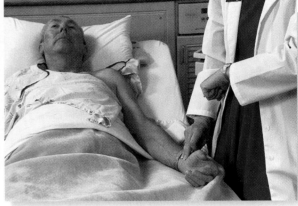

12 Palpate peripheral pulses.

■ Radial pulse

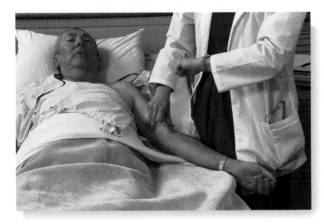

■ Brachial pulse

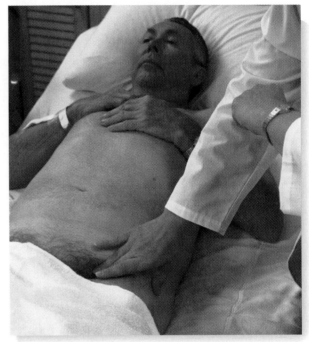

■ Femoral pulse

■ Dorsalis pedis pulse

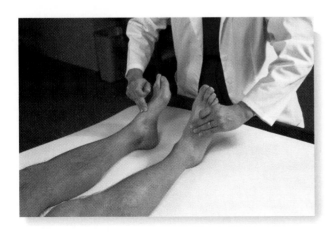

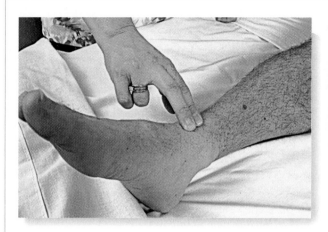

13 Assess for peripheral edema.

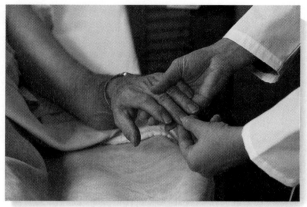

14 Assess fingernail bed for capillary refill time.

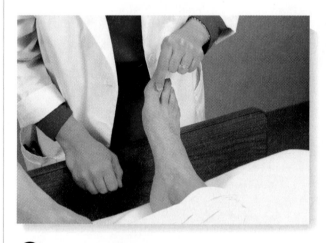

15 Assess toenail bed capillary refill time (normal is within 2 to 3 sec).

CLINICAL NOTE

Assess for edema using an approved scale, for example:

+0	no pitting
+1	0 to ¼ in pitting (mild)
+2	¼ to ½ in pitting (moderate)
+3	½ to 1 in pitting (severe)
+4	greater than 1 in pitting (severe)

TABLE 8-6	RESPIRATORY ASSESSMENT	

System	Objective Examination: Inspection, Auscultation, Palpation, and Percussion	Subjective Examination: Questions to Ask the Client
Respiratory	■ Breath sounds ■ Rate ■ Rhythm ■ Depth ■ Effort ■ Subcutaneous emphysema ■ Presence of supplemental oxygen ■ Assess correct use of incentive spiro- meter or coughing and deep breathing technique	■ Are you now, or do you ever feel, short of breath? ■ Do you have a cough? ■ Do you bring up any phlegm or sputum? ■ What is the amount, color, consistency, odor? ■ Are there any positions that are more/less com- fortable for your breathing? ■ How many pillows do you use to sleep? ■ Smoking history

CLINICAL NOTE

Auscultate the lungs:

- ■ Proceed in organized manner.
- ■ Complete anterior examination, then proceed to posterior fields.
- ■ Progress from upper to lower and lateral fields.
- ■ Compare sides.
- ■ Avoid placing stethoscope over bony areas.
- ■ Have client breathe through mouth.
- ■ Listen through entire inspiratory and expiratory phase.
- ■ Move stethoscope to next location just before client takes next inhalation.
- ■ Client should sit as upright as possible for maximum lung expansion.

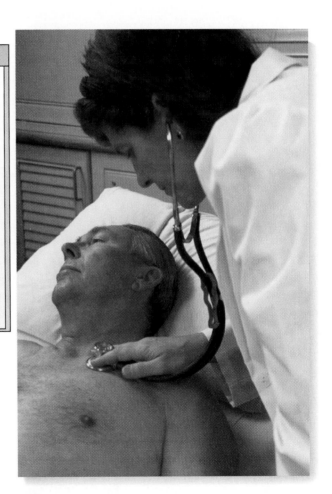

16 Auscultate lung sounds.

■ Complete anterior examination, then proceed to posterior fields.

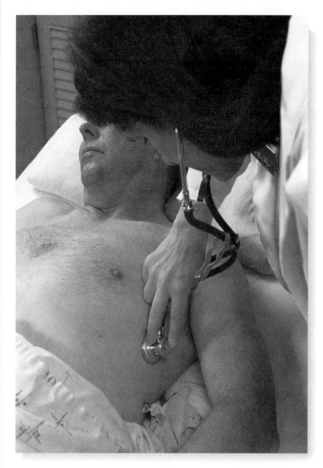

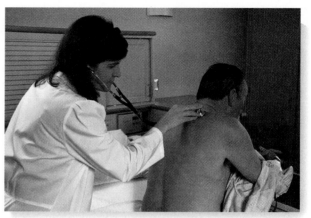

- Avoid placing stethoscope over bony areas.

- Progress from upper to lower and lateral fields.

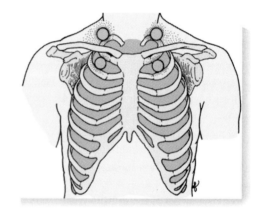

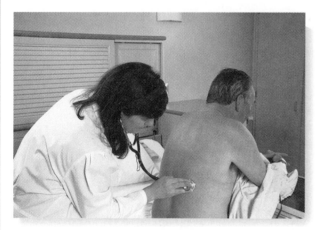

- Ascultate posterior lung fields from upper to lower lobes, moving stethoscope gradually down the back.
- Compare breath sounds on each side.

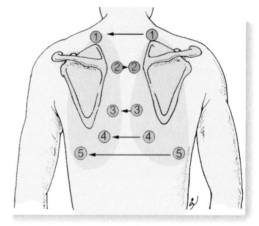

● **FIGURE 8-3** *Place stethoscope at correct sites to auscultate breath sounds.*

CLINICAL NOTE

In each lung field, check for the following adventitious lung sounds. (Remember that inspiration should be twice as long as expiration.)

Sound	Characteristics	Lung Condition
Crackles	Popping, crackling, bubbling moist sounds on inspiration	Pneumonia, pulmonary edema
Rhonchi	Rumbling sounds on expiration	Pneumonia, emphysema, bronchitis
Wheezes	High-pitched musical sounds during both inspiration and expiration (louder)	Emphysema, asthma, foreign body

TABLE 8-7	GASTROINTESTINAL ASSESSMENT

System	Objective Examination: Inspection, Auscultation, Palpation, and Percussion	Subjective Examination: Questions to Ask the Client
Gastrointestinal	■ Abdominal size, shape, contour ■ Skin appearance (veins, bruising) ■ Bowel sounds ■ Soft, firm, tender ■ Swallowing difficulty ■ Dentition ■ Nausea ■ Appearance of stool ■ Dressings ■ Drains and tubes (input, output, color, amount) ■ Colostomy or ileostomy site and output ■ Incontinence of stool	■ How is your appetite? ■ Do you have any difficulty swallowing? ■ Do you ever choke? ■ Do you have any nausea? ■ What is your regular bowel movement pattern? Has there been a change? ■ Are you having any constipation or diarrhea? ■ What type of laxative do you use and how frequently? ■ Is there ever blood in your stool? ■ Have you vomited recently? ■ What was the color, consistency, amount? ■ Does your abdomen look like it usually does? ■ Are you passing gas? ■ Recent weight gain/loss? ■ Are there any foods that you can't eat? Why?

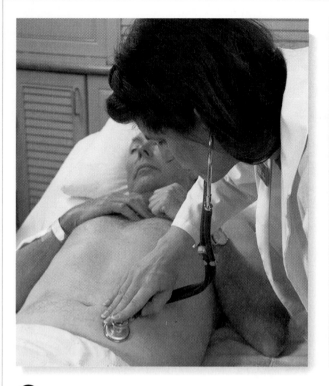

17 Auscultate all four quadrants of abdomen to determine presence of bowel sounds.

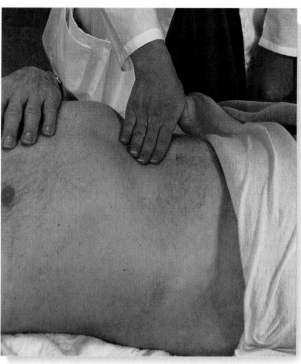

18 Lightly palpate abdomen to assess for firmness.

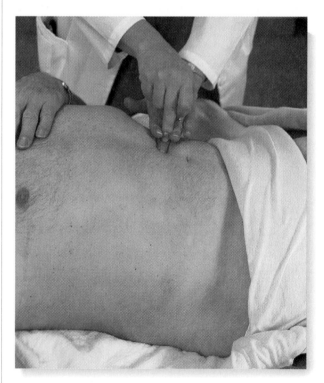

19 Percuss abdomen to assess for normal tympany.

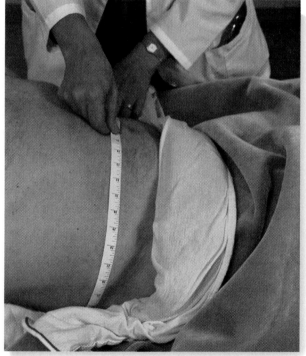

20 Measure abdominal girth at largest diameter.

■ Mark abdomen in exact location for consistent measurements.

	TABLE 8-8	**URINARY ASSESSMENT**

System	**Objective Examination:** **Inspection, Auscultation, Palpation,** **and Percussion**	**Subjective Examination:** **Questions to Ask the Client**
Urinary	■ Urinary output amount ■ Clarity, color, odor, sediment ■ Bladder distention ■ Catheter site (meatus or urostomy) ■ Incontinence of urine	Do you ever have ■ Urgency, frequency, burning, hesitation? ■ Incomplete emptying? ■ Difficulty starting your flow? ■ Blood in the urine? ■ Pain in lower abdomen (suprapubic area) or flanks? ■ How many times do you get up at night to urinate? ■ Do you ever have trouble getting to the bathroom in time?

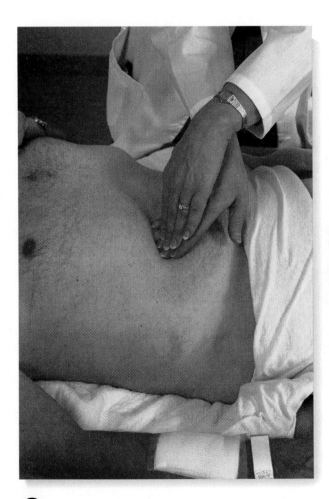

21 Palpate bladder to check for distention.

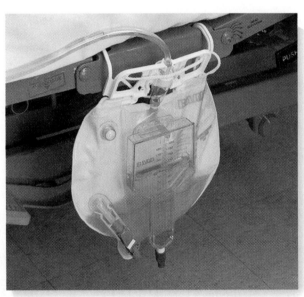

22 Inspect all urinary output (voided or catheter) for amount, clarity, color, odor, or sediment.

TABLE 8-9	MUSCULOSKELETAL ASSESSMENT	
System	**Objective Examination: Inspection, Auscultation, Palpation, and Percussion**	**Subjective Examination: Questions to Ask the Client**
Musculoskeletal	■ Limb range of motion, strength, and equality ■ Atrophy of any muscle mass ■ Posture (include significant scoliosis, kyphosis, or lordosis) ■ Transfer ability and gait stability ■ Ability to position and reposition self in bed ■ Correct use of mobility aids	Do you have ■ Joint stiffness? ■ Pain in any limb? ■ Cramps or spasms? ■ Problems getting out of chairs, up stairs, etc.? ■ Do you use a cane, walker, etc.?

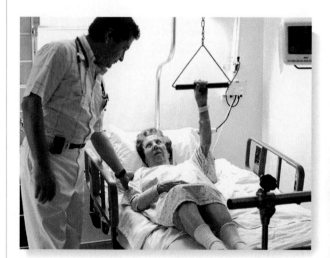

23 Assess range of motion and client's ability to reposition self in bed.

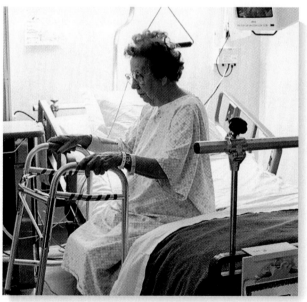

24 Assess safe and correct use of mobility aids such as walkers.

TABLE 8-10	REPRODUCTIVE ASSESSMENT

System	Objective Examination: Inspection, Auscultation, Palpation, and Percussion	Subjective Examination: Questions to Ask the Client
Reproductive	**Female** ■ Menses regularity, duration, pain ■ Vaginal discharge ■ Breast exam (lumps, thickening, discharge, pain) ■ Frequency of Pap exams ■ Obstetrical history **Male** ■ Penile discharge ■ Impotence ■ Testicular exam ■ History of prostate problems	**Female** ■ Are your menses (periods) regular? ■ How long do they last? ■ Are they painful? ■ How many pads/tampons do you typically use? ■ Review sexual history (if appropriate) ■ Do you do breast self-exam? **Male** ■ Testicular pain? ■ Do you do testicular self-exam? ■ Review sexual history (if appropriate)

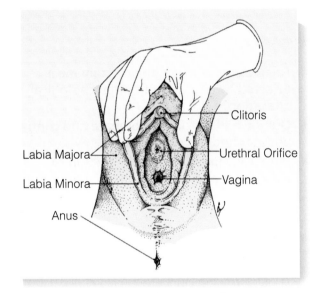

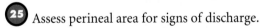

25 Assess perineal area for signs of discharge.

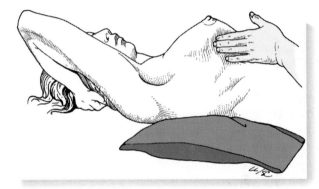

26 Breast examination may be done in some facilities.

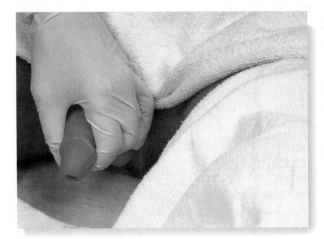

27 Check penis for discharge.

■ Check scrotum for alterations in testicles.

CHARTING

- All abnormal assessment data charted in nurses's notes
- System findings that are normal in physical assessment flow sheet
- Interventions done for abnormal physical assessment findings
- Documentation of notification of findings to physician

SECTION FOUR

FOCUS ASSESSMENT

The admission assessment is completed within 1 to 2 hrs of admission to the health care facility. A focus assessment is one that is performed at the beginning and ending of the shift. The focus assessment concentrates on the vital assessment parameters for each client and tracks the changes from shift to shift. It should take no more than 5 min to complete. Several activities in the assessment can be completed at the same time. Usually, it is individualized to fit the client's condition, diagnosis, and level of acuity. More attention is given to the system(s) associated with the client's condition. For example, if the client has a cardiovascular condition, a more in-depth heart, lung, and peripheral vascular assessment is completed. When an alteration in client status or condition occurs, it may necessitate a complete assessment.

As the assessment is performed, observe all dressings and drainage tubes. Check all IV sites as well as bag number, amount, type, and rate of IV solution infusing.

RATIONALE

- To determine client's physical or psychological changes within shift
- To make timely changes in client's plan of care based on assessment changes
- To identify potential complications in a timely manner
- To compare and contrast physical and psychological changes from admission assessment findings

ASSESSMENT

- Focus assessment on body system most affected by disease state or psychological alteration.
- Quickly and efficiently compare and contrast physical findings within shift.
- Effectively monitor client's reaction to treatments and medications.

CLINICAL NOTE

The frequency with which a physical examination is performed depends on:

- The severity of the client's condition
- Agency policy
- State laws and regulations
- Changes in the client's condition
- The examiner's scope of practice and/or job description

Equipment

- Stethoscope
- Penlight

SKILL

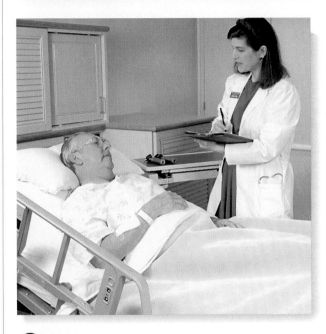

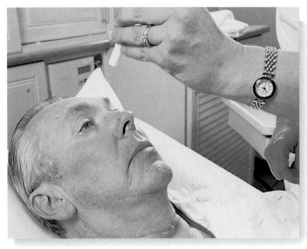

1 As you enter room, evaluate client's position in bed, level of consciousness, eye contact and responsiveness, color and texture of skin, and any IVs, dressings, or tubes. Ask appropriate questions to determine orientation to time and place.

- Establish nurse-client relationship at this time.

2 After these routine assessment areas, individualize the assessment and pay close attention to assessment findings based on body system involved in the disease process. For example, if the client has a neurological condition, check pupils for equality, size, and reaction to light. If the client has a respiratory condition, check nailbeds for presence of cyanosis or clubbing.

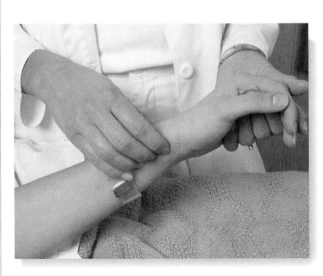

3 Assess vital signs. While taking pulse, feel skin temperature and moisture. Check bilateral radial pulses. Observe for edema in face or neck.

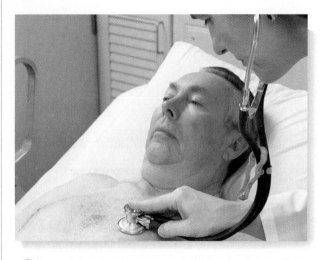

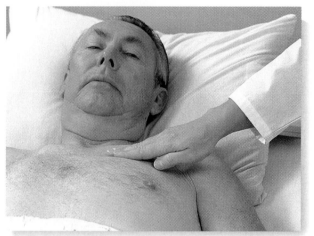

4 Remove client's gown. Use stethoscope to listen to heart sounds, apical pulse, and breath sounds bilaterally. If cardiac or respiratory system is involved, a more in-depth evaluation needs to be done, such as monitoring all four heart sounds, heart murmurs, apical-radial pulse, or abnormal breath sounds.

5 Observe breathing patterns, symmetry of chest movement, and depth of respirations.
- Observe shape of chest.
- Check for skin turgor by pinching fold of skin and noting how quickly it returns to original position.

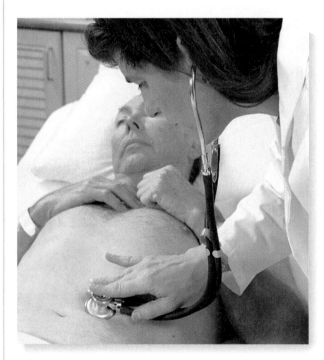

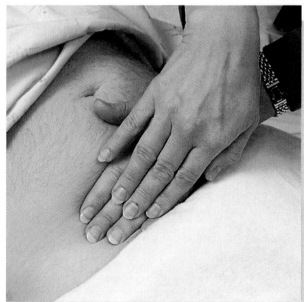

6 Auscultate abdomen for bowel sounds. All four quadrants will be auscultated and palpation and percussion techniques will be used only if appropriate to diagnosis.

7 Palpate bladder if necessary (based on urine output). If catheter is in place, observe urinary output for color, odor, consistency and amount.
- Observe urinary meatus for signs of exudate.
- Ask client about bowel movement.

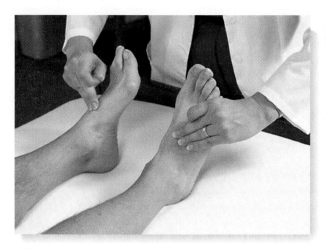

8 Assess lower extremities for warmth, color, moisture, presence of pedal or popliteal pulses, muscle tone, and sensation. Assess for pedal edema or general edema in lower extremities.

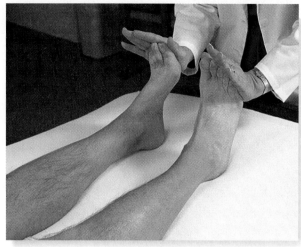

9 Check for a positive Homan's sign for high-risk clients.

- Check traction or casted areas for alignment, placement, and skin breakdown.

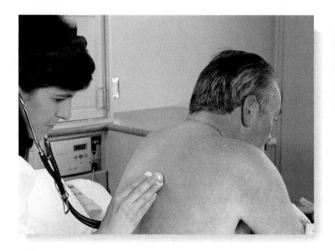

10 Turn client onto side or have client sit at side of bed. Assess posterior lung fields and check for symmetry of chest movement with inspiration.

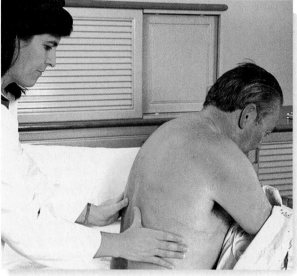

11 Assess skin for pressure areas, particularly at coccyx and heels. When client returns to side-lying position, complete skin assessment, especially at heels.

- Evaluate client's ability to move in bed and ambulate, if appropriate.

CHARTING

- Assessment findings (document on assessment flow sheet)
- Abnormal findings and interventions provided (chart in nurses' notes)

- Changes in client's condition since previous assessment

CRITICAL THINKING FOCUS

SECTION ONE ▪ Admission of Client

Unexpected Outcomes

- Client is unable to adapt to hospital environment.

- Client refuses to have laboratory or diagnostic work done.

Alternative Nursing Actions

- Assess physiological and emotional basis for maladaptation. Request consultation with nurse manager, client advocate, physician.

- Explain that tests are necessary to determine condition and treatment plan.
- Discuss reason for refusal. Client may be afraid of tests. Explanation of purpose for tests will be required.

SECTION TWO ▪ Obtain Height and Weight

Unexpected Outcomes

- Weight varies excessively from one day to the next.

- Client is too critically ill to be weighed accurately because of mechanical devices used to sustain life.

Alternative Nursing Actions

- Check if same scale was used for both weights.
- Check what clothing or linen was on client when he or she was weighed on both days.
- Check that scale was balanced appropriately.
- Reweigh client to determine if an error was made in weight.

- If in-bed scale is not available, estimate weight loss or gain by assessing other factors such as changes in skin turgor, output, or presence of edema.
- Weigh client on bed scale and note equipment in place when weighed.
- Weigh client each day with same equipment to provide good estimate of weight changes.

SECTION THREE ▪ Admission Assessment

Unexpected Outcomes

- Assessment findings are different from earlier findings.

- Client refuses assessment.

Alternative Nursing Actions

- Recheck assessment data. If it is the same, note change in nurses' notes or assessment flow sheet.
- Ask another nurse to verify your findings.
- Ask client if he or she has experienced any physical or emotional changes since last assessment.
- Notify physician if changes are critical and intervention needs to be done.

- Explain rationale for assessment.
- Have client explain reason for refusal.
- If client continues to refuse assessment, note refusal on chart and indicate those findings that can be observed.

SECTION FOUR ▪ Focus Assessment

Unexpected Outcomes	Alternative Nursing Actions
▪ Client condition has changed since earlier focus assessment.	▪ Complete more in-depth assessment to determine all changes in client condition. ▪ Document all changes clearly on assessment flow sheet or nurses' notes. ▪ Notify physician if change is critical or intervention must be done.
▪ Client becomes anxious when more complete assessment is done.	▪ Explain to client that you just want to check every system very thoroughly. ▪ Reassure client that it is necessary to complete entire assessment if there is a change in findings, even if it is a positive change. ▪ Do not discuss an abnormal finding with client until you have discussed it with physician.

SELF-CHECK EVALUATION

PART 1 ▪ Matching Terms

Match the definition found in column B with the correct term in column A.

	Column A	Column B
_____	a. Admission	1. Information, both subjective and objective, gathered on admission
_____	b. Client plan of care	2. Comprehensive physical assessment completed by RN
_____	c. Identaband	3. Process of signing client into health care facility
_____	d. Baseline data	4. Assessment that monitors changes in affected body systems
_____	e. Admission assessment	5. Plan of care for a specific client based on client needs and problems.
_____	f. Focus assessment	6. Biographical client data found on a bracelet

PART 2 ▪ Multiple Choice Questions

1. All of the following information is provided to the client on admission to the nursing unit except:

a. Telephone.
b. Bed controls.
c. Tests that will be performed.
d. Meal times.

2. The Client's Bill of Rights contains all of the following information except the right to:
   a. Refuse treatment.
   b. Participate in one's own care.
   c. Have visitors at any time.
   d. Receive courteous care.

3. The rationale for using the same scale each time you weigh a client is:
   a. The client becomes familiar with one particular method.
   b. You know that the scale is balanced correctly.
   c. The same scale gives consistency in weight from day to day.
   d. The physician orders a particular scale and the nurse must follow orders.

4. A client's weight has increased by 5 lb since yesterday. All of the following interventions should be implemented except:
   a. Check client's I&O record.
   b. Check if the scale is balanced correctly.
   c. Check what clothing the client wore on both days.
   d. Use a different scale to check the weight.

5. To prevent hearing abnormal sounds, such as bowel sounds, the normal sequence of the physical examination should be:
   a. Palpation, percussion, inspection, auscultation.
   b. Inspection, auscultation, palpation, percussion.
   c. Percussion, auscultation, palpation, inspection.
   d. Auscultation, palpation, percussion, inspection.

6. Percussion is best defined as:
   a. The art of striking one object with another to create a sound.
   b. The process of examining the surface of the body.
   c. The technique of using touch to gather data.
   d. The act of listening to sounds produced by the body using a stethoscope.

7. A focus assessment is best defined as an assessment that:
   a. Comprises all body systems.
   b. Is completed on admission.
   c. Is done whenever a client's condition changes.
   d. Is concentrated on specific measurements.

8. Vesicular breath sounds are best described as:
   a. Loud, harsh, high-pitched sounds.
   b. Blowing sounds, moderate intensity and pitch.
   c. Soft, low-pitched sounds with a breezy quality.
   d. Soft, high-pitched harsh sounds.

9. Which one of the following lung sounds is considered normal?
   a. Crackles.
   b. Rhonchi.
   c. Rales.
   d. Bronchovesicular.

10. Bronchovesicular breath sounds are heard normally over the:
   a. Lung base.
   b. Trachea above the sternal notch.
   c. Mainstem bronchi below the clavicle.
   d. Entire lung parenchyma.

11. An S_2 heart sound represents:
   a. Closure of the aortic valve.
   b. Closure of the mitral valve.
   c. An atrial gallop.
   d. A ventricular gallop.

12. The tricuspid valve sound is best heard at the:
   a. 2nd intercostal space, left sternal border.
   b. 2nd intercostal space, sternal border.
   c. Midclavicular line, 5th intercostal space.
   d. Left 5th intercostal space, sternal border.

13. If you identify that a client has +3 edema, you estimate it as:
   a. Mild.
   b. Moderate.
   c. Severe.
   d. Absent.

PART 3 ▪ Critical Thinking Application

Mrs. Smiley has had a history of hypertension for several years and has recently experienced the inability to use her right arm and leg and the loss of ability to express herself. She has been admitted to your unit with the diagnosis of r/o left CVA and has been placed on a continuous heparin drip.

1. Based on admitting data, make a judgment about the deviations from normal you would find in the physical assessment.

2. List appropriate nursing diagnoses based on the client's physical state and immobility status. (This affects virtually all systems.)

3. In view of all these existing and potential problems, identify priority concerns (all are important concerns) for this client.

9

VITAL SIGNS

INTRODUCTION

Vital signs, also termed *cardinal signs,* reflect the body's physiologic status and provide information critical to evaluating homeostatic balance. Vital signs include four critical assessment areas: temperature, pulse, respirations, and blood pressure. The term *vital* is used because the information gathered is the clearest indicator of overall status. These four signs form baseline assessment data necessary for an ongoing evaluation of a client's condition. If the nurse has established the normal range for a client, deviations can be more easily recognized.

Vital signs should be taken at regular intervals. The more critical the client's condition, the more often these signs need to be taken and evaluated. They are not only indicators of a client's present condition, but also provide clues to a positive or negative change in status.

Obtaining the total picture of a client's health status is a major objective of client care. Although vital signs yield important information, they gain even more relevance when compared with the client's diagnosis, laboratory tests, history, and records.

(continued on next page)

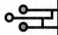

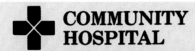

CLINICAL RECORD

DATE																						
HOSP DAY/POSTOP DAY																						
TIME				0200	0600	1000	1400	1800	2200	0200	0600	1000	1400	1800	2200	0200	0600	1000	1400	1800	2200

KEY	PULSE	TEMP	
		C	F
	140	40.6	105
	130	40.0	104
	120	39.4	103
	110	38.8	102
	100	38.3	101
	80	37.7	100
	80	37.2	99
	70	36.6	98
	60	36.1	97
	50	35.5	96

BLACK – PULSE & RESPIRATIONS
RED – TEMPERATURE

RESPIRATIONS																						
BLOOD PRESSURE																						

HEIGHT		WEIGHT			WEIGHT			WEIGHT		
		BREAKFAST	LUNCH	DINNER	BREAKFAST	LUNCH	DINNER	BREAKFAST	LUNCH	DINNER
DIET – TYPE										
% CONSUMED										
	INTAKE & OUTPUT	0600-1400	1400-2200	2200-0600	0600-1400	1400-2200	2200-0600	0600-1400	1400-2200	2200-0600
INTAKE	HOURS									

● **FIGURE 9-1** *Clinical record.*

PREPARATION PROTOCOL: FOR VITAL SIGNS SKILLS

Complete the following steps before each skill.

1. Check physician's order and client plan of care.
2. Gather equipment.
3. Check client's identaband.
4. Introduce yourself to client and explain nursing care you will be giving.
5. Provide privacy as necessary for client.
6. Wash hands.
7. Don gloves as indicated.

COMPLETION PROTOCOL: FOR VITAL SIGNS SKILLS

Make sure the following steps have been completed.

1. Remove gloves (if used) and discard appropriately, then wash hands.
2. Return client to position of comfort.
3. Return equipment to appropriate location.
4. Wash hands.
5. Document pertinent data and report as indicated.

SECTION ONE

TEMPERATURE

Temperature control of the body is a homeostatic function regulated by a complex mechanism involving the hypothalamus. The temperature of the body's interior (core temperature) is maintained within ±1°F, except in the case of febrile illness. The surface temperature of the skin and tissues immediately under the skin rises and falls when there is a change in the temperature of the surrounding environment. Core temperature is maintained when heat production equals heat loss. The temperature-regulating center in the hypothalamus keeps the core temperature constant. Temperature receptors, which determine if the body is too hot or too cold, relay signals to the hypothalamus. When the body becomes overheated, heat-sensitive neurons stimulate sweat glands to secrete fluid, which enhances heat loss through evaporation. The vasoconstrictor mechanism of the skin vessels is reduced, thereby conducting heat from the core of the body to the surface. Heat loss occurs through radiation, evaporation, and conduction. When the body temperature falls below the normal range, the client experiences hypothermia and complains of being cold, shivers, and has cool extremities. Hypothermia may be caused by accidental exposure, frostbite, or GI hemorrhage. Medically induced hypothermia is used for some surgical interventions. The ability of the hypothalamus to regulate body temperature is greatly impaired when the body temperature falls below 94°F (34.4°C) and is lost below 85°F (29.4°C). Cellular metabolism and heat production are also depressed by a low temperature.

When the body's core is cooled below 98.6°F (37°C), heat conservation is affected. Intense vasoconstriction of the skin vessels results. There is also piloerection and a decrease in sweating to conserve heat. Heat production is stimulated by shivering and increased cellular metabolism.

The *set point* is the critical temperature level at which the regulatory mechanisms attempt to maintain the body's core temperature. Above the set point, heat-losing mechanisms are brought into play, and below that level, heat-conserving and heat-producing mechanisms are set into action.

RATIONALE

- To determine if core temperature is within normal range
- To provide baseline data for further evaluation
- To determine alterations in disease conditions

ASSESSMENT

- Determine most appropriate method for obtaining temperature, i.e., oral, rectal, axillary, or tympanic.
- Determine number of times temperature is to be taken daily.
- Track temperature fluctuation relative to time of day and age of client.
- Compare with other vital signs to establish baseline data.
- Determine amount of time since client has ingested hot or cold liquids or has smoked.

CLINICAL NOTE

Fever is considered to be any abnormal elevation of body temperature (over 100.8°F). The most common signs and symptoms are:

- Perspiration over the body surface
- Body warm to the touch
- Chills and shivers
- Flushed face
- Client complaints of feeling alternately cold and hot
- Increased pulse and respirations
- Complaints of malaise and fatigue
- Parched lips and dry skin
- Convulsions, especially in children

DIGITAL THERMOMETER

Equipment

- Client's own oral or digital thermometer
- Tissues
- Clean gloves

SKILL

Oral Temperature

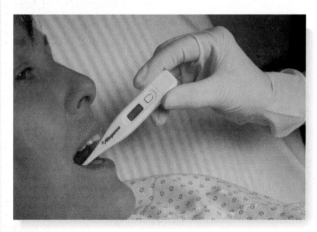

① Place thermometer in client's mouth under tongue. **RATIONALE:** Location ensures contact with large vessels under tongue.

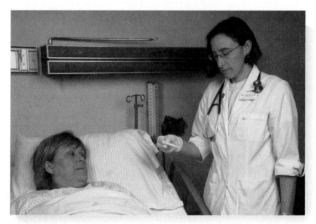

③ Remove thermometer and read temperature displayed in digital window.

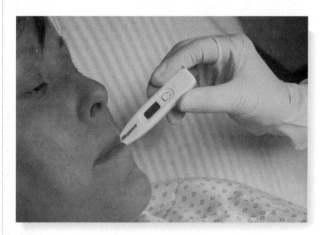

② Ask client to hold lips closed and leave thermometer in place 3 to 5 min. **RATIONALE:** Open-mouth breathing produces abnormally low readings. This is the optimum time to record accurate temperature.

TABLE 9-1	COMPARING CELSIUS AND FAHRENHEIT TEMPERATURES
Celsius (C)	**Fahrenheit (F)**
36.0	96.8
36.5	97.7
37.0	**98.6**
37.5	99.5
38.0	100.4
38.3	101.0
39.0	102.2
39.5	103.1
40.0	104.0

To convert °F to °C, subtract 32, then multiply by ⅚.
To convert °C to °F, multiply by ⅚, then add 32.

Source: Smith, S. F., Duell, D. J., and Martin, B. C. *Clinical Nursing Skills: Basic to Advanced Skills* (5th ed.). Upper Saddle River, NJ: Prentice Hall Health, 2000, p. 219.

Axillary Temperature

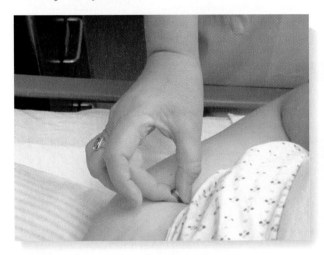

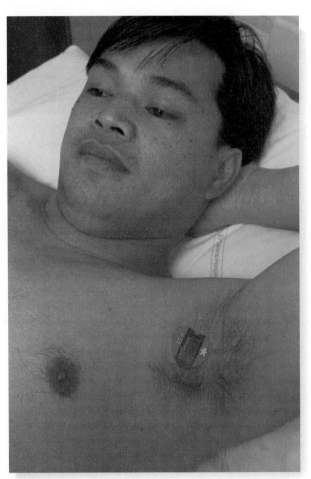

1 If axillary temperature is ordered, place thermometer in center of axilla and lower client's arm down and across chest.

- Hold thermometer in place 8 to 9 min, because axillary temperature recordings take a longer time to register accurately.

SAFETY ALERT

The Centers for Disease Control (CDC) has recently notified facilities that mercury (glass) thermometers are unsafe and should no longer be used. If they are broken, the mercury content is very dangerous and could result in mercury poisoning.

2 Place TraxIt, a continuous-reading wearable thermometer, deep in client's axilla. Last dot to turn from green to black indicates correct temperature. May be used for 2 days.

ELECTRONIC THERMOMETER

Equipment

- Electronic thermometer unit with digital probe (separate probe unit for oral or rectal)
- Disposable cover for thermometer
- Clean gloves
- Lubricant on tissue (for rectal temperature)

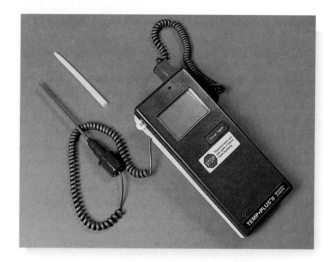

SKILL

Oral Temperature

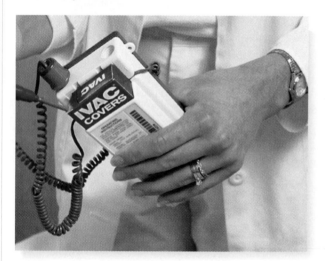

1 Remove thermometer from charger unit and, using your thumb and forefinger, grasp probe around top of stem. Firmly insert probe in disposable probe cover. **RATIONALE:** If pressure is directly on top, ejection button is activated.

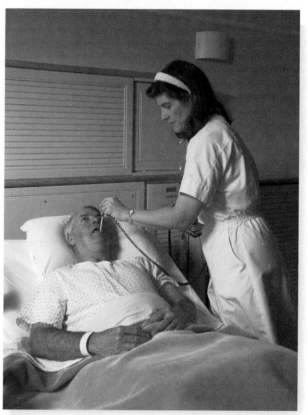

2 Place thermometer in client's mouth under tongue, and ask client to hold lips closed. **RATIONALE:** Larger blood vessels under tongue reflect accurate core temperature; open-mouth breathing produces an abnormally low temperature reading.

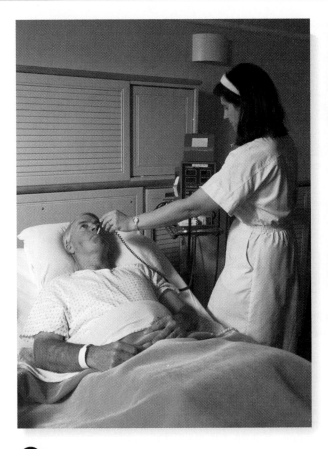

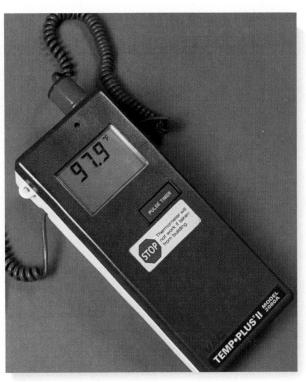

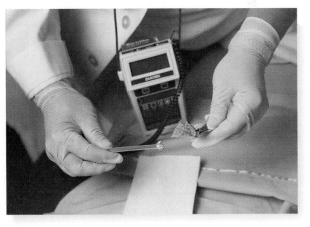

4 Read temperature on monitor unit.

- Discard probe cover into trash by pushing ejection button.
- Return probe to storage.

3 Hold thermometer in place; remove probe when audible signal occurs.

Rectal Temperature

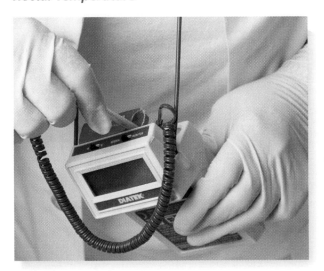

2 Lubricate tip of thermometer with lubricant on paper tissue.

1 Remove thermometer from charger unit and, using thumb and forefinger, grasp probe at top of stem. Firmly insert probe into disposable probe cover. **RATIONALE:** Probe cover must be securely attached.

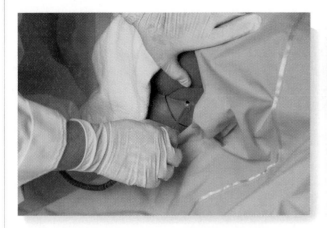

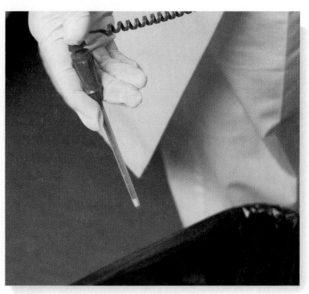

 Separate buttocks with one hand so anal sphincter opening is visible and insert thermometer approximately 1 to 1½ in into rectum. **RATIONALE:** Insertion too far into anal canal could damage tissue.

■ Hold in place until audible signal occurs (about 2 to 5 min). **RATIONALE:** Holding thermometer prevents potential injury to client.

 Remove thermometer, read temperature on monitor unit, and discard probe cover into trash by pushing ejection button. Return probe to storage.

> **SAFETY ALERT**
>
> Only use client's own dedicated electronic rectal thermometer if diagnosis includes *Clostridium difficile*–associated diarrhea because of the potential for spreading bacteria and increasing the risk of nosocomial infection to other clients.

TYMPANIC MEMBRANE TEMPERATURE

Equipment

■ Infrared thermometer unit
■ Disposable probe cover

Preparation

> **SAFETY ALERT**
>
> Do not use thermometer in infected or draining ear, or if adjacent lesion or incision exists.

① Position client so that probe can be safely inserted in ear.

② Select mode on tympanic thermometer: CORE, ORAL, RECTAL, or UNADJUSTED. **RATIONALE:** When code is ORAL, reading will correlate to an oral temperature taken with a glass thermometer.

SKILL

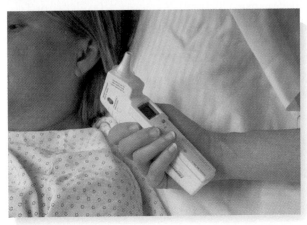

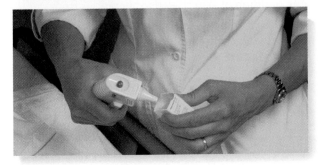

1 Attach disposable cover, centering probe on film, and press firmly until backing frame of probe cover engages base of probe. **RATIONALE:** Cover protects client from transmission of microorganisms.

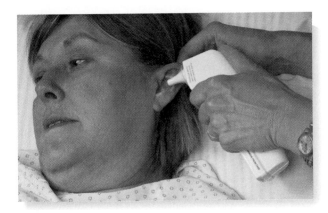

2 Position client so ear canal is easily seen and pull pinna back and up. **RATIONALE:** Position straightens ear canal's natural curve and provides access to tympanic membrane.

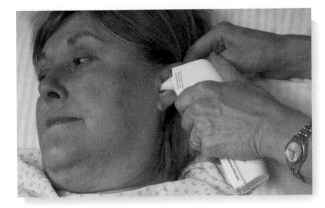

3 Place probe in client's ear and advance into ear canal to make a firm seal. **RATIONALE:** Pressure close to tympanic membrane seals ear canal and allows for accurate reading.

4 Press and hold temperature switch until green light flashes and temperature reading displays (approximately 3 sec). **RATIONALE:** Method records core body temperature.

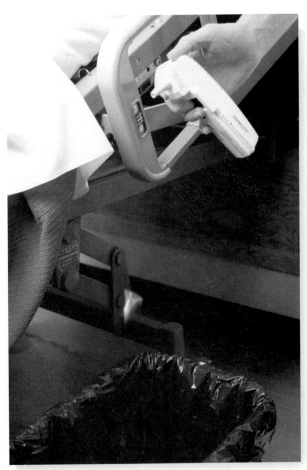

5 Remove thermometer and discard probe cover.

- Site designated: O (oral), R (rectal), A (axillary), or T (tympanic)
- Temperature recorded on temp sheet and graph (clinical record)
- Nursing interventions used for alterations in temperature

- Condition of skin related to alterations from normothermia (e.g., diaphoresis)
- Signs and symptoms associated with alterations in temperature (e.g., shivering, dehydration)

SECTION TWO

PULSE

The pulse is an index of the heart's rate and rhythm. The apical pulse rate is the number of heartbeats per minute. With each beat, the heart's left ventricle contracts and forces blood into the aorta. Closure of the heart valves creates the sounds heard. The forceful ejection of blood by the left ventricle produces a wave that is transmitted through the arteries to the periphery of the body. The pulse is a transient expansion of peripheral arteries resulting from internal pressure changes. If cardiac output is reduced (such as with a premature or irregular heartbeat), the peripheral pulse is weak, if felt, or skipped so that the radial pulse rate is less than the apical rate (called a *pulse deficit*). The pulse wave is influenced by the elasticity of the larger vessels, blood volume, blood viscosity, and arteriolar and capillary resistance.

A normal adult heart rate is from 60 to 100 beats per minute (BPM); the average rate is 72 BPM. Rates are slightly faster in women, and more rapid in children and infants. The resting heart rate usually does not change with age. Tachycardia is a pulse rate over 100 BPM. Bradycardia is a pulse rate below 60 BPM.

Heart rhythm is the time interval between each heartbeat. Normally the heart rhythm is regular. Slight irregularities do not necessarily indicate cardiac malfunction, however. An irregular cardiac rhythm, labeled either a *dysrhythmia* or an *arrhythmia,* especially if sustained, requires cardiac evaluation because it may be indicative of cardiac disease.

Variance in heart rate, either increased or decreased, may be attributed to many factors, such as drug intake, lack of oxygen, loss of blood, exercise, and body temperature. When evaluating a pulse rate, it is important to ascertain the normal baseline for each client and then determine variances from normal for that particular client. The heart normally pumps about 5 liters of blood through the body each minute. This cardiac output is cal-

culated by multiplying the heart rate per minute by the stroke volume (the amount of blood ejected with one contraction). Increasing the heart rate is one of the first compensatory mechanisms the body employs to maintain cardiac output.

The pulse should be taken frequently (every 5 to 15 min to 1 to 2 hrs) on acutely ill hospitalized clients and less frequently (every 4 to 8 hrs) on more stable hospitalized clients. Once a day or even once a week is adequate for clients in long-term care facilities. Do not wait to take vital signs until the next routine vital sign check if the client develops unexpected symptoms or has experienced a trauma.

RATIONALE

- To determine if pulse rate is within normal range and if rhythm is regular
- To evaluate quality of corresponding arterial pulses
- To monitor and evaluate amplitude and contour of pulse wave and artery elasticity
- To monitor and evaluate changes in client's status
- To reflect functioning of vital organs

ASSESSMENT

- Determine appropriate site to obtain pulse.
- Track rate, rhythm, pattern, and volume variation when client's health status changes.
- Determine apical pulse for clients with irregular rhythms or those taking heart medications.

- Obtain baseline peripheral pulses for cardiac or vascular surgery or medical clients with diabetes or arterial occlusive diseases.
- Obtain apical-radial pulse when deficits occur between apical and radial measurements.
- Determine need to monitor pulses with an ultrasound or electronic device.

CLINICAL NOTE

Pulse quality is determined by the amount of blood pumped through the peripheral arteries. The amount of pumped blood usually remains fairly constant; when it varies, it is also indicative of cardiac malfunction.

- **Bounding pulse:** Occurs when the nurse is able to feel the pulse by exerting only a slight pressure over the artery. May occur with increased stroke volume.
- **Weak or thready pulse:** Occurs if, by exerting firm pressure, the nurse cannot clearly determine the flow. May be associated with decreased stroke volume.
- **Pulsus alternans:** A regular pulse that the nurse feels as strong alternating with weak beats. May be related to left ventricular failure.
- **Bigeminal pulse:** Every second beat has a decreased amplitude. May be due to premature contractions.

Normal pulse

Hypokinetic (weak) pulse

Pulsus alternans

Hyperkinetic (bounding) pulse

Bigeminal pulse

Source: LeMone, P., and Burke, K.M. *Medical-Surgical Nursing: Critical Thinking in Clinical Care* (2d ed.). Upper Saddle River, NJ: Prentice Hall Health, 2000, p. 1186.

TABLE 9-2   **CAUSES OF PULSE ABNORMALITY**

Possible Causes of Tachycardia
- Sympathetic nervous system stimulation: fear, anger, anxiety, stress, pain
- Decrease in cardiac output
  —Congestive heart failure
  —Low blood volume (hypovolemia)
  —Shock
- Increased need for oxygen and other tissue nutrients
  —Exercise
  —Coitus
  —Fever (heart rate increases 8 BPM for every 1°F rise in temperature)
  —Increased thyroid activity (thyrotoxicosis)
- Inadequate oxygenation by the lungs (hypoxemia)
- Hypoxia
  —Anemia
  —Pulmonary emboli
- Certain drugs, such as atropine, isoproterenol, aminophylline, epinephrine

Possible Causes of Bradycardia
- Well-conditioned athletes
- Sleep
- Parasympathetic nervous system stimulation: Valsalva maneuver, carotid sinus massage
- Ischemia to sinus node
- Decreased thyroid activity (myxedema)
- Increased intracranial or intraocular pressure
- Stokes-Adams attacks
- Hyperkalemia
- Drugs, such as digitalis or propranolol

BEYOND THE SKILL

PULSE CHARACTERISTICS

When counting pulse rate, pay attention to:

- **Rate:** Average is 72 BPM. The normal adult heart rate range is 60 to 100 BPM.
- **Rhythm:** The pattern of beats, either regular or irregular. Nurse may note early or skipped beats.
- **Volume or amplitude:** The force of blood with each beat; can range from absent to bounding (see Clinical Note on pulse quality).
- **Symmetry:** Bilateral uniformity of pulse.

RADIAL PULSE

Equipment

- Watch with sweep second hand

SAFETY ALERT

If pulse rate is below 60 or above 100 (outside normal parameters), notify team leader or physician.

SKILL

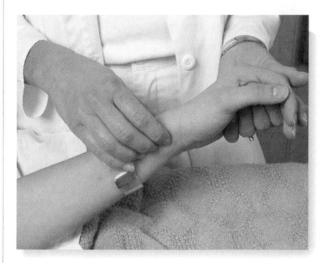

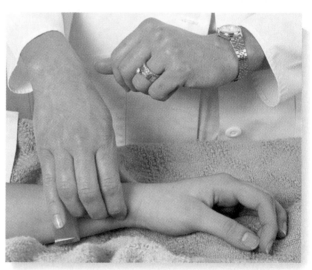

1 Locate radial artery on each wrist by using pads of middle three fingers. **RATIONALE:** Nurse may feel own pulse if palpating with thumb.

- Press artery against firm surface to occlude vessel, then gradually release pressure. **RATIONALE:** Too much pressure obliterates pulse.

2 Count pulse for 30 sec, and multiply by 2 to obtain per minute pulse rate. **RATIONALE:** This is sufficient time for rate determination if pulse rhythm is regular.

BEYOND THE SKILL

PALPATING THE PULSE

- The radial artery is usually used because it lies close to the skin surface and is easily accessible at the wrist.
- Press the artery against bone or underlying firm surface to occlude the vessel, and then gradually release pressure.
- Note quality (strength) of the pulse. This is an indication of stroke volume.
- If the pulse is difficult to palpate, try exerting more pressure on the most distal palpating finger.

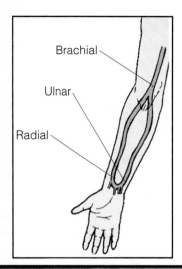

Brachial
Ulnar
Radial

APICAL PULSE

Equipment

- Watch with sweep second hand
- Stethoscope

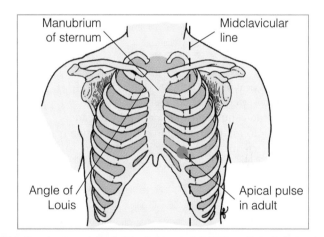

Manubrium of sternum

Midclavicular line

Angle of Louis

Apical pulse in adult

SKILL

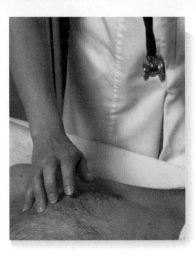

① Place client in supine position with chest exposed. Locate angle of Louis by palpation. It is just below suprasternal notch (angle between top and bottom of sternum).

- Palpate 2nd intercostal space with index finger. **RATIONALE:** Heart sounds are enhanced when examiner is at client's right side.

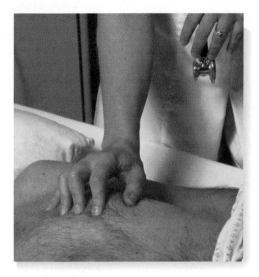

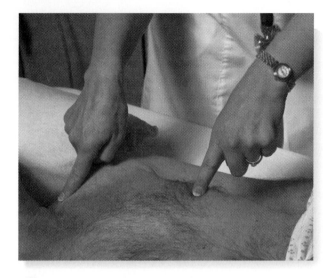

 Place middle finger in 3rd intercostal space and continue to move downward to 5th intercostal space.

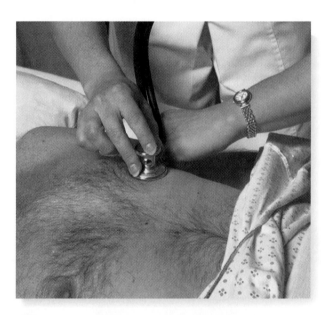 Move index finger horizontally along 5th intercostal space to midclavicular line, tricuspid area, or Erb's point. **RATIONALE:** Accurate apical pulse is heard at this position.

SAFETY ALERT

Count apical pulse for at least 1 min if radial rhythm is irregular or difficult to count. An apical-radial pulse measurement provides additional information regarding cardiac function if pulse is irregular. It may take a minute or so to detect the irregularity. This method allows an accurate pulse count.

After warming diaphragm in your hand, place it over apical area and auscultate for normal S_1 and S_2 heart sounds ("lub-dub"). **RATIONALE:** Heart sounds are high-pitched and most clearly heard with diaphragm of stethoscope.

■   Count rate for 1 min minimum when taking apical pulse. **RATIONALE:** More accurate readings are obtained over 1 min, especially if pulse is irregular.

APICAL-RADIAL PULSE

Equipment

- Watch with sweep second hand
- Stethoscope
- Second nurse to assist with procedure

SKILL

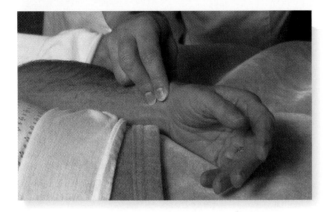

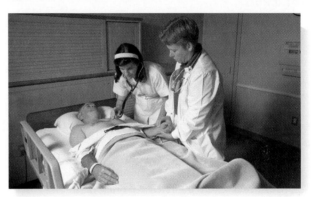

1 First nurse locates radial pulse. Place tips of first two fingers lightly over radial area on client's inner wrist. **RATIONALE:** Fingertips (not thumb) are the most sensitive to palpate for arterial pulse.

2 Second nurse locates apical pulse at the 5th intercostal space and midclavicular line, and firmly places diaphragm of stethoscope (that has been warmed in nurse's hand) on site. **RATIONALE:** Firm application of diaphragm helps transmit high-pitched heart sounds.

- Place watch where clearly visible to both nurses. **RATIONALE:** Both nurses must count pulse rates within the same time span, using one watch.
- Select number on watch to start counting; both nurses simultaneously auscultate apical and palpate radial pulse.

BEYOND THE SKILL

EXPERIENCE IS IMPORTANT

An experienced nurse may be able to assess radial and apical rates simultaneously without an assistant.

Note pulse deficit between apical and radial pulses when rhythm is irregular.

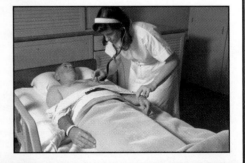

PERIPHERAL PULSE
Equipment

- Felt-tip pen
- Watch with second hand

SKILL

Carotid Pulse

1 Place client in reclining position at a 30° angle and inspect neck for presence of pulsation. **RATIONALE:** This position allows for easier accessibility for carotid artery.

2 Palpate carotid artery along sternocleidomastoid muscle by pressing middle two fingers on underlying firm surface. **RATIONALE:** This occludes vessel, and, when pressure is gradually released, pulse is felt.

3 Gradually release pressure until pulse is felt.

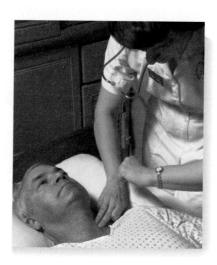

Dorsalis Pedis Pulse

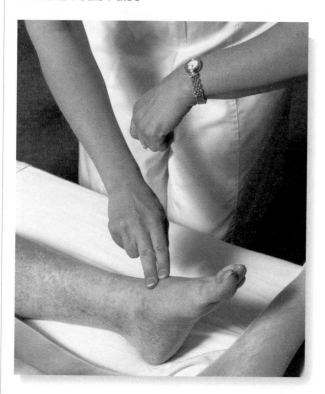

1 Place client in supine position with foot relaxed.

2 Palpate top of foot between large and second toe with middle two fingers.

Posterior Tibial Pulse

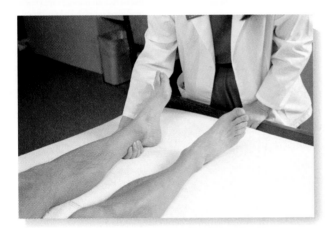

1 Place client in supine position with foot relaxed or knee bent. **RATIONALE:** Either position provides accessibility to artery.

2 Palpate area behind and slightly below medial malleolus (ankle bone).

Brachial Pulse

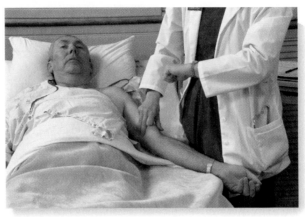

1 Place client in supine position with arm exposed.

2 Palpate brachial artery by placing first two fingers above and slightly behind antecubital fossa.

Femoral Pulse

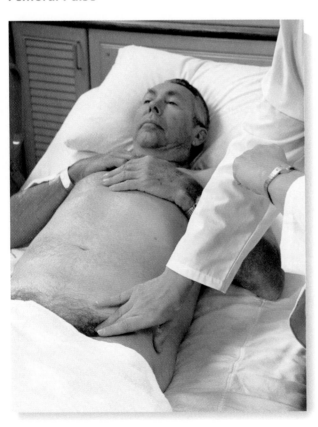

1 Place client in supine position with leg slightly flexed. **RATIONALE:** This position exposes inguinal area.

2 Palpate femoral pulse by placing first two fingers between pubic symphysis and anterosuperior iliac spine over inguinal area.

BEYOND THE SKILL

UNDERSTANDING PHYSIOLOGY

Carotid Artery

When the carotid pulse is palpated, take care not to exert too much pressure, because this could stimulate a vagal response and slow the heart rate. Avoid pressing on the carotid sinus in the upper neck area, near the jaw. Also, do not palpate both carotids simultaneously, because this decreases blood flow to the brain.

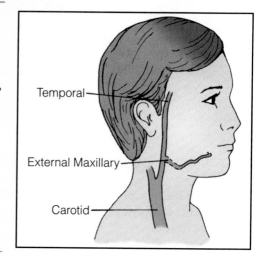

Palpation

- The arterial pulse can be felt over arteries that lie close to the body surface and over a bone or firm surface that can support the artery when pressure is applied.
- The radial artery is palpated most frequently because it is the most accessible.
- The femoral and carotid arteries are used in cases of cardiac arrest to determine the adequacy of perfusion.
- When peripheral pulses cannot be palpated, a Doppler ultrasound stethoscope is used to confirm the presence or absence of the pulse.

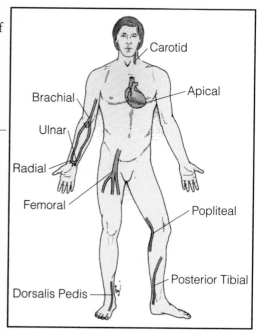

Pulse Sites

- If the pulse is not immediately palpable, examine the adjacent area. This identifies where interruption or alteration in circulation occurs in an extremity.
- Pulse locations differ; therefore, mark locations with a felt-tip pen, especially when they are difficult to palpate. Marking the site allows the next nurse to find the location without spending extra time.
- Compare the presence and characteristics of peripheral pulses with previous findings. This facilitates early identification of alterations in peripheral circulation.

PERIPHERAL PULSE WITH DOPPLER

Equipment

- Doppler ultrasound stethoscope
- Conductive gel (not K-Y)

SKILL

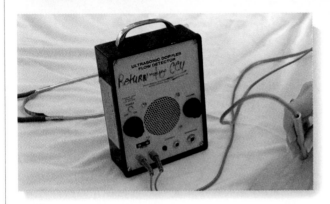

1 Plug headset (stethoscope) into one or two outlet jacks located near volume control. If not using a stethoscope, plug probe into monitor.

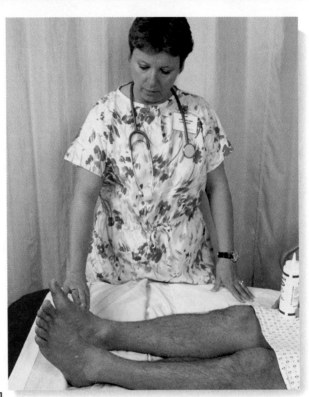

2 Uncover extremity to be assessed and place client in a comfortable position. Locate peripheral pulse with fingers.

CLINICAL NOTE

Peripheral pulses may be absent or weak. The *size* (amplitude) of a pulse depends on the degree of filling of the artery during systole (ventricular contraction) and emptying during diastole (ventricular relaxation). The *amplitude* of a pulse is described as being large or small and determines the pulse pressure (the difference between systolic and diastolic pressure). The *type* (contour) of pulse felt by the fingers depends on how fast the pulse pressure changes and is described as being quick or prolonged.

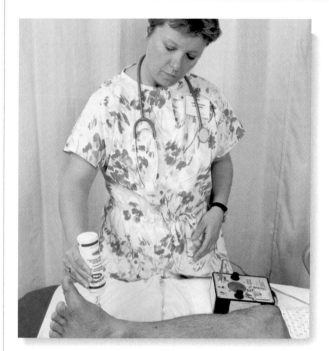

3 Apply conductive gel to client's skin. **RATIONALE:** Ultrasound beam travels best through gel and requires an airtight seal between probe and skin.

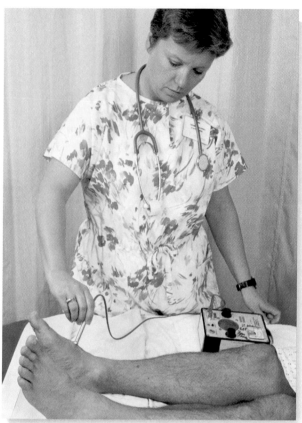

4 Position probe over pulse site. Keep in direct contact with skin at a 90° angle to the blood vessel being assessed. **RATIONALE:** This position facilitates detection of swooshing pulse sounds.

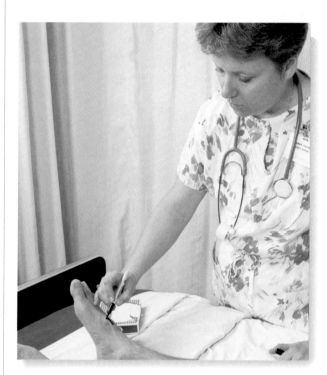

5 Clean area and mark site where pulsations were heard. **RATIONALE:** Leaving marks on site will facilitate future assessments.

■ Clean gel from skin and Doppler probe and return to original location.

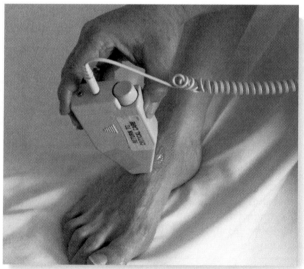

6 Alternate equipment for Doppler probe. Skill steps are the same.

CHARTING

- Method of pulse reading
- Rate and rhythm of pulse
- Pulse volume
- Pulse deficit, if any present

- Characteristics of all peripheral pulses—use rating scale
- Use of Doppler stethoscope, if needed
- Effects of nursing or medical treatments on abnormal pulse rates or rhythms

SECTION THREE

RESPIRATION

Respiration is the process of bringing oxygen to body tissues and removing carbon dioxide. The lungs play a major role in this process. Another respiratory function is to maintain arterial blood homeostasis by maintaining the pH of the blood. The lungs accomplish this by the process of breathing.

Breathing consists of two phases, inspiration and expiration. Inspiration is an active process in which the diaphragm descends, the external intercostal muscles contract, and the chest expands to allow air to move into the tracheobronchial tree. Expiration is a passive process in which air flows out of the respiratory tree.

The respiratory center in the medulla of the brain and the level of carbon dioxide in the blood both control the rate and depth of breathing. Peripheral receptors in the carotid body and the aortic arch also respond to the level of oxygen in the blood. To some extent, respiration can be voluntarily controlled by holding the breath or hyperventilating. Talking, laughing, and crying also affect respiration.

The diaphragm and the intercostal muscles are the main muscles used for breathing. Other accessory muscles, such as the abdominal muscles, the sternocleidomastoid, the trapezius, and the scalene, can be used to assist with respiration if necessary.

After assessing the pattern, type, and depth of breathing, it is important to observe the physical characteristics of chest expansion. The chest normally expands symmetrically without rib flaring or retraction. In addition, observation of chest deformities should also be made, as all of these signs yield information about the respiratory process and overall health status of the client.

RATIONALE

- To note respiratory rate, rhythm, and depth
- To establish baseline information upon admission of client to unit
- To note labored, difficult, or noisy respirations or cyanosis
- To identify alterations in respiratory pattern resulting from disease conditions

ASSESSMENT

- Note respiratory rate, depth, and position.
- Assess for abnormalities during inspection and palpation or by percussion and auscultation.
- Assess for alterations in breathing and presence of dyspnea or cyanosis.
- Assess for presence of abnormal sounds, such as stertorous or sonorous breathing.

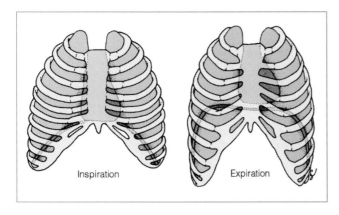

Inspiration   Expiration

CLINICAL NOTE

RATE, DEPTH, AND PATTERN OF RESPIRATIONS

- Normal breathing is almost invisible, effortless, quiet, automatic, and regular. When the breathing pattern varies from normal, evaluate thoroughly.

- Bronchial sounds heard over large airways are fairly loud. There is normally a pause between inspiration and expiration.

- Softer sounds are heard over peripheral lung areas, and there are no pauses between inspiration, which is a long sound, and expiration, which is a short sound.

- Breathing that is noisy, labored, or strained indicates an obstruction may be affecting the breathing pattern, which could lead to major alterations in homeostasis.

- The normal rate of breathing for a resting adult is 12 to 18 breaths per minute.

- A rate of 24 or above is considered tachypnea, and a rate of 10 or less is considered bradypnea.

- The ratio of pulse to breathing is usually 5:1 and remains fairly constant.

- Depth of breathing (tidal volume) is the amount of air that moves in and out with each breath. The tidal volume is 500 mL in the healthy adult.

- Alveolar air is only partially replenished by atmosphere air with each inspiratory phase. Approximately 350 mL (tidal volume minus dead space) of new air is exchanged with the functional residual capacity volume during each respiratory cycle.

- Accurate tidal volume can be measured by a spirometer, but a nurse can judge the approximate depth by placing the back of the hand next to the client's nose and mouth and feeling the expired air.

- Another method of estimating volume capacity is to observe chest expansion and to check both sides of the thorax for symmetrical movement.

- *Apnea* (absence of breathing) may be intermittent.

- *Bradypnea* is a rate slower than normal (<10 breaths per minute).

- *Tachypnea* is a rate faster than normal (>24 breaths per minute) and more shallow.

- *Hyperpnea* is increased depth of respirations.

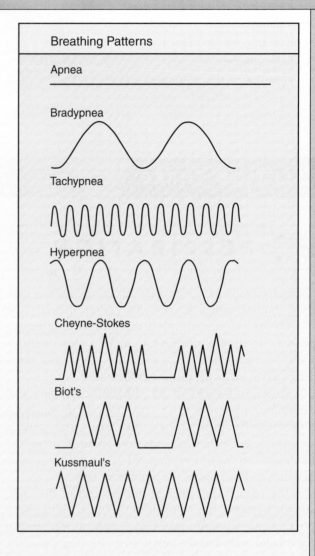

Breathing Patterns

Apnea

Bradypnea

Tachypnea

Hyperpnea

Cheyne-Stokes

Biot's

Kussmaul's

- *Cheyne-Stokes* respirations are a respiratory cycle in which respirations increase in rate and depth, then decrease, followed by a period of apnea.

- *Biot* respirations are an irregular pattern—slow and deep or rapid and shallow, followed by apnea.

- *Kussmaul* respirations are deep and gasping (hyperventilation); 20 breaths per minute.

Note: For assessing normal breath sounds, see Chapter 8, "Admission and Assessment," for discontinuous/continuous (adventitious) breath sounds, *see* Respiratory chapter.

RESPIRATORY RATE

Equipment

- Watch with second hand

SKILL

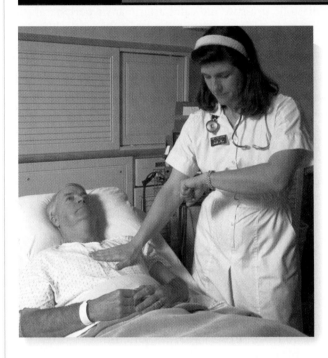

1 Place hand on client's chest or observe chest rise and fall when client is unaware respirations are being counted. **RATIONALE:** When client is aware of being observed, respirations may be altered.

- Note relationship of inspiration to expiration. Note also depth and effort of breathing.
- Count respirations for 30 sec and multiply by 2. Note abnormal patterns. **RATIONALE:** 30 sec is adequate for normal breathing patterns. One full minute is more accurate for abnormal breathing patterns.

CHARTING

- Rate and rhythm of respirations
- Abnormal sounds associated with breathing
- Effectiveness of therapy, if needed, to correct respiratory problems
- Alterations from baseline respiratory patterns

BLOOD PRESSURE

The heart generates pressure during the cardiac cycle to perfuse the organs of the body with blood. Blood flows from the heart to the arteries, into the capillaries and veins, and then back to the heart. Blood pressure in the arterial system varies with the cardiac cycle, reaching the highest level at the peak of systole and the lowest level at the end of diastole. The difference between the systolic and diastolic blood pressure is the pulse pressure, which is normally 30 to 50 mm Hg. There are many factors that affect blood pressure: cardiac output, peripheral vascular resistance, elasticity and distensibility of arteries, blood volume, blood viscosity, hormones and enzymes, chemoreceptors, and methods of measuring blood pressure.

Normal blood pressure in an adult varies between 100 and 140 mm Hg systolic and between 60 and 90 mm Hg diastolic. As blood moves toward smaller arteries and into arterioles where it enters the capillaries, pressure falls to 35 mm Hg. It continues to fall as blood goes through the capillaries, where the flow is steady and not pulsatile. As blood moves into the venous system, pressure falls until it is lowest in the venae cavae.

Blood pressures vary widely. A blood pressure of 100/60 mm Hg may be normal for one person, but hypotensive for another. Hypotension (90 to 100 mm Hg systolic) in a healthy adult without other clinical symptoms is little reason for concern.

Blood pressure readings are recorded in association with Korotkoff sounds. These sounds are described as *K phases.* The systolic, or first, pressure reading occurs with the advent of the first Korotkoff sound. The systolic reading represents the maximal pressure in the aorta following contraction of the left ventricle and is heard as a faint tapping sound.

According to American Heart Association standards, the diastolic, or second, reading should be taken at the time of the last Korotkoff sound (phase V) for adults. The diastolic reading represents the minimal pressure exerted against the arterial walls at all times.

Measuring Blood Pressure

Measuring arterial blood pressure provides important information about the overall health status of the client. For example, the systolic pressure provides a database about the condition of the heart and great arteries. The diastolic pressure indicates arteriolar or peripheral vascular resistance. The pulse pressure, or difference between the systolic and diastolic pressure, provides information about cardiac function and blood volume. A single blood pressure reading, however, does not provide adequate data from which conclusions can be drawn about all of these factors. Rather, a series of blood pressure readings should be taken to establish a baseline for further evaluation.

RATIONALE

- To note any major changes from prior assessments
- To determine size of cuff needed for accurate reading to be taken
- To note beginning and disappearance of Korotkoff sounds during a blood pressure reading
- To note presence of factors that can alter blood pressure readings

ASSESSMENT

- Determine if arterial blood pressure is within normal range for individual client.
- Assess condition of heart and arteries, blood vessel resistance, and stroke volume.
- Establish a baseline for further evaluation.
- Identify alterations in blood pressure resulting from a change in disease condition.
- Correlate blood pressure readings with pulse and respirations.

BLOOD PRESSURE

Equipment

- Sphygmomanometer with properly sized cuff
- Stethoscope

SKILL

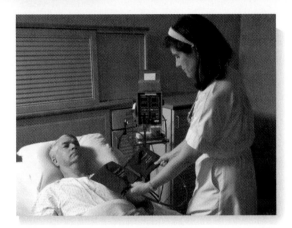

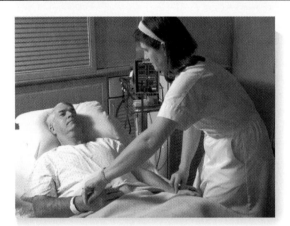

1 Choose cuff size appropriate for client. Cuff width should be about 4½ to 5½ in for the average adult. **RATIONALE:** When cuff is too narrow, it results in erroneously high readings. If cuff is too wide, reading will be falsely low.

2 Palpate radial pulses simultaneously on both arms if both are accessible. If pulses are equal, either arm may be used to measure blood pressure. Choice may be dictated by accessibility or nurse comfort. **RATIONALE:** Evaluation of both arms allows nurse to determine stronger pulse site.

CLINICAL NOTE

BLOOD PRESSURE CUFF SIZES

- Standard (12 to 14 cm wide) for the average adult arm.
- Narrower cuff for infant, child, or adult with thin arms.
- For children (younger than 13 years), the bladder should be large enough to encircle the arm completely (100%).
- Wider cuff (18 to 22 cm) for clients with obese arms or for thigh pressure readings.

The width of the cuff's inflatable bladder should be 40 percent of the circumference of the limb on which it is used. The length of the bladder should be twice its width.

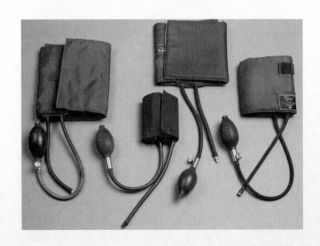

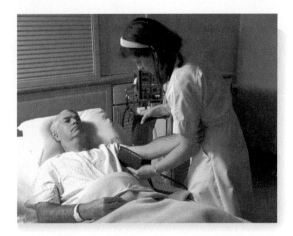

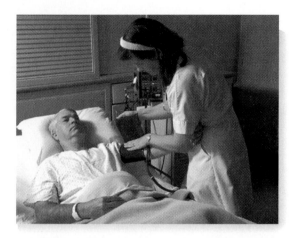

(3) Expose upper part of client's arm and position with arm slightly flexed and supported at heart level. **RATIONALE:** If arm is below level of heart, blood pressure reading will be higher than normal. If arm is above level of heart, reading will be lower than normal.

(4) Wrap totally deflated cuff snugly and smoothly around upper part of arm (lower border of cuff 1 in above antecubital space) with center of cuff bladder over brachial artery (pressure dial or mercury meniscus at zero). **RATIONALE:** Position of cuff allows space for bell placement.

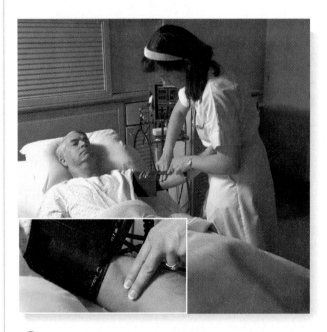

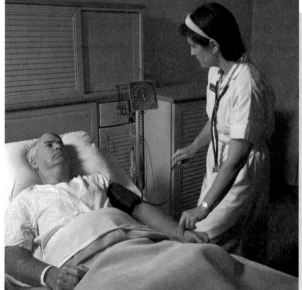

(5) Locate and palpate brachial artery pulsations on cuffed arm. **RATIONALE:** Locating artery before inflating cuff will identify most audible site for hearing pulsations.

(6) Close valve on sphygmomanometer pump while palpating radial artery and inflate to level 30 mm Hg above level at which radial pulsations are no longer felt.

- Note level and rapidly deflate, and wait 60 sec for venous congestion to decrease. **RATIONALE:** Level (palpated systolic blood pressure) provides parameters to measure blood pressure. *Note:* Clinical practice protocol varies, and this step may or may not be included with every blood pressure reading.

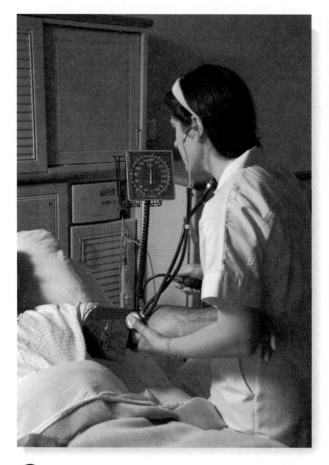

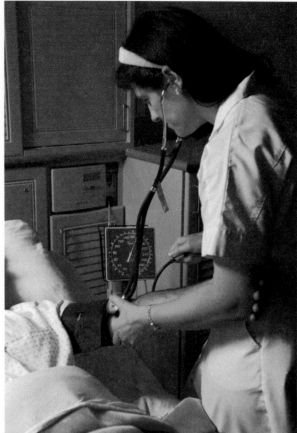

7 Place bell (or diaphragm) of stethoscope lightly on medial antecubital fossa where brachial artery pulsations are located and rapidly inflate cuff to 30 mm Hg above palpated systolic pressure (see step 6). **RATIONALE:** This assures that cuff is inflated to pressure exceeding client's systolic pressure.

8 Deflate cuff gradually at a constant rate by opening valve on pump (2 to 4 mm Hg/sec) until first Korotkoff sound is heard. This is systolic pressure, or phase I, of Korotkoff sounds. **RATIONALE:** Slower or faster deflation yields false readings.

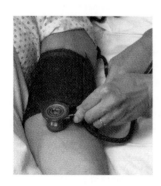

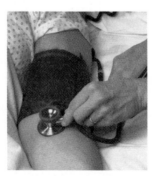

SAFETY ALERT

Routinely, blood pressure for an acutely ill client should be taken every 1 to 2 hrs, and blood pressure for more stabilized clients should be taken every 4 to 8 hrs. Clients with severe hypotension or hypertension, with low blood volume, or on vasoconstrictor or vasodilator drugs may require checking every 5 to 15 min.

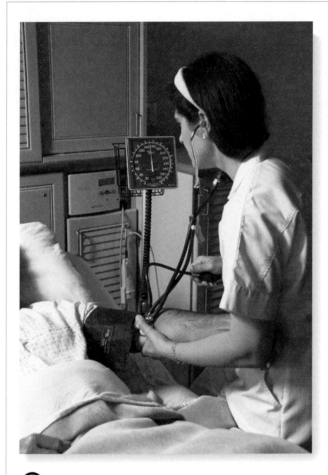

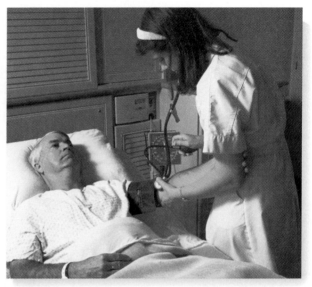

10 Continue to completely deflate cuff while reading pressure with mercury at eye level when using manometer filled with mercury. **RATIONALE:** If mercury meniscus is below eye level, reading is false low.

9 Note at which level Korotkoff sounds begin (phase I), and when they disappear completely (phase V). **RATIONALE:** Disappearance of sounds (phase V) is regarded by the American Heart Association as the best index of diastolic pressure in individuals over age 13. The best index of diastolic pressure in children is distinct muffling of sounds at phase IV.

CLINICAL NOTE

KOROTKOFF SOUND PHASES
The American Heart Association recommends routine use of the bell of the stethoscope for blood pressure (Korotkoff sounds) auscultation.

- **Phase I:** The pressure level at which the first faint, clear tapping sounds are heard. The sounds gradually increase in intensity as the cuff is deflated. This phase coincides with reappearance of a palpable pulse.
- **Phase II:** That time during cuff deflation when a murmur or swishing sounds are heard.
- **Phase III:** The period during which sounds are crisper and increase in intensity.
- **Phase IV:** That time when a distinct, abrupt, muffling of sound (usually a soft, blowing quality) is heard.
- **Phase V:** That pressure level when the last sound is heard and after which all sound disappears.

Source: American Heart Association, 1996.

In persons with hypertension, an auscultatory gap may be present. This gap is an absence of sounds after the first Korotkoff sounds appear and then the reappearance of the sounds at a lower level. This condition can be avoided if the brachial artery is palpated first and the cuff is inflated above the level where the pulsations disappear.

BEYOND THE SKILL

TYPES OF MANOMETERS

The *indirect method* of taking a blood pressure using a sphygmo-manometer (mercury or anaeroid) and a stethoscope is accurate for most clients. New electronic blood pressure devices constantly monitor systolic, diastolic, and mean readings at preset time intervals and are helpful in measuring blood pressure trends in clients who are at risk for hypertension or hypotension. These devices also provide a printout if needed for documentation. If a stethoscope is unavailable or the brachial artery amplitude is decreased, the brachial or radial artery can be palpated as the blood pressure cuff is inflated to determine the systolic blood pressure (palpated pulse disappears at this point). The *direct method* is continuous and measures mean arterial pressures. A needle or catheter is inserted into the brachial, radial, or femoral artery. An oscilloscope displays arterial pressure waveforms.

1. **Tube manometer:** Has a tube filled with mercury. The pressure reading is taken by observing the meniscus of mercury at eye level as it travels down the tube.
2. **Cuneroid manometer:** Has a calibrated dial with a needle that points to the pressure level.
3. **Continuous-monitoring electronic robotic unit:** Records a digital number as blood pressure.

1.

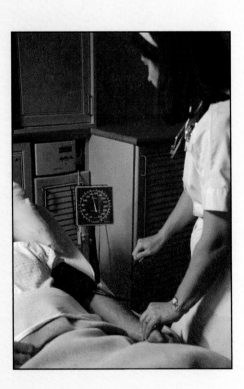

2.

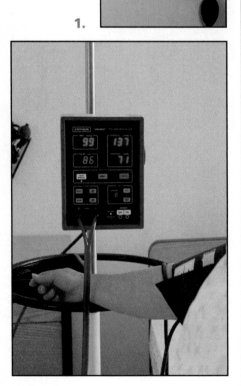

3.

LOWER-EXTREMITY BLOOD PRESSURE

Equipment

- Sphygmomanometer with standard-size cuff

Preparation

SKILL

Thigh Pressure

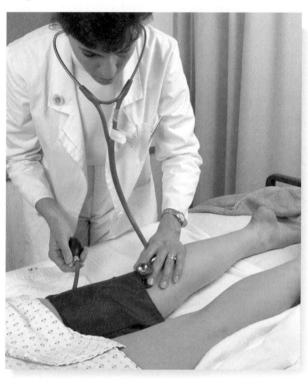

1 Measure blood pressure in thigh by using large cuff with bladder placed over posterior midthigh. Listen at popliteal fossa with client in prone position.

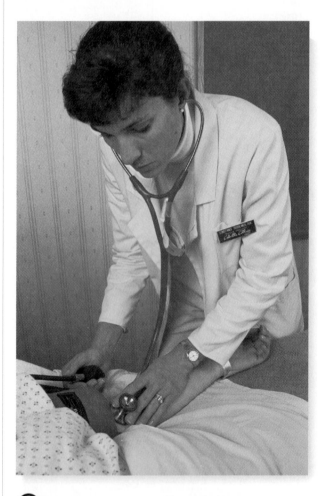

1 Measure brachial blood pressure and record. **RATIONALE:** Measurement will be baseline for comparison with leg pressure. (See previous procedure.)

Lower Leg Pressure

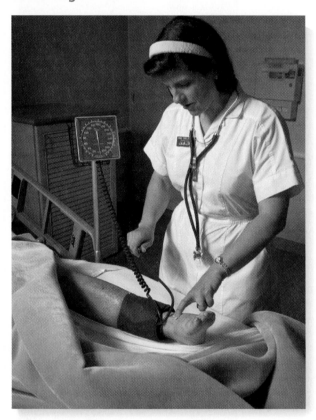

1 Wrap cuff snugly and smoothly around lower leg with cuff's distal edge at malleolus and locate dorsalis pedis. **RATIONALE:** Main artery in foot is used to palpate and measure blood pressure.

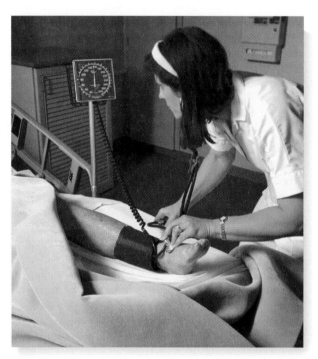

2 Place diaphragm of stethoscope quickly on pulse site and inflate cuff rapidly to a level 30 mm Hg above level at which artery pulsations were no longer felt. **RATIONALE:** Comparing brachial and foot measurements will yield assessment data of vascular system. *Note:* Systolic pressure is 20 to 30 mm Hg higher than in the brachial artery. Diastolic pressure is the same in the dorsalis pedis and brachial arteries.

- Deflate cuff slowly.
- Record level at which pulsations start and stop.

BEYOND THE SKILL

ALTERNATE METHODS FOR BLOOD PRESSURE

By Palpation

1. Palpate brachial artery while inflating cuff to 30 mm Hg above level at which radial artery pulsations are no longer felt.

2. Slowly release pressure, noting first palpated beat. **RATIONALE:** First palpated beat is systolic pressure and should be same point at which last pulsation was felt when inflating cuff.

3. Remove cuff and note palpated systolic pressure.

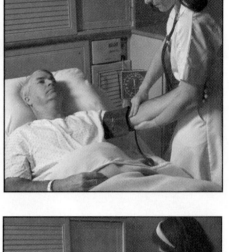

By Electronic Robotic Unit

Follow steps 1 to 5 for taking a blood pressure.

6. Inflate cuff (while palpating radial artery) to level 30 mm Hg above level at which radial pulsations are no longer felt. Note reading on manometer. **RATIONALE:** This procedure assures that cuff is inflated to pressure exceeding client's systolic pressure.

7. Deflate cuff and wait 60 sec to clear venous congestion (often, steps 6 and 7 are not done in clinical practice).

8. Inflate cuff to level 30 mm Hg above palpated systolic pressure.

9. Deflate cuff gradually at constant rate by opening valve on pump (2 mm Hg/sec). Systolic and diastolic readings will register digitally on readout panel. **RATIONALE:** Slower or faster deflation may yield false readings.

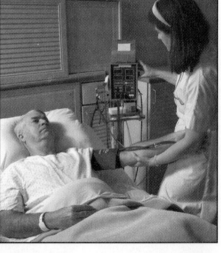

By Continuous-Monitoring Device

1. Attach cuff to air hose by firmly pushing valve from cuff into air hose and twisting to secure fit.

2. Wrap cuff securely around extremity (usually arm).

3. Position extremity at level of heart. **RATIONALE:** Allows for accurate reading; if arm is below heart level, reading will be higher than normal.

4. Turn power switch ON. Set arterial pressure alarm limits by pushing *alarm* button to ON and both HIGH and LOW parameters by depressing *alarm* button until parameters read out on digital display. **RATIONALE:** Alarm parameters provide safety factor by alerting nurse when reading exceeds parameters.

5. Press *start* button for approximately 4 sec. **RATIONALE:** Activates printer for readout of blood pressure, including systolic, diastolic, mean arterial pressure, and heart rate.

6. Press *start* button again to begin timed blood pressure reading.

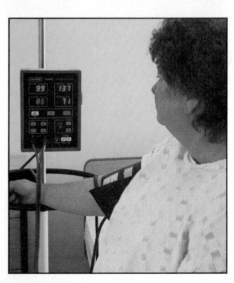

CHARTING

- Two phases of Korotkoff sounds (e.g., 120/80 and site)
- Response to position changes
- Systolic blood pressure

- Diastolic blood pressure
- Level of muffled Korotkoff sounds and their disappearance (for example: 126/80/72 mm Hg)
- Presence of pulsus paradoxus or pulsus alternans

CRITICAL THINKING FOCUS

SECTION ONE ▪ Temperature

Unexpected Outcomes

- Fever develops.

- Temperature dangerously elevated.

- Despite initial cooling measures, temperature remains elevated due to hypothalamus damage from brain disease or injury.
- Temperature remains elevated because of bacterial-produced pyrogens.

Alternative Nursing Actions

- Check possible sources of infection, and take preventative measures.

- Employ cooling methods such as tepid sponge bath, cool oral fluids, ice packs, alcohol sponge bath, or antipyretic drugs (as ordered).

- Notify physician, and request cooling blanket.
- Monitor temperature every 15 to 30 min.
- Continue to administer antipyretic drugs as ordered.

- Check for order to obtain culture of possible sources of infection.
- Give antipyretic drugs as ordered.
- Decrease room temperature and remove excess covers.
- Give tepid sponge bath.

SECTION TWO ▪ Pulse

Unexpected Outcomes

- Abnormal heartbeats are present.

- Tachycardia (pulse rate over 100 BPM in adults or 140 in children) is present.

- Bradycardia (pulse rate less than 60 in adults or less than 70 in children) is present.

Alternative Nursing Actions

- Relieve anxiety, fear, or stress through communication and pertinent information.
- If client has pain, relieve with change of position, back rub, or analgesic.

- Decrease heart rate by reducing an elevated temperature to normal.
- Take vital signs every 15 min to 2 hrs until condition stabilizes and pulse is within normal limits.
- Determine significance of pulse rate as it affects blood pressure, sensorium, and client comfort.
- Notify physician if persistent tachycardia continues.

- Notify physician for electrocardiogram request to determine if heart block is present.

- If client is on digitalis, hold the drug and notify the physician.
- Have atropine and temporary pacemaker available for physician if pulse is consistently slow (less than 50).
- Continue monitoring pulse rate every 15 min to 2 hrs until pulse is within normal limits.

- Doppler stethoscope is unable to detect sounds.

- Check that conductive jelly is used (salt in K-Y Jelly can damage the probe).
- Check that batteries are less than 6 mo old. The date should be indicated on all batteries.
- Check that abnormal pressure is not applied, as this obliterates pulse.

SECTION THREE ▪ Respiration

Unexpected Outcomes

- Apnea (absence of breathing) occurs—may be intermittent.

- Tachypnea (rate faster than normal [>24 breaths per minute] and more shallow) occurs.

- Bradypnea (rate slower than normal [<10 breaths per minute]) occurs.

- Hyperpnea (increased depth of respiration) occurs.

- Cheyne-Stokes respirations (respiratory cycle in which respirations increase in rate and depth, then decrease, followed by a period of apnea) occur. One of the indicators that death is approaching.

Alternative Nursing Actions

- Summon help immediately.
- Begin artificial ventilation by mouth-to-mouth, mouth-to-nose, or other airway adjunct method at the rate of 12 per minute for an adult or 20 per minute for a child.

- Relieve anxiety, fear, and stress through communication and relaxation methods.
- Relieve fever if that is the cause.
- Correct respiratory insufficiency with low-flow oxygen administration, good pulmonary toilet, and deep breathing and coughing exercises as ordered.

- If due to respiratory depressant drugs, such as opiates, barbiturates, and tranquilizers, be prepared to assist respirations or administer mouth-to-mouth resuscitation.
- Administer oxygen at 6 L/min via nasal cannulae as ordered. If client has COPD, use 2 L/min.
- Stimulate client to take breaths at least 10 times per minute.

- Provide rest after period of exertion.
- Relieve fear, anxiety, or stress.
- May be indicative of respiratory distress or cardiac disease.

- Follow physician's orders to treat underlying disease state (e.g., heart failure, increased intracranial pressure).
- Monitor respirations every 15 min to hourly, depending on client's status.
- Be prepared to administer CPR if apnea occurs.

SECTION FOUR ▪ Blood Pressure

Unexpected Outcomes	Alternative Nursing Actions
▪ Blood pressure reading is abnormally high without apparent physiologic cause.	▪ Check if arm was unsupported. ▪ Check if cuff was too narrow. ▪ Check if cuff was not snug. ▪ Check if cuff was deflated too slowly or reinflated during deflation, causing venous engorgement and abnormally high diastolic readings. ▪ Observe if mercury column, if used, was above eye level. ▪ Ask if client has pain, is anxious (white coat syndrome), or has just exercised, eaten, or smoked. ▪ Recheck pressure as indicated. ▪ Check blood pressure on both arms. The normal difference from arm to arm is usually no more than 5 mm Hg. ▪ Check if client had insufficient rest before assessment.
▪ Blood pressure reading is very low and there are no significant clinical indicators.	▪ Assess if cuff is too wide. ▪ Check if mercury column was below eye level. ▪ Check if client's arm was above heart level. ▪ Check if inflation was too slow. This reduces intensity of Korotkoff sounds. ▪ Assess if Korotkoff sounds were barely audible. Raise client's arm and then recheck. Sounds should be louder. ▪ Identify if stethoscope was was not placed on brachial artery.
▪ Hypotension (systolic pressure is less than 90 mm Hg) develops.	▪ Take blood pressure 3 min after client rises from supine to standing position if postural hypotension is suspected. ▪ Take vital signs more frequently (every 15 min to 2 hrs) until condition has stabilized. ▪ Place client in supine position with lower extremities elevated 45° and head on pillow. ▪ Assess cause of hypotension, and notify physician. ▪ Increase or administer fluids as ordered by physician. ▪ Observe postoperative clients for signs of bleeding. ▪ Administer oxygen.
▪ Korotkoff sounds cannot be heard due to hypotension.	▪ Use the palpation method or ultrasound technique. Client may be candidate for intraarterial (direct method) pressure monitoring.
▪ Hypertension (blood pressure consistently over 140/90 mm Hg) develops.	▪ For client with severe, acute hypertension, take vital signs more frequently (every 15 min to 2 hrs) until condition has stabilized. ▪ If client is anxious or excited, institute relaxation techniques to lower blood pressure. ▪ Allow client to rest after strenuous exercise.

- Relieve pain with reassurance, change of position, and analgesia as ordered by physician.
- For clients with essential hypertension, administer antihypertensive and diuretic drugs as ordered by the physician.
- Evaluate response by checking blood pressure in reclining, sitting, and standing positions. Instruct client in diet therapy, such as low salt, low fat, and inclusion of vitamins and garlic.
- For client with hypoxia, relieve with oxygen administration by most effective mode.

SELF-CHECK EVALUATION

PART 1 ▪ Matching Terms

Match the definition in column B with the correct term in column A.

Column A	Column B
a. Apnea	1. Difference between apical and radial pulse with irregular rhythm
b. Bradypnea	
c. Cheyne-Stokes respirations	2. Index of diastolic blood pressure
d. Vital signs	3. Slow, regular respirations
e. Systolic blood pressure	4. Absence of breathing
f. Set point	5. Increased rate (faster than normal)
g. Tachypnea	6. Information about condition of the heart and great arteries
h. Pulse	
i. Korotkoff sounds	7. Deep, fast respirations followed by slow rate and apnea
j. Pulse deficit	8. Index of the heart's rate and rhythm
	9. Reflects the body's physiologic status
	10. Level at which regulatory mechanisms maintain the body's core temperature

PART 2 ▪ Multiple Choice Questions

1. There are many factors that may alter vital signs. Which one of the following is the most common?

a. Pain.
b. Stress.
c. Age.
d. Exercise.

2. The normal range for an oral temperature is:

a. 96 to 105°F.
b. 97 to 99.5°F.
c. 98.6 to 99.6°F.
d. 97.6 to 98.6°F.

3. Which of the following statements is true regarding temperature?

    a. It is higher in the aged.
    b. It is highest in the early morning.
    c. It increases with exercise.
    d. It increases with colder environments.

4. The most accurate and safe method for taking a rectal temperature for a child or an adult is to insert the thermometer how many inches and hold in place for how many minutes?

    a. ½ to 1 in, 5 to 10 min.
    b. 1 to 2 in, 2 to 3 min.
    c. ½ to 1 in, 1 to 2 min.
    d. ½ to 1 in, 2 to 5 min.

5. The rationale for positioning the probe of the electronic thermometer in the sublingual pocket at the base of the tongue is that the:

    a. Client can more easily close his or her mouth, and thus an accurate temperature is obtained.
    b. Client's teeth do not rest on the probe, which can lead to an inaccurate temperature reading.
    c. Larger blood vessels in the pocket more accurately reflect the core temperature.
    d. Blood supply is limited in that area, so it does not cause a false temperature reading.

6. The appropriate method for obtaining an apical pulse is to use the:

    a. Bell of the stethoscope; listen at the 2nd intercostal space, right side of sternum.
    b. Bell of the stethoscope; listen at the 5th intercostal space, left sternal border.
    c. Diaphragm of the stethoscope; listen at the 2nd intercostal space, left sternal border.
    d. Diaphragm of the stethoscope; listen at the 5th intercostal space, midclavicular line.

7. The most accepted method of obtaining an apical-radial pulse is:

    a. One nurse counts the pulse for 1 min, first at the brachial site and then at the apical site.
    b. One nurse counts the pulse for 1 min at the brachial and apical sites simultaneously.
    c. Two nurses count the pulse for 1 min simultaneously, one at the apical site and one at the radial site, using one watch.
    d. Two nurses count the pulse for 1 min, first one at the apical site and second one at the radial site, each using her or his own watch.

8. Conductive gel is applied to the client's skin before performing Doppler ultrasound to facilitate the movement of the ultrasound beam. To assist with this process, the nurse must ensure that:

    a. The old gel is removed before applying new gel.
    b. An airtight seal is maintained between the probe and skin.
    c. The Doppler machine is turned to the OFF position until it is placed on the skin.
    d. The gel is liberally spread over a 2 × 2 cm area on the client's skin.

9. The bladder of the blood pressure cuff should be what percentage of the circumference of the limb?

    a. 40 percent.
    b. 50 percent.
    c. 60 percent.
    d. 70 percent.

10. If the client's arm is positioned below the level of the heart when taking the blood pressure, the reading will be:

    a. Lower than normal.
    b. No different than if the arm were positioned above the level of the heart.
    c. Higher than normal.
    d. Altered if the client has peripheral vascular disease only.

11. The blood pressure cuff is wrapped snugly and smoothly around the upper arm:

    a. ½ in above the antecubital space.
    b. 1 in above the antecubital space.
    c. 1 in down from the axilla.
    d. 2 in down from the axilla.

12. When using the stethoscope for taking a blood pressure reading, the nurse needs to remember that:

    a. The bell detects high-pitched sounds best.
    b. The diaphragm detects low-pitched sounds best.
    c. Korotkoff sounds are best heard by the portion of the stethoscope that detects low-frequency sounds.
    d. Either bell or diaphragm can be used, as frequency sounds are not detected with blood pressure readings.

13. The blood pressure cuff is deflated:

    a. Quickly at 5 mm Hg/sec.
    b. Slowly at 2 mm Hg/sec.
    c. Gradually at 2 mm Hg/sec.
    d. At a rate that does not exceed 5 mm Hg/sec.

14. A client who requires peripheral pulses to be monitored using Doppler can be assigned to which member of the team?

    a. CNA/UAP.
    b. RN.
    c. RN or LVN/LPN.
    d. All of the above.

PART 3 ▪ Critical Thinking Application

An elderly client (age 90) has just been admitted to your medical floor. The client's vital signs are temperature 103.4°F, blood pressure 140/90, pulse 114, and respirations 30 and labored. He reports a history of 3 days of diarrhea and fever, and asks you, the nurse, for something to drink. After analyzing the admission data, respond to the following parameters using your critical thinking skills.

1. What is the appropriate nursing diagnosis for this client?

2. What are the metabolic effects of fever on pulse and respiration?

3. Consider the other assessment findings that would be indicative of the diagnosis you established from the admission data.

4. How does the client's age contribute to the existing problems?

5. What is a plan of care for this client?

6. What would you look for in terms of the evaluative outcomes for resolution of the client's problems?

10

HEAT AND COLD

INTRODUCTION

Heat and cold receptors adapt rapidly to temperature changes in the body's environment. Tolerance to changes in heat and cold depends on the part of the body affected. The perineum, the inner aspect of the forearm, and the wrist are very sensitive to changes in heat and cold. The foot and the back of the hand are not very sensitive to these changes. In addition to these sensitive areas of the body, several other factors play a role in the body's reaction to temperature changes. Clients with altered skin integrity are more sensitive to changes in temperature than clients whose skin is intact. For example, burn clients are very sensitive to changes in temperature due to loss of skin and, perhaps, subcutaneous tissue. This is because fewer receptors are available to warn the client of tissue damage. Clients with subcutaneous and visceral tissue damage are the most sensitive to temperature alterations because they have the fewest available receptors.

Individuals react differently to temperature changes based on age, size of the exposed body part, and length of exposure. The very young and the very old have more difficulty adjusting to temperature variations. Young children have immature thermoregulation control and cannot easily communicate pain or discomfort. In elderly clients, altered

(continued on next page)

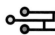

nerve conduction may affect pain sensation, or alterations in circulation may prevent identification of complications. Clients with a mental status impairment, such as confusion or altered level of consciousness, or those with a sensory deficit, such as a spinal cord injury, are unable to determine when a negative response to heat or cold occurs.

In addition to age and physiological alterations, there are other factors involved in client reactions to temperature. The larger the involved area, the lower the tolerance will be to changes in temperature. The longer an application of heat or cold lasts, the more tolerant the client becomes. This can lead to complications associated with prolonged heat and cold applications. Individuals feel the change in temperature when the application is first applied and alters the temperature of a particular body part. It does not make a difference whether the application is hot or cold.

Therapeutic use of heat or cold applications is vital for many clients. Heat applications are used to resolve inflammation, improve healing of soft tissues, and relieve muscle pain and joint stiffness. Cold applications are usually used immediately following soft tissue trauma or for clients with joint involvement. Cold promotes vasoconstriction; therefore it is used to control local bleeding, edema, and pain. When blood flow to an injury site is reduced, edema is avoided.

Client safety must be considered when choosing heat and cold applications. Either heat or cold can damage tissues or alter thermoregulation control. Systemic effects can also occur with either of these therapies. Extensive use of heat over a large body surface

CLINICAL NOTE

Follow these guidelines when applying heat and cold applications:

- Evaluate client's physical status before initiating therapy to prevent systemic complications.
- Determine if there are any contraindications present to prevent use of these therapies.
- Determine client's understanding of treatment and ability to inform you of any untoward effects.
- Assess integrity of skin where application is to be applied.
- Explain purpose of and procedure for heat or cold application.
- Determine type of application most appropriate for client's condition.
- Determine length of time most therapeutic for client, keeping time parameters in mind.
- Take client's vital signs, if appropriate.
- Assess client 10 to 15 min after application is begun; determine if untoward effects are occurring.
- Assess client's skin after removing application.
- Determine client's response to treatment.
- Document findings.

may cause peripheral vasodilation, leading to hypotension and fainting. This occurs more in clients with circulatory or pulmonary disease. Cold therapy leads to vasoconstriction with a resultant increase in blood pressure as blood is shunted from the periphery to the core of the body. Shivering is a manifestation of this effect. A rebound phenomenon occurs when heat or cold applications are left on the area beyond the prescribed time. This phenomenon occurs at the time the maximum therapeutic effect of the hot or cold application is achieved and causes the opposite effect to take place. For example, when cold applications are applied, vasoconstriction occurs when the skin temperature reaches 60°F (15.7°C). When the temperature drops below 60°F (15.7°C), the opposite action—vasodilation—occurs. This is the body's protective mechanism to prevent freezing of delicate tissues. Heat produces maximum vasodilation in 20 to 30 min. Beyond 30 to 45 min, vasoconstriction and tissue congestion occur and the client is at risk for complications associated with the inability to dissipate heat via the circulatory system.

The physiological effects of heat and cold are in opposition to one another. Beneficial effects related to thermal treatment include the following:

- Heat produces vasodilation.
- Cold produces vasoconstriction.
- Heat decreases pain through its relaxation effect on muscles.
- Cold decreases pain through slowing nerve impulse conduction, thus increasing the pain threshold.
- Cold also acts as an anesthetic by numbing the affected area, thus decreasing pain.
- Heat increases capillary permeability and cellular metabolism, which can lead to loss of fluids into the tissue, causing edema.
- Cold decreases capillary permeability and cellular metabolism, thus preventing a transfer of fluids and reducing the risk of edema.

PREPARATION PROTOCOL: FOR HEAT AND COLD

Complete the following steps before each skill.

1. Check physician's orders and client's plan of care.
2. Gather appropriate equipment, based on client's condition.
3. Check client's identaband.
4. Introduce yourself to client and explain nursing care you will be giving.
5. Provide privacy for client as needed.
6. Wash hands.
7. Don gloves if there is risk of contact with blood or body fluids.
8. Assess client's skin at site where application is to be applied.

COMPLETION PROTOCOL: FOR HEAT AND COLD

Make sure the following steps have been completed.

1. Remove heat or cold application.
2. Assess area for signs of redness, cyanosis, disrupted skin, or excessive temperature.
3. Return client to position of comfort.
4. Clean and/or dispose of equipment in appropriate location.
5. Remove gloves and discard in appropriate receptacle.
6. Wash hands.
7. Document pertinent data and report as indicated.

SECTION ONE

HEAT THERAPY

The physiologic effects of heat application include vasodilation, increased metabolism leading to growth of new tissue, increased capillary permeability, activation of the autonomic nervous system, and increased muscle relaxation.

As stated earlier, heat dilates blood vessels and increases capillary permeability. This physiologic response increases the blood flow to a specific area of the body. Capillary permeability and increased blood supply provide a mechanism by which nutrients and oxygen reach tissues while at the same time toxins and wastes are removed. Heat also decreases venous congestion and pain at an injury site. As fluid is removed through vasodilation, pain is decreased as a result of decreased pressure on the nerve endings. There is a potential complication associated with capillary permeability. Increased capillary permeability can lead to the formation of edema, third spacing, or pain due to pressure on the nerve endings from the excess fluid.

Heat stimulates metabolism and growth of new tissue through increased blood supply to the injured area. The increased permeability that occurs with heat application assists in clearing debris from an infected area through suppuration. Heat also reduces blood viscosity, allowing leukocytes and antibodies to reach the affected area more readily.

Dry heat therapy using Aqua K pads, commercial heat packs, and heating pads is most often used to relieve pain and support suppuration. Moist heat administered via hot moist compresses, sterile moist compresses, and sitz baths is used to promote muscle relaxation, reduce edema and inflammation, debride wounds, and apply medication to wounds.

RATIONALE

- To produce local vasodilation
- To increase circulation to affected area
- To promote comfort for injured area
- To improve tissue metabolism in infected area
- To increase mobility of leukocytes
- To hasten suppuration and soften exudate from wound

ASSESSMENT

- Assess skin condition before and after heat application; observe for redness, burns, or blisters related to application.
- Check for appropriate type of heat application.
- Check for appropriate length of time for application.
- Determine if client's vital signs need to be monitored.

HOT MOIST PACK

Equipment

- 4 × 4 gauze pads for hot packs
- ABD pads
- Aqua K pad (optional)
- Absorbent pad for moisture barrier
- Container for warming solution bottle
- Petroleum jelly (optional)
- Towel for securing pack (if Aqua K pad is not used)
- Safety pins
- Clean gloves (optional)
- Sterile gloves (for open wound)

SKILL

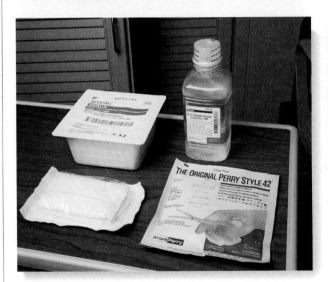

1 Gather equipment and warm solution bottle in pan of hot water for 10 to 15 min. Solution is warmed to 105 to 110°F. **RATIONALE:** Temperatures higher than 105 to 110°F may cause burns.

- Place absorbent pad under area where pack will be applied. **RATIONALE:** To prevent bed from getting wet. Absorbent pad can be used as outside covering for hot pack if Aqua K pad is not used. It will keep pack warm and intact.

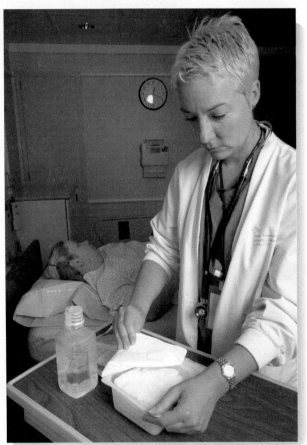

2 Open all containers and packages, including gloves if they are to be used. **RATIONALE:** Clean gloves are worn if there is risk of contact with blood or body fluids.

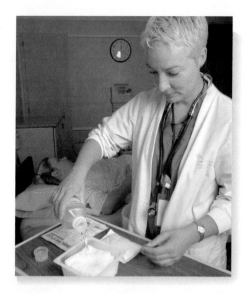

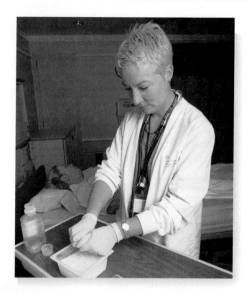

(3) Pour solution into gauze pad container. This container is waterproof and sterile.

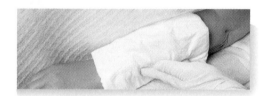

(5) Place an ABD pad over the gauze pads. **RATIO-NALE:** To maintain position of pads and to absorb excess solution. Check client's comfort level and application site after 30 sec to determine if temperature of pack is satisfactory.

- Discard disposable items in appropriate containers.

(4) Put gloves on as needed. Wring excess moisture from gauze pads.

- Place 4 × 4 gauze pads over area. Number of pads is dependent on extent of area to be covered. Ensure there is a sufficient number of pads to maintain moist environment for at least 20 min.
- A light layer of petroleum jelly may be placed over the affected area if there is not an open wound. **RATIONALE:** To protect skin from excoriation due to extended periods of moisture.

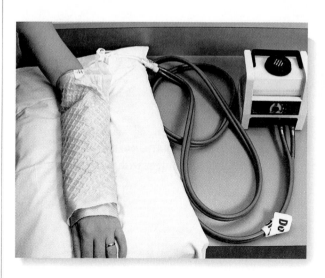

(6) Place absorbent pad over area and tape securely or apply Aqua K pad to area (see Aqua K pad skill on page 257).

- Check client after 5 min to determine comfort level.
- Remove pack after 20 to 25 min. Leave pack off at least 4 hrs before reapplying. **RATIONALE:** To prevent local or systemic effects of treatment.
- Put on clean gloves, if needed for removing pack.
- Dry area and remove petroleum jelly, if used.
- Check area for adverse signs from heat application.

HOT STERILE MOIST COMPRESS

Equipment

- Sterile 4 × 4 gauze pads
- Sterile ABD pads
- Sterile absorbent pad
- Sterile bowl or clean bowl
- Aqua K pad
- Sterile towel (optional)
- Sterile solution
- Sterile gloves

SAFETY ALERT

If the client has a circulatory or respiratory condition, vital signs should be assessed before hot compresses are placed. **RATIONALE:** Systemic effects can occur when hot compresses are used. Hypotension can result from vasodilation in clients with these conditions.

SKILL

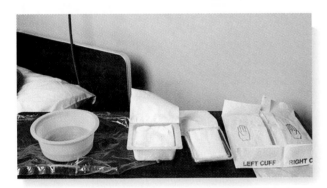

1 Warm sterile solution by placing bottle for 15 min in pan of hot water (not to exceed 110°F [43.7°C]).

- When solution is warm, open sterile supplies and place on over-bed table in preparation for application.
- Pour sterile solution into gauze pad container. **RATIONALE:** Container is sterile and leakproof.
- Expose area for application of compresses and check skin for altered integrity.

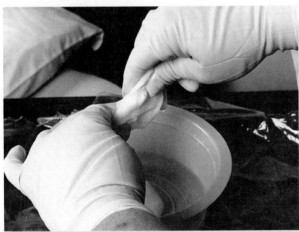

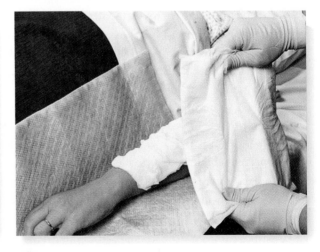

2 Don sterile gloves.

- Wring out gauze pads as dry as possible, maintaining sterility.
- Place gauze dressings over site. Place sufficient number of pads to ensure adequate coverage of area.

3 Cover area with ABD pads.

- Wrap sterile absorbent pad or towel over dressings and tape or pin in place.
- Check client's comfort level after 30 sec. **RATIONALE:** To determine if temperature of hot compresses is comfortable.

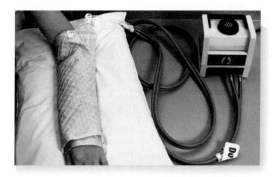

4 Apply Aqua K pad over pad or towel. Set temperature to 105 to 110°F (40.9 to 43.7°C). **RATIONALE:** This temperature setting will prevent trauma to tissue.

- Check with client in 5 min to determine comfort level.
- Remove pack in 20 to 25 min and check client's skin. **RATIONALE:** To prevent rebound vasoconstriction from occurring.

BEYOND THE SKILL

Sitz Bath

Equipment

- Portable sitz bath or bathroom sitz bath
- Towels (three to four)
- Inflatable tub ring (optional)
- Bath blanket
- Clean gown
- Clean gloves (if needed)

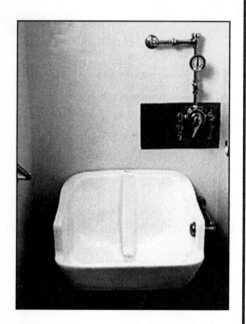

Skill

1. Take linen to bathroom for sitz bath, or place linen on chair in room if using portable sitz bath.
2. Fill sitz bath about one-third full of water between 105 and 110°F (40.8 and 43.7°C). *Note:* A bathtub can be used if a sitz tub is not available. Follow same steps when using a bathtub.
3. Place inflatable ring or towel in sitz bath. **RATIONALE:** Provides for comfort. Place towel on floor in front of sitz bath.
4. Assist client with undressing as needed.
5. Check temperature of water.
6. Assist client into sitz bath. Ensure water temperature is comfortable for client.
7. Place towel or bath blanket over client's shoulders. **RATIONALE:** To prevent chilling and provide privacy.
8. Close curtain or door. Place call bell within easy reach of client.
9. Check on client frequently during the 20- to 25-min procedure.
10. Don clean gloves, if needed.
11. Assist client from sitz bath and assist with drying and dressing as needed.
12. Clean sitz bath and discard linen into hamper.
13. Remove gloves and discard. Wash hands.
14. Assist client back to bed or into chair.

AQUATHERMIC (AQUA K) PAD

Equipment

- Aquathermic reservoir container
- Aquathermic pad (disposable)
- Distilled water

CLINICAL NOTE

It is not necessary to cover the Aqua K pad; the nonwoven surface can be placed directly against the client's skin. The pads are for one-client use only and are disposed of after completion of therapy. Either side of the pad can be used for dry heat therapy. The pad can be used for moist heat therapy by moistening the nonwoven fabric side of the pad.

SKILL

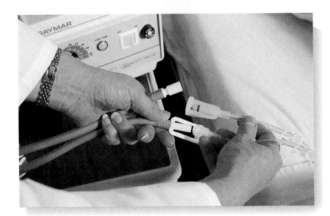

1 Check equipment for frayed cords, water leaks, etc.

- Fill reservoir container two-thirds full with distilled water.
- Place reservoir container on bedside stand and plug into electrical outlet. **RATIONALE:** Reservoir needs to be at bed level to allow for water circulation throughout system.
- Place temperature control at low setting.
- Connect pad to reservoir by inserting male fittings into female fittings with a twisting motion.
- When fittings are fully inserted, snap locking ring into place. Ensure that fittings are snug. **RATIONALE:** To prevent leaking from system.
- Turn on switch and allow water to circulate through pad. Ensure temperature does not exceed 105°F (40.9°C).

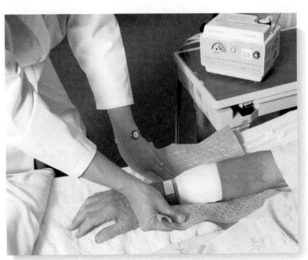

2 Fold pad to size/shape desired. Ensure that pad surface with tubes is placed against client's extremity.

- Assess skin before application of pad and 2 to 3 min after pad is applied. **RATIONALE:** To ensure that skin is not reddened or exhibiting any untoward reaction to heat.
- Check that temperature is comfortable for client.

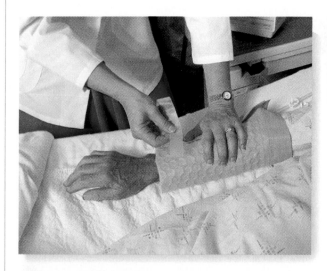

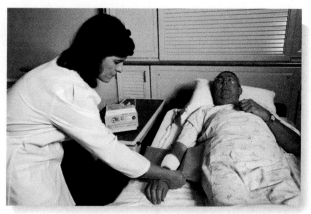

③ Secure pad with tape. Do not use safety pins. **RATIONALE:** Safety pins can pierce coils in pad, leading to leak in system.

④ Remove pad after 20 min. Observe area for redness, pain, or any untoward effects.

- Place pad on overbed table for next use. (The pad is for use by a single client only. Each client has his or her own disposable pad.)
- Reposition client for comfort.

CLINICAL NOTE

Commercial disposable hot packs are available. Read the manufacturer's directions carefully. Each brand is activated differently; some are heated in the microwave, some are heated in boiling water, and others are activated by striking or kneading the pack. The pack should be covered with a towel and placed on the affected area. Use tape (do not use safety pins) to secure the pack in place.

CHARTING

- Appearance of skin before and after application
- Length of time of application
- Specific type of application used
- Client's response to application

SECTION TWO

COLD THERAPY

The physiologic effects of cold treatments to the body are mainly vasoconstriction and decreased metabolism. Vasoconstriction of blood vessels and the resulting decreased supply of blood to an injured area prevent edema. Decreased metabolism and decreased cellular activity reduce inflammation by reducing the amount of oxygen and nutrients available to the tissue. Cold therapy acts like a local anesthetic, blocking pain receptors and slowing nerve impulse conduction, which reduces pain. Increased blood coagulation at the injury site occurs as a result of increased blood viscosity from cold therapy. Some forms of cold therapy are also used to reduce fever and temperature.

Cold therapy, like heat therapy, can be either moist or dry. Moist therapy is given in the form of tepid baths or cold compresses. Tepid baths reduce fever by promoting heat loss through conduction and vaporization. A tepid bath is one in which the temperature is 90°F (32°C). A fan may be used in conjunction with a tepid bath. The increased air movement aids in lowering the body temperature through convection. The application of an ice pack or ice collar is also considered dry therapy. These applications provide cold to a localized area. Full-body hypothermia is sometimes used when a client has a very high fever that is not controlled with medication or if there is a risk of cerebral edema following head injury or cranial surgery. It can also be used in some surgical procedures in which the body temperature needs to be lowered.

RATIONALE

- To promote vasoconstriction
- To decrease edema
- To reduce pain
- To decrease temperature
- To reduce fever
- To decrease bleeding

ASSESSMENT

- Assess client's condition to determine if cold therapy can be tolerated.
- Check if antipyretic medications have been administered.
- Assess condition of client's skin before and after application to determine if alterations have occurred.
- Assess client's vital signs and determine if any contraindications to cold therapy exist.

SAFETY ALERT

A mixture of alcohol and water may be ordered for the tepid bath, although it is ordered less frequently than water. It should be used cautiously, as alcohol has a drying effect on the skin. Alcohol removes body heat quickly and evaporates at a lower temperature than does water, thus decreasing the body's temperature more quickly than water alone.

TEPID SPONGE BATH

Equipment

- Basin filled with water at 70 to 90°F
- Thermometer
- Washcloths (four to six) and towels
- Bath blanket or sheet

SKILL

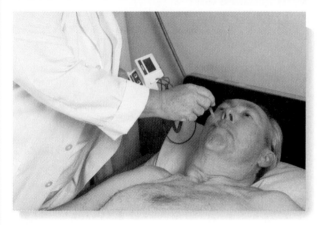

1 Take client's vital signs before beginning bath and every 15 min during and after completion of bath. **RATIONALE:** To monitor effectiveness of bath.

- Place absorbent pads under client to protect bed from becoming wet.

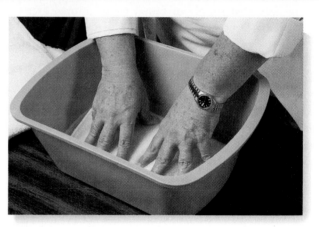

2 Place washcloths in basin of water.

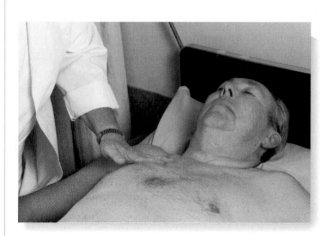

3 Feel client's skin temperature, check turgor, and observe skin color for assessment database. Assessments are completed throughout sponge bath. If client's skin becomes pale or cyanotic or pulse is rapid or irregular, stop bath.

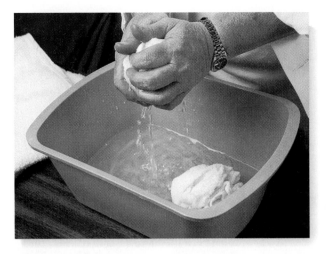

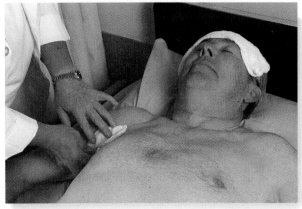

4 Wring excess water from washcloths and sponge client's face, arms, legs, back, and buttocks. Each area is sponged gently. **RATIONALE:** Rubbing the skin can lead to heat production.

- Sponge one part of client's body at a time. The bath should take about 30 min. **RATIONALE:** If bath is done more quickly, shivering may occur and will increase the body's heat production. Stop bath immediately if shivering occurs.
- If desired, leave area wet and place damp towel over area to decrease temperature more quickly.

5 Place cool cloth on head, axilla, and groin during bath. **RATIONALE:** These areas contain large superficial blood vessels that aid in dissipating heat.

- Cool room air to 68 to 72°F (20 to 22.2°C) if possible.
- Promote movement of air with fan, if possible.

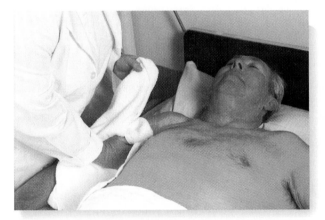

6 Replace washcloths every 5 min. **RATIONALE:** This prevents washcloths from holding onto body heat.

- Once body temperature reaches ideal point (based on physician's order), remove washcloths and towel, dry client, and place sheet over client. Do not place heavy linens on client as this could cause client's temperature to rise again.
- Discard linen into hamper.

CLINICAL NOTE

Follow these steps when using a noncommercial ice application:

- Follow tepid sponge protocol for monitoring client's vital signs and physical condition.
- Fill ice container (ice cap, ice glove, ice collar, or freeze bag) two-thirds full with crushed ice. Express all air and shut top securely.
- Cover ice pack with towel and tape towel shut.
- Place ice pack on designated area.
- Secure pack with gauze strip or tape.
- Remove pack every 10 min during 30-min application. Check client's skin for redness, mottled or gray color, or blisters. Remove ice pack if skin shows any abnormal effects of application.
- Discard towel in hamper; save ice container if additional applications will be necessary.

INSTANT COLD PACK

Equipment

- Commercial cold pack
- Towel
- Tape

SKILL

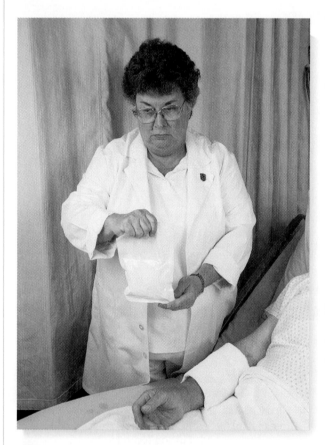

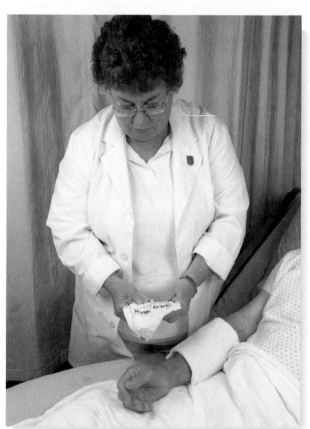

① Remove outer wrap from cold pack. If packs come in different sizes, choose appropriate size to cover site.

- Check client's skin site before, during, and following application.

② Following manufacturer's directions, squeeze cold pack to break inner pouch and activate chemical response. **RATIONALE:** This releases alcohol-based solution that produces cold effect.

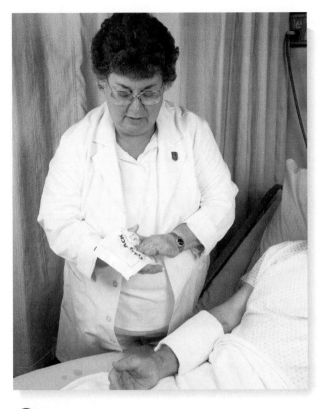

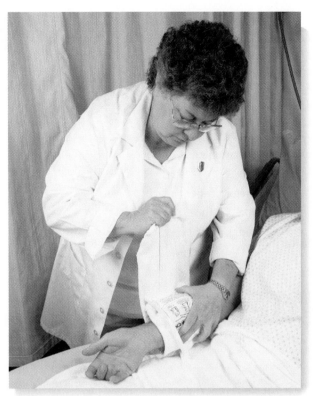

3 Pat cold pack to gently mix chemicals together.

■ Check that pack is not broken or punctured. **RATIONALE:** If solution touches skin, chemicals can burn skin.

4 If pack has a protective cover, it can be placed directly on site. Otherwise, wrap pack in a towel.

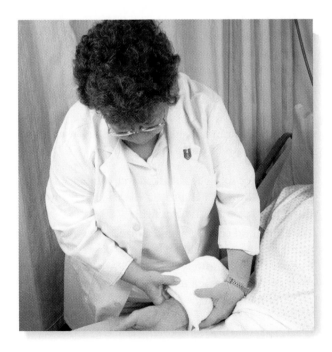

5 Stabilize pack by wrapping a towel around it and securing with tape or gauze.

■ Remove pack after 5 min to check skin for untoward effects.

■ Leave pack in place for 20 to 25 min. Check skin area every 10 min. **RATIONALE:** The temperature is about 59°F (15°C); therefore alteration in skin integrity can occur with some clients.

HYPOTHERMIA BLANKET

Equipment

- Disposable cooling blanket, top or bottom (or both)
- Cooling machine
- Thermometer
- Sphygmomanometer
- Stethoscope
- Thermometer probe
- Thin blanket or sheet
- Towels (four)

CLINICAL NOTE

CLASSIFICATION OF HYPOTHERMIA

Mild	89.6 to 98.6°F (32 to 37°C)
Moderate	82.4 to 89.6°F (28 to 32°C)
Deep	68.0 to 82.4°F (20 to 28°C)
Profound	0 to 68.0°F (0 to 20°C)

SKILL

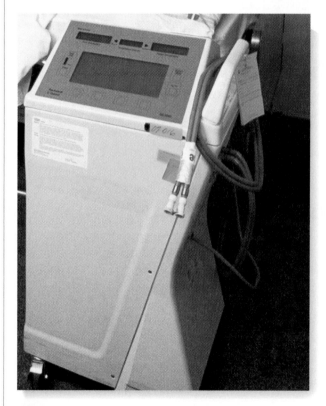

1 Bring cooling blanket and machine to client's bedside.

- Check that all solution levels are full or adequate; if not, return to CSR.
- Take baseline vital signs before starting treatment. **RATIONALE:** Baseline temperature is essential to determine effects of treatment.

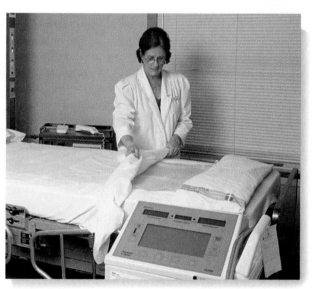

2 Place hypothermia blanket on bed. Blanket usually fits entire length of bed.

- Place sheet or thin bath blanket over cooling blanket. **RATIONALE:** To protect client's skin from direct contact with cold blanket.
- Place client on cooling blanket. Place sheet or top cooling blanket on client, if ordered. Wrap client's feet and hands in towels if needed. **RATIONALE:** To prevent frostbite when temperature is set at maximum low setting.

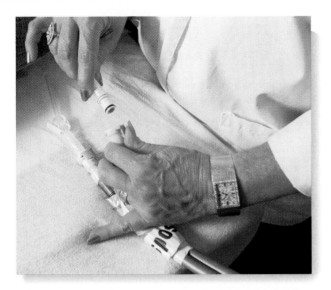

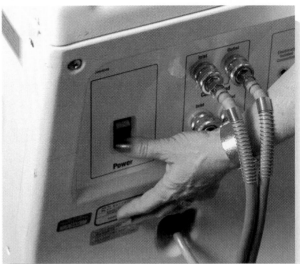

3 Connect cooling blanket to machine:

- Push connector tab down. Insert male tubing connector of cooling pad into inlet opening. Release tab.
- Repeat connection using outlet opening.
- Ensure that fittings are tight.

4 Turn unit on by pushing power switch.

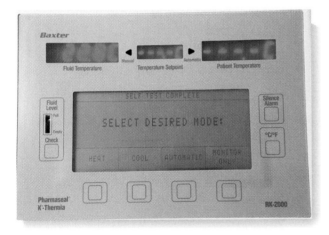

5 Set master temperature control to either automatic or manual operation. *Note:* The same machine can be used to cool or heat. Be careful you select the correct application for the machine.

Automatic Control

- Insert probe into client's rectum. Remove and clean probe every 4 hrs.
- Set temperature control at desired temperature (fluid temperature set point).
- Observe that automatic mode light is on.
- Check that pad temperature limits are set at desired safety limits.
- Press START when fluid set point is correct.

Manual Control

- Insert probe into client's rectum.
- Observe that manual mode light is on.
- Monitor fluid set point, which indicates temperature of pad. **RATIONALE:** This ensures pad temperature is maintained at desired level.

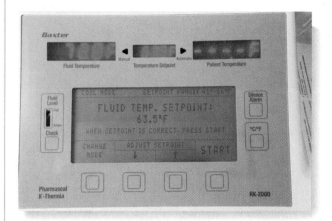

6 Set temperature control at 98.6°F (37°C). Lower temperature 2 to 3°F every 15 min until 90°F is reached (or set temperature according to physician's order or hospital policy). Keep blanket on at set temperature until client's body temperature is close to normal. Gradually increase blanket temperature over 6 hrs or turn machine off and monitor client's temperature. **RATIONALE:** Determines client's ability to maintain body temperature without use of cooling blanket.

■ Remove cooling blanket when client's temperature is stabilized.

SAFETY ALERT

Maintain safety measures for clients on hypothermia blankets by using these guidelines:

■ Monitor client's body temperature every 15 min. (This is automatically recorded when rectal temperature probe is used.)

■ Check automatic temperature control for accuracy every 4 hrs by taking client's temperature with external thermometer. Use appropriate type of thermometer (oral, rectal, axillary) based on client's condition.

■ Monitor all vital signs every 30 min during hypothermia treatment. Monitor every 2 hrs for 24 hrs after treatment is discontinued.

■ Monitor with ECG if client has cardiac condition.

■ Observe client closely for signs of shivering (ECG muscle tremor artifact, visible facial muscle twitching, hyperventilation, verbalized sensations). If shivering occurs, obtain order for IV medications (usually chlorpromazine). **RATIONALE:** Shivering increases heat production by thermogenesis.

■ Observe obese clients for fluid balance alterations.

■ Check physician's orders for and apply thigh-high support stockings, because stockings prevent venous stasis.

■ Monitor client's skin condition and bony prominences every 2 hrs. **RATIONALE:** Client is at risk for altered tissue integrity when skin temperature is low and skin is moist.

■ Observe client for signs of edema, particularly dependent edema. **RATIONALE:** Edema can be caused by increased cellular permeability, acidotic shock due to shivering, fluid imbalance, or hypothermia.

CHARTING

■ Client's vital signs, particularly temperature
■ Untoward effects of treatment and actions taken

■ Settings on cooling blanket
■ Condition of skin

CRITICAL THINKING FOCUS

SECTION ONE ■ Heat Therapy

Unexpected Outcomes

- Affected limb throbs with increased circulation.

- Pain occurs in affected site or is increased in intensity.

- Client's core temperature rises above normal or desired value.

- Altered tissue integrity occurs.

Alternative Nursing Action

- Elevate extremity above level of heart to increase venous return.
- Assess if application is too heavy and putting excess pressure on vessel.
- Check peripheral pulses.

- Evaluate if temperature of application is too hot for client comfort. Reduce temperature of application to one of comfort for client.
- Ensure that temperature is not over 110°F (43.7°C).
- Check surrounding tissue for erythema or signs of burning.

- Remove heat source immediately.
- Avoid chilling client; place bath blanket or blanket over client.
- Monitor vital signs frequently until they return to normal or desired levels.

- If client's skin is reddened but not blistered or open, remove heat application and notify physician.
- If nonblanchable erythema of intact skin occurs, obtain order for adhesive transparent film dressing (e.g., Tegaderm).
- If blisters or open lesion are present, obtain order for hydrocolloid dressing (e.g., DuoDerm).

SECTION TWO ■ Cold Therapy

Unexpected Outcomes

- Local edema is not reduced.

- Internal (core) temperature drops too low.

- Skin becomes irritated or macerated from sponging or cooling measures.

Alternative Nursing Action

- Elevate extremity above level of heart.
- Ensure affected area is covered entirely to provide for vasoconstriction.
- Apply cold treatment for first 24 hrs until edema has dissipated, as ordered.

- Place blanket over unaffected areas.
- Monitor vital signs, particularly temperature, frequently.

- Remove cold application from area.
- Use alternate site, if appropriate.
- Apply petroleum jelly to area and use alternative surface site for treatment.

- Do not massage or rub area, as this action can cause tissue damage.

- Total numbness occurs at site of cold application.
  - Warm area immediately by placing extremity in 110°F (43.7°C) water.
  - Remove extremity from water when red flush appears.
  - Apply loose, dry dressing if area appears broken down.
  - Observe circulation closely for any abnormal findings.
  - Observe for signs of frostbite.

- Pain occurs at site of cold application.
  - Remove pack immediately.
  - Warm site a few degrees.
  - Assess for tissue damage.

- Client's core temperature decreases rapidly and falls below 98.6°F (37°C) when using hypothermia blanket.
  - Turn cooling blanket off.
  - Remove top blanket, if used.
  - Place blanket over client.
  - Set blanket at higher temperature when treatment is resumed.
  - Monitor vital signs every 15 min until temperature increases to 98.6°F (37°C).
  - If temperature continues to fall, blanket can be set for warming.

- Client's core temperature is not reduced.
  - Check master temperature control to see what limits are set. Limit may need to be decreased or lowered. Do not set below 86°F (30°C) without checking with physician.
  - Place top cooling pad on client to provide greater body surface area in contact with cold therapy.

- Altered skin integrity occurs with use of cooling blanket.
  - After treating any skin lesions, begin preventative treatment when restarting cooling blanket.
  - Turn client every 30 min while on cooling blanket.
  - Lubricate skin with petroleum jelly to provide protection.
  - Wrap client's hands and feet in towels to prevent frostbite.
  - Check bony prominences at least every hour.
  - Ensure that master control temperature is not set too low.

- Cooling blanket does not function properly.
  - Check that plug is connected tightly to outlet.
  - Check that connectors are tight.
  - Check that fluid level is sufficient and that unit freezing has not occurred.
  - Check that cool limit on pad is not set too high.
  - Check that there is no constriction through pads or tubing.

SELF-CHECK EVALUATION

PART 1 ▪ Matching Terms

Match the definition in column B with the correct term in column A.

Column A

_____ a. Conduction
_____ b. Hypothermia
_____ c. Evaporation
_____ d. Convection
_____ e. Erythema
_____ f. Thermogenesis

Column B

1. Heat production by the body
2. Increased red color of skin due to vasodilation of capillaries
3. Transfer of heat by air
4. Conversion from a liquid state to a gaseous state
5. A body temperature lower than normal
6. Transfer of heat by direct contact through fluids, solids, or any suitable substance

PART 2 ▪ Multiple Choice Questions

1. Heat conservation is accomplished by:

a. Shivering.
b. Vasomotor constriction.
c. Nonshivering thermogenesis.
d. Peripheral vasodilation.

2. The most effective mechanism for heat loss is:

a. Evaporation.
b. Shivering.
c. Decreased metabolic activity.
d. Vasoconstriction.

3. Application of heat for short intervals produces which of the following effects?

a. Vasodilation of all vessels.
b. Decrease in general heat production.
c. Decrease in leukocyte mobility.
d. Increase in peripheral heat production.

4. Which one of the following actions would not be included in applying heat or cold applications?

a. Place a protective layer of petroleum jelly on the skin.
b. Observe the skin for color and integrity.
c. Maintain temperature below 86°F (30°C) for cold therapy.
d. Take vital signs before, during, and after therapy.

5. Nursing assessments that should be completed during a tepid bath include all of the following except:

a. Extent of the client's ability to assist in treatment.
b. Vital signs.
c. Condition of the skin.
d. Presence of shivering.

6. While you are administering a tepid bath, the client begins to shiver. Your immediate intervention is to:

   a. Continue with the bath, as this helps dissipate the heat.
   b. Stop the bath for a few minutes and place a warm blanket on the client to stop the shivering.
   c. Stop the bath, as the body is attempting to produce heat.
   d. Warm the solution, continue the bath, and change the location of the washcloth.

7. During an assessment, you find the client's skin is irritated from the continuous use of an ice application. Your nursing action is to:

   a. Massage the skin directly over application site to bring blood to the area.
   b. Massage the whole area to warm it.
   c. Place a towel between the body area and the ice application.
   d. Place the ice application on an alternative body surface.

8. When applying hot, moist packs, your next action, after lubricating the skin with petroleum jelly, is to:

   a. Check the skin for redness.
   b. Place the moist pack over an unaffected area to check for heat tolerance.
   c. Place a moistureproof pad under the affected area.
   d. Place towels over the affected area.

9. For proper functioning of an Aqua K pad, which one of the following actions must be carried out?

   a. The reservoir container is kept full at all times.
   b. The reservoir container is kept below the bed for adequate water circulation.
   c. The pad is covered with a bath blanket to maintain heat to the specified area.
   d. The pad is placed on an extremity with gauze or tape to secure it in place.

PART 3 ■ Critical Thinking Application

During the morning assessment you identify that one of your clients has a temperature of 101°F (38.6°C). The client had abdominal surgery 2 days ago and has had IVs since surgery.

1. What priority actions will you take? State a rationale for your actions.
2. What clinical manifestations would indicate a call to the physician for a hot moist compress order? Provide a rationale for your answer.
3. State the major safety precautions for hot moist compresses and the scientific rationale for the precautions.
4. After removing the hot moist compress, you assess that the skin is red and blistered. What immediate actions will you take?

11

WOUND CARE AND DRESSINGS

INTRODUCTION

In order for a wound to occur, there must be a disruption in skin integrity. This can be caused by a surgical incision, invasive technique, chronic peripheral vascular disease, restricted mobility, or trauma. Age influences skin integrity relative to fragility and susceptibility to injury and breakdown, with the very young and the very old being most affected. Clients who have chronic illnesses and are undergoing specific treatments for these conditions have increased problems with skin integrity. Clients with peripheral vascular disease are commonly affected by altered skin integrity, particularly lower extremity ulcers. The use of corticosteroids for long-term respiratory or immune system disorders predisposes clients to fragile skin and poor wound healing.

Factors to be considered in order to prevent disruption in skin integrity include awareness of preventative measures to promote healthy skin and prevent skin breakdown, requirements for nutritional support, and teaching of high-risk clients. A diet high in protein, carbohydrates, vitamins A and C, and iron is essential for collagen synthesis during wound healing.

Nurses must also be aware of the physiology of wound healing so they can more

(continued on next page)

effectively care for clients with wounds and plan wound care management. There are three types of wound healing: primary intention, the simplest form of healing when the skin has been cleanly incised through surgical incision or laceration; secondary intention, when the wound heals by granulation; and tertiary intention, when the wound is left open to heal due to infection and the need for frequent irrigations and dressing changes.

There are several different classification systems used to describe wounds. These systems categorize wounds by cause (intentional or unintentional), cleanliness (clean, contaminated, or infected), depth (superficial, partial thickness, or full thickness), and color. The red-yellow-black (RYB) classification system has been used in wound classification since the late 1980s. This system classifies acute and chronic open wounds that are healing by secondary or delayed primary intention. It is used as an adjunct to other classification systems. The RYB system identifies what phase a wound is in on the continuum of the wound healing process.

Red (R) wounds can be in the inflammatory, proliferative, or maturation phase. Yellow (Y) wounds are infected or contain fibrinous slough and are not ready to heal. Black (B) wounds contain necrotic tissue and are not ready to heal. Treatment options are based on the color of the wound. Red wounds need to be kept clean and moist. Yellow wounds require the removal of slough or fibrinous tissue. Black wounds must have the eschar removed for healing to take place. If the wound has a combination of colors, the rule is that treatment corresponding to the most severe color is used.

TABLE 11-1	RYB WOUND DRESSING GUIDELINES
Red Wounds ■ Biologicals ■ Foam ■ Gauze ■ Hydrocolloid ■ Hydrogel ■ Moist gauze ■ Nonadherent gauze ■ Transparent film	**Yellow Wounds** **(Fibrinous Slough)** ■ Alginate ■ Exudate absorber ■ Foam ■ Hypertonic gauze ■ Hydrocolloid ■ Hydrogel ■ Transparent film
Yellow Wounds **(Infected)** ■ Alginate ■ Impregnated dressings ■ Exudate absorber ■ Foam ■ Hypertonic gauze ■ Wound pouches	**Black Wounds** ■ Alginate ■ Gauze ■ Hydrocolloid ■ Hydrogel ■ Transparent film

PREPARATION PROTOCOL: FOR WOUND CARE AND DRESSINGS

Complete the following steps before each skill.

1. Check physician's order and client plan of care.
2. Gather equipment.
3. Check client's identaband.
4. Introduce yourself to client and explain nursing care you will be giving.
5. Provide privacy as necessary for client.
6. Wash hands.
7. Don gloves as necessary.
8. Place bed in HIGH position.
9. Place absorbent pad under client if wound irrigation or cleaning is to be done.
10. Assess status of wound healing.
11. Evaluate client's laboratory studies.

COMPLETION PROTOCOL: FOR WOUND CARE AND DRESSINGS

Make sure the following steps have been completed.

1. Discard old dressings and supplies in disposal bag.
2. Clean any reusable equipment, bag, and prepare for removal to dirty utility room.
3. Remove gloves and discard appropriately; then wash hands.
4. Return client to position of comfort.
5. Wash hands.
6. Document pertinent data regarding wound assessment and type of dressing change completed. Report abnormal findings.

SECTION ONE

MEASURES TO PREVENT INFECTION

Several interventions are necessary to prevent wound infections. Two major interventions are good handwashing technique and the use of clean or sterile gloves when caring for clients at risk for developing an infection. Nosocomial infections are usually caused by poor handwashing technique. Frequent assessments of a surgical site or trauma area need to be done to detect potential wound infections. Early detection results in immediate treatment of a wound, with a desirable outcome.

RATIONALE

- To prevent clients with impaired resistance from acquiring infections
- To prevent microorganisms from entering wounds
- To prevent the spread of microorganisms between clients

ASSESSMENT

- Identify clients at risk for infection (i.e., diabetic, malnourished, obese, elderly).
- Identify length of time client remained in surgery; the longer the time spent in surgery, the greater the risk for infection.
- Assess incision each shift.
- Assess need for sterile technique when providing client care.
- Assess health care worker compliance with handwashing and gloving technique.
- Assess client's lab results for abnormal values (e.g., WBCs, Hgb, Hct).

STERILE GLOVES

Equipment

- Package of sterile gloves

SKILL

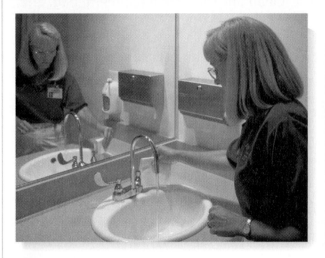

① Wash and dry your hands.

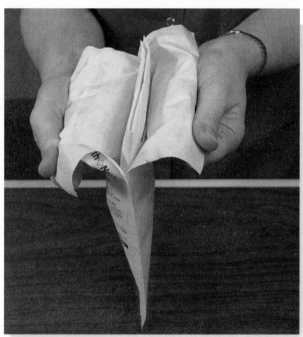

② Remove outside wrapper of glove package by peeling tabs apart and pulling edges laterally to expose glove package. Ensure this step is accomplished over a firm surface at waist height. **RATIONALE:** Objects below waist level are considered to be out of sterile field.

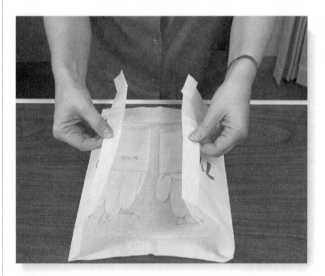

③ Place glove package on firm surface, maintaining sterility of gloves by touching only outside of wrapper.

- Grasp two edges of wrapper and lift wrapper edges up and away from gloves, being careful not to touch gloves as you open package. **RATIONALE:** Lifting edges up and away will prevent accidental touching and contaminating of gloves.

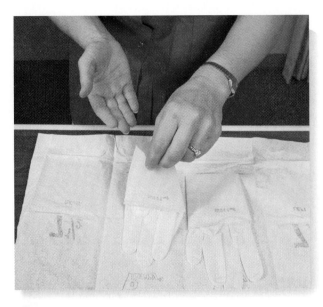

4 With your nondominant hand, pick up opposite glove by grasping section that has folded edge (inside edge of cuff). Lift glove up and away from wrapper. **RATIONALE:** This prevents accidental contamination of glove or inside of glove package.

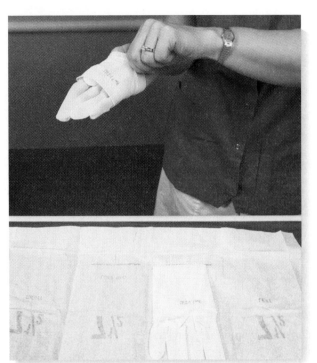

5 Holding your hands above waist level, insert your dominant hand into the glove opening. Gently pull glove into place with your nondominant hand, touching only inside of cuff. Do not attempt to straighten out gloved fingers until both gloves have been put on. **RATIONALE:** It is easy to contaminate glove when attempting to adjust fingers in glove.

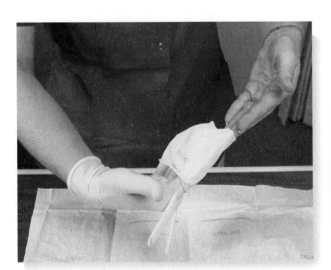

6 With your dominant, gloved hand, remove other glove from package, making sure you touch only inside of folded cuff. Lift glove up and away from wrapper. **RATIONALE:** This prevents gloves from inadvertently touching wrapper and becoming contaminated.

■ Hold your gloved thumb away from your body to prevent touching your skin.

■ Place your ungloved fingers into opening of new glove. Gently pull glove over your hand as before.

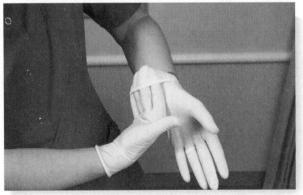

7 Adjust second glove by placing gloved fingers under cuff and gently pulling glove into place.

■ Keep your hands above waist level and adjust both gloves by touching only your fingers. **RATIONALE:** This maintains sterility of gloves.

■ Keep both sterile gloves in front of you and above waist level at all times. **RATIONALE:** This prevents potential contamination of gloves.

LIQUID FROM STERILE CONTAINER

Equipment

- Sterile container
- Nonsterile container
- Solution

Preparation

1 Open sterile package according to procedure.

2 Place sterile cup or container on sterile wrap of package. Be careful not to contaminate site.

3 Take cap off bottle and invert cap on firm surface. Ensure cap is not placed on sterile surface. **RATIONALE:** This keeps inside of cap sterile.

4 Place nonsterile cup away from sterile surface.

SAFETY ALERT

Guidelines for Sterile Field

- Never turn your back on a sterile field.
- Avoid talking, coughing, sneezing, or reaching across a sterile field.
- Keep sterile objects above waist level.
- Do not spill solutions on a sterile field.
- Open all sterile packages away from a sterile field to prevent contaminating the sterile field by crossing over it.

SKILL

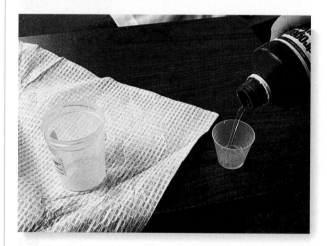

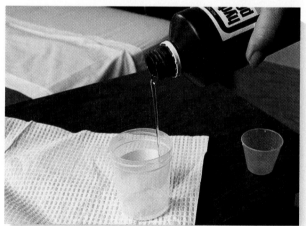

1 Hold bottle with label facing up and pour small amount of liquid into nonsterile container. **RATIONALE:** This action cleans lip of solution bottle, if bottle is being reused.

2 Pour liquid into sterile container while keeping label facing up and not touching container with bottle. Do not reach over sterile field while pouring liquid.

- Replace cap if liquid remains in bottle; if entire contents have been used, dispose of bottle in appropriate container. Replace bottle in storage area if it is to be reused.

DRESSING CHANGE PREPARATION WITH PREPACKAGED KIT

Equipment

- Prepackaged kit

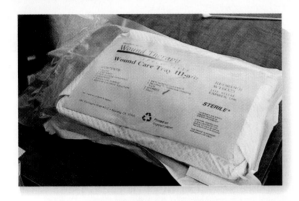

1 Place wound care kit on working surface that is clean and dry. Client's over-bed table is frequently used as preparation area. **RATIONALE:** This prevents contamination of sterile package.

- Remove outer plastic wrap and place in trash.

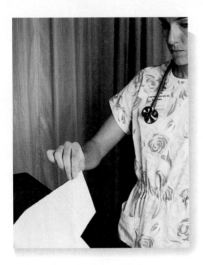

2 Place package in center of work area and position it so that first flap will be opened away from you. **RATIONALE:** This prevents reaching across sterile field as you continue to open package.

- Grasp edge of first flap of wrapper, move it away from you, and let it drop on working surface.
- Grasp first side flap, lift it up, then lift second side flap and move them out together toward sides. Let flaps fall to working surface.

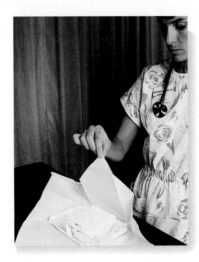

3 Grasp last flap of wrapper and open it toward you, taking care not to touch inside of flap or any of the contents of package.

- Before touching any of the contents of kit, don sterile gloves. **RATIONALE:** This maintains sterility of kit contents.
- If additional supplies need to be added to surface, grasp two sides of package and invert package over edge of sterile field.
- Drop contents onto wrapper. Make sure you do not cross over sterile field or contaminate kit. **RATIONALE:** Inside of wrapper is considered sterile except for 1-in margin at edges of wrapper.

DRESSING CHANGE PREPARATION WITH INDIVIDUAL SUPPLIES

Equipment

- Antiseptic cleaner or solution bottle
- Number and type of dressings needed (i.e., 4 × 4 gauze pads, ABD pads, applicator sticks)
- Tape
- Sterile gloves
- Disposal bag for contaminated dressings and package containers
- Mask, if needed

SKILL

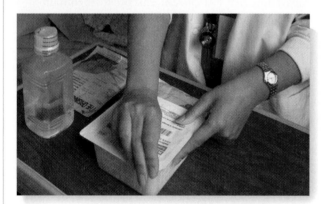

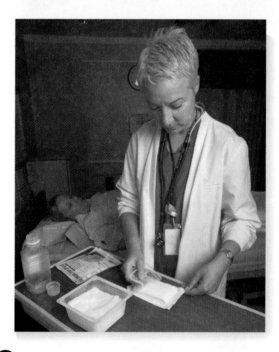

1 Clean off bedside stand and wash thoroughly with antiseptic solution.

- Place supply packages on table in configuration that allows you to open packages without reaching over sterile field. **RATIONALE:** To prevent contamination of supplies.
- Grasp unsealed flap of 4 × 4 pad container and pull back on flap (away from sterile area). Discard cover.

2 Grasp edge of transparent package, peel back top covering, and lay it down on work surface. Do not cross over sterile container when placing it on work surface. Continue to open all supply packages using this method.

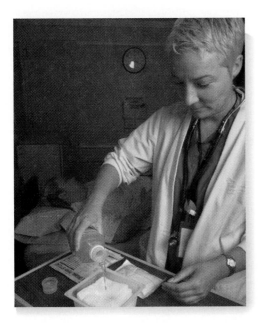

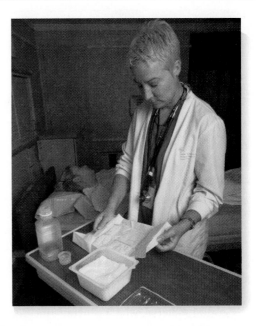

3 Pour solution over pads in container, if ordered.

4 Open sterile gloves. Place in position on table such that you do not cross over sterile field. Tear tape and place on edge of over-bed table.

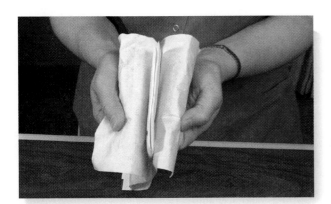

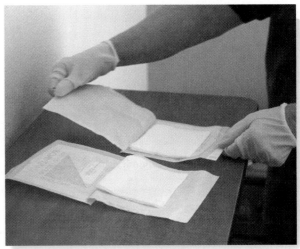

5 Alternate method: Open supply packages with sealed edges by holding each side of package with one hand and gently pulling edges apart.

6 Alternate method continued: Place outer wrap of package on work surface. Lay package open to expose dressing.

CHARTING

■ Type of sterile dressings used
■ Type of solutions used

DRESSING CHANGE

A dressing is a protective covering placed over an incision or wound. Dressings are used to protect surgical sites from infection, to cover infected wounds to prevent contamination of other areas or other individuals, to absorb drainage, or to prevent mechanical injury to wounds. The type of dressing used and the frequency of dressing changes are dependent on wound status, type of dressing, drainage, and need for wound assessments.

Clean, newly created incisions are usually covered with a woven cotton material, which generally includes 4 × 4 gauze pads and ABD pads. These nonocclusive dressings allow oxygen to reach the wound surface. Pressure for hemostasis can be applied using this type of dressing.

Nurses are often responsible for the removal of staples and sutures for clients with uncomplicated wounds or incisions. This is frequently accomplished during a home or clinic visit. Sutures are usually removed 7 to 10 days after surgery, while skin staples are usually removed in 5 to 7 days. The sutures or staples should be assessed during every dressing change.

RATIONALE

- To maintain a sterile incisional area
- To prevent cross contamination of microorganisms
- To absorb drainage
- To prevent wound infection

ASSESSMENT

- Assess wound for drainage or signs of infection.
- Assess sutures and staples for stability and signs of infection.
- Assess extent of healing.
- Assess site to determine type of dressing needed.

CLINICAL NOTE

Check facility policy to determine if routine dressing change includes swabbing the incision. If so, follow these steps:

- Cleanse incision area with swabs soaked in normal saline, according to agency policy.
- Cleanse from incision line outward, cleaning from the top to bottom, using swab only once. Cleaning outward from incision cleans from least to most contaminated area. Cleaning from top to bottom prevents contamination from secretions that accumulate at bottom of wound. Discard swabs in disposal bag.

DRY STERILE DRESSING

Equipment

- Sterile gloves
- Clean gloves
- Mask (as needed)
- Gown (as needed)
- Disposal bag for used dressings

- Dressing supplies (as needed)
- Micropore tape
- Sterile normal saline (optional)
- Package of sterile cotton swabs (optional)

SKILL

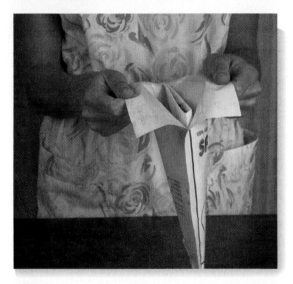

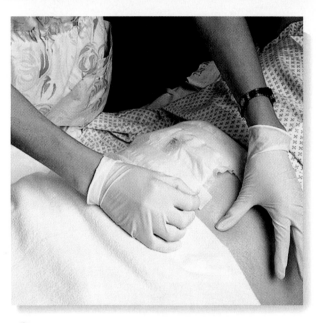

🤚 ① Follow steps in the "Dressing Change" skills.

- Determine type and number of dressings needed for dressing change.
- Determine if gown and mask are needed.

② Remove tape slowly by pulling toward wound. **RATIONALE:** Pulling toward wound decreases pain of tape removal by not putting pressure on incision line.

③ Remove soiled dressings. Assess incision area for erythema, edema, or drainage. **RATIONALE:** Persistent drainage, edema, or temperature above 100.4°F (38.3°C) 2 days postop indicates a complication is occurring.

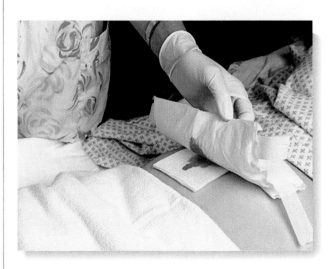

- Assess color of incision. A healing incision looks pink or red. **RATIONALE:** Redness that does not fade 48 hrs after surgery may indicate impaired healing.

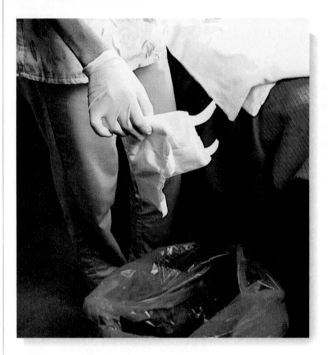

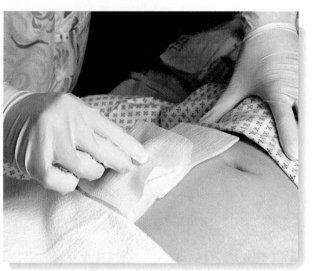

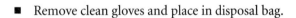

④ Dispose of used dressing in disposal bag.

■ Remove clean gloves and place in disposal bag.

⑤ Don sterile gloves.

■ Place 4 × 4 gauze pads over incision area, being careful not to contaminate dressing.

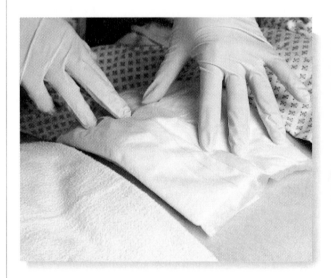

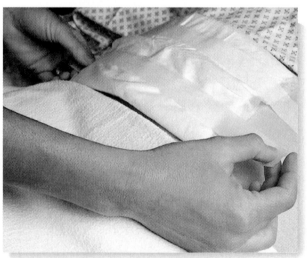

⑥ Place ABD pad over incision, being careful not to contaminate gloves.

⑦ Remove gloves and discard into disposal bag so that dressing can be taped securely.

SUTURE REMOVAL

Equipment

- Suture removal set
- Antiseptic solution (optional)
- Disposal bag for dressings and suture material
- Clean gloves
- Dressings and tape (if necessary)

SKILL

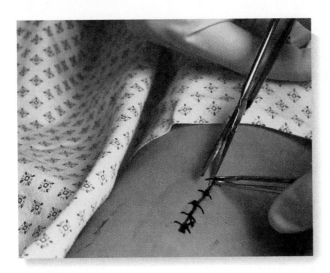

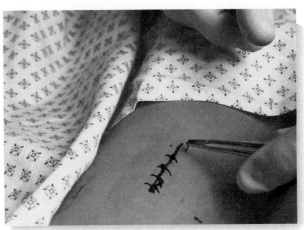

① After opening kit, pick up forceps with non-dominant hand and grasp suture at knot with forceps. Lift suture away from skin.

- Place curved tip of suture scissors under suture, next to knot. Cut suture. *Note:* Check physician's orders to determine if all or half of sutures are to be removed. **RATIONALE:** Some physicians prefer to remove half of sutures only, to prevent dehiscence.

② Use forceps to pull suture through skin in one movement, and continue to remove remaining sutures. Check carefully that all suture pieces are removed.

- Discard sutures in disposal bag.
- Cleanse suture site with antiseptic solution and apply dressing according to facility policy or physician's orders.

STAPLE REMOVAL

Equipment

- Sterile staple remover
- Antiseptic solution (optional)
- Disposal bag
- Clean gloves
- Dressings and tape (as needed)

SKILL

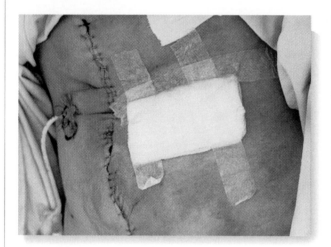

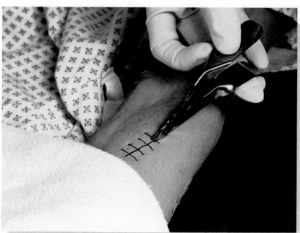

1 Assess incision site and staples to determine appropriateness of staple removal. **RATIONALE:** If incision is healed and there is no drainage or infection, staples can be safely removed.

2 Place lower tip of staple remover under staple.

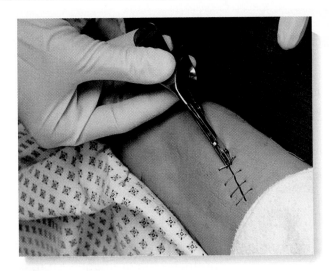

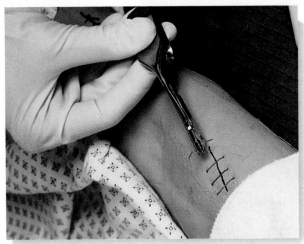

3 Press handles together to depress center of staple.

4 Lift staple remover upward and away from incision site when both ends of staple are visible. This removes staple.

- Place staple removal device over disposal bag and release handles to release staple.
- Continue to remove staples according to physician orders. **RATIONALE:** Some physicians prefer to remove half at one time to prevent dehiscence.
- Cleanse site and apply dressing according to facility policy or physician's orders.

CHARTING

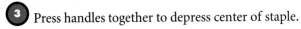

- Wound assessment
- Condition of suture line
- Presence of exudate or erythema at incision site

- Sutures or staples removed
- Cleansing of site (if ordered)
- Dressing applied (if ordered)

WOUND CARE

Wound assessment and measures to treat wounds have changed dramatically over the last 15 years. The major trend is to treat wounds using moisture-retentive dressings rather than drying the wounds. To accomplish the goals for treating wounds, a moist wound environment must be maintained to allow tissue to granulate. Moisture enhances cellular activity in all phases of wound repair, facilitates autolytic debridement of necrotic tissue, enables epithelial cells to migrate into the wound bed, and insulates and protects nerve endings, thus reducing the pain associated with a wound.

A wound bed that is too moist or too dry kills healthy tissue and impairs healing. Drainage from the wound site needs to be contained to protect adjacent healthy skin from maceration. A skin sealant may be helpful to protect the skin around the wound. The skin sealant also keeps the skin intact when dressing changes are frequent, and protects the skin from tearing when tape is removed.

All wounds require a dry dressing on the air-exposed side to prevent bacterial invasion by downward capillary mobility of contaminant; therefore a moisture-retentive dressing is recommended today for many wounds. The dressing should be secured over the wound and taped in place using the "windowpaning" method of taping. Trauma to the wound is prevented by padding the wound with layers of dressing material.

Wound specialists disagree over whether clean or sterile gloves should be used during wound care. All wounds may be considered contaminated, but not necessarily infected. Several microorganisms are responsible for the majority of wound infections. *Staphylococcus aureus* is still a major cause of postoperative infection. *Escherichia coli*, *Streptococcus faecalis*, klebsiella, *Pseudomonas aeruginosa*, and a few others are associated with wound infections.

RATIONALE

- To assess wounds appropriately
- To promote wound healing
- To prevent microorganisms from entering wounds
- To maintain sterility during dressing changes
- To maintain drainage if a drainage system is used

ASSESSMENT

- Assess wound for moisture, debridement, infection, and cleanliness.
- Make sure drainage from wound site is contained and adjacent skin is protected.
- Make sure skin sealant is used appropriately.
- Check that dressing is dry on air-exposed side.
- Make sure drainage system is operating.

CLINICAL NOTE

Document how long client has had wound. Determine previous treatments, if any, and treatment results. Check if client has any known allergies, particularly to wound care products.

WOUND ASSESSMENT

Equipment

- Pliable disposable measuring device/grid
- Cotton-tipped applicator sticks
- Plastic disposal bag
- Clean gloves
- Sterile gloves (if necessary)

SKILL

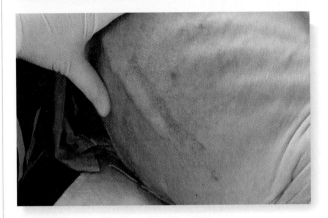

1 Examine wound. Note appearance of wound bed.

- Check for exudate, drainage, necrotic tissue, and signs of infection.

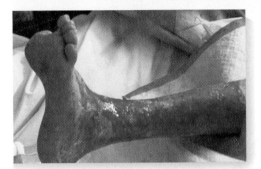

2 Assess surrounding area for problems in skin nutrition.

- Atrophy, loss of hair, thickening of nails
- Edema of skin or scaly skin
- Skin hydration (skin turgor indicates hydration or dehydration)
- Skin integrity or maceration
- Skin color (red [inflammation] surrounding wound, white [arterial insufficiency], blue [cyanosis, severe arterial insufficiency], black [necrosis], brown [venous insufficiency])
- Skin temperature (cool, cold, warm, normal)

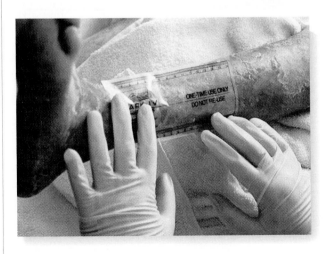

3 Assess extent of wound.

- Measure length and width of wound using a disposable measuring device/grid.
- Measure depth of wound by placing sterile cotton-tipped applicator stick into wound in several areas.
- Measure depth of each area using measuring device/grid.
- Check for tunneling or sinus tracts by placing sterile cotton-tipped applicator stick into suspected areas and advancing stick until resistance is met.

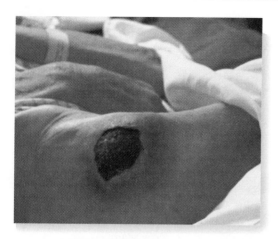

4 Observe color of wound: black (necrotic tissue/ black eschar [inhibits formation of granulation tissue]), yellow (pus, fibrin, debris [will advance to eschar]), red (indicates wound ready to heal [granulation tissue present]).

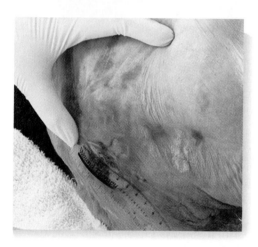

5 Assess wound drainage: type (dry or moist), amount (minimum, moderate, maximum [copious]), color of drainage (clear [serous], brown-brown/yellow [slough], yellow-yellow/green [pus-from strep or staph], blue-green [pseudomonas]).

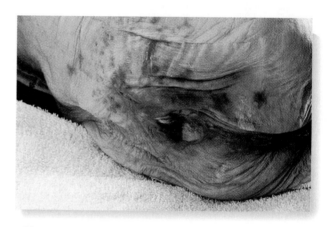

6 Assess level of moisture in wound. A moist environment allows wound to heal without forming a scab.

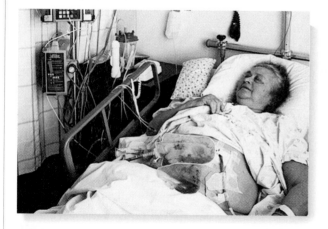

7 Assess odor of wound: foul (infected [necrotic tissue has an odor even if not infected]), sweet (pseudomonas infection).

CLINICAL NOTE

Laboratory values need to be assessed routinely while the wound is healing:

- Increased white blood cell count indicates infection, usually before other signs and symptoms are evident.
- Low hemoglobin and hematocrit indicate anemia, which can decrease oxygen transport to the wound.
- Altered serum glucose levels may indicate the presence of diabetes mellitus, which interferes with normal wound healing.

WOUND CLEANING

Equipment

- Sterile normal saline or noncytotoxic wound cleanser
- Sterile dressings, 4 × 4 gauze pads, ABD pads
- Tape
- Sterile round bowl, if solution not in disposable squeeze bottle
- Sterile emesis basin
- Sterile gloves (two pairs)
- Absorbent pad
- Disposal bag for soiled supplies
- Goggles

SKILL

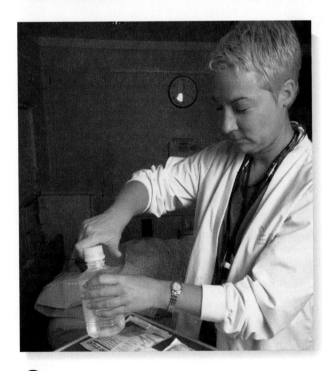

1 Check physician's order for wound cleaning solution. Sterile normal saline or a noncytotoxic wound cleanser should be used. (Common types of cleansing solutions include Comfeel Sea-Clens and ClinsWound.) **RATIONALE:** Other products, such as the long-used Dakin's solution or hydrogen peroxide, should be avoided as they are toxic to cells.

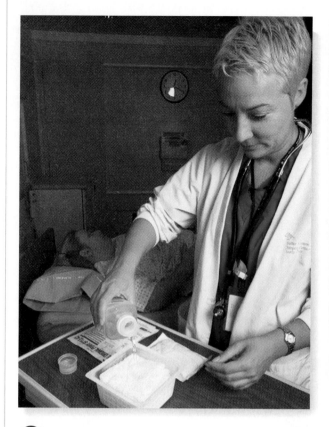

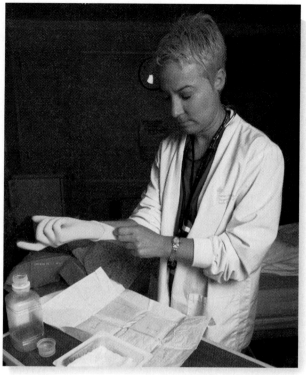

③ Don sterile gloves.

② Pour cleaning solution over gauze pads. Do not use products that can shed cotton fibers. **RATIONALE:** This can lead to a foreign body reaction, thus delaying the healing process as a result of prolonging the inflammatory phase.

- If antimicrobial solutions are used, ensure they are well diluted.
- Warm solution to body temperature. **RATIONALE:** This prevents lowering of wound temperature, which slows the healing process.

- Pick up several gauze pads, pulling edges together. Form a ball with the pads. **RATIONALE:** This action prevents sterile gloves from touching wound during cleaning process and therefore maintains sterility of gloves. Forceps can be used to hold gauze pads during cleansing process.
- Sterile cleansing solution may be poured directly over wound before gauze pads are used for cleaning. Place emesis basin to side of client to catch excess cleansing solution.
- Cleanse wound from cleanest area to dirtiest, starting at wound itself and working out to periphery. **RATIONALE:** This prevents bringing microorganisms into wound bed.
- Clean from top to bottom of wound, using new gauze pad with each stroke.

BEYOND THE SKILL

Wound Irrigation

Equipment

- As in wound cleaning skill
- Warmed irrigation solution
- Syringe: 30- to 60-mL piston syringe, 30- to 60-mL rubber-tipped syringe, or 250-mL squeeze bottle
- Clean gloves and sterile gloves (two pairs)

Skill

1. Check orders for type and amount of irrigating solution to be used. Warm solution.

2. Don clean gloves and remove dressing. Discard dressing and gloves in disposal bag.

3. Open sterile supplies and place on over-bed table. Syringe packages can be opened and placed on open dressing packages to preserve sterility. Pour warmed irrigating solution into sterile basin.

4. Don sterile gloves. Draw up solution into either 60-mL piston syringe, 20-mL syringe with rubber tip, or 250-mL squeeze bottle with irrigation tip. Amount of irrigation solution required depends on extent of wound.

5. Instill solution into wound. Reach into wound with irrigation tip to ensure all areas are irrigated.

6. Place sterile emesis basin next to wound to catch irrigation solution as it drains from wound.

7. Repeat irrigation process until returns are clear and free of debris.

8. Cleanse around wound with moist gauze pads; dry thoroughly with gauze pads.

9. Remove gloves and place in disposal bag.

10. Don sterile gloves and apply dressings.

11. Remove gloves and place in disposal bag.

WET-TO-DAMP DRESSING

Equipment

- 4 × 4 gauze pads in container
- ABD pads
- Dry sterile 4 × 4 pads
- Sterile solution (usually saline)

- Tape
- Clean gloves
- Sterile gloves
- Disposal bag

SKILL

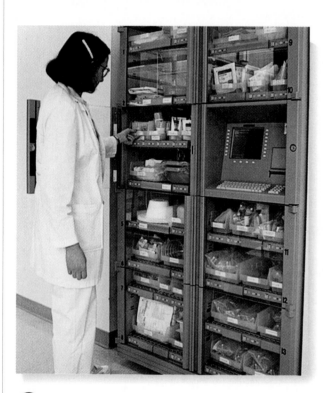

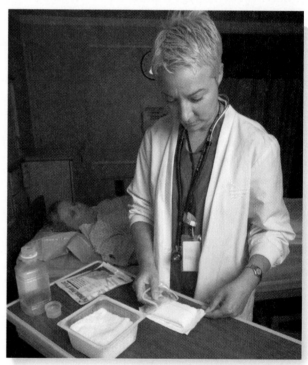

1 Identify type and number of dressings and type of solution needed. Obtain all supplies from supply station such as the Pyxis.

2 Clean over-bed table; open all sterile packages and place on over-bed table. Arrange packages to ensure you do not cross over sterile field.

- Cut tape strips and place on over-bed table. **RATIONALE:** Commercially prepared sterile packages can be opened and used for sterile field; inside of package is considered sterile.

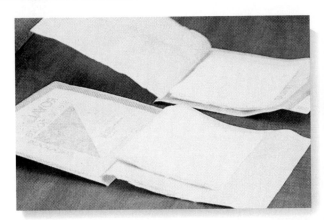

3 Ensure that two packages of dry 4 × 4 gauze pads are open for use in outer dressing.

- Fanfold top linen to foot of bed. Use bath blanket to cover client, exposing only dressing area.
- Place bag for soiled dressings near wound site.

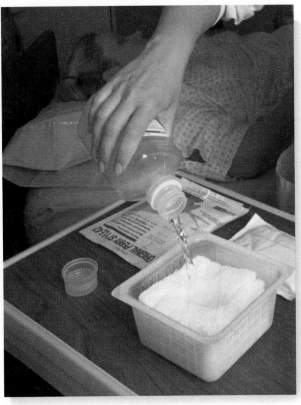

4 Pour sterile solution into 4 × 4 gauze dressing container.

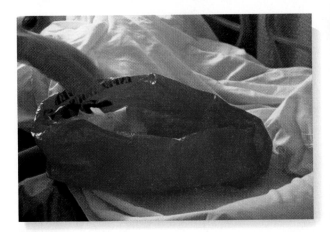

5 Remove dressing and place in disposal bag.

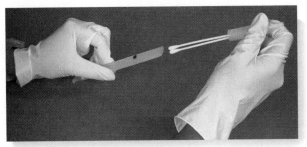

6 Obtain wound specimen for culture, if ordered.

- Remove clean gloves and dispose in appropriate container.

CLINICAL NOTE

Obtain a wound culture using the following steps:

- Rinse wound thoroughly with sterile normal saline.
- Use non-cotton-tipped swab.
- Rotate swab while obtaining specimen.
- Swab wound edges starting at top; crisscross wound to bottom.
- Do not take specimen from exudate or eschar.
- Remove gloves and place in disposal bag.
- Wash your hands.

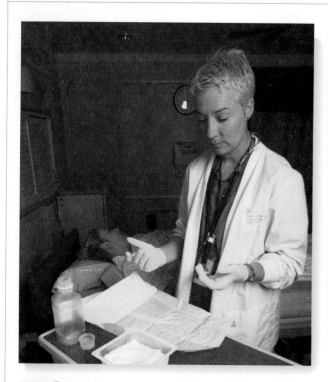

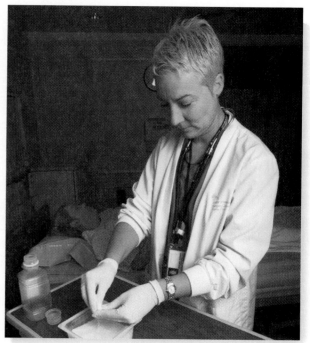

 7 Don sterile gloves and have materials needed for dressing change available.

8 Wring out several gauze pads until slightly moist. **RATIONALE:** If dressing is too moist when applied to wound bed, risk of bacterial invasion and maceration of surrounding skin is increased.

- Fluff moistened dressings and lightly pack them into all crevices and depressions in wound. Necrotic tissue is usually in deep crevices. **RATIONALE:** If packed too tightly, dressings can inhibit wound edges from contracting and may compress capillaries.

- If wound is grossly contaminated by foreign material, bacteria, slough, or necrotic tissue, wound must be cleaned or irrigated with each dressing change. **RATIONALE:** Necrotic tissue or foreign material acts as a conduit for wound infection (see wound cleaning skill).

SAFETY ALERT

A skin barrier, such as skin sealant, may be applied to the skin surrounding a wound to prevent it from becoming macerated.

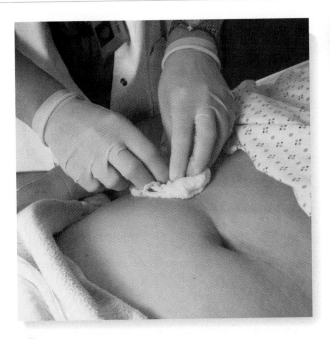

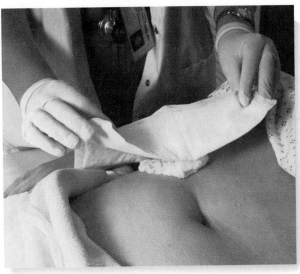

10 Place sterile ABD pad over wound site. **RATIO-NALE:** Pad protects wound from trauma and external contamination.

- Remove gloves and place in disposal bag.

9 Apply sterile, dry gauze pads over moist dressing. **RATIONALE:** This will assist in absorbing excess exudate.

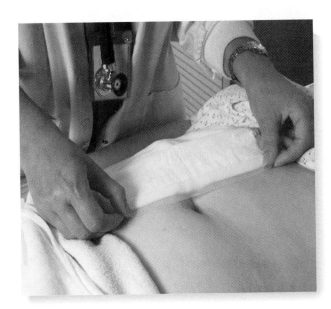

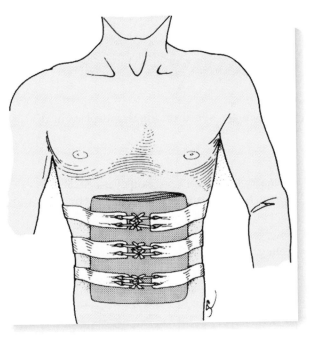

11 Tape wound securely. Tape should be long and wide enough to adhere to several inches of skin in order to prevent dressing from slipping off wound. After taping lengthwise, tape across dressing at top and bottom.

Alternative Method
Using Montgomery tie tapes

Montgomery tie tapes are used when frequent dressing changes are required. The tapes prevent skin irritation and trauma to the skin. Tapes are not replaced unless they are soiled and there is a risk of infection. Tincture of benzoin can be applied to skin under tapes to prevent skin irritation in clients with sensitive skin.

OPEN WOUND DRAINAGE SYSTEM

Equipment

- Dressings (4 × 4 gauze pads, ABD pads)
- Precut sterile 4 × 4 gauze pads (two)
- Sterile premoistened cotton applicator sticks or forceps and cotton balls
- Sterile cleansing solution and sterile container
- Sterile safety pin
- Sterile scissors
- Sterile gloves
- Clean gloves
- Disposal bag

CLINICAL NOTE

ADVANCE PENROSE DRAIN
To advance a Penrose drain, complete the following steps:

- Using sterile forceps, pull drain out of wound number of centimeters ordered.
- Reposition safety pin so it is at level of skin. Pin prevents drain from slipping back into wound.
- Cut off excess tubing with sterile scissors. Leave at least 2 in of tubing on outside. This prevents drain from being drawn back into wound opening.

SKILL

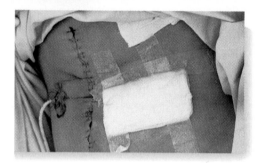

1 Remove soiled dressings and place in disposal bag.

- Remove clean gloves.
- Open sterile packages; place on over-bed table. Pour sterile cleansing solution into container or open premoistened applicator sticks.
- Observe wound closely for signs of infection or healing.

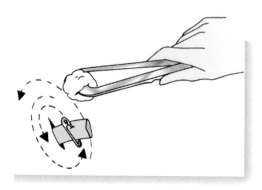

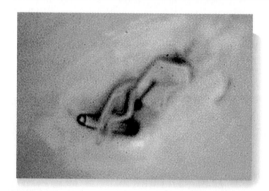

2 Don sterile gloves, and closely observe pin in Penrose drain. If drain is crusted, replace pin with new sterile pin. Be careful not to dislodge drain.

3 Cleanse drain site with cleansing solution. Use applicator sticks or forceps with cotton balls soaked in cleansing solution. Start cleansing at drain site, moving in circular motion toward periphery. **RATIONALE:** This prevents contamination of drain site area.

- Discard applicator sticks or cotton balls in disposal bag.
- Advance drain, if ordered.

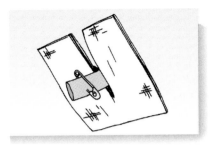

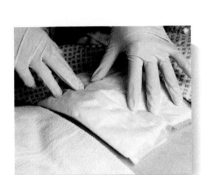

4 Place precut 4 × 4 gauze under Penrose drain.

- Place several 4 × 4 gauze pads around drain site.
- Apply 4 × 4 gauze pads over drain. **RATIONALE:** Pads absorb drainage and prevent drainage from accumulating on skin.

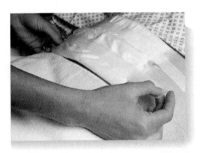

5 Place ABD pads over sterile gauze pads. Remove gloves and place in disposal bag.

6 Tape ABD pads securely to skin. Montgomery tie tapes should be used if frequent dressing changes are required or client has sensitive skin.

BEYOND THE SKILL

Drainage Pouches for Wounds

Pouches or drainage bags are used for the following purposes:

1. Collecting drainage, particularly if it is excessive
2. Measuring drainage
3. Protecting skin from drainage
4. Containing drainage
5. Containing microorganisms to decrease their spread to other areas
6. Decreasing frequency of dressing changes

Care for clients with drainage bags includes the following:

1. Don clean gloves.
2. Remove dressings and place in disposal bag.
3. Measure drainage from pouches, as ordered.
4. Remove clean gloves and don sterile gloves.
5. Clean drain site with sterile cleansing solution and cotton applicator sticks or forceps and cotton balls. Use new applicator sticks or cotton balls for each site.
6. Apply sterile dressings as ordered. Drainage pouches may be left open for assessment.

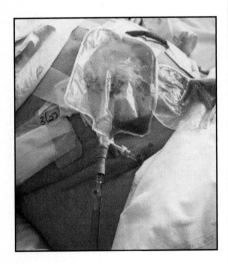

CLOSED WOUND DRAINAGE SYSTEM

Equipment

- Specimen cup for measuring drainage
- I&O bedside record
- Absorbent pad
- Clean gloves

SKILL

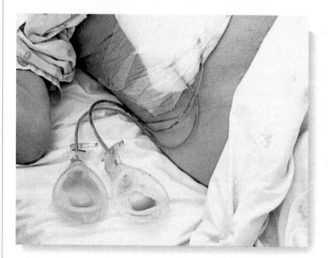

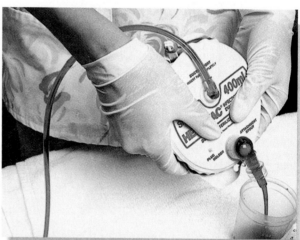

1 Expose catheter insertion site while keeping client draped.

- Place drainage system on absorbent pad or towel. **RATIONALE:** To protect bed from becoming soiled.
- Examine Jackson-Pratt pump or Hemovac catheter for patency, seal, and stability. If catheter is occluded, notify physician.

2 Empty Hemovac drainage system by removing Hemovac plug from pouring spout. Pour drainage into specimen container.

SAFETY ALERT

To maintain drainage, compress Jackson-Pratt bulb or Hemovac container every 4 hrs.

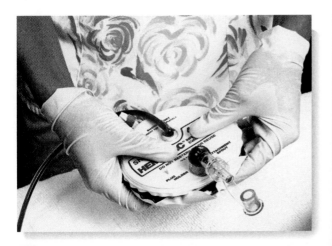

3 Compress Hemovac by pushing top and bottom together with your hands. Keep pump tightly compressed while you reinsert plug.

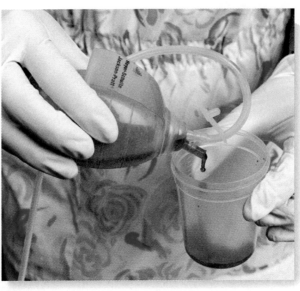

4 Disconnect tubing from Jackson-Pratt system. Pour drainage into specimen container.

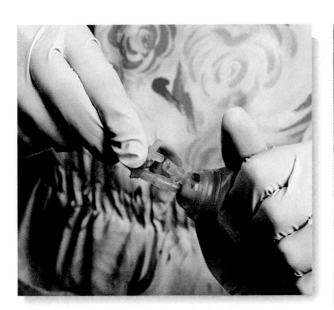

5 Compress bulb on Jackson-Pratt system.

■ Hold bulb tightly compressed and connect to tubing.

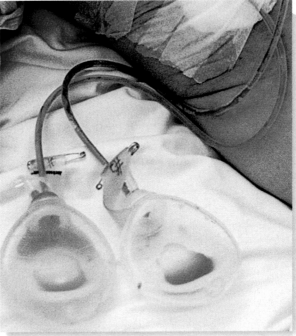

6 Place drainage system on bed. **RATIONALE:** This allows for easy observation of system and facilitates drainage from wound.

■ Measure and record amount of drainage.
■ Observe color, consistency, and odor of drainage.

- Wound assessment: amount, color, and odor of drainage; appearance of site
- Observation of granulating tissue and redness
- Observation of surrounding skin
- Client's response to dressing change
- Condition of suture or staples

- Amount, color, and odor of drainage from wound drainage systems
- Penrose drain: amount, color, and odor of drainage; advancement of tube
- Wound irrigation: type and amount of solution, characteristics of drainage
- Type and amount of dressings applied to wounds

SECTION FOUR

VASCULAR INSUFFICIENCY WOUNDS

There are three types of wounds caused by vascular insufficiency: venous insufficiency ulcers, arterial insufficiency ulcers, and pressure or capillary insufficiency ulcers. Five major factors contribute to vascular insufficiency ulcer formation: (1) poor nutrition and a lack of blood flow causing inability of nutrients to diffuse through the intestinal spaces; (2) continuous pressure on certain areas of the body, such as bony prominences; (3) mechanical, thermal, or chemical insults to vascularized limbs, resulting in a lack of nutrients reaching the limbs; (4) decreased sensation in the lower extremities; (5) excess moisture from incontinence.

Venous ulcers result from a diminished ability of nutrients to diffuse through the interstitial space from the capillaries. The etiology of this condition is usually calf pump failure as a result of outflow tract obstruction, pregnancy, obesity, tumor, or deep vein thrombosis. Other causes include insufficient valves (either deep venous valve incompetence or superficial vein incompetence), peripheral neuropathy, and musculoskeletal disorders resulting from calf muscle disuse.

Arterial ulcers are often seen in clients with diabetes mellitus and hypertension. Clients with a history of smoking or who sustain mechanical trauma are also prone to arterial ulcers. In this condition there is diminished oxygenation and thus flow of nutrients to the periphery. Drug therapy with vasodilators, anticoagulants, or thrombolytic agents is part of the treatment plan for these clients. Surgical intervention is sometimes necessary when drug therapy is ineffective.

Pressure ulcers are caused by mechanical factors including pressure, friction, shearing, and moisture. Pressure ulcers are usually located over a bony prominence, where normal tissue is squeezed between the bone and pressure or friction caused by a bed or chair. External pressure that results in decreased blood flow causes altered oxygenation and nutrition of the tissue and leads to formation of a pressure ulcer.

Vacuum-assisted wound closure (VAC) is the newest and most effective nonsurgical technique for healing both acute and chronic wounds. This system accelerates wound healing by promoting granulation of tissue. Granulation tissue completely closes or improves the health of a wound before a skin graft is performed. The VAC is a negative suction pressure system whose pressure is lower than that of the atmosphere at sea level. The VAC pump applies 75 mm Hg of pressure initially and is increased to a target pressure of 125 mm Hg. At this pressure, blood flow is increased fourfold. The system can be programmed to deliver an amount of negative pressure appropriate to a client's level and type of wound.

RATIONALE

- To determine extent of wound healing
- To promote circulation in vascular insufficiency
- To prevent infection of wound
- To promote wound healing
- To prevent microorganisms from entering wound
- To prevent formation of pressure ulcer
- To identify appropriate treatment for specific ulcer stage
- To apply medication to wound

ASSESSMENT

- Assess vascular insufficiency wounds to determine type of treatment required.
- Determine extent of wound healing.
- Determine presence of infection.
- Identify type and number of dressings required for wound care.
- Identify clients at risk for pressure ulcer formation.
- Assess stage of pressure ulcer.
- Assess other bony prominences for potential formation of pressure ulcers.

SAFETY ALERT

Compression dressings are contraindicated in clients with phlebitis, diminished sensation, or arterial insufficiency, as they will exacerbate the insufficiency. Assess peripheral circulation every 4 hrs to ensure that compression dressings are not too tight.

VENOUS DRESSING

Equipment

- Cleansing solution
- Normal saline
- Sterile 4 × 4 gauze dressings
- Translucent dressing
- Gel
- Compression dressing

- Clean gloves
- Sterile gloves
- Biohazard bag
- Scissors
- Absorbent pad

SKILL

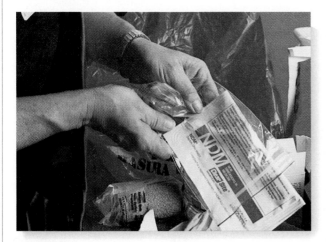

1 Open sterile packages; arrange supplies on over-bed table.

- Place absorbent pad under wound.
- Don clean gloves.

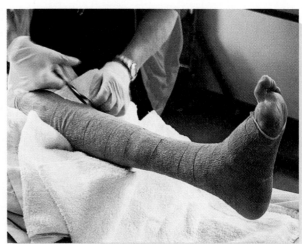

2 Remove compression bandage and old dressing and place in biohazard bag. Compression dressings may be left in place for 3 to 7 days depending on amount of drainage and type of dressing.

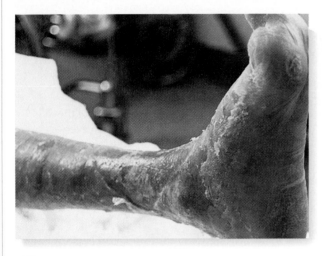

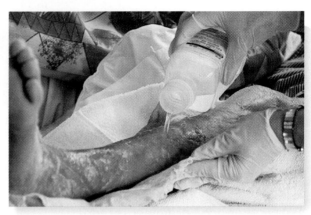

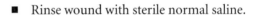

4 Pour cleansing solution over wound. **RATIONALE:** To cleanse wound of debris.

■ Rinse wound with sterile normal saline.

3 Assess wound to determine effectiveness of treatment (Stage II).

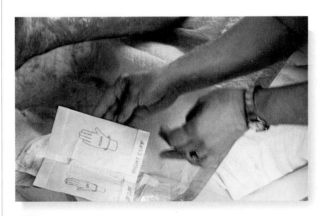

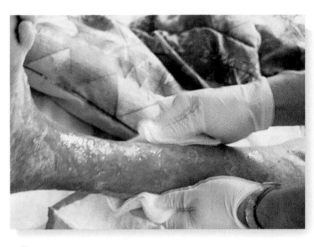

5 Remove clean gloves and discard into biohazard bag.

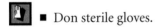 ■ Don sterile gloves.

6 Dry wound using sterile 4 × 4 gauze pads. Place used pads in biohazard bag.

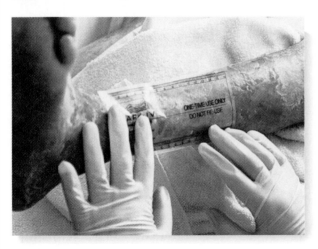

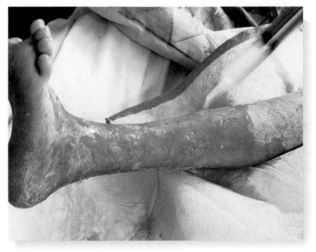

7 Measure wound to evaluate effectiveness of treatment.

8 Apply medicated moisturizer over wound.

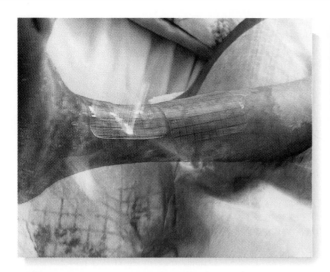

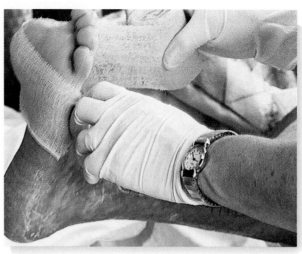

9 Remove backing on transparent dressing, and place dressing over open wound site.

10 Palpate arterial system (dorsalis pedis, posterior, or tibial pulse). If pulses are palpable, obtain an ankle-brachial index (ABI). ABI is not reliable in clients with diabetes. **RATIONALE:** Arterial calcification causes false high readings.

- Apply compression dressing if ABI is greater than 0.6. **RATIONALE:** Effective compression bandages generate 40 to 70 mm Hg of pressure. If arterial insufficiency is present, another ulcer can occur.

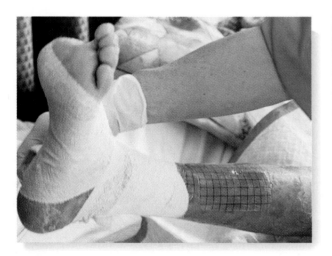

11 Apply even pressure when placing compression dressing over extremity.

- Reposition leg in elevated position. **RATIONALE:** This prevents venous stasis and promotes healing.

CLINICAL NOTE

ABI INDEX

Normal	0.6–1 ABI
Moderate disease	0.75–0.9 ABI
Severe disease	0.5–0.75 ABI
Limb-threatening disease	>0.5 ABI

BEYOND THE SKILL

Assessing Ankle-Brachial Index (ABI)

1. Place client in supine position.
2. Obtain blood pressure readings in both arms. Use the higher systolic pressure as the brachial pressure in the ratio.
3. Wrap leg cuff around leg just above malleoli.
4. Place Doppler probe at a 45° angle to the dorsalis pedis or posterior tibial artery.
5. Inflate cuff until Doppler sound stops.
6. Deflate cuff slowly while maintaining Doppler probe in place over artery.
7. Record number on sphygmomanometer when Doppler sound returns. **RATIONALE:** This is the ankle systolic pressure.
8. Divide ankle systolic pressure by arm systolic pressure to obtain ABI.

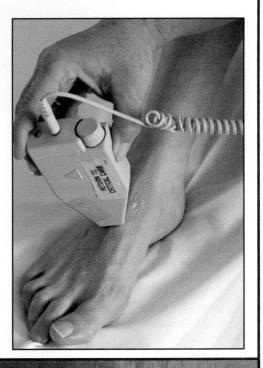

CLINICAL NOTE

ARTERIAL ULCERS

Arterial insufficiency ulcers are treated similarly to venous ulcers except for the dressing material.

Assessment
■ Assess arterial flow (dorsalis pedis, femerol, popliteal, or posterior tibial).
■ Use Doppler to assess pulses if necessary.
■ Assess ankle-brachial index; below 0.5 indicates severe arterial insufficiency.
■ Assess temperature of skin.
■ Observe color of extremities.
■ Assess for presence of pain when client is resting.

Treatment
■ Keep ulcer moist.
■ Use saline-moistened gauze and hydrocolloid dressings.
■ Use petroleum jelly on skin surrounding wound to prevent skin maceration.
■ Secure dressing with gauze; do not use tape as skin is fragile and tears easily.

PREVENTION OF PRESSURE ULCERS

Equipment

- Turning sheet as needed
- Norton or Braden scale

SKILL

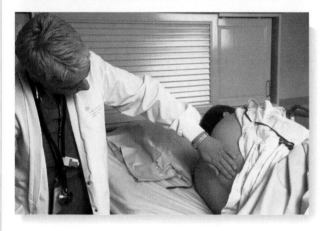

1 Inspect skin at least daily, particularly over bony prominences.

- Identify clients at risk for pressure ulcer formation.
- Complete pressure ulcer risk assessment using either Norton or Braden scale.

CLINICAL NOTE

NURSE'S GUIDE FOR ASSESSMENT OF CLIENTS AT RISK FOR PRESSURE ULCERS

Factors that contribute to development of pressure ulcers are pressure, friction, shearing, and moisture. Identify at-risk individuals needing preventative measures:

- Bed- and chairbound individuals
- Clients with impaired ability to reposition themselves
- Clients who are immobilized
- Clients who are incontinent
- Clients with nutritional deficits, such as inadequate dietary intake or malnutrition
- Clients with altered level of consciousness
- *Note:* Identification of stage I pressure ulcer may be difficult in a dark-skinned client.

A risk assessment tool (Braden scale or Norton scale) should be used for all clients admitted to long-term care facilities, or acute care settings, or receiving home care. Systematic reassessments should be done at designated intervals.

TABLE 11-2	PRESSURE ULCER RISK ASSESSMENT SCALES

Norton Scale

Physical Condition		Mental Condition		Activity		Mobility		Continence	
Good	4	Alert	4	Walks	4	Full	4	Good	4
Fair	3	Apathetic	3	Walks with help	3	Slightly limited	3	Occasional incontinence	3
Poor	2	Confused	2	Sits in chair	2	Very limited	2	Frequent incontinence	2
Very poor	1	Stuporous	1	Remains in bed	1	Immobile	1	Urine and fecal incontinence	1
Total ____		Total ____		Total ____		Total ____		Total ____	

Grand total = ____

A score of 14 or less indicates risk of pressure ulcer; a score under 12 indicates high risk.

Braden Scale

Sensory Perception		Moisture		Activity		Mobility		Nutrition		Friction and Shear	
No impairment	4	Rarely moist	4	Walks frequently	4	No limitations	4	Excellent	4		
Slightly limited	3	Occasionally moist	3	Walks occasionally	3	Slightly limited	3	Adequate	3	No apparent problems	3
Very limited	2	Moist	2	Chairfast	2	Very limited	2	Probably inadequate	2	Potential problem	2
Completely limited	1	Constantly moist	1	Bedfast	1	Immobile	1	Very poor	1	Problem	1
Total ____		Total ____		Total ____		Total ____		Total ____		Total ____	

Grand total = ____

Assign a score of 1 to 4 in each category. Total the score; if it is 16 or less, the client is at high risk for pressure ulcer development.

SOURCE: Adapted from *Pressure Ulcers in Adults: Prediction and Prevention*, Rockville, MD, U.S. Department of Health and Human Services, Public Health Service, Agency for Health Care Policy and Research Publication No. 92-0047, May 1992. Norton Scale, p. 15; Braden Scale, p. 16–17.

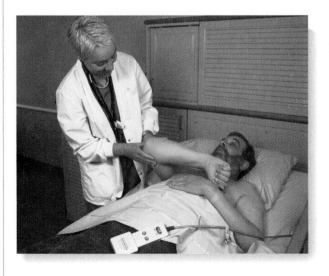

2 Avoid massaging over bony prominences. **RATIONALE:** Massaging can lead to deep tissue trauma.

- Keep bony prominences from direct contact with one another.
- Use pillows, foam wedges, or other positioning devices.

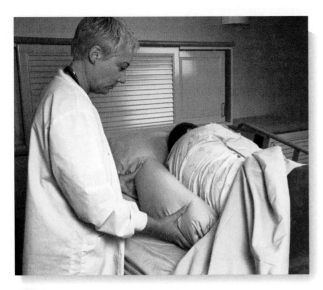

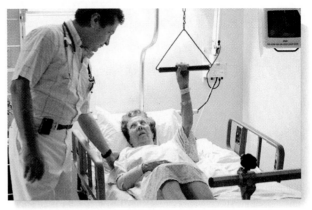

4 Use trapeze or turning sheet to reposition client. **RATIONALE:** This will prevent friction on skin.

3 Reposition bedridden client every 2 hrs. **RATIONALE:** To prevent decreased blood flow to dependent area. Altered oxygenation and nutrition to tissue results in pressure ulcers.

- Do not position client directly on trochanter.
- Raise client's heels off bed by placing pillow under legs; allow heels to hang over edges.

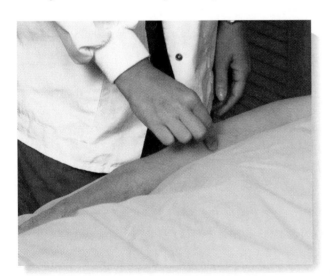

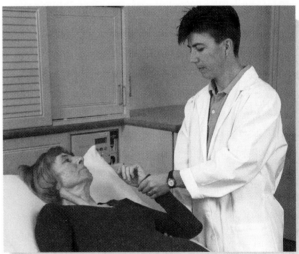

6 Encourage mobility or provide range-of-motion exercises.

5 Check hydration and nutrition status daily.

- Promote adequate dietary intake of protein, calories, and nutrients. **RATIONALE:** Adequate protein intake in addition to vitamins and minerals helps prevent pressure ulcer formation.

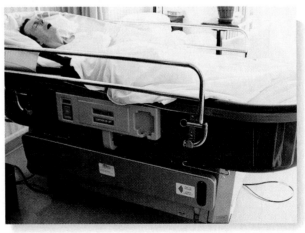

7 Place high-risk clients on pressure-reducing devices such as air-fluidized mattresses.

BEYOND THE SKILL

Pressure Ulcer Staging and Treatment*

Stage†

Stage I: Nonblanchable erythema of intact skin, the heralding lesion of skin ulceration.

Stage II: Partial-thickness skin loss involving epidermis or dermis. The ulcer is superficial and presents clinically as an abrasion, blister, or shallow crater.

Stage III: Full-thickness skin loss involving damage or necrosis of subcutaneous tissue that may extend down to, but not through, underlying fascia. The ulcer presents clinically as a deep crater with or without the undermining of adjacent tissue.

Stage IV: Full-thickness skin loss with extensive destruction, tissue necrosis, or damage to muscle, bone, or supporting structures (tendon or joint capsule are examples). Undermining and sinus tracts may be associated with this stage ulcer.

Treatment Protocol for Pressure Ulcer Stages

Stage I: Apply an adhesive film dressing over the red area. These dressings are semipermeable to oxygen and prevent bacterial invasion. Healing can occur in 24 hrs.

Stage II: Apply a transparent adhesive film dressing if ulcer is not draining. If wound is draining, irrigate with normal saline and apply a hydrocolloid dressing. These occlusive dressings remain in place for 5 to 7 days, creating a moist environment that promotes epithelialization and restoration of the epidermis.

Stage III: Irrigate with normal saline and cover with a hydrocolloid dressing. With excessively draining wounds, absorptive products are placed in the wound for absorption, and then the dressing is applied.

Stage IV: Chemical debridement, autolysis, or surgery is required for treatment of this stage. Wet-to-damp or wet-to-tacky dressing changes are used for small wounds; surgical interventions are used for larger wounds.

*SOURCE: *Pressure Ulcers in Adults: Prediction and Prevention,* Rockville, MD, U.S. Department of Health and Human Services, Public Health Service, Agency for Health Care Policy and Research.
†Pressure ulcers are classified in stages by the degree of tissue damage observed.
Accurate staging of pressure ulcers is not possible until eschar has sloughed or wound is debrided.

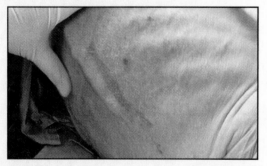
Stage I

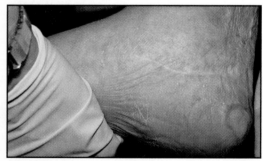
Stage II

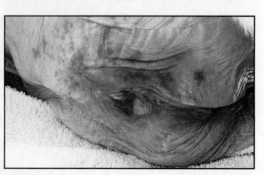
Stage III

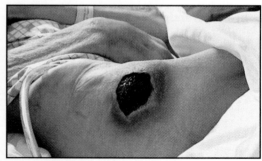
Stage IV

TEGADERM TRANSPARENT ADHESIVE FILM DRESSING

Equipment

- Sterile normal saline
- Tegaderm transparent dressing
- Sterile 4 × 4 gauze pads
- Cleansing solution (optional)
- Hypoallergenic tape
- Clean gloves or sterile gloves
- Skin prep (optional)
- Disposal bag

Preparation

1 Remove old dressing and place in disposal bag.

2 Cleanse wound if needed.

CLINICAL NOTE

- Tegaderm is used as a primary dressing for Stage I and II pressure ulcers or other wounds with minimal to moderate amounts of drainage.
- Tegaderm is used for clients at risk for skin breakdown.
- Tegaderm is used as a moist dressing for autolytic debridement.

SKILL

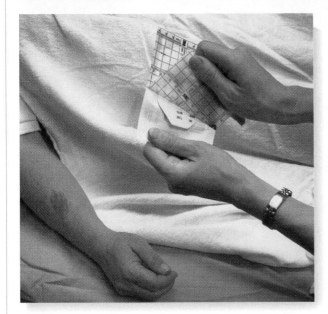

1 Remove transparent dressing from outer wrap.

- Assess wound site.

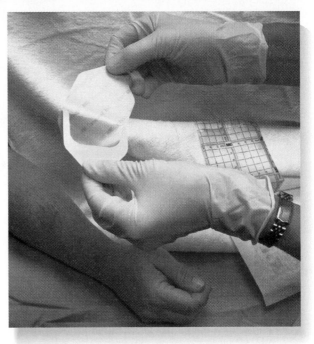

2 Don clean gloves or sterile gloves if condition warrants. Remove backing from sterile dressing.

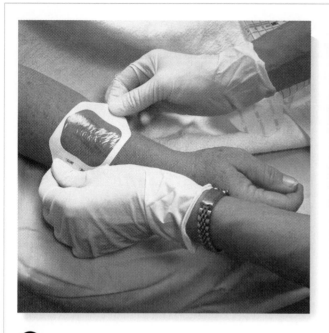

3 Position dressing over wound site. Ensure that entire wound site is covered.

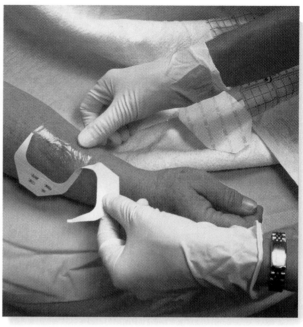

4 Remove backing from edge of transparent tape.

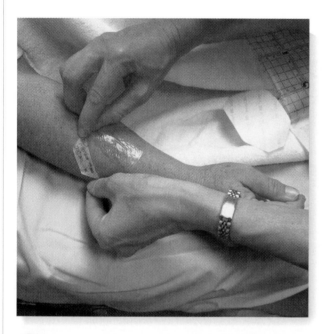

5 Press down edges of dressing securely to skin.

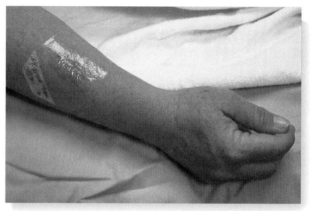

6 Label dressing with date and time applied.

SAFETY ALERT

Transparent film dressings remain in place for 5 to 7 days. It is imperative to observe the ulcer area daily to determine if a large amount of secretions or serous fluid has accumulated under a dressing. If fluid has increased, aspirate with a 26-gauge needle. These dressings are not used for infected areas.

TABLE 11-3	MOISTURE-RETENTIVE DRESSINGS		
	Advantages	**Disadvantages**	**Clinical Use**
Transparent Adhesive Film	■ Transparency allows wound visualization. ■ Conforms to area of application. ■ Can reduce friction of area. ■ Promotes autolysis of dry eschar. ■ Semipermeable; vapor can escape and environmental oxygen can enter to reduce chance of anaerobic bacterial growth. ■ Barrier to bacterial invasion; can aspirate fluid and patch. ■ Does not require secondary dressing.	■ Does not absorb exudate. ■ Exudate may macerate skin around wound. ■ Edges will roll in friction area. ■ May be difficult to apply. ■ May be too tightly applied. ■ Removal may tear underlying skin. ■ May increase bacterial growth in infected wounds.	■ Stage I and II pressure ulcers. ■ Donor sites. ■ Abrasions. ■ Extend edge to minimum 1¼ in beyond wound; skin around wound must be dry for adhesion; apply without tension. ■ Change when fluid build-up and leaking occurs and when edges are loosening to potentially expose wound.
Hydrogel	■ Comes in sheets or gel to conform to wound. ■ May be soothing. ■ Absorbs some exudate. ■ Provides moist wound healing. ■ Rehydrates dry wound beds.	■ Expensive. ■ Held in place with gauze dressing or transparent film. ■ May have transparent film on both sides (film next to wound must be removed).	■ Wounds with necrosis and slough. ■ Partial thickness (use sheets). ■ Gel can be used to fill wound cavity. ■ Change every day or twice a day, based on wound exudate.
Hydrocolloids	■ Use on acute and chronic wounds. ■ Absorbs exudate. ■ Conforms to area. ■ Prevents bacterial invasion.	■ Not transparent. ■ Melts down with exudate. ■ Characteristic drainage and odor. ■ Edges may need to be taped to prevent rolling. ■ Most do not allow environmental oxygen, so growth of anaerobic bacteria may be a problem.	■ Noninfected dermal ulcers. ■ May leave in place up to 7 days. ■ Change if leaking. ■ Change in clinical signs of infection. ■ Cleanse wound before application. ■ Roll dressing over wound. ■ Do not stretch; press securely.

SOURCE: Adapted from Frommhagen, J., *Current Management of Wounds.* Cabrillo College Syllabus, Level 1. Used with permission.

OP-SITE TRANSPARENT ADHESIVE FILM DRESSING

Equipment

- Sterile normal saline
- Op-Site transparent dressing
- Sterile 4 × 4 gauze pads
- Hypoallergenic tape

- Clean gloves or sterile gloves
- Skin prep (optional)
- Disposal bag

Preparation

1 Remove old dressing by "walking off" dressing from one edge to other and discard in disposal bag.

2 Assess wound.

3 Clean wound with sterile gauze pads moistened with sterile normal saline. Dry thoroughly.

SKILL

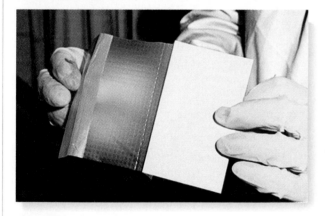

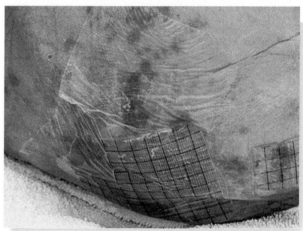

1 Measure wound using pliable device.

- Apply skin prep, if ordered. *Note:* Do not apply directly on ulcer as agent contains alcohol, which will burn area.
- Loosen transparent dressing from one side of backing paper.
- "Walk on" dressing: Start at one edge of site and gently lay dressing down, keeping it free of wrinkles. Allow at least a 1¼-in margin of dressing beyond ulcer margins. **RATIONALE:** This ensures coverage of entire wound area.

2 Ensure dressing is wrinkle free.

- Cut off tabs after wound is completely covered.
- Tape edges with hypoallergenic tape, if needed.

BEYOND THE SKILL

Hydrocolloid Dressing

Equipment

- Sterile normal saline
- Hydrocolloid dressing (e.g., DuoDerm, Restore, Ultec, ClearSite)
- Hydrocolloid gel, if needed
- Sterile 4 × 4 gauze pads
- Hypoallergenic tape
- Clean gloves

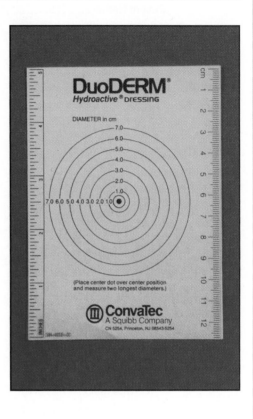

Skill

1. Select dressing size to ensure coverage 1¼ in beyond ulcer margin. **RATIONALE:** This ensures complete covering of wound.

2. Don clean gloves.

3. Cleanse skin with gauze pad moistened with sterile normal saline and pat dry with gauze pad.

4. Measure wound using pliable device.

5. Fill ulcer area with gel if ordered (usually used when exudate is present). Do not overfill wound with gel. **RATIONALE:** Gel absorbs exudate.

6. Remove silicone release paper backing from dressing. Minimize finger contact with adhesive surface. **RATIONALE:** Dressing is sterile and contamination should be avoided.

7. Center dressing over affected area. Gently roll dressing over pressure ulcer; do not stretch dressing. **RATIONALE:** Stretching dressing may cause wrinkling of dressing, which allows air to enter wound.

8. Mold dressing gently to skin, and hold down with hand for approximately 1 min.

9. Apply skin prep to area that is to be covered by tape if ordered. Allow to dry. Do not apply skin prep under hydrocolloid dressing. **RATIONALE:** Hydrocolloid dressings are placed over broken skin; skin prep may cause damage to skin.

10. Picture-frame sides of hydrocolloid dressing with hypoallergenic tape.

11. Check dressing daily for signs of leaking. **RATIONALE:** Dressings should not be left on more than 7 days.

SAMPLE PRESSURE ULCER ASSESSMENT GUIDE

Patient Name: _____ Date: _____ Time: _____

Ulcer 1:   Ulcer 2:
Site _____   Site_____
Stage[a] _____   Stage[a] _____
Size (cm)   Size (cm)
   Length _____   Length _____
   Width _____   Width _____
   Depth _____   Depth _____

Sinus Tract   Sinus Tract
Tunneling   Tunneling
Undermining   Undermining
Necrotic Tissue   Necrotic Tissue
   Slough   Slough
   Eschar   Eschar
Exudate   Exudate
   Serous   Serous
   Serosanguineous   Serosanguineous
   Purulent   Purulent
Granulation   Granulation
Epithelialization   Epithelialization
Pain   Pain

Surrounding Skin:
Erythema   Erythema
Maceration   Maceration
Induration   Induration

Description of Ulcer(s):
_____

_____

Indicate Ulcer Sites:

Anterior   Posterior
(Attach a color photo of the pressure ulcer[s] [Optional])

● **FIGURE 11-1** *Sample pressure ulcer documentation form.*

CHARTING

- Type, location, and extent of wound
- Results of ankle-brachial index measurement
- Complete pressure ulcer assessment guide
- General condition of skin surrounding wound

- Wound assessment, drainage, evidence of tissue granulation for vascular wound
- Type of wound care provided; type and size of dressings used
- Skin prep, if applied

CRITICAL THINKING FOCUS

SECTION ONE ▪ Measures to Prevent Infection

Unexpected Outcomes

- Hole develops in glove while sterile technique is being performed.

- Sterile field becomes wet or damp.

Alternate Nursing Actions

- Discard gloves and replace with sterile gloves.
- Examine hands for cuts if hole is caused by sharp object.
- If hands are cut, scrub hands and replace sterile gloves.

- Discard supplies on sterile field.
- Set up new sterile field.

SECTION TWO ▪ Dressing Change

Unexpected Outcomes

- Wound becomes infected with microorganisms.

- Wound does not heal.

- Skin appears red and broken.

Alternate Nursing Actions

- Notify physician about changes in color or odor of drainage.
- Obtain culture and sensitivity if physician orders one.
- Wash hands thoroughly after removing gloves and caring for client to prevent spread of infection.
- Pay strict attention to changing dressings.

- Evaluate use of dressing and perhaps choose different type of dressing.
- Assess nutritional status. Increase protein and carbohydrates if not contraindicated.
- Determine availability of vacuum-assisted closure machine.

- Clean area with sterile saline and dry thoroughly with sterile 4 × 4 pads.
- Apply moisture-retentive dressing.

SECTION THREE ▪ Wound Care

Unexpected Outcomes	Alternate Nursing Actions
▪ Wound drainage increases.	▪ Decrease time between dressing changes to every 4 hrs. ▪ Obtain order for culture and sensitivity to determine if different microorganism is present or if organism is not sensitive to antibiotic medication.
▪ Dressings dry between changes.	▪ Moisten dressing with sterile normal saline before removal to prevent debridement of granulation tissue. ▪ Ensure that dressing is moist when applied to wound and cover with dry dressing. ▪ Moisten and change dressing more frequently.
▪ Edges of wound split open (wound dehiscence).	▪ Place client in supine position. Apply butterfly tape to wound edges. Cover opening with sterile dressings. ▪ Apply binder for abdominal incision after obtaining order. ▪ Notify physician if signs of infection are present. ▪ Obtain culture of drainage if physician orders one. ▪ Observe client for signs of shock. If client is in shock, notify physician immediately. ▪ Encourage high-protein diet.
▪ Evisceration (protrusion of bowel contents) occurs.	▪ Institute emergency measures. Place client in supine position. Cover bowel with sterile gauze, moisten with sterile saline. Have IV-certified nurse insert IV catheter and infuse normal saline. Reassure client. Obtain vital signs, and treat for shock if present.
▪ Wound is too extensive for application of drainage bag or ABD pads cannot contain drainage.	▪ Obtain adhesive 8 × 8 adhesive sheets (e.g., Stomahesive or Hollihesive) cut on diagonal ⅛ to ¼ in larger than wound. ▪ If larger barrier is needed, Stomahesive may be pieced together to form larger barrier, reinforcing juncture points with Karaya paste. ▪ A superadhesive pouch may then be applied. If dressings are used, they may be secured with Montgomery straps (tie tapes).
▪ Abdominal binder is not effective in supporting incisional area.	▪ Evaluate effectiveness of abdominal binder. ▪ Assess if binder is properly positioned at hip level and waist level to provide support. ▪ Assess if binder is too loose.
▪ Client is too large for abdominal binder.	▪ Fold a draw sheet in half lengthwise and place under client. Position edges at waist and pubic area. ▪ Pull tightly on drawsheet, and secure edges with safety pins.
▪ Drainage system expands quickly after being reconnected.	▪ Check all connections for air leak; properly functioning reservoirs expand slowly.

SECTION FOUR ▪ Vascular Insufficiency Wounds

Unexpected Outcomes

- Client does not get sufficient exercise; appetite is decreased.

- Client's wound does not heal with traditional types of treatments.

Alternate Nursing Actions

- Encourage small, frequent feedings.
- Offer high-calorie drinks like eggnog or Isocal.

- In client care conference, discuss the following: Is everyone following the same treatment? Are causative agents preventing healing? Should treatment be adjusted or changed? Would use of a flotation or pressure-relieving mattress be useful? Is surgical debridement and grafting necessary for healing?

SELF-CHECK EVALUATION

PART 1 ▪ Matching Terms

Match the definition in column B with the correct term in column A.

Column A

_____ a. Dehiscence
_____ b. Evisceration
_____ c. Exudate
_____ d. Granulation
_____ e. Necrosis
_____ f. Pressure ulcer
_____ g. Tertiary healing
_____ h. Primary healing
_____ i. Second intention

Column B

1. Opening up of an incision
2. Protrusion of the viscera
3. Wound debris resulting from an inflammatory process
4. Outgrowth of new capillaries that become fibrous scar tissue
5. Death of a portion of tissue
6. Break in skin caused by decreased blood flow over a bony prominence
7. Open method of healing
8. Inflammatory reaction developing at wound site
9. Process involving wound granulation

PART 2 ▪ Multiple Choice Questions

1. The first stage in healing is best described as:
   a. Healing by use of retention sutures.
   b. Inflammatory reaction occurring at the wound site.
   c. Scar tissue formation.
   d. Wound healing using wet-to-damp dressings.

2. Which of the following factors usually affects wound healing?
   a. Sex of client.
   b. Type of surgery.
   c. Low-fat diet.
   d. Weight of client.

3. Which of the following clinical manifestations indicates a wound infection?

a. Temperature of 100.9°F (38.9°C).
b. Edema surrounding incision.
c. Decreased tenderness surrounding incision.
d. Increased urine output.

4. When putting on sterile gloves, the most appropriate concept to remember is:

a. Place your nondominant hand in the glove first.
b. The edges of the gloves are considered clean.
c. You can readjust the fingers of the first glove once the gloves have been donned.
d. When opening supplies, one glove can be contaminated, leaving the remaining glove to place dressings on the wound.

5. When cleaning a wound, the most important principle is to:

a. Start at the periphery and work toward the center of the wound.
b. Start at the bottom of the wound and work toward the top.
c. Start anywhere at the wound site, but do not contaminate the wound.
d. Start at the wound and work outward.

6. When placing sterile 4 × 4 gauze pads on the client's incision, you did not cover the incision as you intended. You should:

a. Remove the gauze pads and replace them with new pads.
b. Adjust the pads to cover the incision.
c. Place an additional pad over the exposed section of the incision.
d. Leave the gauze pads in place and apply an ABD pad over them.

7. Several days after surgery the physician orders removal of the client's staples. The most appropriate action to accomplish this is to place the staple-removing device:

a. On one side of the staple; depress device and lift off staple.
b. On both ends of the staple, one side at a time; depress device and lift off staple.
c. Under the center of the staple; press down on the handle to clip the staple.
d. Under the center of the staple; lift the staple, then depress the device.

8. You are ambulating a client down the hallway 5 days after surgery when he suddenly coughs and dehiscence occurs. Your first action is to:

a. Place the client in a supine position.
b. Call the doctor.
c. Obtain vital signs.
d. Cover the wound with a sterile dressing.

9. A client has a score of 12 on the Norton Scale for assessing the risk of developing a pressure ulcer. What does this indicate?

a. No risk for ulcer development.
b. High risk for ulcer development.
c. Some risk for ulcer development.
d. Low risk for ulcer development.

10. Which of the following interventions is most beneficial in preventing formation of a pressure ulcer?

a. Keep skin dry by applying benzoin or alcohol around reddened areas.
b. Ensure fluid intake of at least 2000 mL each day.
c. Elevate the head of the bed to prevent pressure on the coccyx and heels.
d. Change chux under the client each shift.

11. The most effective wound dressing for a Stage III pressure ulcer is:

  a. Wet-to-damp.
  b. Hydrocolloid.
  c. Transparent film.
  d. Dry dressing.

12. Goals of wound healing include which one of the following principles?

  a. Maintain a wet wound bed.
  b. Decrease granulation tissue at the wound site.
  c. Promote air circulation to the wound through application of loose dressings.
  d. Choose dressings based on the type of wound.

13. Transparent film dressings are best used with _____ wounds.

  a. Nondraining.
  b. Draining.
  c. Infected.
  d. Full-thickness.

14. The dressing most commonly used to treat a yellow wound is:

  a. Moist gauze.
  b. Transparent film.
  c. Exudate absorber.
  d. Dry gauze.

PART 3 ▪ Critical Thinking Application

Mrs. James is an 84-year-old client with diabetes mellitus admitted to the unit for treatment of a Stage III pressure ulcer on her coccyx. This occurred as a result of being on bed rest for the past 2 wks.

1. Describe the pressure ulcer findings you expect to observe in your assessment.
2. Identify the type of dressing most appropriate for this client and discuss the scientific basis for using this type of dressing.
3. Describe the steps in applying this type of dressing.
4. What is the relationship between the diagnosis and clinical picture of this client?

12

BODY MECHANICS AND POSITIONING

INTRODUCTION

Alterations in mobility can result from problems in the musculoskeletal system, the nervous system, or the skin. A primary cause for alterations in muscles is inactivity. Alterations in joints result when mobility is limited by changes in the adjacent tissues. When muscle movement decreases, the connective tissue in the joints, tendons, and ligaments becomes thickened and fibrotic. Chronic flexion or hyperextension can also cause joints to become contracted in one position so that they are unmovable. Alterations in bone are caused by disease processes, decalcification and breaks due to trauma, or twisting.

Encouraging clients to stand and to walk is important because the body functions best when in a vertical position. Physical activity forces muscles to move and increases blood flow, which improves metabolism and facilitates such body functions as gastrointestinal peristalsis.

Body mechanics is best defined as using alignment, balance, and correct posture when lifting, moving, or bending while providing client care. These movements are performed in a coordinated effort to promote safe musculoskeletal functions. These

(continued on next page)

coordinated movements prevent undue strain on muscles, thus preventing injury to health care workers. In addition to using coordinated movements, it is important to provide a wide base of support to give stability when changing body positions. The weight-bearing joints and skeletal muscles of the legs provide this wide base of support.

PREPARATION PROTOCOL: FOR BODY MECHANICS AND POSITIONING SKILLS

Complete the following steps before each skill.

1. Determine if client or object to be moved is too heavy or unwieldy for one person to move.
2. Determine best method for moving object or client.
3. Gather appropriate equipment for positioning or moving client.
4. Check physician's orders or client plan of care for positioning or moving client.
5. Check client's identaband.
6. Introduce yourself to client and explain nursing care you will be giving.
7. Provide privacy for client as needed.
8. Wash hands.
9. Don gloves as indicated.

COMPLETION PROTOCOL: FOR BODY MECHANICS AND POSITIONING SKILLS

Make sure the following steps have been completed.

1. Position client as ordered.
2. Return equipment to appropriate location.
3. Remove gloves, if used, and wash hands.
4. Document pertinent data and report as indicated.
5. Complete unusual occurrence forms if injury occurs while moving client or object.
6. Report any injury to nurse manager.

SECTION ONE

BODY MECHANICS

Proper use of body mechanics promotes safety for all health care workers and clients. Nurses are required to use their bodies throughout the day as they assist clients with moving, turning, and ambulating. Nurses often need to move equipment that could lead to injury to themselves or others if proper body mechanics is not used.

Body mechanics includes a center of gravity, line of gravity, and base of support. As you move, your center of gravity shifts in the direction of the moving body parts. Balance is dependent on the interrelationship of these three components. To maintain balance and stability as the person is moved, you must maintain the line of gravity at the center of the base of support.

Review the principles of body mechanics associated with maintaining good posture, body alignment, and balance. A simple task can lead to an injury if proper body mechanics is not maintained. Incorrectly lifting a pan of water or stretching to reach something on a shelf can cause a serious back injury. Incorrect lifting puts most of the pressure on the muscles of your lower back. Because these muscles are not strong enough to handle the stress, injury can occur.

RATIONALE

- To promote nurse and client safety through proper use of body mechanics
- To maintain good posture, thereby promoting optimum musculoskeletal balance
- To prevent injuries to clients and nurses when proper body mechanics is maintained

ASSESSMENT

- Determine your ability to move client or object without assistance.
- Assess your knowledge and use of proper body mechanics when providing client care.
- Assess client's ability to help with moving or positioning.

SAFETY ALERT

The most common back injury is strain on the lumbar muscle group. Follow these steps to protect your back:

- Establish firm base of support by placing both feet flat on floor with one foot slightly in front of the other.
- Distribute weight evenly on both feet.
- Maintain broad base of support: The broader the base of support and the lower the center of gravity, the greater the stability and balance.
- Slightly flex both knees; this allows strong muscles of legs to do the lifting.

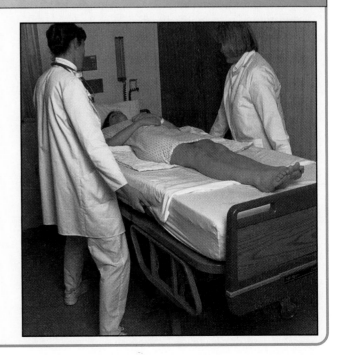

ESTABLISH BODY ALIGNMENT

SKILL

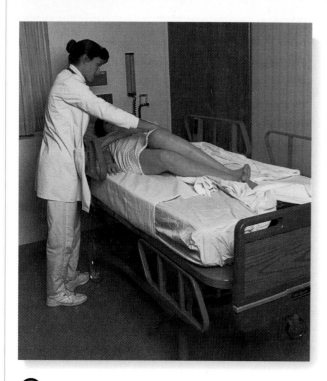

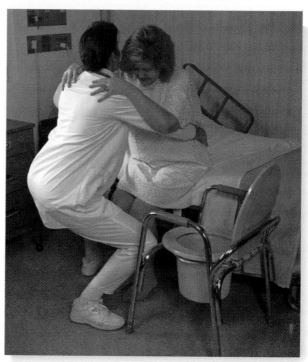

① Determine need for assistance in moving or turning client. **RATIONALE:** Back injury is often associated with lifting or turning clients.

- Face in direction of movement when sliding, pushing, or pulling objects. This helps prevent twisting of spine and acute flexion of back. **RATIONALE:** To prevent back injury.

② Hold abdomen firm and tuck buttocks in so that spine is in alignment as seen in safety alert. **RATIONALE:** This position protects back.

- Hold head erect and secure firm stance. Use this stance as basis for all actions in moving, turning, and lifting clients.
- Keep weight to be lifted as close to your body as possible. **RATIONALE:** This position maintains center of gravity.

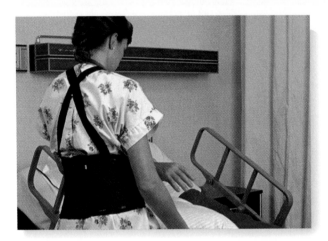

3 Wear back brace for moving, lifting, or turning if you have potential for back injury or client assignment dictates need for back support. **RATIONALE:** Brace protects and supports back and keeps body in alignment.

CLINICAL NOTE

GUIDELINES FOR MAINTAINING PROPER BODY MECHANICS

- Assume proper stance before moving or turning clients; position feet for broad base of support.
- Distribute workload evenly before moving or turning clients.
- Establish comfortable height when working with clients.
- Maintain balanced center of gravity (pelvis slightly anterior to sacrum).
- Keep spine in vertical alignment.
- Keep hips and knees flexed when moving clients.

- Maintain strong grip with arms and keep elbows slightly flexed.
- Push and pull objects when moving them to conserve energy.
- Use large muscle groups of legs for lifting and moving, not back muscles.
- Avoid leaning and stretching.
- Request assistance from others when working with heavy clients to avoid back strain.
- Avoid twisting your body.

PROPER BODY ALIGNMENT

SKILL

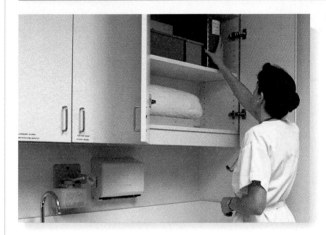

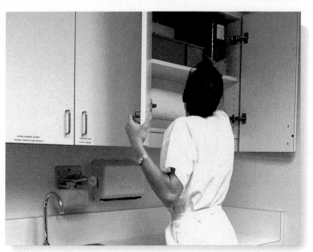

① Begin with proper stance as outlined in skill for establishing body alignment.

- Evaluate working height necessary to achieve objective.
- Establish comfortable height at which to work (usual height is between waist and lower level of hip joint).
- Check that this level minimizes muscle strain by extending your arms, and make sure your body maintains proper alignment.

② Do not stretch or twist when you need to reach for objects out of close proximity to your body.

- Flex your knees if you need to work at a lower level.

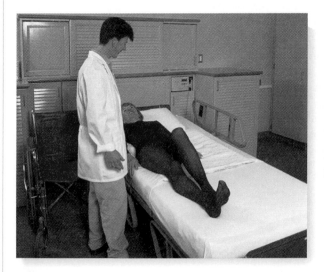

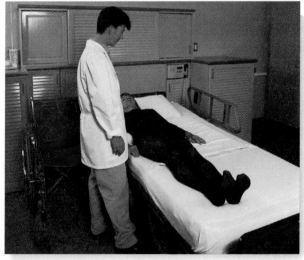

④ Do not bend over or reach for an object. **RATIONALE:** This can cause back strain.

③ Work close to your body so that your center of gravity is not misaligned and your muscles are not hyperextended.

- Use your longest and strongest muscles (biceps, quadriceps, and gluteals) when moving and turning clients.

BASIC PRINCIPLES OF BODY MECHANICS

SKILL

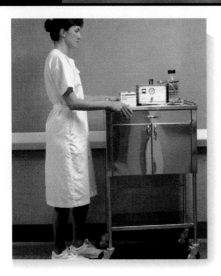

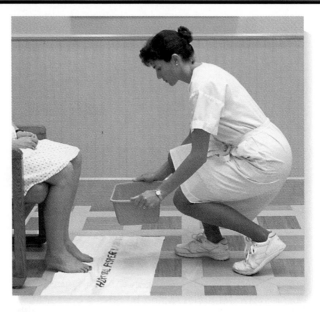

1 Move objects by pushing or pulling them. Stand close to object.

- Place your body in proper body alignment stance.
- Tense muscles and prepare for movement.
- Push away from you by leaning toward object, using body weight to add force.
- Pull toward you by leaning away from object and letting hips, arms, and legs do the work.

2 When working at lower surface levels, flex body at knees and, keeping back straight, use thigh and gluteal muscles to accomplish task.

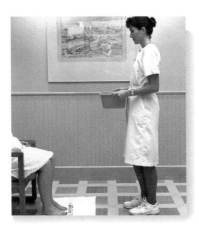

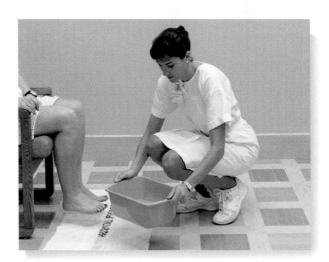

3 Hold objects close to your body when carrying them. **RATIONALE:** This prevents muscle strain and back injury.

- Place yourself in proper body alignment stance.
- Lift object by lifting with arms or stooping and using leg and thigh muscles.

4 Move muscles as a unit and in alignment rather than twisting your body.

- When changing direction, use pivotal movement—move muscles as a unit and in alignment, rather than rotating or twisting upper part of body.

- Devices needed for turning or moving client
- Number of staff members required to turn or move client
- Injury incurred by client with improper turning or moving

SECTION TWO

BODY POSITIONING

Nursing care measures to preserve the joints, bones, and skeletal muscles should be carried out for all clients who require bed rest. Positions in which clients are placed and methods of moving and turning clients should all be based on the principles of maintaining the musculoskeletal system in proper alignment. Frequent positioning is necessary for clients who are unable to move themselves. Whether the position is correct or incorrect, if the client remains in one position for a protracted period of time, complications of immobility can occur. The use of trochanter and hand rolls may be necessary to maintain correct positioning for some clients. The nurse must also use good body mechanics when moving or turning clients to preserve her or his own musculoskeletal system from injury.

If at all possible, clients should sit in a chair or ambulate at least two to three times each day. This will help preserve the client's musculoskeletal system and prevent formation of pressure ulcers.

RATIONALE

- To prevent contractures
- To promote optimal joint movement
- To prevent injury due to improper movement
- To prevent pressure ulcer formation

ASSESSMENT

- Observe client's bony prominences when turning client.
- Determine client's ability to help with positioning.
- Determine client's ability to maintain certain positions for specified time.
- Assess client's alignment after positioning or moving into chair.

POSITION CHANGES

Equipment

- Pillows for positioning
- Turning sheet (optional)

- Draw sheet or bath blanket for trochanter roll

Preparation

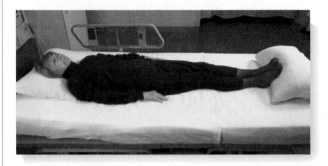

1 Lower head of bed completely or to as low a position as client can tolerate. Elevate bed to comfortable working height.

- Move client to opposite side of bed.

SKILL

Lateral Position

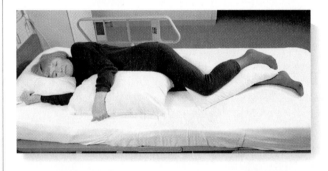

1 Place one hand on client's hip and one hand on client's shoulder; flex knees and roll client onto side facing you.

- Position pillow to maintain proper alignment.
- Be sure to position client's arms so they are not under client's body.

Prone Position

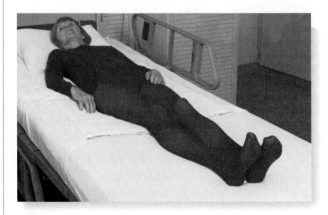

1 Move client to side of bed away from side where she will finally be positioned.

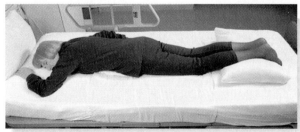

2 Roll client onto pillows, making sure client's arms are not under her body.

- Position pillows for client's head and feet.

BEYOND THE SKILL

Position Changes

1. Clients may be positioned in a semi-Fowler's or supine position. The semi-Fowler's position is frequently used for clients following surgery. It allows the lungs to expand and thus prevents pneumonia or atelectasis. Pillows are used to support the arms, under the head, and at the feet, to prevent the client from sliding down the bed and as a foot rest.

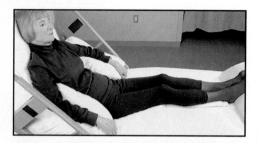

2. The supine position is used infrequently, mainly for spinal surgery clients or following myelography. Many of these clients may be placed in a low Fowler's position, however. A small pillow under the head and one at the feet are the usual support in this position.

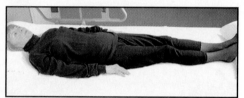

MOVE CLIENT UP IN BED

Equipment

- Draw sheet, folded to use as lift sheet (as noted)

One Assistant

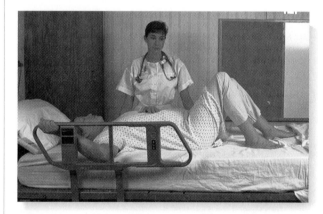

1 Lower head of bed so it is flat or as low as client can tolerate.

- Raise bed to comfortable working height.
  RATIONALE: Allows your center of gravity to assist in turning.

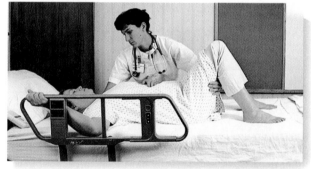

2 Place one arm under client's shoulders and other arm under client's thighs.

- Flex your knees and hips. Move feet close to bed.
- Place your weight on your back foot.
- Instruct client to put arms across chest, flex legs, and put feet flat on bed. If client is able, she can hold onto side rails to assist in moving.

SKILL

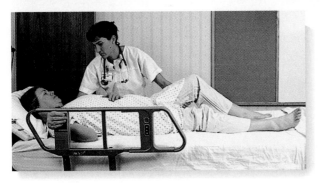

3 Shift your weight from back to front foot as you lift client up in bed. **RATIONALE:** Shifting weight reduces force needed to move client up in bed.

■ Ask client to push with feet as you move her.

■ Position client comfortably, replacing pillow and arranging bedding as necessary.

Two Assistants

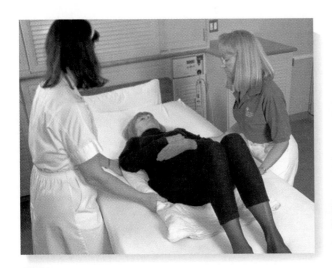

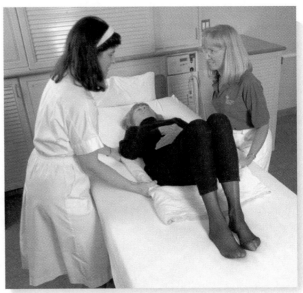

1 Remove pillow and place it at head of bed. **RATIONALE:** This prevents striking client's head against bed and makes it easier to move client.

■ Instruct client to flex knees. **RATIONALE:** This allows client to assist nurse in moving by pushing with feet.

2 Position one nurse on each side of client.

■ Place folded draw sheet under client's body extending from shoulder line to just below buttocks.

■ Roll up sides of lift sheet as close as possible to sides of client; have client flex knees, if possible.

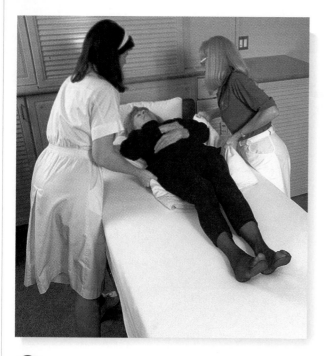

3 Grasp draw sheet at level of client's upper back with one hand and at level of buttocks with other hand.

- Assume broad base of support with feet; flex knees.
- Place weight on back foot. With one firm, coordinated rocking movement (shifting weight from back to front foot), lift client toward head of bed.

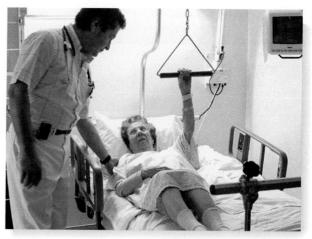

4 Alternate method: A trapeze is often used for clients with orthopedic injuries.

- Instruct client to grasp trapeze with both hands and flex knees.
- Follow steps for assuming proper stance.
- Place your arm under client's thighs; as you move client, instruct her to lift and pull herself toward head of bed.

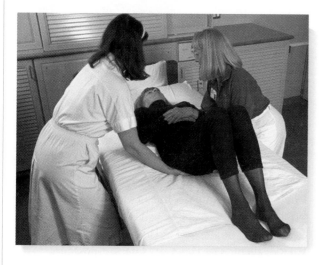

5 Alternate method for moving without draw sheet: After placing client flat in bed, use two nurses to move client.

- Position one nurse on each side of client.
- Assume broad base of support and position front foot facing head of bed, body slightly turned toward head of bed.
- Instruct client to bend knees.
- Each nurse places one arm under client's shoulders and other arm under client's buttocks. Then each nurse places weight on back foot in readiness for moving.

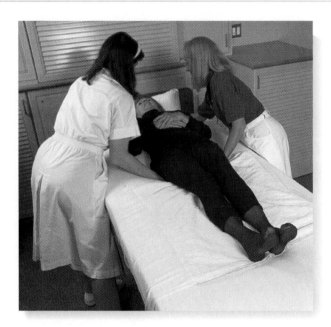

6 Alternate method continued: On count of three, have client push with feet and legs while you pivot weight from back foot to front foot and lift client toward head of bed. **RATIONALE:** Client can help move up in bed by pushing with feet and legs.

Three Assistants

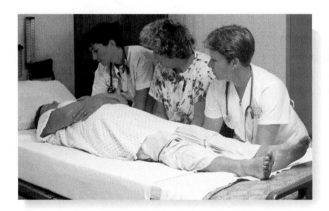

1 Position all three nurses at same side of bed. First nurse supports client's head and shoulders; second nurse supports waist and buttocks; third nurse supports thighs and lower legs.

- Each nurse assumes broad base of support with one foot slightly in front of the other, flexing knees and straightening back.

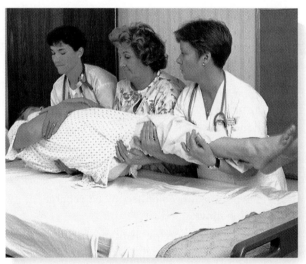

2 Nurse at head of bed counts to three; nurses lift client up and toward their chests. Using large muscles of legs, nurses move sideways in a coordinated movement to move client to head of bed.

- Nurses then place client on bed by flexing knees and using thigh muscles to lower client to bed. Pillow is placed under client's head and positioned for comfort.

LOGROLL CLIENT

Equipment

- Pillows, towels, blankets for positioning
- Turning sheet

SKILL

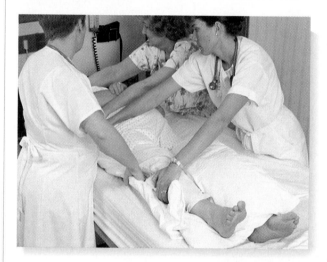 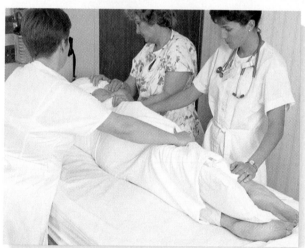

① Obtain sufficient assistance to complete procedure with ease. Three nurses are preferable.

- Place pillow between client's knees before moving client. **RATIONALE:** To prevent adduction of hip; this will prevent spinal torque.
- Position two nurses on side of bed to which client will be turned. Position third nurse on opposite side of bed.
- Designate person at head of bed to be in charge of coordinating move.
- Assume correct position for client move: Nurse at head supports client's head by placing arm under neck; other arm is placed over client's chest, keeping arm straight when reaching over client.
- Second nurse grasps client's upper hip with one hand and places other hand and arm around client's lower thigh or knee, again keeping arms straight when reaching over client.
- Third nurse, on opposite side of bed, holds draw sheet firmly and close to client's body to support torso. **RATIONALE:** This maintains body alignment.

② Move client in one coordinated movement when nurse at head of bed counts to three. **RATIONALE:** To maintain proper alignment, all body parts must be moved at same time to prevent torque to spinal cord.

- Instruct client to place arms across chest.
- Assume broad stance with one foot ahead of the other.
- Flex knees and maintain center of gravity.
- As client is turned, rock onto back foot, using leg and arm muscles.

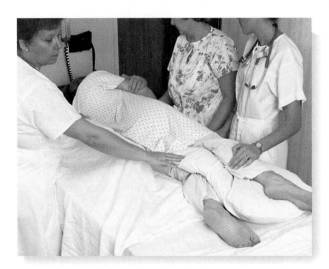

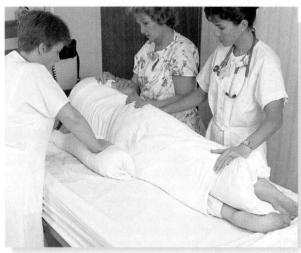

3 Place pillows behind client's back.

- Adjust pillow between client's legs.
- Flex client's upper leg slightly over pillow.
- Place client's head on a pillow.

4 Instruct client to lean back into pillow for support.

- Pillow can be placed in front of client with client's upper arm placed on pillow. **RATIONALE:** This allows client to maintain body alignment and prevent client from falling forward and placing torque on spine.
- Tuck pillow tightly at client's body.

TROCHANTER ROLL PLACEMENT

Equipment

- Bath blanket

SKILL

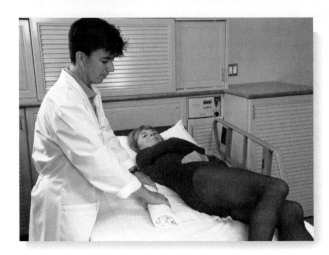

1 Place client in supine or prone position.

- Place folded bath blanket on bed next to client. Extend blanket from greater trochanter to thigh or knee.
- Place blanket edge under leg and buttocks to anchor.
- Roll bath blanket by rolling it toward you (each turn is rolled under earlier roll) until it reaches client's body.

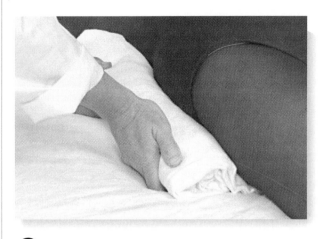

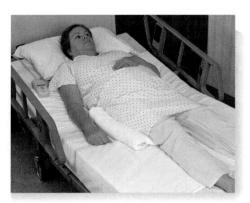

2 Rotate affected leg to slight internal hip rotation. **RATIONALE:** This prevents external rotation of head of femur in the acetabulum.

- Tighten roll by tucking roll under hip joint.
- Allow affected leg to rest against trochanter roll.

3 Check that hip is in normal alignment, not internally or externally rotated. Patella should be facing upward. **RATIONALE:** This is used most commonly for clients with muscle weakness due to paralysis of one side of body.

BEYOND THE SKILL

Hand Rolls

Hand rolls can be made from folded washcloths. The hand roll is used to position and maintain the wrist and fingers in a functional position. The purpose is to prevent deformity and contractures.

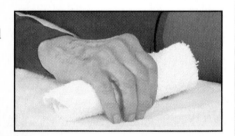

SAFETY ALERT

Footboards are used to maintain dorsiflexion of the feet and keep linens off the feet of clients on long-term bed rest. Footboards are also used to maintain a Fowler's or semi-Fowler's position for clients on bed rest. Prolonged periods of plantarflexion can lead to footdrop. Ensure that clients' feet and ankles are put through range-of-motion exercises when a footboard is being used. Many rehabilitation facilities place clients in high-top sneakers or Unna boots while on bed rest, because both help to prevent footdrop and keep the feet in a functional position.

TRANSFER FROM BED TO GURNEY

Equipment

- Gurney
- Sheets to cover gurney and client

SKILL

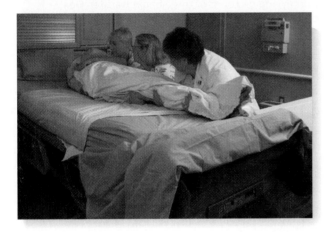

1 Position gurney at right angle (90°) to bed and lock brakes. Elevate bed slightly higher than gurney. **RATIONALE:** Makes it easier to transfer client.

- Place bed in flat position and lower side rails.
- Cover client with sheet or bath blanket.
- Place nurses (two or three, depending on size of client) on same side of bed; one nurse is at head and shoulders, one at hips, and one at thighs and ankles of client. **RATIONALE:** These positions will distribute client's weight evenly.
- Place client's arms across chest.

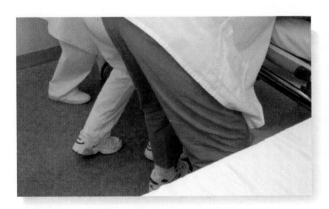

2 Place one foot toward gurney, using wide stance. **RATIONALE:** This position is more balanced when pivoting and gives broad base of support.

- Flex knees. **RATIONALE:** This position reduces back strain and lowers center of gravity.

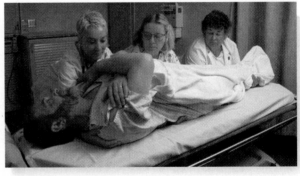

3 Place arms under client so that fingers are wrapped around client's body.

- Lift client on count of three and bring close to nurses' chests.
- Pivot and step toward gurney on count of three. **RATIONALE:** Counting to three ensures that nurses will move together and keep client in alignment.
- Lower client gently to center of gurney by flexing knees and hips. **RATIONALE:** This position prevents back strain from bending at waist.
- Check client's alignment, fix safety straps on gurney, and put up side rails.

CLINICAL NOTE

ALTERNATIVE METHOD FOR TRANSFERRING CLIENT
- Place draw sheet under client as needed. Cover client with sheet or bath blanket.
- Raise bed a little higher than gurney height. **RATIONALE:** To facilitate move to gurney.
- Move client to edge of bed. Undo draw sheet from sides of bed and roll close to client's side.
- Move gurney next to bed and lock wheels on gurney. **RATIONALE:** Prevents gurney from moving during transfer.
- Roll draw sheet tightly against client.
- Instruct client to place arms across chest and flex neck during transfer.
- Instruct all assistants to press their bodies tightly against gurney and on count of three begin transfer. Flex hips and pull client on pull sheet directly toward you onto gurney.
- Raise side rails and straighten draw sheet. **RATIONALE:** To prevent client from lying on wrinkled sheet and thus causing pressure on coccyx and sacrum.

MOVE TO GURNEY USING TRANSFER BOARD

Equipment

- Smooth polyethylene board about 18 to 22 in wide by 72 in long (45 to 55 cm by 182 cm)
- Sheets to cover board, gurney, and client (three)
- Bath blanket (optional)
- Gurney

SKILL

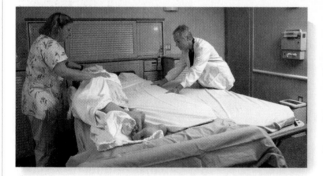

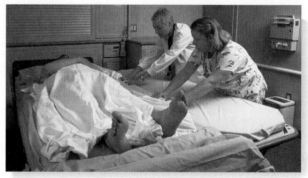

1 Cover turning board and gurney with sheet.

- Cover client with sheet or bath blanket.
- Position client on side of bed away from gurney in lateral position.
- First nurse supports client while second nurse places board as close to client as possible. **RATIONALE:** This allows client to be positioned on entire board after turn.

2 Instruct client to turn onto back, directly onto board. Client may need assistance to turn.

- After client is on board, nurse moves to other side of bed to assist with transfer.

SAFETY ALERT

Be sure to lock wheels on both bed and gurney.

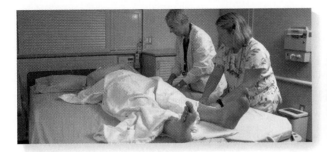

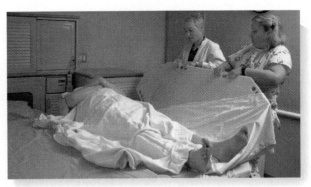

3 Assume appropriate stance (broad base of support, one foot in front of the other); flex knees and hips.

- On count of three, transfer weight from front to back foot as you lift board and pull it toward you.

4 Center client on gurney and remove board by pulling board out and up using handholds along edge of board.

- When removing board, maintain proper body mechanics.
- Place all side rails in UP position.

DANGLE CLIENT AT BEDSIDE

SKILL

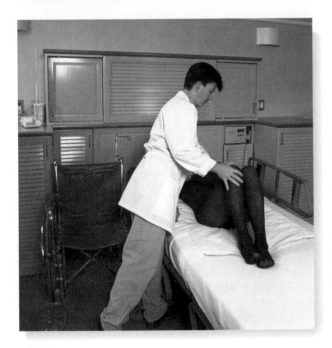

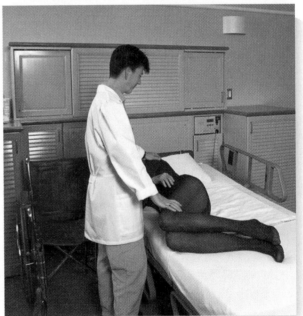

1 Lower bed to lowest position.

- Move client to edge of bed. **RATIONALE:** This allows client to easily move legs and feet over side of bed onto floor.
- Instruct client to flex knees.

2 Turn client onto side, keeping knees flexed, or place bed in Fowler's position (head elevated at 45° angle). **RATIONALE:** This position is sometimes preferred; it is easier for nurse to pivot client to sitting position.

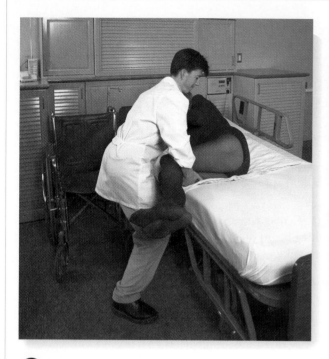

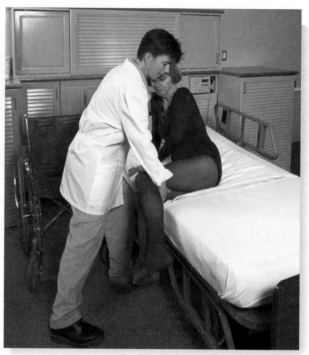

3 Stand at client's hip level. Assume broad base of support with forward foot closest to client. Flex your knees, hips, and ankles.

- Place one of your arms under client's shoulders and other arm beneath both of client's thighs near knees. **RATIONALE:** This will prevent client from falling backward onto bed.

4 Lift client's thighs slightly and pivot on balls of your feet as you move client into sitting position.

- Use your gluteal, abdominal, leg, and arm muscles to move client to sitting position.
- Stand in front of client until client is stable in upright position. **RATIONALE:** Clients may experience orthostatic hypotension if they have been on bed rest for a period of time.
- Vital signs may be taken when client is first dangled.
- Client should be dangled for a few minutes before being transferred to chair or wheelchair.

MOVE CLIENT FROM BED TO CHAIR

Equipment

- Wheelchair or bedside chair

SKILL

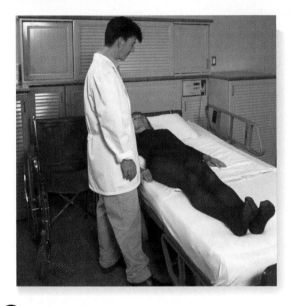

1 Place chair or wheelchair at head of bed. Set brake on wheelchair by pulling lever backward to lock wheels.

- Move client to side of bed.

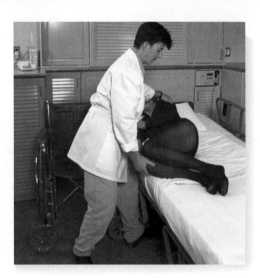

2 Place client in lateral position with knees flexed.

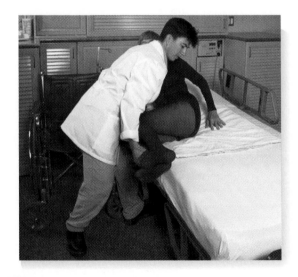

3 Follow steps 3 and 4 in skill for dangling client at bedside.

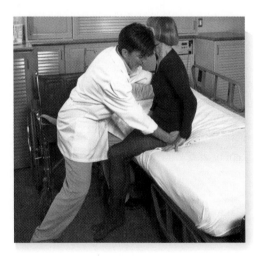

4 Place hands on client's hips and pull client toward edge of bed until client's feet touch floor.

- As you move client toward edge of bed, shift your weight to back foot and keep your knees and hips flexed. Use large muscles of legs for pulling client to edge of bed.
- Dangle client until stable.

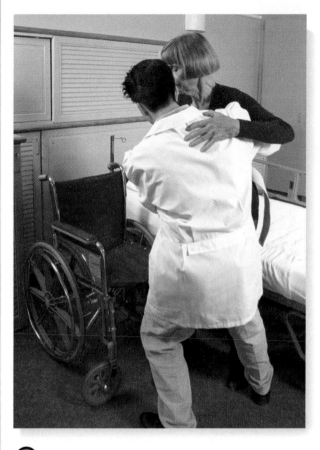

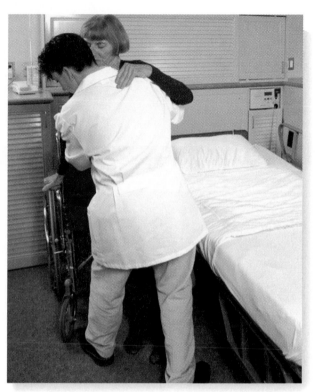

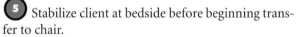

6 Instruct client to grasp handrail on chair as you pivot client into chair.

- Move your back foot toward wheelchair as you pivot client toward chair.
- Keep both feet on outside of client's feet. **RATIONALE:** This provides more stability as you pivot client because broad base of support is maintained.

5 Stabilize client at bedside before beginning transfer to chair.

- Instruct client to place arm (away from chair) over your shoulder. **RATIONALE:** This will help stabilize client when pivoting into chair.
- Place your hands under client's axillae or around client's back.
- Assume broad-based stance with foot closest to bed slightly in front of back foot; place your foot on outside of client's foot.
- Rock client and, on count of three, pivot client into chair.

SAFETY BELT TRANSFER

Equipment

- Transfer belt
- Wheelchair or chair

SKILL

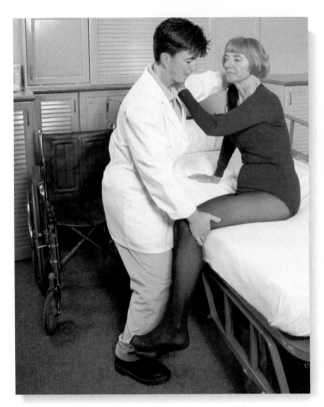

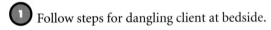

① Follow steps for dangling client at bedside.

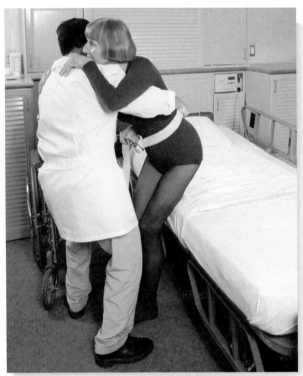

② Place safety belt around client's waist. Follow directions from manufacturer on how to secure belt.

- Instruct client to place arm away from chair over your shoulder.
- Assume broad-based stance with your feet on outside of client's feet and place forward foot in front of wheelchair and back foot facing bed.
- Stabilize client by holding onto safety belt.

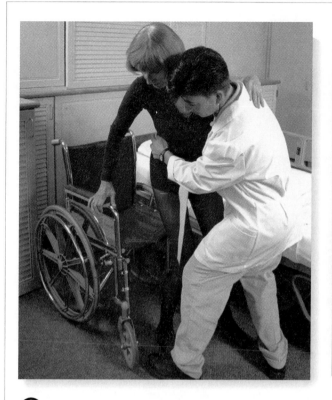

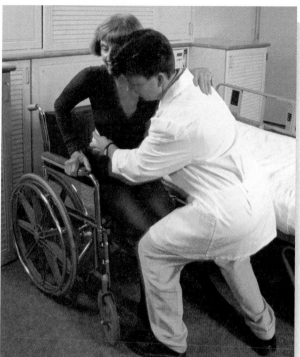

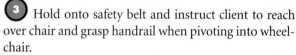 Hold onto safety belt and instruct client to reach over chair and grasp handrail when pivoting into wheelchair.

- Guide client into chair using safety belt while keeping your feet on outside of client's feet, maintaining broad base of support.

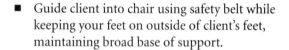 Lower client into chair by flexing your knees and hips and using large muscles in your thighs, not your back, as you move client.

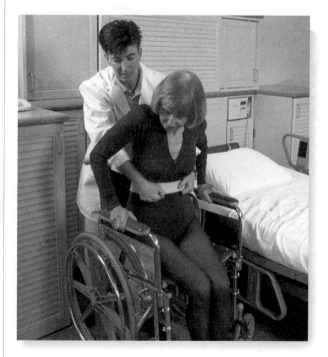

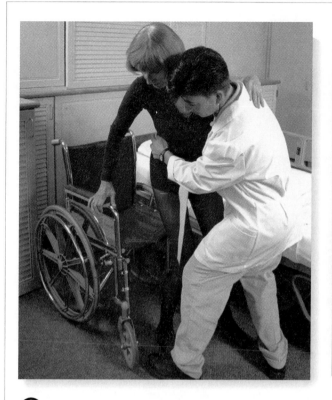 Stand behind wheelchair and instruct client to push with feet as you pull up on safety belt to move client back in wheelchair.

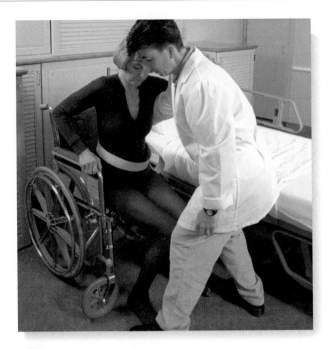

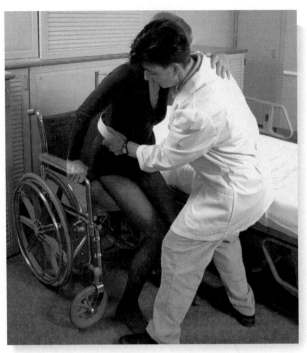

6 Move client back into bed; instruct client to place arm nearest bed over your shoulder.

- As you pull on safety belt, have client push forward using side rail for leverage.
- Assume broad base of support with both feet outside client's feet.

7 Rock client and, on count of three, pull client to standing position using safety belt.

- Flex knees and hips and shift weight backward as you pull client into standing position.

8 Pivot client onto bed. Shift your weight to back leg, keeping your knee flexed, as you pivot client.

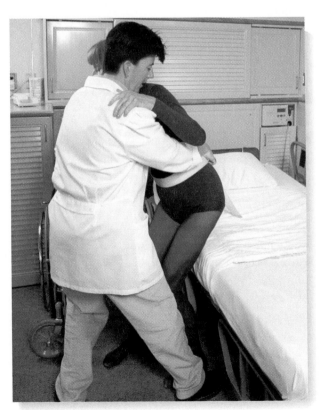

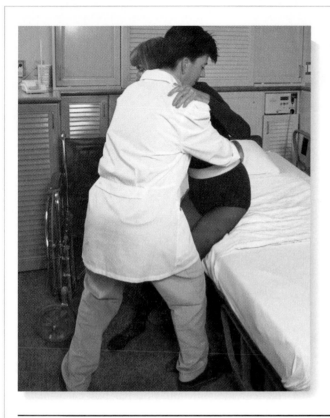

9 As you lower client down on bed, flex your knee and shift your weight toward leg nearest bed.

■ Remove belt and assist client to reclining position.

HOYER LIFT MOVE

Equipment

■ Hoyer frame
■ Canvas pieces (one large, one small)

■ Canvas straps (two sets)

SKILL

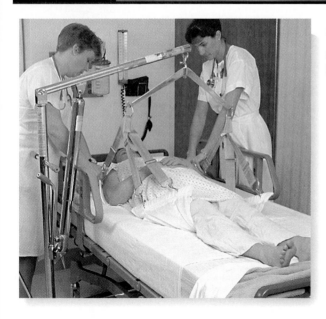

1 Obtain assistance, if possible, to complete procedure with ease. Two nurses are preferable for hospitalized clients.

■ Bring Hoyer frame to bedside.
■ Place client's chair nearby for easy access.
■ Raise bed to HIGH position and adjust head and knee gatch so that mattress is flat.
■ Roll client to one side and place lower edge of wide canvas piece under client's thighs.
■ Place upper edge of narrow canvas piece under client's shoulders.
■ Roll client to other side; straighten out canvas pieces. Turn client to supine position.

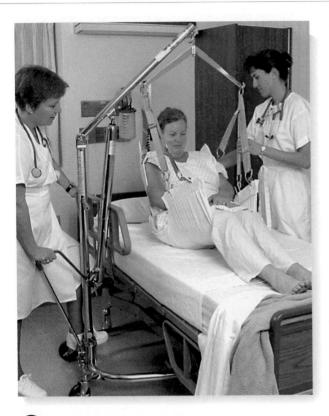

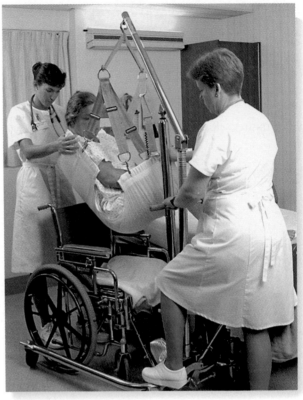

2 Place U base of frame under bed on side where chair is positioned.

- Lock wheels on frame.
- Attach canvas straps from swivel bar to each canvas piece using hooks.
- Be sure straps are evenly placed on canvas pieces. Sling extends from client's shoulders to knees. **RATIONALE:** This supports client's weight evenly.
- Assist client to raise head.
- Raise client by turning release knob clockwise to close pressure valve.
- Pump lift handle until client is lifted clear of bed.

3 Place chair under lift.

- Maneuver client over chair. Lower client by turning release knob slowly counterclockwise.
- Guide client into chair.
- Align client in chair.
- Remove straps from bar; move lift out of way.
- Check client's comfort in chair; place call bell close at hand.

CHARTING

- How often client is turned or moved
- Condition of skin and joint movement
- Unexpected problems with moving or positioning client and solutions to problems
- Client's acceptance of and feelings about procedure

- Number of staff members needed to complete procedure
- Use of assistive devices in transfer—safety belt, transfer belt, Hoyer lift
- Time client is in chair or dangled at bedside
- Use of footboard, trochanter roll, hand roll

CRITICAL THINKING FOCUS

SECTION ONE ▪ Body Mechanics

Unexpected Outcomes

Alternative Nursing Actions

- Nurse injures self while giving client care.

- Wear back brace to support back.
- Report any back strain immediately to supervisor.
- Complete unusual occurrence form.
- Go to health service or emergency room for evaluation and immediate care.
- Evaluate any activities that led to injury to determine incorrect use of body mechanics.
- Prevent additional injury by obtaining assistance when needed.
- Use devices such as turning sheets to assist in turning difficult clients.

- Nurse uses poor body mechanics and injures client.

- Assess extent of client's injury.
- Notify client's physician.
- Complete unusual occurrence form.
- Carry out physician's orders for follow-up treatment.

- Due to staffing shortage, nurse is unable to obtain sufficient assistance with turning and moving clients.

- Place turning sheets under all clients who are difficult to move.
- Use principles of leverage in moving clients.
- Turn and position clients from side to side at least every 2 hrs.
- Use Hoyer lift to move heavy clients.

SECTION TWO ▪ Body Positioning

Unexpected Outcomes

Alternative Nursing Actions

- Client is unwilling to move due to fear of pain or discomfort.

- Explain rationale and need for procedure more thoroughly.
- If possible, check if client can be medicated before procedure.
- Obtain additional assistance to decrease client's apprehension.

- Client is unable to assist with moving.

- Use draw sheet to provide more support for client.
- Obtain additional assistance to help with moving.

- Client is unable to maintain positions without assistance.

- Use trochanter roll to prevent external rotation of client's hip.
- Use foam bolsters to maintain lateral positions.
- Use pillows to maintain alignment.

- Client's skin begins to break down.

- Change client's position every 2 hrs.
- Check with physician for therapeutic mattress or treatment plan for pressure ulcer.

SELF-CHECK EVALUATION

PART 1 ▪ Matching Terms

Match the definition in column B with correct term in column A.

Column A

_____ a. Strain
_____ b. Trochanter
_____ c. Musculoskeletal
_____ d. Line of gravity
_____ e. Alignment
_____ f. Body mechanics
_____ g. Center of gravity
_____ h. Dangle
_____ i. Dorsiflexion
_____ j. Fowler's position
_____ k. Footdrop
_____ l. Flexion

Column B

1. Midpoint or center of the body weight
2. Movement of the body in a coordinated and efficient way
3. An imaginary line that goes from the center of gravity to the base of support
4. Pertaining to muscles and bones
5. Injury caused by excessive force or stretching of muscles or tendons around a joint
6. Head of bed at a 45° angle
7. Either of two bony prominences below the neck of the femur
8. Referring to posture, the relationship of body parts to one another
9. The act or condition of being bent
10. A falling or dragging of the foot; paralysis of the flexors of the ankle
11. Flexion of the foot or ankle joint
12. Position in which client sits at edge of bed with feet in a dependent position

PART 2 ▪ Multiple Choice Questions

1. Body mechanics is best described as:

a. Maintaining the body in an erect position.
b. Using alignment, balance, and correct posture when providing client care.
c. Using flexion and extension when moving clients.
d. Maintaining a wide base of support during moving and turning.

2. Balance is dependent on the interrelationship of all of the following components except:

a. Center of gravity.
b. Line of gravity.
c. Degree of flexion of knees and hips.
d. Base of support.

3. Which one of the following concepts is *not* correct in maintaining body alignment?

a. Distribute weight evenly on both feet.
b. Maintain a broad base of support.
c. Keep both feet on the same plane.
d. Maintain knee flexion when lifting.

4. When working at a surface that is lower than ideal height, which one of the following actions will *not* be used?

a. Keeping knees bent when moving objects.
b. Keeping back straight when moving objects.
c. Using thigh muscles to move objects.
d. Using arm muscles to move objects.

5. The primary rationale for the nurse to use proper body mechanics is to:
   a. Protect the client.
   b. Prevent injuries.
   c. Establish body alignment.
   d. Maintain body alignment.

6. To perform the skill for turning to the lateral position, you lower the head of the bed, elevate the bed to working height, move the client to your side of the bed, and flex the client's knees. The next step is to:
   a. Roll the client onto his or her side.
   b. Reposition the client.
   c. Place one hand on client's hip and the other on his or her shoulder.
   d. Position client's arms so they are not under his or her body.

7. When moving the client up in bed, remove the pillow and place it at the head of the bed. The rationale for this action is to:
   a. Get the pillow out of the way.
   b. Prevent the client from striking his or her head.
   c. Facilitate completing the procedure.
   d. Enable the client to push from his or her knees.

8. You are assigned to move a client from the bed to a chair. What is the first appropriate intervention?
   a. Dangle the client at the bedside.
   b. Put slippers on the client.
   c. Rock the client and pivot.
   d. Position the client so that he or she is comfortable.

9. Which type of client is *not* appropriate to move with a Hoyer lift?
   a. CVA.
   b. Immobilized.
   c. Obese.
   d. Back-injured.

10. Which one of the following guidelines is *not* appropriate when implementing body mechanics?
   a. Use large muscles for lifting and moving clients.
   b. Hold head erect and slightly bend back.
   c. Push and pull objects to conserve energy when moving clients.
   d. Assume a broad-based stance when moving clients.

PART 3 ■ Critical Thinking Application

You are assigned to care for a client who weighs 300 lb. The client was out of bed for lunch and now insists on getting back into bed. There are no male staff members available to help you.

1. Suggest some creative resolutions to this problem.

2. What other problems would you anticipate with this client?

13

EXERCISE AND AMBULATION

INTRODUCTION

Exercise and ambulation activities are used to preserve and restore mobility. Preservative methods, such as exercises and assisted ambulation, include those interventions that are needed to help clients maintain their normal mobility. Because the changes that occur in the human body when a person is hospitalized are varied and subtle, preservative methods are used with every client. Restorative methods, such as crutch walking and using canes or walkers for ambulation, are used with clients who have decreased mobility caused by such factors as debilitating illness or major surgery. The purpose of applying restorative methods is to assist the client in achieving the level of mobility he or she enjoyed before becoming ill.

The general goals for using these methods are to assist the client in gaining optimal function, to prevent further injury, and to restore normal function. Being hospitalized and immobile seriously affects a person's body image, behavior, and overall adaptation and adjustment. The greater the disability, the more these aspects of a person's life are affected.

(continued on next page)

PREPARATION PROTOCOL: FOR EXERCISE AND AMBULATION

Complete the following steps before each skill.

1. Check physician's order and client plan of care.
2. Gather equipment and check for safety aspects (i.e., rubber stoppers on crutches are intact).
3. Check client's identaband.
4. Introduce yourself to client and explain nursing care you will be giving.
5. Instruct client on steps required to participate in skill.
6. Provide privacy as necessary for client.
7. Wash hands.

COMPLETION PROTOCOL: FOR EXERCISE AND AMBULATION

Make sure the following steps have been completed.

1. Return client to bed, chair, or position of comfort.
2. Return equipment to appropriate location.
3. Wash hands.
4. Document pertinent data and report changes or unusual findings as indicated.

SECTION ONE

RANGE OF MOTION

Muscles that are not used become weak and shortened. During prolonged bed rest, strength and endurance decrease rapidly. Clients can regain muscle strength and mobility by practicing specific groups of exercises daily. Promoting exercise, both passive and active, is one of the most important nursing functions. The purpose of exercising is to promote good body alignment, prevent contractures, stimulate circulation, prevent thrombophlebitis, and decrease the opportunity for formation of pressure ulcers. Exercise can also prevent edema of the extremities and promote lung expansion.

Passive exercises are carried out by the physical therapist and the nurse without assistance from the client. These exercises enable the client to retain as much joint range of motion as possible, as well as stimulate circulation. Range-of-motion exercises are the most common form of exercises for maintaining joint mobility and increasing maximal motion of a joint when the client is totally or partially immobilized. During the exercises, the extremity is put through its full range so that the joint is moved through all the appropriate planes.

RATIONALE

- To improve or maintain joint function
- To improve or maintain muscle tone and strength
- To prevent contractures
- To prepare client for ambulation

ASSESSMENT

- Assess client's condition and baseline range-of-motion capabilities.
- Establish extent of range of motion to be carried out.
- Assess client's understanding of exercises and role in completing exercises.

RANGE-OF-MOTION EXERCISES

Preparation

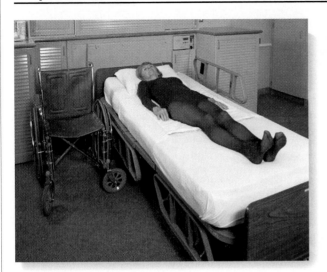

1 Position client on back with bed as flat as possible. Put all joints through range of motion slowly and gently. Provide cradling support above and below joint while performing exercises. All joints should be exercised at least twice daily for clients on bed rest. Encourage clients to do active exercises as soon as possible. **RATIONALE:** Passive exercises only help prevent contractures, but do not maintain muscle.

SAFETY ALERT

Discontinue all range-of-motion exercises if the client complains of pain, because at this point the exercises become counterproductive.

SKILL

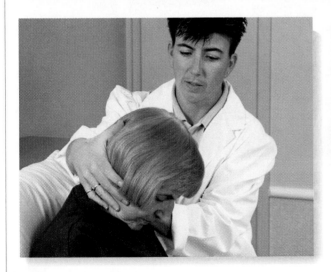

1 Flex head by moving from upright position until chin rests on chest.

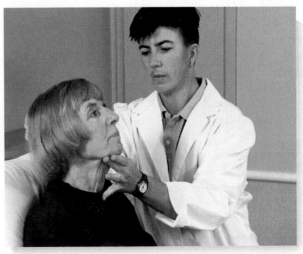

2 Hyperextend head by moving head as far back as possible.

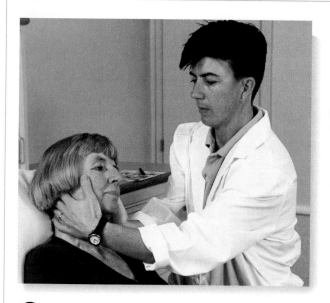

3 Promote lateral flexion by moving head toward right shoulder and then left shoulder.

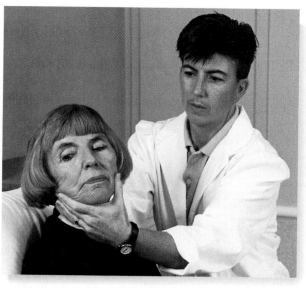

4 Rotate head to right and left.

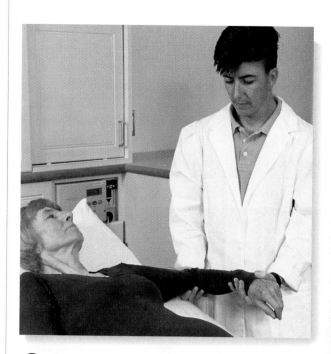

5 Move forearm so palm of hand touches mattress (internal rotation of shoulder).

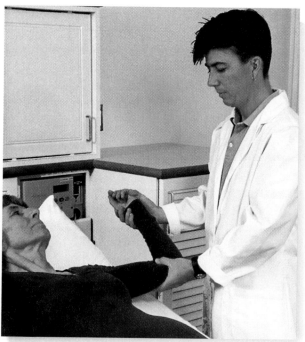

6 Flex elbow and move arm so back of hand touches mattress (external rotation of shoulder).

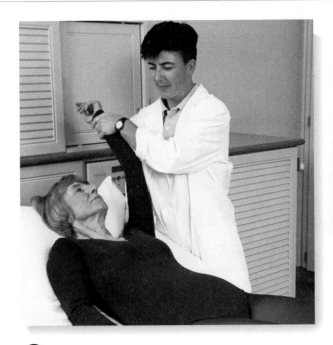

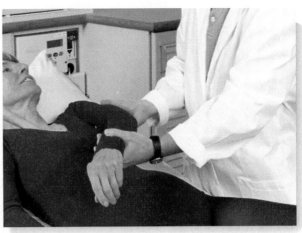

8 Adduct shoulder: Move arm toward midline of body.

7 Abduct shoulder: Rotate shoulder by raising arm from side position to alongside head.

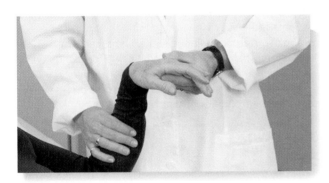

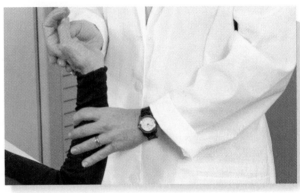

9 Flex wrist: move hand downward.

10 Extend wrist: Bend dorsal surface of hand backward.

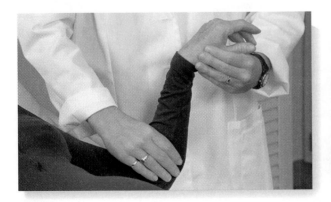

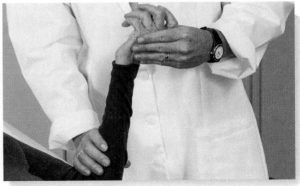

11 Pronate wrist and forearm: Bend elbow 90° and turn hand so palm is facing down.

12 Supinate wrist and forearm: Bend elbow 90° and turn hand so palm is facing up.

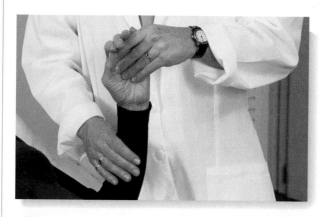

13 Abduct wrist by bending toward thumb (radial deviation of wrist).

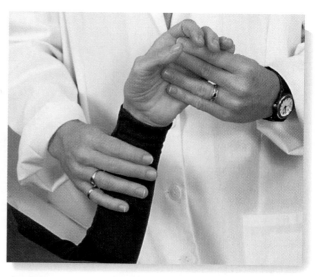

14 Adduct wrist by bending toward 5th finger (ulnar deviation of wrist).

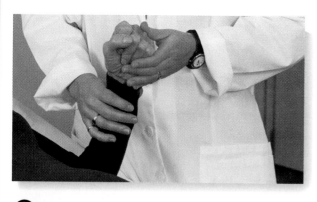

15 Flex fingers: Have client make fist.

SAFETY ALERT

Some facilities advocate extending the fingers at the metacarpal-phalangeal joints when flexing the interphalangeal joints. When extending the interphalangeal joints, flex the fingers at the metacarpal-phalangeal joints to decrease pressure on surrounding structures.

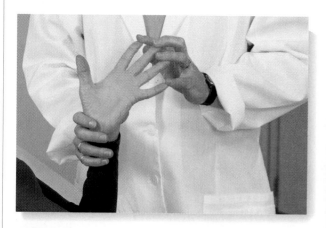

16 Extend fingers: Have client spread fingers apart and then bring them back together.

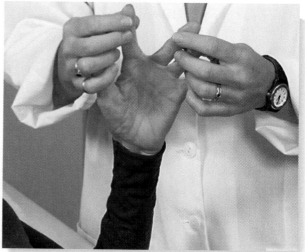

17 Abduct fingers: Spread client's fingers as much as possible.

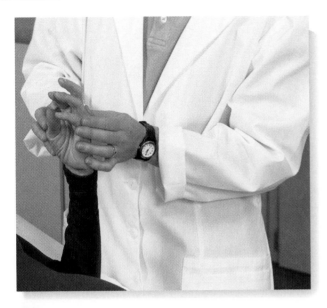

18 Move thumb out and around to touch 5th finger (opposition of fingers).

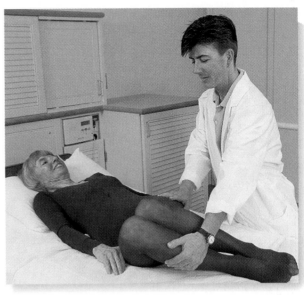

19 Rotate lower trunk: Flex knees and move hips and legs together to one side.

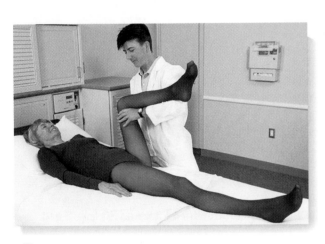

20 Flex hip and knee: Bend hip as far as possible.

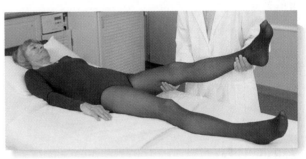

21 Perform straight leg raises: Support leg by placing hands under thigh and ankle.

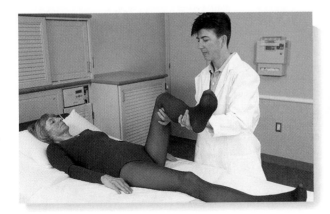

22 Rotate hip externally: Support leg under thigh and ankle.

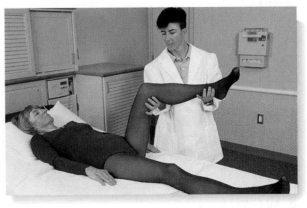

23 Rotate hip internally: Move knee and lower leg outward as hip rotates internally.

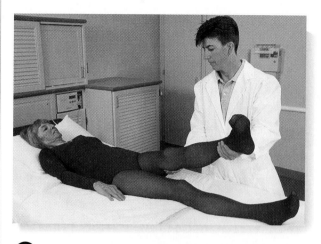

24 Adduct hip: Move leg toward midline of body with foot pointed inward.

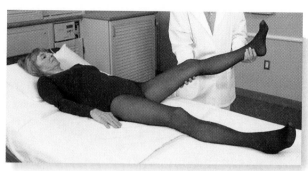

25 Abduct hip: Move leg away from center of body with foot pointed outward.

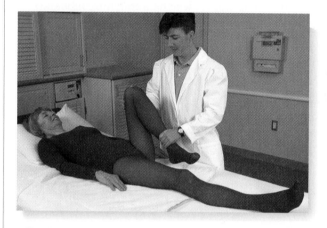

26 Flex knee: Bend knee and bring leg as close to thigh as possible.

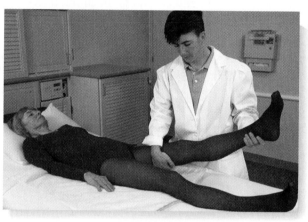

27 Extend knee: Straighten knee and lift leg off bed.

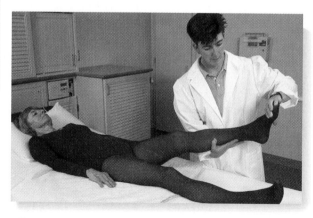

28 Bend toes toward ball of foot (plantarflexion).

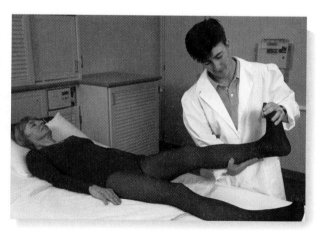

29 Move foot toward leg (dorsiflexion).

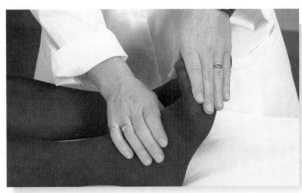

30 Flex toes: Bend toes toward ball of foot.

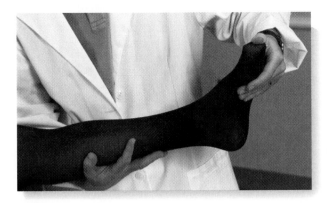

31 Extend toes: Bend toes toward leg.

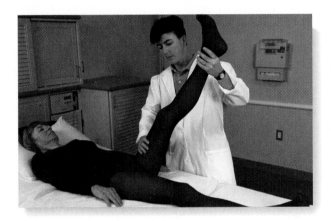

32 Stretch hamstring: Flex hip and bring leg up as far as it can be lifted.

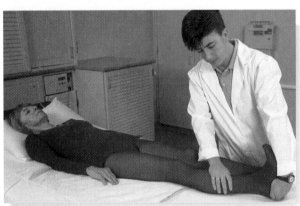

33 Stretch gastrocnemius: Flex toes and lift heel slightly.

CLINICAL NOTE

To preserve joint mobility, joints are placed through passive range-of-motion exercises when clients are on bed rest. Joints are put through the following movements:

Abduction	Movement of a bone away from the midline of the body or body part, as in raising the arm or spreading the fingers.
Adduction	Movement of a bone toward the midline of the body or part.
Eversion	Turning outward; movement of the foot at the ankle joint so that the sole faces outward.
Extension	Movement that increases the angle between two bones, straightening a joint.
Flexion	Movement that decreases the angle between two bones, bending a joint.
Hyperextension	Continuation of extension beyond the anatomic position, as in bending the head backward.
Inversion	Turning inward; movement of the foot at the ankle joint so that the sole faces inward.
Pronation	Rotation of the forearm so that the palm faces backward or downward; movement of the whole body so that the face and abdomen are downward.
Rotation	Movement of a bone around its own axis, as in moving the head to indicate "no" or turning the palm of the hand up and then down.
Supination	Rotation of the forearm so that the palm faces forward or upward; movement of the whole body so that the face and abdomen are upward.

CHARTING

- Amount of time taken to complete exercises
- Any changes in condition of joint or joint mobility
- Movements that caused unusual pain or discomfort

- Amount of client participation
- Specific joints put through exercises

SECTION TWO

AMBULATION

Ambulation, or walking, is an important function that most of us accomplish automatically. When a person is immobilized—either confined to bed following surgery or an injury or unable to ambulate due to another cause—reestablishing mobility can present a major hurdle. The longer the client does not ambulate, the more difficult it is to regain mobility. Early ambulation decreases hospitalization time and prevents complications such as paralytic ileus, respiratory complications, or thrombophlebitis. Ambulation increases muscle strength and joint mobility. Without stress on bones, calcium deposits occur and renal problems increase due to calcium-based calculi.

Balance, coordination, and good body alignment are important aspects of walking. The major muscle groups used for walking are the thigh and leg muscles. If these muscles have not been used or exercised because the client has been in bed for a long time, ambulation must be accomplished step by step. The first step is muscle-strengthening exercises, including quadriceps-setting and gluteal-setting exercises. These exercises restore muscle strength and prepare the legs for weight bearing, and should be done several times a day.

In preparation for ambulation, the client should be helped to dangle his or her feet at the edge of the bed until stable. Vital signs should be within normal range and the client should not experience vertigo when sitting up. Determine if the client needs an assistive device, such as a walker or cane, to ambulate. If not, have the client walk by taking short steps and walk only as long as he or she can tolerate.

RATIONALE

- To increase strength and promote exercise tolerance
- To prevent complications of immobility
- To promote healing by increasing circulation to muscles
- To restore independence and a feeling of self-worth

ASSESSMENT

- Assess client's strength and readiness for ambulation.
- Assess client for signs of vertigo when dangling at side of bed.
- Assess need for safety belt or assistive devices when ambulating client.
- Assess stability of client when standing at bedside before ambulation.

SAFETY ALERT

Observe the client for signs of orthostatic hypotension if the client has been on bed rest for a prolonged period of time. Complaints of vertigo, lightheadedness, fainting, pallor, nausea, or a sudden drop in blood pressure (25 mm Hg systolic or 10 mm Hg diastolic) when moving the client from a horizontal to a vertical position are indicative of orthostatic hypotension. To evaluate the client for this condition, place client in supine position for 5 min and take pulse and blood pressure. Then assist client to stand, wait 1 min, and recheck pulse and blood pressure. Vital signs will be within normal limits if orthostatic hypotension is not present; a drop in blood pressure will occur if it is present.

AMBULATION

Equipment

- Robe or second gown (put on backward so client is not exposed)
- Nonslip slippers or shoes
- Safety belt, if indicated

Preparation

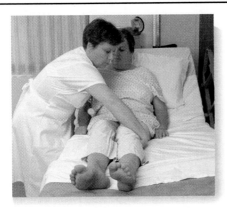

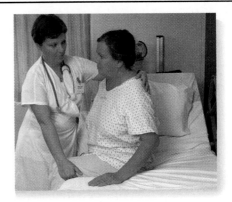

① Move client to side of bed after placing bed in LOW position.

② Assist client to sit at edge of bed.

- Assess for vertigo or faintness. **RATIONALE:** Keeping client in this position until able to stand without experiencing vertigo will prevent client from falling when standing up.
- Place safety belt around client if indicated.

SKILL

One Assistant

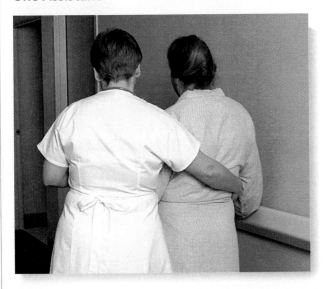

① Assist client to stand and observe balance.

- Grasp client around waist to stabilize, and grasp arm with other hand to guide client.
- If handrail is available, instruct client to hold onto handrail when first ambulating. **RATIONALE:** This will help stabilize client and provide support during ambulation.

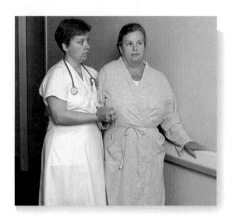

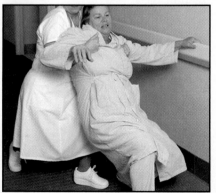

2 Encourage client to maintain good posture and to look straight ahead. **RATIONALE:** Tendency is for client to look down, which may increase vertigo.

- Instruct client to lift each foot to take a step, not to shuffle.
- Walk client as far as he or she is capable of walking without becoming exhausted.

SAFETY ALERT

Stand on client's weaker side (except for CVA clients—then stand on unaffected side). **RATIONALE:** The flaccid muscles on the affected side do not provide sufficient muscle strength for you to grasp and support client.

BEYOND THE SKILL

Prevent Client Injury

1. If client is collapsing, try to break fall with your body and guide client to floor.

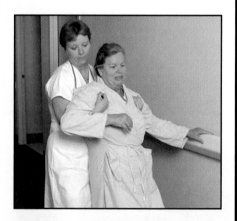

2. If client is unsteady or appears to be falling, support his or her body, especially head and trunk, maintaining your body in good alignment with line of gravity within your base of support. Guide client to floor if necessary. **RATIONALE:** This alignment prevents injury to yourself, while giving client adequate support.

Two Assistants

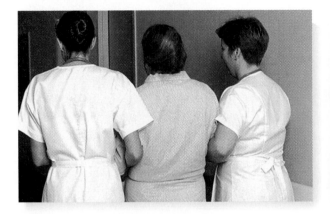

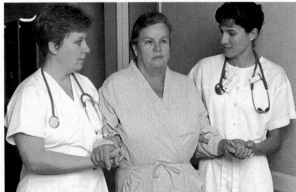

1 Position one nurse on each side of client and have each nurse grasp client's upper arm with hand closest to client.

■ Have each nurse grasp client's hand with other hand.

2 Encourage client to maintain good posture and look straight ahead, not down.

■ Instruct client to lift each foot to take a step, not to shuffle.
■ Walk client only as far as he or she is capable of walking without getting exhausted.

AMBULATION WITH WALKER

Equipment

■ Walker with safety tips and handle grips
■ Nonslip slippers
■ Robe or second gown (put on backward so client is not exposed)

SAFETY ALERT

Make sure that the walker is adjusted to the client's height. The height is based on allowing for 20 to 30° of flexion of the elbows when grasping the hand grips of the walker.

SKILL

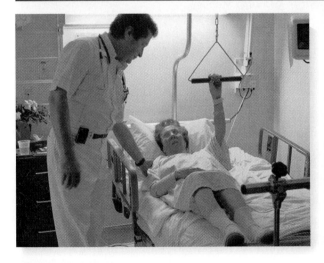

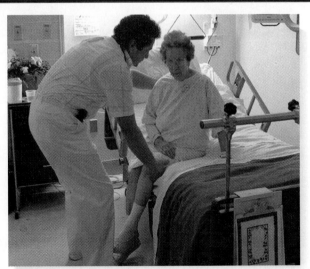

1 Instruct client to move to edge of bed, using trapeze if appropriate.

2 Assist client to sitting position at edge of bed.

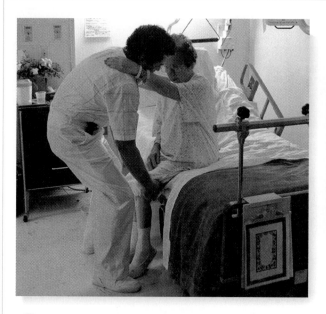

3 Move client to edge of bed so feet touch floor.

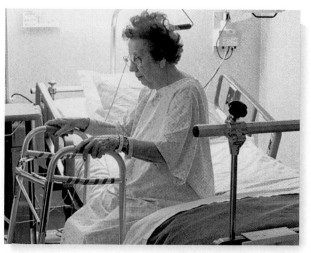

4 Place walker directly in front of client. Instruct client to push self off bed. Instruct client to hold onto hand grips. **RATIONALE:** To provide stability when moving walker.

- After standing, have client move walker forward 6 to 8 in by leaning into walker and keeping all four feet of walker on floor.

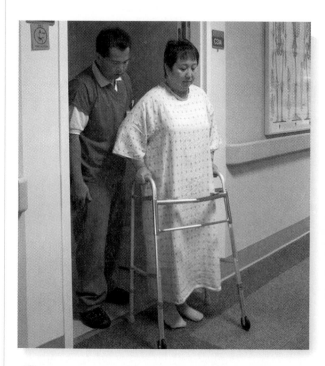

5 Instruct client to bend elbows slightly and move walker forward.

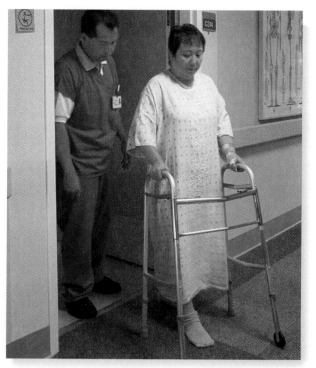

6 Instruct client to move weaker side first by supporting body weight on hands and advancing weaker leg. Partial weight bearing on affected side may be allowed; check physician's orders.

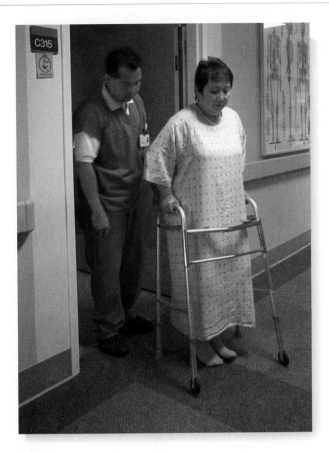

 Instruct client to balance self and then move unaffected side by placing foot even with first foot.

- Move walker forward and continue same pattern of ambulating.

AMBULATION WITH CANE

Equipment

- Appropriate type of cane (straight-legged or standard, tripod, quad)
- Nonskid slippers or sturdy shoes
- Robe or second gown (put on backward so client is not exposed)

SAFETY ALERT

A properly sized cane extends from the greater trochanter to the floor, allowing 20 to 30° of elbow flexion. If the cane is too short, the client cannot support his or her weight and may injure his or her back.

SKILL

Quad Cane

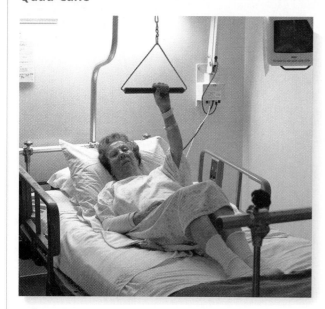

1 Instruct client to move to side of bed using trapeze if appropriate.

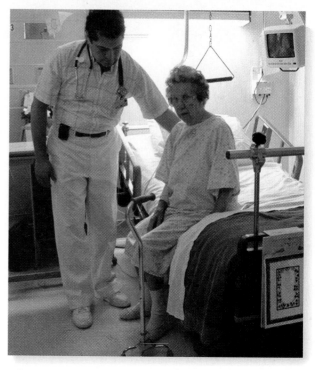

2 Assist client to sit at edge of bed; ensure that feet are placed flat on floor.

■ Assist client to put on slippers or shoes.

3 Determine appropriate type of cane. **RATIONALE:** To provide adequate support for client during ambulation.

■ Assist client to standing position with feet firmly on floor.
■ Instruct client to place cane on stronger side of body and grasp cane about 12 inches in front of foot and slightly to outside. **RATIONALE:** This position provides best balance, because client's center of gravity is within base of support.

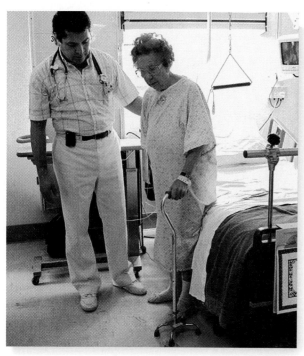

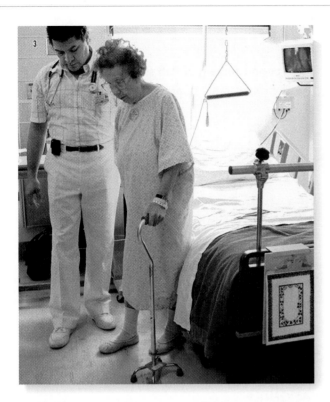

4 Assist client to move cane and weaker side at same time. **RATIONALE:** This allows client's weight to be distributed on unaffected leg and is method used when less support is needed for affected side.

- Accompany client by walking beside him or her on affected side. **RATIONALE:** If client loses balance, supporting client on affected side is most effective.
- When ambulation is completed, assist client back to bed.

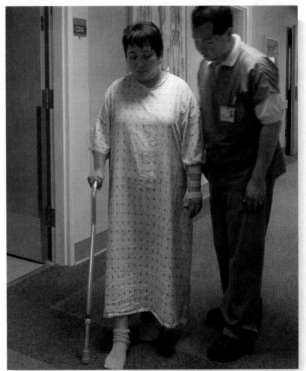

6 Move weak side forward to cane. Weight is borne by cane and stronger side.

- Move stronger leg forward ahead of cane and weaker leg. Weight is borne by cane and weak leg.
- Continue this procedure until ambulation is completed. This pattern of movement ensures that at least two points of support are always bearing weight.

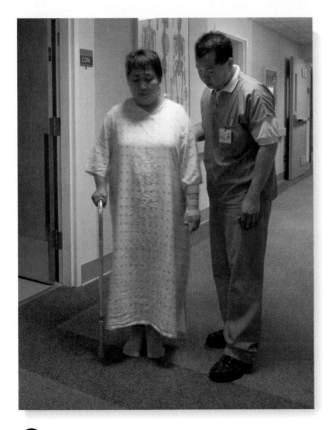

5 Alternate method: When maximum support is needed, move cane forward about 12 in or a distance that is comfortable for client. Client's body weight is borne by both legs.

- Client's ability to maintain balance using assistive devices
- Time and distance of ambulation

- Type and amount of staff support required
- Client's tolerance of procedure

SECTION THREE

CRUTCH WALKING

Crutches are an assistive device used to support ambulation when the lower extremities are unable to support body weight. Crutches allow independence of movement whether the client has a permanent or temporary condition.

There are three main types of crutches: the axillary or underarm; the Lofstrand, a forearm crutch with a metal band and handle; and the shelf crutch, used with a client unable to use his or her wrists to bear weight. The axillary or underarm crutch is the type most commonly used for short-term assistance.

Keep in mind the principles of crutch walking when instructing clients: Crutches must be accurately measured to ensure proper support; an erect posture is necessary to prevent strain on muscles and joints; the weight of the body should be borne by the arms, not the axillae; crutch tips should be clean and in good repair.

Before clients attempt to use crutches, they should practice muscle-strengthening exercises. These include quadriceps-setting and gluteal-setting exercises, pushups in the sitting position, and pushups in the prone position.

RATIONALE

- To support ambulation
- To promote mobility and independence
- To increase muscle strength, especially in arms and legs
- To promote feeling of well-being

ASSESSMENT

- Assess ability of client to maintain balance when on crutches.
- Assess appropriate gait for client.
- Determine appropriate length of crutches.
- Determine client's ability to understand and use crutches.

BEYOND THE SKILL

MEASURING FOR CRUTCHES

Equipment

- Measuring tape
- Crutches
- Shoes used during crutch walking

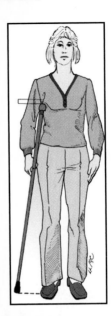
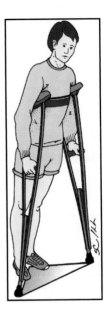

Skill

1. Instruct client to put on shoes that will be used during walking.
2. Place client flat in bed with arms at side.
3. Measure distance from client's axilla to a point 6 to 8 in out from heel.
4. Adjust hand bars on crutches so that client's elbows are slightly flexed at 30°.
5. Instruct client to stand at bedside with crutches under arms.
6. Measure distance between client's axilla and arm pieces on crutches. There should be two to three fingerwidths between axilla and shoulder rest of crutch.

SAFETY ALERT

The proper standing position for clients using crutches is termed a tripod position. The crutches are placed 6 in in front and 6 in out laterally to form a wide base of support. The feet are slightly apart, knees and hips slightly extended, and the back is straight.

FOUR-POINT GAIT

Equipment

- Properly fitted crutches
- Hard-soled shoes
- Safety belt (optional)

SKILL

Four-Point Gait

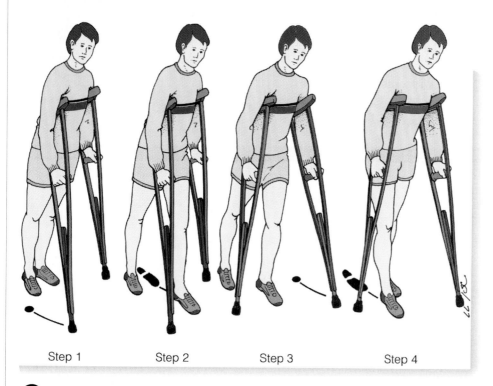

Step 1   Step 2   Step 3   Step 4

1 Demonstrate and have client return demonstration of crutch-foot sequence.

- Move right crutch.
- Move left foot.
- Move left crutch.
- Move right foot.

Three-Point Gait

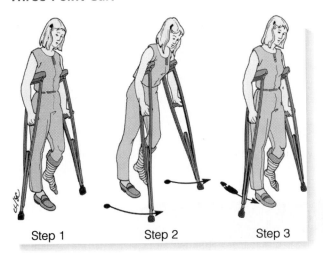

Step 1   Step 2   Step 3

1 Demonstrate and have client return demonstration of crutch-foot sequence.

- Two crutches support weaker extremity.
- Balance weight on crutches.
- Move both crutches and affected leg forward.
- Move unaffected leg forward.

CLINICAL NOTE

The three-point gait is fairly rapid and requires strong upper extremities and good balance. This gait can be performed when the client can bear little or no weight on the affected leg or the client has only one leg.

Two-Point Gait

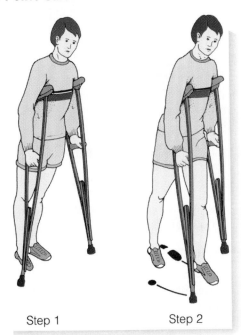

Step 1   Step 2

1 Demonstrate and have client return demonstration of crutch-foot sequence.

- Advance right foot and left crutch simultaneously.
- Advance left foot and right crutch simultaneously.

CLINICAL NOTE

The two-point gait requires more balance than the four-point gait. It is a rapid version of the four-point gate.

Swing-to and Swing-Through Gaits

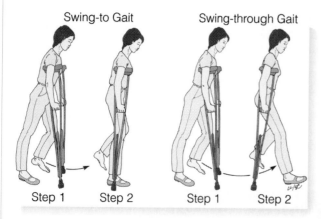

Swing-to Gait   Swing-through Gait

Step 1   Step 2   Step 1   Step 2

1 Demonstrate and have client return demonstration of swing-to or swing-through gait.

- Move both crutches forward.
- Swing-to gait: Lift and swing body to crutches.
- Swing-through gait: Lift and swing body past crutches.
- Bring crutches in front of body and repeat gait.

CLINICAL NOTE

The swing-to and swing-through gaits are usually used when the client's lower extremities are affected by weakness or when the client has paralysis of the hips or legs.

SKILL

Walking Up and Down

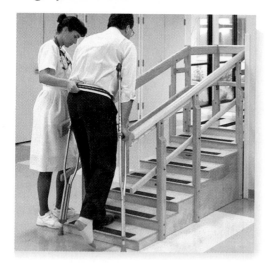

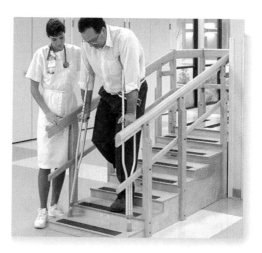

1 Demonstrate and have client return demonstration for going up stairs.

- Place safety belt on client before instruction begins.
- Start with crutches and unaffected extremity on same level.
- Put weight on crutch handles and lift unaffected extremity onto first step of stairs.
- Put weight on unaffected extremity and lift other extremity and crutches to step.
- Repeat until client understands procedure.

2 Demonstrate and have client return demonstration for going down stairs.

- Place safety belt on client before instruction begins.
- Start with weight on unaffected leg and crutches on same level.
- Put crutches on first step.
- Put weight on crutch handles and transfer unaffected extremity to step where crutches are placed.
- Repeat until client understands procedure.

CHARTING

- Time and distance of ambulation on crutches
- Type of crutch gait used
- Use of safety belt or assistance needed
- Unusual problems associated with use of crutches

CRITICAL THINKING FOCUS

SECTION ONE ▪ Range of Motion

Unexpected Outcomes

- Client continues to lose mobility and strength despite nursing interventions.

- Client experiences pain or discomfort during range-of-motion exercises.

Alternative Nursing Actions

- Discuss with health team need for additional interventions to improve joint range.
- Assess client's need for splints or braces to maintain physiological position.

- Assess amount and type of pain and report findings to physician.
- Evaluate your techniques to ensure exercises are being performed correctly.
- Determine need for pain management when performing exercises.

SECTION TWO ▪ Ambulation

Unexpected Outcomes

- Client complains of vertigo and feels faint.

- Client complains of being too weak to ambulate.

- Client has poor balance.

- Client is fearful.

Alternative Nursing Actions

- Assist client to nearest chair or return client to bed.
- If in hallway, ease client down wall to floor. Do not attempt to hold client.
- Summon help.

- Provide active and passive range-of-motion exercises.
- Dangle client at side of bed several times before attempting ambulation again.

- Use two assistants to ambulate.
- Use safety belt if necessary.

- Medicate 1 hr before ambulation if client is experiencing pain.
- Discuss why client is afraid of ambulation.
- Ambulate only short distance at first.

SECTION THREE ▪ Crutch Walking

Unexpected Outcomes

▪ Client states he or she is frightened of crutches.

Alternative Nursing Actions

▪ Explain that you will stay with client until he or she feels comfortable and is safe using crutches.

▪ Use safety belt when assisting client.

▪ Determine client's strength and ability to use crutches properly.

▪ Have client take only a few steps and allow to sit in chair for a few minutes before attempting to continue to use crutches.

▪ If fear persists, request that physician order walker for client until he or she feels less frightened.

SELF-CHECK EVALUATION

PART 1 ▪ Matching Terms

Match the definition in column B with the correct term in column A.

Column A

_____ a. Abduction
_____ b. Adduction
_____ c. Pronation
_____ d. Supination
_____ e. Flexion
_____ f. Extension
_____ g. Hyperextension
_____ h. Plantarflexion

Column B

1. Rotation of forearm so palm faces upward
2. Movement of a bone away from the midline of the body
3. Movement that increases the angle between two bones, straightening a joint
4. Extension of the foot at the ankle joint, foot and toes turned downward
5. Rotation of the forearm so palm faces downward
6. Movement of a bone toward the midline of the body
7. Extension of the head beyond the anatomic position
8. Movement that decreases the angle between two bones

PART 2 ▪ Multiple Choice Questions

1. Before having any client ambulate, it is important to:
   a. Ensure that the client wants to ambulate at this time.
   b. Medicate the client 1 hr before ambulation.
   c. Have client dangle at bedside for a few minutes.
   d. Place a safety belt on the client.

2. While you are ambulating a client down the hall, the client feels faint and begins to fall. It is best to:

  a. Return the client to his or her room immediately.
  b. Guide the client to the floor without letting him or her fall.
  c. Call for help and hold the client up by pressing his or her body into you.
  d. Move the client near the wall or a handrail and instruct him or her to hold onto it until you obtain assistance.

3. Instructions given to clients when ambulating include the following:

  a. Always walk with your eyes toward the floor to prevent tripping.
  b. Look up when walking and slide your feet forward with each step.
  c. Look straight ahead and focus on an object nearby.
  d. Look straight ahead and stand erect when walking.

4. Active exercises are best explained as:

  a. Exercises that are done using special equipment.
  b. Exercises performed by the client without support of a nurse.
  c. Exercises in which both client and nurse participate.
  d. Exercises provided by the nurse for the client.

5. Passive range-of-motion exercises are most often provided with the client in a:

  a. Semi-Fowler's position.
  b. Supine position.
  c. Chair.
  d. Position of comfort.

6. Abduction refers to which one of the following movements?

  a. Moving a bone toward the midline of the body or part.
  b. Moving a joint beyond the anatomic position, as in bending the head.
  c. Turning the foot or ankle joint so the sole faces inward.
  d. Moving a bone away from the midline of the body or body part.

7. Instructions for a client using a walker include the following:

  a. Have the client move the walker forward before moving his or her feet.
  b. Instruct the client to move both feet toward the walker before moving the walker.
  c. Have the client pick up the walker, move it forward, and then move the affected leg.
  d. Have the client move first the unaffected leg, then the affected leg, toward the walker and then move the walker forward.

8. Clients are instructed in the following actions when using a cane:

  a. Always move the unaffected side before moving the cane and affected side.
  b. Hold the cane on the affected side of the body.
  c. Place the cane about 12 in in front of and slightly toward the side of the foot.
  d. Move the weaker side ahead of the cane and then the unaffected side.

9. When measuring the client for crutches, it is important to:

  a. Measure the distance from the client's axilla to a point 6 to 8 in out from the bed.
  b. Measure the client without shoes.
  c. Ensure that crutches and arm pieces just touch the axilla when the client is standing.
  d. Ask the client to stand with crutches close to the feet so you can measure them properly.

10. When teaching the four-point gait to a client, you will instruct the client to move the:
   a. Foot first, then move the opposite crutch.
   b. Crutch and then the same-side foot.
   c. Crutch and then the opposite foot.
   d. Crutch and the same-side foot.

11. Instruct the client when walking up stairs to:
   a. Do so only when someone is accompanying him or her.
   b. Start with both crutches and the affected extremity on the same stair.
   c. Put weight on the crutch handles and lift the unaffected extremity onto the next step.
   d. Place affected foot on step and then move crutches and unaffected leg to step.

PART 3 ▪ Critical Thinking Application

You are assigned to a 70-year-old client. She is about to be discharged following a laparoscopic cholecystectomy. She refuses to exercise at all and has not ambulated without a great deal of encouragement from the staff. When questioned why she is not up and moving, she states, "I am old and at my age I can be a couch potato, and that is what I am going to do."

1. Based on this statement, what generalizations can you make about the general health and projected health of this client?

2. What is the primary danger to the health of this client? How would you explain this to the client?

3. What will you include in your discharge plan and teaching for this client that would have a positive effect?

14

ORTHOPEDIC MEASURES

INTRODUCTION

Orthopedic nursing involves the prevention and correction of alterations in the musculoskeletal system. To help clients achieve and maintain optimal mobility, nurses use preventive, restorative, and rehabilitative methods. Preventive and restorative measures include the use of bandages, positioning, splints, traction, and casts. Rehabilitative treatments include the use of special beds and halo traction.

The usual cause of injury to the musculoskeletal system is trauma from accidents. Accidents can result in soft tissue injuries, fractures, and dislocations. Injuries occurring from falls in the home account for many admissions to health care facilities. Sprains and strains are also common musculoskeletal injuries. The usual treatment for sprains and strains is application of a pressure bandage, elevation, and ice.

Woven cotton, elastic webbing, and gauze are the most common materials used in the treatment of sprains, strains, contusions, and dislocations. Remember the mnemonic RICE: R stands for resting the injured part; I refers to immobilization, usually with a bandage or splinting; C stands for application of cold treatments, such as ice packs applied intermittently for 24 to 48 hrs; and E refers to elevation of the affected

(continued on next page)

extremity. These initial interventions prevent edema and other complications. Avoid heat for at least 24 hrs to prevent edema and pain.

Fractures

The long bones, the type most commonly involved in fractures, are composed of the shaft, or diaphysis, and the flared ends, termed the metaphyses. When a bone is fractured, a specific repair process takes place, beginning with the formation of a blood clot at the site of the fracture. Osteoblasts and osteoclasts remodel the callus area into permanent and strong bone.

Fractures are classified in a variety of ways. One classification system is organized by the type of injury to the bone or surrounding tissue. Examples of these fractures include transverse fractures, which proceed directly across the bone, and comminuted fractures, which result in displacement of more than two fragments of bone.

Fractures can also be classified as open or closed. An open fracture is one in which the skin has been broken due to penetration of a bone fragment or external trauma. An open fracture requires additional treatment to prevent infection as a result of the skin puncture. Surgical debridement and irrigation must be completed within hours of the fracture. A closed fracture is one that is contained under the skin surface.

Soft tissue injury is also a probability with fractures. Immediate splinting and elevation of the extremity can prevent complications.

Fractures can be treated by manipulation or closed reduction to return broken bones to their normal anatomic positions. Casts are generally applied to maintain the reduced fracture in proper alignment. Casts are made from plaster of paris or from synthetic materials such as polyester, polyurethane, fiberglass, or plastic.

Open reduction—the correction of bone alignment through a surgical incision—includes internal fixation of the fracture with rods, wires, screws, pins, or nails. An external fixator apparatus, usually used when casts or traction are not appropriate, is employed to compress fracture fragments and immobilize reduced fractures. The fixator is attached to the bone by the use of percutaneous pins.

Traction

Traction is another method of treating fractures. It is most effective and useful when reduction of a bone fracture is required. Two types of traction are used: skin traction and skeletal traction. Skeletal traction is usually more reliable and effective than skin traction because it maintains the reduction of the fractured limb.

Neuromuscular function must be assessed every 4 hrs, because clients requiring traction devices usually have extensive soft tissue, nerve, and vessel damage. Extensive client teaching needs to be accomplished because the clients go home with devices in place.

Many types of skin traction are seen in hospital settings. The oldest and simplest type is Buck's traction. This type of traction is usually applied for short periods of 48 to 72 hrs.

Halo Traction and Back Braces

Clients who require more sophisticated orthopedic procedures may be immobilized by the use of several types of equipment. Halo traction, the Jewett-Taylor brace, and the Stryker frame or kinetic therapy Rotorest bed are used to immobilize clients with spinal cord injury. Clients are immobilized to prevent further complications and to promote healing. Skeletal traction may be necessary and is applied by placing tongs through burr holes in the outer layer of the skull. Weights are applied to ropes connected to the tongs to provide constant hyperextension of the head.

Continuous Passive Motion Device

This device is widely used for clients following knee surgery. It provides flexion and extension movements for the knee joint. There are several types of these devices on the market; however, they function using the same principles of physics.

PREPARATION PROTOCOL: FOR MOBILITY

Complete the following steps before each skill.

1. Check physician's order and client plan of care.
2. Gather equipment.
3. Check client's identaband.
4. Introduce yourself to client and explain nursing care you will be giving.
5. Provide privacy as necessary for client.
6. Wash hands.
7. Don gloves as indicated.

COMPLETION PROTOCOL: FOR MOBILITY

Make sure the following steps have been completed.

1. Remove gloves (if used) and discard appropriately; wash hands.
2. Return client to position of comfort.
3. Return equipment to appropriate location.
4. Wash hands.
5. Document pertinent data and report as indicated.

SECTION ONE

BANDAGES AND SLINGS

Bandages are used for applying pressure over an area, immobilizing a body part, preventing or reducing edema, correcting a deformity, or securing splints in place. Woven cotton, elastic webbing, and gauze are the most common bandage materials. Many kinds of elasticized bandages are applied to provide pressure to an area. They are commonly used as tensor bandages or as partial stockings to provide support and improve venous circulation in the legs.

Nurses must know the purpose and specific assessment parameters for monitoring a client with a bandage. Regardless of the purpose, all bandaged limbs need to be assessed for the presence of edema, circulation, and pain. If the bandage is used to hold a dressing, additional assessment for drainage and wounds is instituted.

RATIONALE

- To immobilize joint or extremity
- To provide support to injured extremity or surgical site
- To prevent edema in injured extremity
- To secure dressing in place

ASSESSMENT

- Determine need for bandage or sling.
- Assess area surrounding bandage to ensure bandage is not restrictive.
- Assess limb for circulation, sensation, and movement.

ARM SLING APPLICATION

Equipment

- Commercial arm sling
- Triangular bandage

SKILL

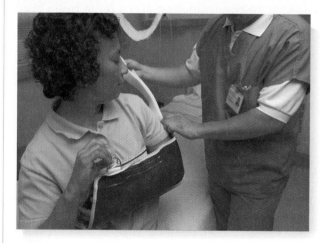

1 Instruct client to sit or lie down.

- Position forearm across client's chest with thumb pointing upward. **RATIONALE:** This position flexes elbow.
- Place affected arm into canvas sling so that elbow fits flush with corner of sling.

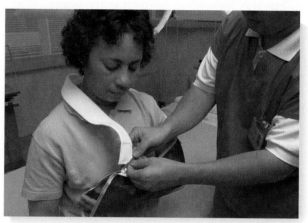

2 Bring strap around opposing shoulder and pull strap through metal loops on sling. Pad neck area if client is uncomfortable.

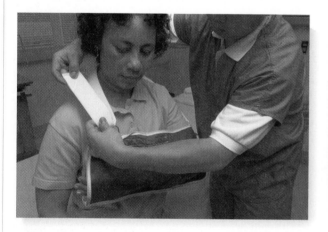

3 Pull strap up toward shoulder until sling is at right angle to body. Wrist should be slightly elevated above arm and elbow should be flexed. **RATIONALE:** To prevent edema formation in dependent areas and facilitate adequate circulation.

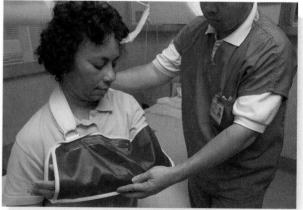

4 Check client's comfort level and position of wrist and elbow.

- Assess for adequate circulation after 20 min and then every 2 to 4 hrs.

CLINICAL NOTE

ALTERNATE METHOD FOR SLING APPLICATION
- Place one end of triangular cloth over shoulder on unaffected area.
- Place cloth against body and under affected arm.
- Place apex, or point, of triangle toward elbow.
- Bring opposite end of triangle around affected arm and over affected shoulder.
- Tie sling at side of client's neck.
- Fold apex of triangle over elbow in front, and secure with safety pin.

FIGURE EIGHT BANDAGE

Equipment

- Roller bandages (number depends on length of bandage)
- Metal clip or safety pin

SKILL

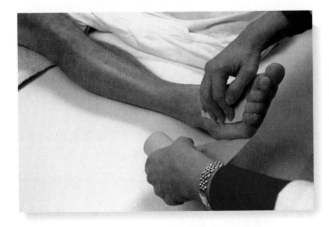

1 Anchor bandage around distal end of extremity using circular turns.

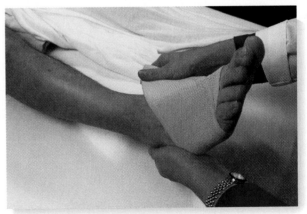

2 Make circular turn around foot and ankle.

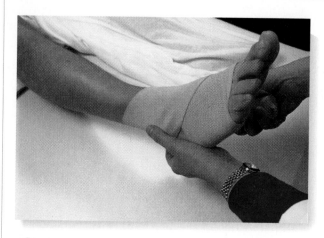

3 Make spiral turn down over ankle and around foot.

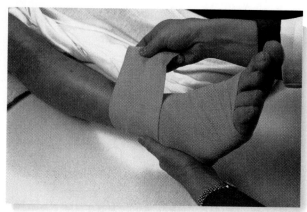

4 Continue to make alternate turns around ankle and foot. Overlap preceding turn by at least one-half to two-thirds of bandage width.

CLINICAL NOTE

If heel is not encased in the bandage, check for edema every 2 to 4 hrs.

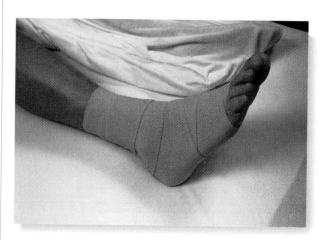

5 Wrap entire area below and above involved point. **RATIONALE:** This immobilizes affected area.

- Rewrap bandage every 4 to 8 hrs.

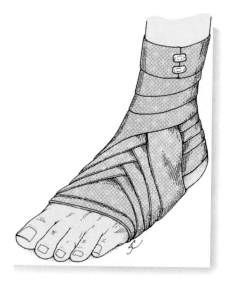

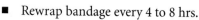

6 Anchor bandage using two metal clips or safety pins.

SAFETY ALERT

Check for adequate circulation 20 min after the application and then every 2 to 4 hrs. Ensure bandage is wrinkle free. If not, redo bandage.

CIRCULAR BANDAGE

Equipment

- Roller bandages (number depends on length of application)
- Metal clips or safety pins

SKILL

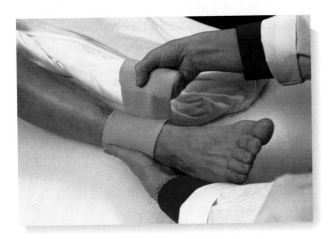

1 Anchor bandage at distal end with two circular turns. Maintain moderate amount of tension on bandage during application.

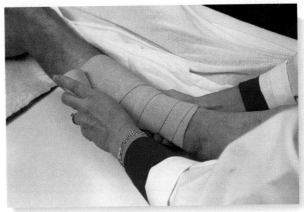

2 Continue to unroll bandage and overlap previous turn until designated area is covered.

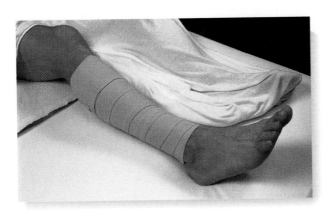

3 Observe for even, tight fit of bandage, and ensure that bandage is not occluding circulation.

- Secure bandage with safety pin or metal clips.
- Assess extremity for circulation after 20 min and then every 2 to 4 hrs.
- Rewrap bandage every 4 to 8 hrs.

CHARTING

- Type of bandage or sling applied
- Condition of extremity following application
- Assessment findings every 2 to 4 hrs
- Effectiveness of bandage
- Pain, if any

SECTION TWO

CAST CARE

The traditional cast material is plaster of paris. As plaster of paris is placed in cool water and applied to the extremity, a heat reaction occurs. The heat can be uncomfortable and alarm the client; therefore clients should be told about this sensation before the cast application begins. Usually the sensation lasts about 15 min. The crystallization process that occurs when the plaster is placed in cool water provides a very rigid dressing. After the plaster sets, the cast remains wet and somewhat soft. No pressure should be placed on the cast until it is dry. The appearance of the cast will change from dull and gray to white and shiny when the cast is dry.

Synthetic casts are used frequently for immobilizing arms, legs below the knee, and feet. These casts are usually made of polyurethane materials. They weigh less, dry more quickly, can get wet, and result in fewer skin problems than plaster casts. However, they have several disadvantages: They cost more, and they cannot be used to immobilize severely displaced bones or unstable fractures.

RATIONALE

- To increase client's level of activity following injury or disease
- To maintain normal sensation, movement, and circulation in casted extremity
- To improve muscle tone and joint flexibility
- To strengthen muscles weakened by immobility, trauma, or surgery

ASSESSMENT

- Check circulation, motion, and sensation of affected extremity.
- Check for edema of affected limb.
- Assess condition of cast: cracks, dents, and presence of drainage.
- Assess client's knowledge of cast care.

TABLE 14-1	COMPARISON OF CASTS	
	Plaster	**Synthetic**
Material	Plaster of paris, composed of powdered calcium sulfate crystals impregnated into the bandages.	Polyester and cotton, fiberglass or plastic. Polyester and cotton is impregnated with water-activated polyurethane resin.
Drying time	24–48 hrs.	7–15 min for setting.
	No weight bearing until dried, 48–72 hrs.	60 min for weight bearing.
Advantages	Less costly.	Less likely to indent into skin.
	More effective for immobilizing severely displaced bones.	Lighter in weight.
		Less restrictive.
	Smooth surface.	Does not crumble.
	Does not require expensive equipment for application.	Nonabsorbent.

WET CAST CARE

Equipment

■ Pillows covered with plastic

SKILL

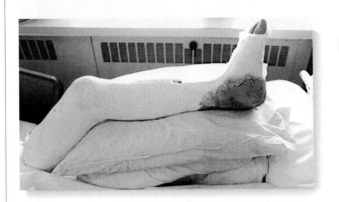

1 Support cast with pillows as necessary.

■ Keep casted extremity above level of heart. **RATIONALE:** This position decreases venous pooling and edema.
■ Maintain angles that were built into cast.
■ Prevent cast from cracking from undue pressure.
■ Prevent flat spot in cast caused by pressure on bed.

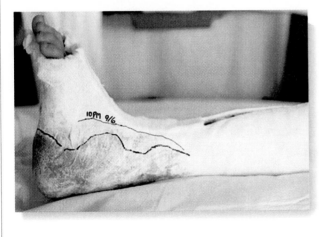

2 Keep cast uncovered. **RATIONALE:** This allows heat and moisture to dissipate and air to circulate.

■ If cast edges are rough or crumbling, pull stockinette over edge of cast and tape down.
■ Turn client according to facility policy, usually every 2 hrs. **RATIONALE:** Turning promotes even drying of cast and prevents pressure areas from developing.
■ Use only palms of hands when handling casted area for first 24 hrs. **RATIONALE:** Fingers can cause dents in cast, which may create pressure areas on inside of cast.
■ Mark and date drainage area on cast, if drainage is present.

BEYOND THE SKILL

Synthetic Cast Client Teaching

1. Instruct client in neurovascular checks of casted extremity.
2. Check cast daily for:
   - Odor or drainage
   - Cracks or position change
3. Instruct client to avoid overly rigorous activities to prevent altering cast alignment.
4. Instruct client in bathing procedures.
   - Place two layers of plastic over cast.
   - Use only mild soap and water when bathing; avoid getting soap on cast.
   - Place nonslip mat on floor to prevent slipping when getting out of bathtub.
   - Remove excess water from cast by blotting with towel.
   - Set blow dryer on cool setting and dry cast by moving dryer along all aspects of cast.

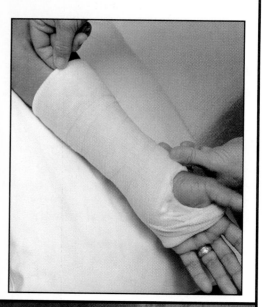

ASSESSMENT OF CASTED EXTREMITY

SKILL

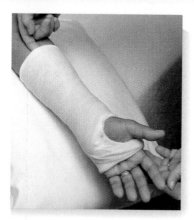

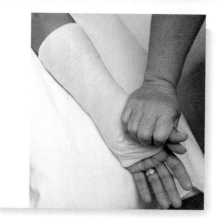

1 Check cast for tightness. You should be able to insert one or two fingers between cast and skin.

- Check for redness or skin breakdown around casted area.
- Instruct client to notify you if there is pain or itching under cast. Remind client not to place anything under cast to scratch skin. **RATIONALE:** Skin breakdown can occur, leading to infection.

2 Check fingers or toes for warmth.

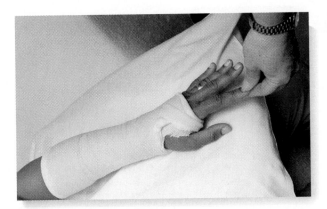

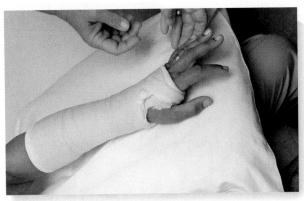

3 Check fingers or toes for color; ensure they are pink in color.

- Press fingertips and check for capillary refill. After stopping pressure, observe nail to see how rapidly color returns to nail bed. **RATIONALE:** Color should return immediately unless a complication has occurred.

4 Ask client to move fingers or toes. Ensure client does not have any unusual sensations such as tingling. **RATIONALE:** This indicates cast is too tight and neurovascular complication can occur.

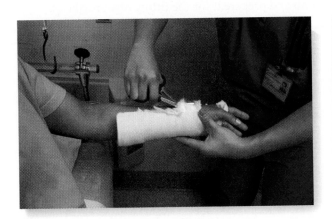

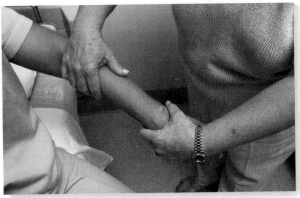

5 If any neurovascular complication occurs, notify physician. Cast may need to be removed and new cast applied.

6 After cast is removed, check skin and bony prominences for any sign of skin breakdown.

SAFETY ALERT

Remember to observe the casted extremity frequently for the four Ps: pulse, pallor, pain, and paresthesia.

BEYOND THE SKILL

Amputee Care

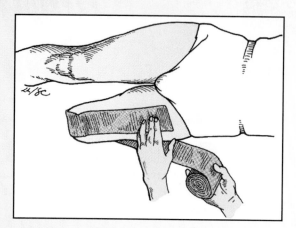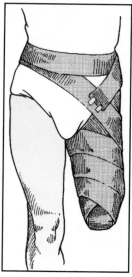

A shrink wrap using elastic compression bandage is used to help shrink the stump and to provide pressure on the surgical site. *Note:* Today most clients with amputation undergo a synthetic casting procedure termed immediate postoperative procedure/prosthesis (IPOP). The fiberglass casting is done on the stump immediately after the surgical procedure. The goal is to help shrink the limb and prepare it for the fitting of a prosthesis.

CHARTING

- Type of cast applied
- Positioning of cast, pillows, etc.
- Client complaints and nursing responses
- Color, warmth, movement, and sensation in casted extremity
- Presence, location, and amount of drainage from wound
- Condition of cast (wet or dry)

TRACTION

Traction is defined as the application of a pulling force to an extremity or another part of the body while countertraction pulls in the opposite direction. Traction is used for several reasons: to prevent or reduce muscle spasm; to immobilize a joint or other body part; to correct and maintain skeletal length and alignment; to promote healing; and to prevent and help correct permanent joint pathologies.

Skeletal traction involves the use of steel pins or wires inserted through the distal fragment and attached to the traction apparatus. The tractive force is applied directly to the bone. The affected limb is maintained in an elevated position, which decreases edema and promotes healing. The most common type of skeletal traction is the Thomas splint with Pearson attachment. Other types are Dunlop's traction, sidearm traction, and tongs, such as Crutchfield and Vinke devices. External fixation devices are commonly used for stabilizing a bone or joint. An external device has a metal frame with attached percutaneous pins that are held rigidly in place on the frame. These devices may be applied to various bones, such as the femur, elbow, knee, or pelvic ring.

Skin traction, such as Buck's traction, is used frequently before hip surgery for elderly clients. Bucks's traction uses a boot with Velcro straps, strips of tape, moleskin, or commercial skin traction strips. Force is applied directly to the client's skin; therefore skin assessment and care are crucial.

RATIONALE

- To maintain correct alignment of bone ends
- To prevent unnecessary injury to soft tissue
- To provide temporary management of fractures in elderly adults
- To maintain pin site free of infection
- To control muscle spasm and to immobilize an area prior to surgery

ASSESSMENT

- Check the amount of weight ordered. No more than 4.5 to 8 lb of traction is used on an extremity.
- Assess circulation, movement, and sensation of affected extremity.
- Assess pin site for signs of infection.
- Assess neurovascular status with external fixation devices.

SKIN TRACTION APPLICATION

Equipment

- Bed with overhead frame and trapeze
- Weights
- Velcro straps or other straps
- Rope and pulleys

- Foot plate
- Boot
- Elastic hose

SKILL

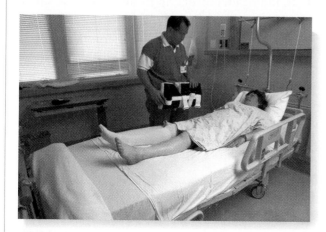

1 Ensure traction apparatus is attached to bed.

- Place elastic hose on affected limb.
- Explain procedure to client.
- Place client in supine position with foot of bed elevated slightly.

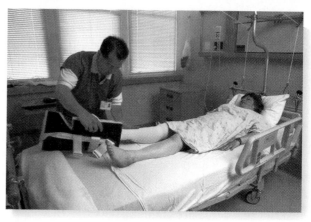

2 Slip Buck's traction boot over client's leg.

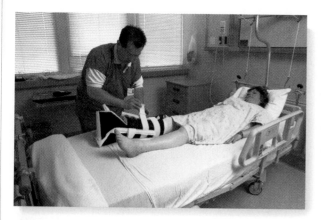

3 Secure boot by closing the three Velcro straps.

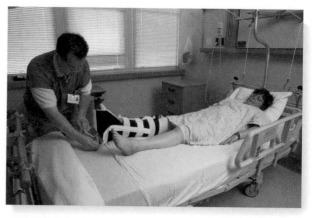

4 Attach traction cord to foot plate of boot.

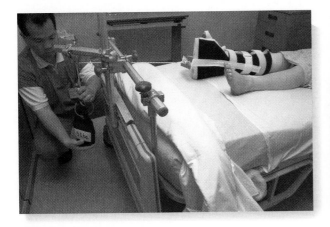

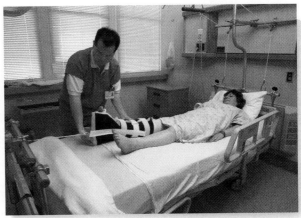

5 Ensure cord is running through pulley system without difficulty.

- Hang prescribed amount of weight on hook—usually 5 to 10 lb for adults.
- Gently let go of weight. **RATIONALE:** To prevent quick pull on extremity.

6 Check client's alignment with traction.

- Complete skin traction assessment according to guidelines in skill for assessment of skin traction.

BALANCED SKIN TRACTION

Equipment

- Elastic hose
- Toweling or cover material for splint
- Weights

SKILL

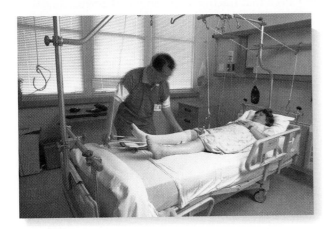

1 Place elastic hose on affected leg.

- Place material on lower splint and secure tightly. Ensure that material is wrinkle free. **RATIONALE:** To prevent skin irritation.
- Place affected leg on splint.

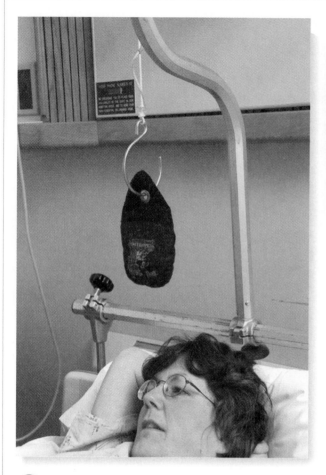

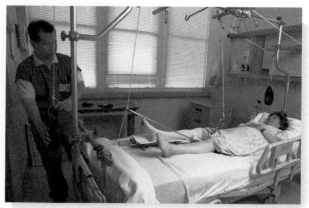

③ Place ordered amount of weight on foot end of traction. Lower weight slowly so that there is no pull on affected leg.

■ Ensure affected leg is positioned appropriately on splint without pressure under popliteal space. **RATIONALE:** To prevent pressure on nerve and potential paralysis.

② Ensure weight is hanging at head of bed. **RATIONALE:** To maintain appropriate traction.

■ Check all ropes and pulleys to ensure ropes slide through pulley system without difficulty.

④ Check that traction apparatus is at correct angle to provide appropriate traction.

■ Complete neurovascular checks immediately and then every 2 to 4 hrs.

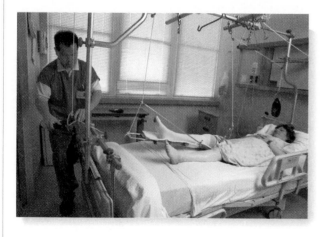

ASSESSMENT OF SKIN TRACTION

SKILL

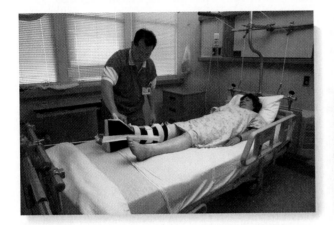

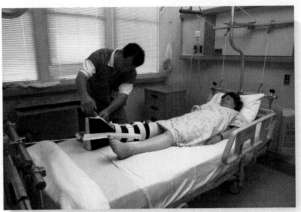

1 Check boot for placement and alignment.

- Remove boot every 8 hrs.
- Check all bony prominences for skin breakdown, abrasions, or pressure areas.
- Check that ropes are going through pulley system without disruption.
- Remove Velcro straps every 4 hrs. **RATIONALE:** To prevent compression of superficial peroneal nerve.

2 Examine extremity distal to traction.

- Note any presence of edema.
- Take and record peripheral pulses.
- Check temperature and color of extremity and compare with unaffected limb.
- Check for neurological impairment, presence of numbness or tingling. **RATIONALE:** These symptoms indicate pressure on a nerve.
- Ask client to move extremity. Note if full range of motion is present.
- Ask client to indicate presence of pain. If client indicates pain, ask where pain level is on scale of 1 to 10.

SAFETY ALERT

Check agency policy or physician's orders to remove Buck's traction. Depending on the procedure or purpose of traction, nurses may not be allowed to remove traction.

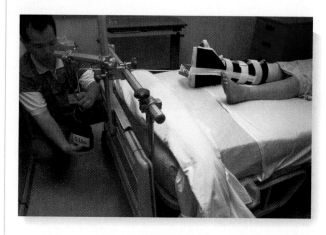

3 Ensure client is positioned in center of bed with affected leg aligned with trunk of body. **RATIONALE:** Misalignment is the leading cause of complications for clients in traction.

- Examine weights and pulley system. Ensure that pull goes directly through long axis of fractured bone.
- Check traction apparatus for safety.
- Weights should hang freely, off floor and bed.
- Knots should be secure in all ropes.
- Ropes should move freely through pulleys.
- Pulleys should not be constrained by knots.

TABLE 14-2	SKIN TRACTION	

Type	Purpose	Bed Position
Buck's extension	Preop for fractured hip; to prevent muscle spasms and dislocation	Flat in bed; head elevated 10–20° for ADLs
Cervical	Degenerative or arthritic conditions of cervical vertebrae; neck strain	Flat in bed or head can be elevated 15–20°
Dunlop	Fractured humerus	Flat in bed
Pelvic girdle	Low back pain; muscle spasm; ruptured or herniated disc	Head of bed and knee gatch raised so hips flexed at 45° angle (Williams position)
Russell's	Fractured shaft of femur in adolescents; lower leg and some knee injuries	Head of bed elevated 30–45°
Bryant's	Preop for fractured femur; children weighing less than 40 lb	Flat in bed with hips flexed at 90° angle to body and buttocks raised 1 in from mattress

SKELETAL TRACTION CARE

Equipment

- Sterile cotton-tipped applicators
- Prescribed cleaning agent
- Sterile gloves

SKILL

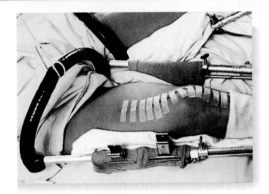

1 Check surgical site, if present, and surrounding pin site.

- Pin should be immobile.
- Pin site should be clean and dry.
- Check for signs of infection at pin site.

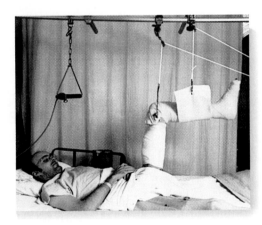

3 Check traction mechanism.

- Check that ropes and weights function properly, pull goes directly through long axis of fractured bone, ropes move freely through pulleys, pulleys are not constrained by knots.
- Weights should hang freely, off floor and bed.
- Knots should be secure in all ropes.

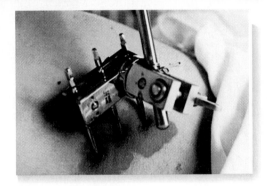

2 Provide pin site care.

- Open applicator sticks and appropriate cleansing agent.
- Clean area with prescribed cleansing agent. Soak cotton-tipped applicators. Dip stick into solution bottle or pour solution over sticks.
- Clean pin site starting at insertion area and working outward (away from pin site). **RATIONALE:** To cleanse site from cleanest to dirtiest area.
- Use new applicator stick for each pin site. **RATIONALE:** This prevents cross contamination of sites.
- Discard sticks.

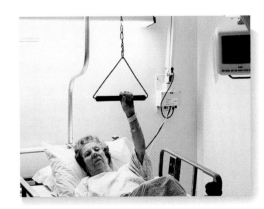

4 Instruct client to use trapeze to assist in moving and turning in bed during linen change and back care.

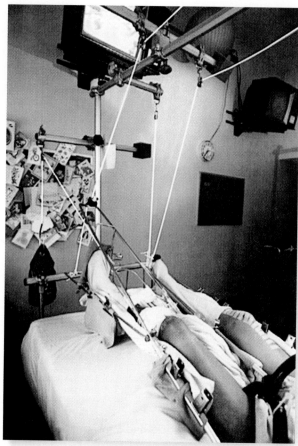

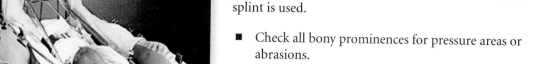

6 Check groin area for skin irritation when Thomas splint is used.

- Check all bony prominences for pressure areas or abrasions.
- Assess distal extremity for pulses, temperature, color, and edema.

5 Ensure client is positioned correctly in bed. **RATIONALE:** If client is pulled down to foot of bed, traction is negated.

- Check placement of foot rest. Client's foot should be correctly positioned to prevent footdrop.

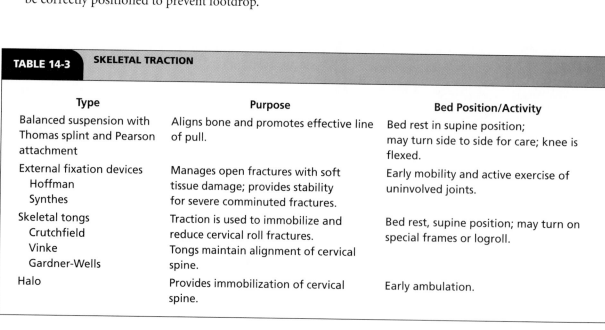

TABLE 14-3	SKELETAL TRACTION	

Type	Purpose	Bed Position/Activity
Balanced suspension with Thomas splint and Pearson attachment	Aligns bone and promotes effective line of pull.	Bed rest in supine position; may turn side to side for care; knee is flexed.
External fixation devices Hoffman Synthes	Manages open fractures with soft tissue damage; provides stability for severe comminuted fractures.	Early mobility and active exercise of uninvolved joints.
Skeletal tongs Crutchfield Vinke Gardner-Wells	Traction is used to immobilize and reduce cervical roll fractures. Tongs maintain alignment of cervical spine.	Bed rest, supine position; may turn on special frames or logroll.
Halo	Provides immobilization of cervical spine.	Early ambulation.

BEYOND THE SKILL

Assessment of External Fixation Devices

External fixation devices are treated very much like skeletal traction. Pin sites are checked frequently and pin site care is done exactly like that for skeletal traction. Neurovascular status of the affected limb is checked every 4 hrs. The security of the pins and stability of the frame are checked every 4 hrs. Pins are retightened by the physician at 24 hrs and at 1 wk after placement. **RATIONALE:** This prevents pin site infections and complications.

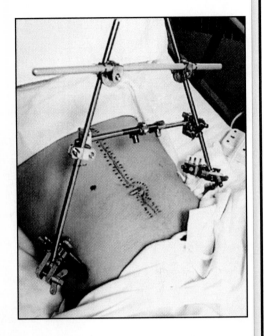

CLINICAL NOTE

Client teaching is critical for clients who will be discharged with pins still in place. The client needs to be able to demonstrate neurovascular checks and pin site care to ensure he or she is using aseptic technique.

TURNING WEDGE FOR POSITIONING

Equipment

- Turning wedge
- Velcro straps (two)

SKILL

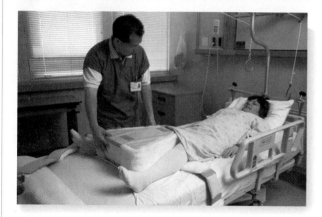

① Place turning wedge with short side of wedge toward client.

- Place Velcro straps under turning wedge, one at top of wedge and one at bottom of wedge.

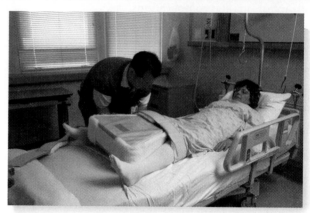

② Place Velcro strap across top of turning wedge first. Ensure strap is around client's thigh, not directly over popliteal space. **RATIONALE:** This will prevent pressure on peroneal nerve.

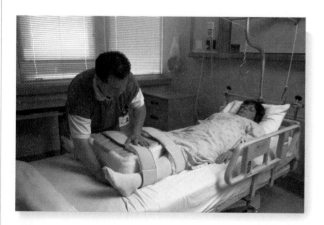

③ Place lower Velcro strap over calf of leg and above ankle. **RATIONALE:** To prevent pressure over bony prominences.

⚠ SAFETY ALERT

The turning wedge is used to prevent adduction and internal rotation of the hip.

CHARTING

- Type of traction used
- Alignment of traction
- Integrity of skin
- Temperature, color, pulse, and range of motion in extremity

- Specific complaints by client and nursing actions
- Neurovascular check
- Client teaching

SECTION FOUR

HALO TRACTION AND BACK BRACE

Halo traction is popular because this form of immobilization allows early mobility of clients with spinal cord injury. Positioning a client into a wheelchair early after injury prevents complications such as pneumonia and circulatory impairment. Some clients with spinal cord injury can be immobilized with the halo brace, but most clients require surgical intervention followed by halo application to stabilize the spinal cord.

The Jewett-Taylor brace is a hyperextension brace used for anterior vertebral body fractures. It extends the spine and takes pressure off the vertebrae.

RATIONALE

- To maintain cervical alignment
- To provide back support for clients following spinal cord surgery
- To maintain pin site free of infection
- To prevent orthostatic hypotension

ASSESSMENT

- Check for respiratory impairment (absence of breath sounds or adventitious sounds).
- Check pin sites for potential infection.
- Assess alignment and position of traction.
- Check for signs of orthostatic hypotension while placing client in sitting position.

HALO TRACTION

Equipment

- Allen wrench
- Prescribed cleansing solution
- Sterile cotton-tipped applicators
- Synthetic fleece lining for vest, as needed

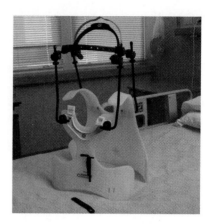

SKILL

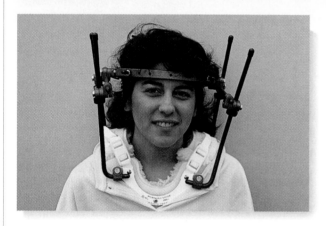

1 Monitor alignment of cast and vest. If traction is intact, client's neck should not be flexed or extended. **RATIONALE:** Traction is maintained by anterior metal bars. Do not pull on anterior bars; use posterior bars for positioning clients.

- Check every bolt on halo superstructure and vest at least daily while client is hospitalized.
- Change vest liner only if necessary. If fleece liner gets wet, it can be dried using hair dryer on cool setting. **RATIONALE:** Loosening of vest or superstructure carries risk of loss of position of cervical spine.
- Wash skin under vest by wringing out bath towel soaked in hot water. Pull towel back and forth in drying motion beneath front and back portions of vest. Do not use soap or lotion under vest. **RATIONALE:** This can cause skin irritation.

SAFETY ALERT

Evaluate respiratory status every 2 to 4 hrs the first 24 to 48 hrs.

- Observe respiratory excursion.
- Monitor breath sounds every shift for presence of adventitious sounds or absence of breath sounds. **RATIONALE:** Pulmonary embolus is a common complication associated with spinal cord injury.
- Keep Allen wrench and tracheostomy tray at bedside. **RATIONALE:** Allen wrench is used to remove screws from vest in order to perform CPR.

CLINICAL NOTE

To prevent orthostatic hypotension when placing a halo traction client in sitting position:

- Apply antiembolic stockings. **RATIONALE:** Stockings promote venous return to heart.
- Apply abdominal binder. **RATIONALE:** Binders increase venous return to heart.
- Raise client to 90∞ sitting position over period of 20 to 30 min. Take vital signs with each incremental change in position.
- Administer medications if hypotension persists or keep client in bed and try to sit client up after 1 hr.

BEYOND THE SKILL

Changing Halo Traction Vest Liner

To change the liner with minimum risk of displacement, three principles must be followed:

1. Proceed slowly and patiently.
2. Do not loosen any of the straps if it can be avoided.
3. Do not loosen any bolts or screws at all.

To replace the fleece liner:

1. Place client face up on firm, flat surface without pillows or other support under head.
2. Place pillowcase between anterior portion of vest and liner to separate liner from hook and loop fasteners that hold liner to vest shell.
3. Pull out liner. Pillowcase protects client's skin from hook material inside vest shell.
4. Work new liner under vest shell between client's skin and pillowcase.
5. Carefully remove pillowcase when vest is in position.
6. Turn client face down and repeat procedure to replace vest liner on posterior shell.

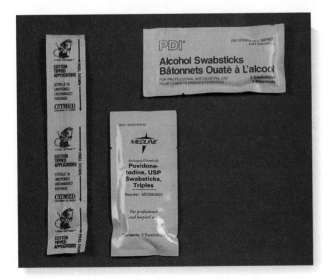

2 Prevent pin site infection.

- Cleanse site areas at least daily and observe for drainage, edema, or erythema.
- Cleanse around pin sites with alcohol swab or with soap and water, using gauze squares or cotton-tipped applicators. Povidone iodine is usually not used as it can corrode pins. Check facility policy for use.
- Remove scabbing with hydrogen peroxide or alcohol, using cotton-tipped applicators. If hydrogen peroxide is used, rinse site with sterile saline.
- Check facility policy if ointments or antiseptics are to be applied to pin sites. This is not usually considered part of routine care.
- Shave hair around pin sites to allow for easy observation and cleaning.

JEWETT-TAYLOR BACK BRACE

Equipment

- Front and back brace with Velcro straps
- T-shirt
- ABD dressings

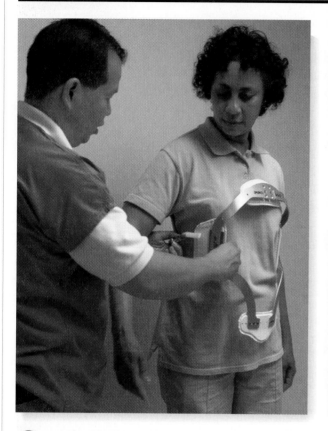

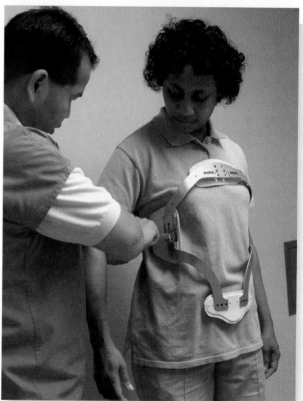

1 Place T-shirt on client. **RATIONALE:** This protects skin from brace rubbing on bare skin.

- Place back of brace first. Ensure it does not rub on vertebrae or surgical incision.

2 Place front section of brace by positioning brace above breast and at top of symphysis.

- Hook back of brace to front using strap.
- Adjust the two pieces to ensure they fit snugly.

- Pin site assessment and interventions
- Pin site care
- Stability of traction
- Presence of orthostatic hypotension signs and symptoms

- Nursing measures to prevent orthostatic hypotension
- Respiratory assessment
- Vest fleece removal

SECTION FIVE

CONTINUOUS PASSIVE MOTION (CPM) DEVICE

Clients undergoing knee surgery, and, in some cases, hip surgery are placed in the continuous passive motion (CPM) machine right after surgery. The amount of flexion and extension of the knee joint is ordered by the physician, and the physical therapist adjusts the machine to the appropriate degrees of flexion and extension. The client's cycle rate (number of revolutions per minute) is ordered by the physician as well. Nurses are responsible for turning the CPM on and off and placing the client in and out of the apparatus. Nurses do not adjust the cycles per minute or the degree of flexion and extension.

RATIONALE

- To increase joint mobility following knee surgery
- To promote circulation in surgical extremity
- To put knee through extension and flexion exercises

ASSESSMENT

- Assess client's pain status.
- Assess client's tolerance to ordered degree of flexion and extension provided by CPM device.
- Assess client's ability to tolerate ordered time for CPM treatment.
- Assess for proper alignment of knee in CPM device.

Equipment

- CPM frame (stored on post bolted to bed)
- Sheepskin slings
- Sequential stockings
- Trapeze

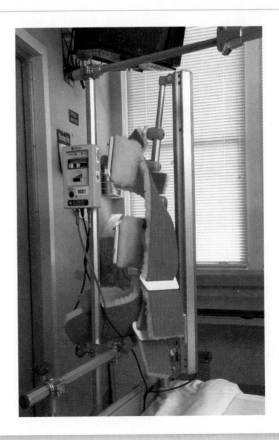

SKILL

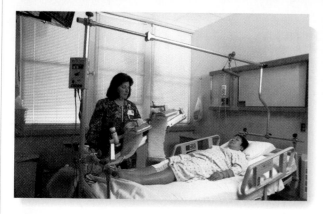

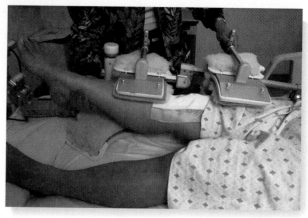

1 Lower CPM unit onto bed. PT obtains correct measurement of client. Measurement is from greater trochanter to knee. **RATIONALE:** To ensure knee is in anatomically correct position for flexion and extension.

2 Place affected extremity on frame and align knee to gauge on bar. When placing leg on frame, support leg by placing hand under client's ankle.

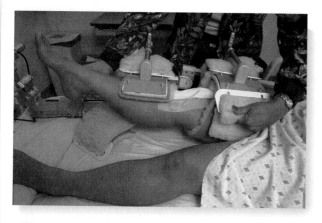

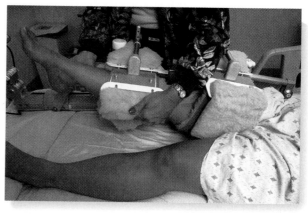

3 Place Velcro sheepskin sling around thigh. Pull sling through plastic frame and attach strap to frame.

4 Place sheepskin sling around calf; bring strap through plastic frame and secure straps by tightening and clipping sling in place.

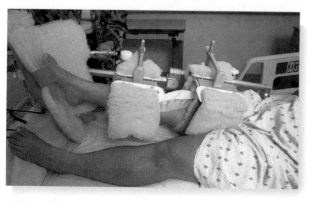

SAFETY ALERT

Clients under 4 ft, 11 in and over 6 ft, 2 in require a nonstandard CPM machine.

5 Attach foot plate to brace.

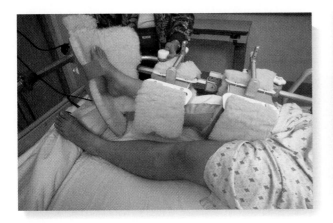

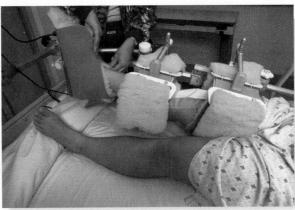

6 Place foot in sheepskin bootie. Tighten foot plate by twisting white knob.

7 Secure bootie by tightening Velcro straps.

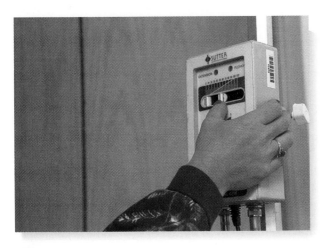

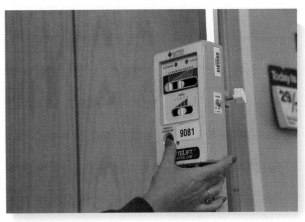

8 Set control panel for degree of extension and flexion according to physical therapist/physician orders or facility policy.

9 Press start button, usually at 2 to 10 cycles/min.

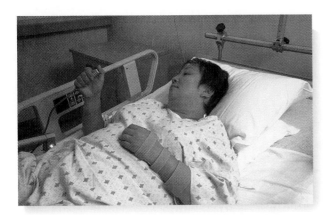

10 Instruct client on use of control button. Client can control start and stop of CPM machine.

SAFETY ALERT

Nurses turn CPM unit on and off and place client in traction only. Physical therapists adjust degree of flexion.

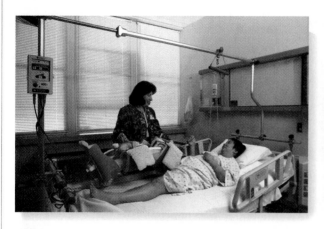

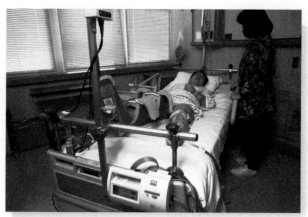

11 Check client's level of comfort and perform neurovascular check every 2 hrs.

- Keep CPM machine on 12 to 14 hrs during the day.

12 Place unaffected leg in sequential compression stocking.

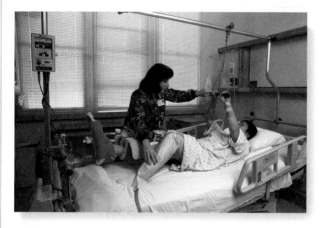

13 Keep side rails up.

- Instruct client on turning using trapeze.

CHARTING

- Time CPM machine applied
- Degree of extension and flexion applied
- Number of cycles per minute
- Neurovascular assessment

- Sequential compression stockings applied
- Client complaints and nursing interventions to alleviate problem

CRITICAL THINKING FOCUS

SECTION ONE ▪ Bandages and Slings

Unexpected Outcomes

- Affected joint or extremity is not immobilized with bandage.

- Edema is noted in area surrounding bandage.

- Distal pulses are diminished or absent.

Alternative Nursing Actions

- Assess if type of bandage is effective or if alternative type of bandage would provide more support.
- Assess need for possible cast immobilizer in place of bandage.
- Evaluate if bandage is applied tightly enough to immobilize extremity.

- Take bandage off; check circulation and skin condition.
- Keep extremity elevated.
- Rewrap bandage after edema has subsided.
- If edema persists, notify physician for orders.

- Take off bandages immediately and reassess pulses. If pulses are present, rewrap bandages, keeping pressure even and bandages loose.
- If pulses remain diminished or absent, notify physician immediately.

SECTION TWO ▪ Cast Care

Unexpected Outcomes

- Client complains of numbness, discomfort, or pain.

- Cast cracks from improper drying procedure or stress.

- Synthetic cast has rough edges.

Alternative Nursing Actions

- Notify physician immediately.
- Reevaluate condition of casted extremity every 15 min.
- Reassess circulation, movement, and sensation (CMS).

- Notify physician immediately.
- Reassure client.
- Do not reposition client until physician assesses.

- Smooth edges by filing with nail file.
- Make sure furniture and clothing are protected from scratches and snags by covering cast with cloth.

SECTION THREE ▪ Traction

Unexpected Outcomes

- There is a change in temperature, color, or pulses of extremity.

Alternative Nursing Actions

- Notify physician at once.
- If client has fractured femur, measure size of thigh with tape measure every 15 to 30 min. Look for areas of

ecchymosis. (It is possible for several units of blood to be sequestered in the thigh if a vessel has been torn.)

- Assess for circulatory shock.

- Countertraction is not maintained for client in Buck's traction.

- Check alignment to ensure client is placed in center of bed and not touching headboard or footboard.
- Instruct client to stay flat on back if turning from waist down or sitting up interferes with countertraction.

- Client has skin abrasions, dermatitis, wounds, impaired circulation, varicose veins, or peripheral neuropathy.

- Notify physician immediately if skin traction is contraindicated with these conditions.

SECTION FOUR ▪ Halo Traction and Back Brace

Unexpected Outcomes	**Alternative Nursing Actions**

- Infection occurs at pin site.

- Monitor neurologic signs closely, as brain abscess is a major complication.
- Obtain culture of drainage.
- Call physician for systemic antibiotic order.
- Cleanse site frequently.
- Apply dressing over pin site to absorb drainage.

- Pins are loose.

- Immobilize client immediately.
- Contact physician.
- Have Allen wrench available for physician.

SECTION FIVE ▪ Continuous Passive Motion (CPM) Device

Unexpected Outcomes	**Alternative Nursing Actions**

- Client complains of pain.

- Medicate for pain every 3 to 4 hrs or as ordered by physician.
- Check degree of extension and flexion and notify physician if client cannot maintain ordered degree.

- Client is unable to maintain cycles per minute without pain.

- Obtain order to decrease number of hours for CPM for first day until client adapts to machine.

SELF-CHECK EVALUATION

PART 1 ▪ Matching Terms

Match the definition in column B with the correct term in column A.

Column A

_____ a. Abduction
_____ b. Adduction
_____ c. Buck's traction
_____ d. Thomas splint
_____ e. Paresthesia
_____ f. Orthostatic hypotension
_____ g. Osteoblast

Column B

1. Low blood pressure in an upright position
2. Abnormal sensation
3. Skeletal traction used for long-term immobilization
4. Movement of a bone away from the midline of the body
5. Cell that plays a role in bone formation
6. Skin traction used primarily in elderly clients
7. Movement of bone toward midline of body

PART 2 ▪ Multiple Choice

1. The repair process following a bone fracture begins with:

a. Laying down of the organic matrix.
b. Formation of a blood clot.
c. Osteoblast formation.
d. Fibroblast development.

2. Clients with bandages applied should have circulatory checks:

a. Every hour for 24 hrs.
b. Every 4 to 8 hrs.
c. 20 min after application, then every hour.
d. 20 min after application, then every 2 to 4 hrs.

3. When applying a circular bandage, begin the wrap by:

a. Anchoring the wrap at the distal end.
b. Anchoring the wrap at the proximal end.
c. Beginning the circular turn at the distal end.
d. Beginning the circular turn at the proximal end.

4. Bandages are rewrapped every _____:

a. 1 to 2 hrs.
b. 2 to 4 hrs.
c. 4 to 8 hrs.
d. 24 hrs.

5. Major differences in synthetic and plaster casts are:

a. Weight-bearing time is about 60 min for synthetic casts.
b. Plaster casts are less restrictive.
c. Synthetic casts are less expensive.
d. Plaster casts are less likely to indent into the skin.

6. A wet cast should be:
   a. Placed on a firm surface.
   b. Handled only with the palms of the hands.
   c. Dry in 3 to 4 hrs.
   d. Kept covered until dried.

7. When applying a sling, place the apex, or point, of the triangle toward the _____ and bring the opposite end around the affected arm and _____:
   a. Wrist, anchor at neck.
   b. Elbow, over affected shoulder.
   c. Wrist, over affected shoulder.
   d. Elbow, anchor at back of neck.

8. When assessing a skeletal traction apparatus, the nurse understands the traction is functioning properly in all of the following situations except when the:
   a. Weights are hanging free.
   b. Rope is on the pulley.
   c. Foot plate is not resting against the pulley.
   d. Pins are movable.

9. While assessing a client in skeletal traction, you observe the distal extremity to be pale with slow capillary refill and palpate a 1+ pulse. Your initial action is to:
   a. Assess the client every 15 min for changes.
   b. Observe for ecchymosis or signs of infection.
   c. Remove the traction.
   d. Notify the physician.

10. Buck's traction is most likely used in which condition?
    a. Elderly client with hip fracture prior to surgery.
    b. Cervical cord injury.
    c. Fractured femur in toddler.
    d. Fractured tibia or fibula in young adolescent.

PART 3 ▪ Critical Thinking Application

Mrs. Jacobson, a 73-year-old retired school teacher, has been admitted to the hospital for a right total hip replacement as a result of osteoarthritis. She has been very active her entire life, playing golf three times a week, bowling on a team, hiking, and gardening. She is very concerned that she will be unable to continue these activities if she doesn't have surgery. Her lab work was completed before her admission. She gave 2 units of autologous blood in case she needs it for surgery. Her vital signs are: BP 148/80, P 88, R 26. She uses a cane, which she says is "for balance."

1. Identify the priority preoperative intervention for Mrs. Jacobson. Provide a rationale for your choice.

2. Develop a client care plan: Identify short- and long-term goals, state three nursing diagnoses in priority order, and provide the rationale for your choices. Describe at least two priority nursing interventions for each nursing diagnosis.

3. Identify two safety issues related to Mrs. Jacobson's care.

4. Describe at least three procedures that need to be discussed prior to Mrs. Jacobson's discharge.

15

NONPARENTERAL MEDICATIONS

INTRODUCTION

Medications or drugs are given to exert specific physiologic effects on the body. Since they play such an important role in preventing, treating, and curing illness, their administration has become one of the most important, complex, and risk-laden aspects of nursing care. While medications are administered for an intended therapeutic effect, they can also have side effects, adverse effects, or even toxic effects. The route of administration influences the drug's effect on the body. Drugs are designed to be administered orally (by mouth); topically (via skin, eye, or ear); mucosally (via mouth, lung, nose, rectum, or vagina); or by parenteral injection (via intradermal, subcutaneous, intramuscular, or intravenous sites). Medications produce either a local effect that is confined to an external or internal part of the body or a systemic, generalized action. It is important to know why a particular drug is being given, why a particular formulation and route are used, and the desired outcome intended.

Four biologic processes—absorption, transportation, metabolism, and excretion—determine a medication's onset, duration, and intensity of action. A medication is absorbed as it moves from the administration site into the bloodstream. Once absorbed

(continued on next page)

into the bloodstream, the medication is transported to the site of action, where it becomes available to the body. The anatomic site of absorption and the individual client's physiologic variables affect this process. Bioavailability is decreased with oral administration because the drug is circulated to the liver and metabolized before reaching the general circulation.

Through metabolism the drug is converted by enzymes into a less active form that can be excreted. Most drugs are metabolized in the liver, where some drugs are converted into metabolites that are more effective. If a drug is metabolized in the liver, some of the active drug is inactivated or diverted before it reaches the circulation and attains its site of action. Once the drug is circulating, some of it is bound to plasma protein while the rest is transported freely through the circulation to all parts of the body. The free drug is pharmacologically active, crossing cell membranes to reach the site of action.

Finally, the drug is excreted or eliminated from the body. The kidneys are the most important route for excretion; other routes include the GI tract, lungs, saliva, sweat, and breast milk. Because the liver is so important to metabolism, and the kidneys are so important to excretion, clients with hepatic or renal dysfunction are at risk for accumulating toxic drug levels.

While the physician prescribes the medication and the pharmacist dispenses it, the nurse is responsible for validating, preparing, and administering medications safely

---

THE FIVE RIGHTS

- **Right Medication:** Compare the medication container label to the medication sheet (MAR) before, during, and after dispensing during preparation. Know the drug's action, side effects, and contraindications. Changing the form of the drug (e.g., crushing) can alter the drug's effect.
- **Right Dose:** Carefully note dosage dispensed (e.g., 10 mg/mL) and dosage to be given (e.g., 8 mg). Some drug dosages are based on the client's weight or body surface area, or may be adjusted by the nurse according to established protocol based on the client's laboratory findings. Always verify calculations of divided or individualized doses with another nurse. Always check heparin, insulin, and digitalis doses with another nurse.
- **Right Route:** Validate the route for administration on the container label (e.g., IV). Request that the physician write a new medication order if a change in route is indicated (e.g., client is NPO).
- **Right Time:** Carefully validate b.i.d., t.i.d., q.i.d., or q8h times for drug administration. Absorption of oral drugs is affected by stomach contents as well as the ingestion of other drugs. Note before-meal and between-meal formulations.
- **Right Client:** Check the room number, bed number, and client's identaband, and have client state name. The client has the right to take or refuse the medication.

● **FIGURE 15-1** *The Five Rights of medication administration.*

and in accordance with agency policies and procedures. In addition, the nurse assesses and documents the client's response to the drug administered. It is important to follow the Five Rights each time you give a medication in order to decrease the risk of medication error.

PREPARATION PROTOCOL: FOR MEDICATION ADMINISTRATION SKILLS

Complete the following steps before each skill.

1. Validate each medication to be given according to skill for medication validation.
2. Wash hands.
3. Prepare medication according to skill for route of administration (e.g., oral, parenteral).
4. Take medication to client's room, validating room and bed numbers.
5. Validate client's identity (check identaband and have client state name). Check for presence of allergy bracelet.
6. Provide privacy.
7. Inform client of drug name, purpose, and procedure for administration.
8. Assess vital signs or other parameters affected by drug to be given to determine safety for administration.
9. Place client in appropriate position for route of administration.
10. Don gloves if indicated.
11. Administer medication according to medication route.

COMPLETION PROTOCOL: FOR MEDICATION ADMINISTRATION SKILLS

Make sure the following steps have been completed.

1. Dispose of equipment appropriately.
2. Reposition client for comfort.
3. Remove and dispose of gloves if used, then wash hands.
4. Document medication on appropriate forms (medication administration record [MAR], client record) and report client responses as indicated.

SECTION ONE

MEDICATION ADMINISTRATION

Medications are prescribed by a physician as a signed written order in the client's chart. If a written order is illegible or is questionable for any reason, the physician should be notified for clarification. The medication order includes the name of the drug, the dose, the route (PO if not specified otherwise), and the number of times the drug is to be given.

Most medications have more than one name: The *generic* name is the patented official name (e.g., acetaminophen), while the *trade* name is created by the particular manufacturer and is capitalized (e.g., Tylenol). Generic formulations are usually less expensive than trade name products.

Routine medications are administered according to instructions (e.g., b.i.d.). PRN drugs are administered when the client needs the medication. (see Appendix B for abbreviations). The pharmacy monitors the client's list of medications and produces the medication administration record (MAR) sheet for each day.

RATIONALE

- To administer medications safely following physician's orders
- To identify potential sources of error
- To administer medications following the Five Rights

ASSESSMENT

- Assess continued validity of order (some medications require renewal orders at specified intervals, e.g., narcotics).
- Check that medication sheet is consistent with original physician's order.
- Check interactive effect of medication with other drugs client is receiving.
- Check compatibility of two medications being physically combined in solution (e.g., in syringe).
- Check that medication is designed for route being used.
- Check laboratory data, serum drug levels, and client assessment data (vital signs, height and weight, allergy) to ensure safe parameters for drug administration.

SAFETY ALERT

- Keep all medicines in locked carts or cupboards.
- Keep all poisonous solutions and materials in a secure area away from medicines.
- Check the drug label of all medications being dispensed three times against the MAR:
  - When taking medication from storage place
  - Before preparing medication
  - Before returning medication to storage place

MEDICATION VALIDATION

Equipment

- Computer access for client data (e.g., recent lab reports)
- Client's medication administration record (MAR) or Kardex
- Medication to be administered
- Client's record
- Pharmacology text or *Physician's Desk Reference* (PDR)
- Calculator as needed

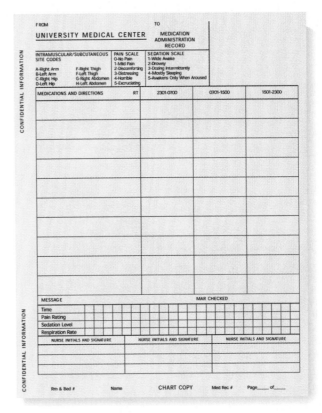

● **FIGURE 15-2** *Medication administration record.*

SKILL

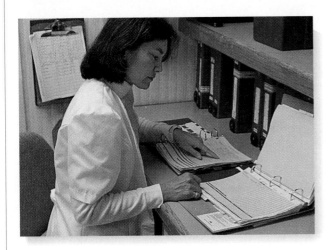

① Validate client's MAR medications to be given with physician's most recent order on client's record (or Kardex).

- Validate drug dose, route, and time to be given.
- Assess for any potential drug interaction of medications being administered. **RATIONALE:** Special monitoring may be indicated.
- Assess client's record for lab results, allergy, or other relevant data. **RATIONALE:** To ensure safe parameters for drug administration.

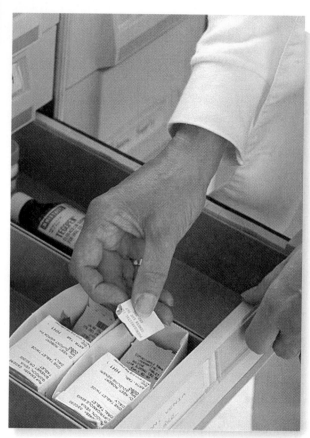

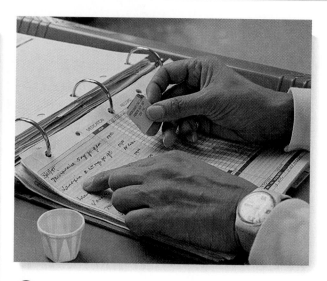

③ Validate each medication with client's MAR for the **right** client, **right** drug, **right** time of administration, **right** dosage, and **right** route.

② Locate the **right** client's medications to be given at a specific time; check medication expiration date.

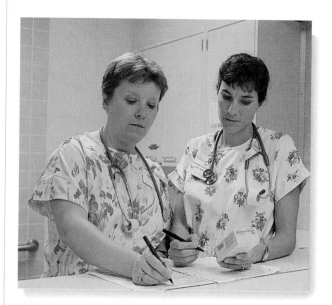

④ Check any necessary drug calculations with another nurse.

 SAFETY ALERT

- Report any errors in the administration of medicines to the charge nurse and the client's physician immediately.
- Document the drug given, and complete a written unusual occurrence report.
- Monitor the client closely for any adverse effects that may occur.

BEYOND THE SKILL

Computerized Access Systems

Many agencies utilize computerized access systems for dispensing and recording drugs. Examples include PYXIS, SURE-MED, and DIEBOLD systems. The purpose of these systems is to:

- Control access to drugs and narcotics
- Eliminate need for shift change narcotic count
- Accurately record medications dispensed
- Facilitate directly billing the client

Computerized Access

- Enter your ID code number and/or user password or scanned fingerprint.

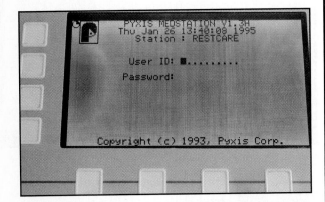

- Input client's ID number to access client's file. Validating with client's MAR, select desired drug and dose on monitor screen; charge will be generated to client.

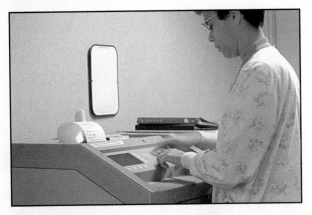

- When drawer opens, open container and remove the prescribed dose.

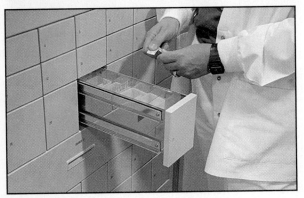

(continued on next page)

- Count and input number of dispensable units remaining.
- Close drawer and sign off system.

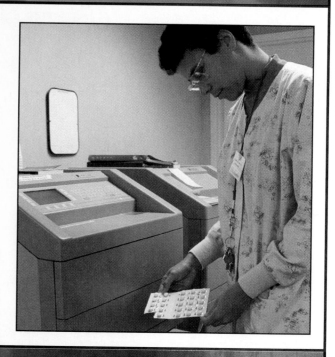

NARCOTIC PREPARATION

Equipment

- Client's MAR
- Narcotic book
- Narcotic drawer keys

SKILL

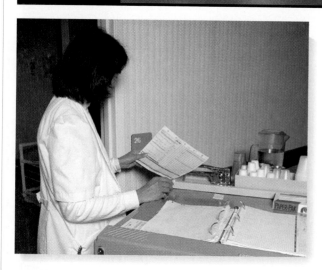

1 Perform skill for medication validation. Check dose and time last narcotic was administered.

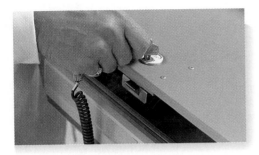

2 Unlock narcotic drawer and find appropriate narcotic container.

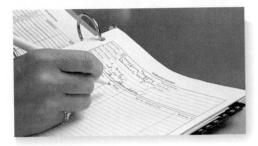

4 Sign out for narcotic on narcotic sheet after taking narcotic out of drawer. **RATIONALE:** It is the nurse's responsibility to account for all controlled substances dispensed.

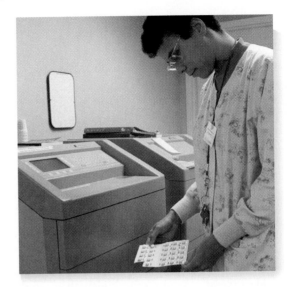

3 Count number of pills, ampules, or prefilled cartridges in container. Check narcotic sign-out sheet and verify that number of narcotics in drawer matches number on specific narcotic sign-out sheet. **RATIONALE:** Discrepancies must be rectified.

■ Lock drawer or cupboard after obtaining medication and keep keys with you at all times. **RATIONALE:** Laws on controlled substances require careful monitoring of narcotics.

CLIENT VALIDATION

Equipment

■ Medication cart with client's MAR (medication cart is taken through hallway to clients' rooms in many agencies)
■ Prepared medication
■ Stethoscope (if indicated)

SAFETY ALERT

■ Follow preparation protocol for medication administration when administering all medications.
■ Never administer a medication that has been prepared by someone else.

SKILL

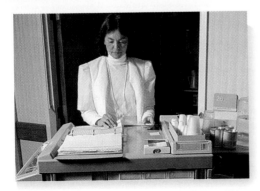

1 Prepare medication according to route of administration.

■ Take medication to client's room and validate room and bed number. Medication cart is taken through hallway to client's room in many agencies. **RATIONALE:** Room and bed number must concur with client's medication record.

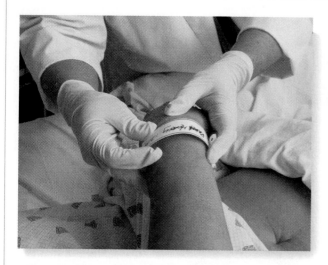

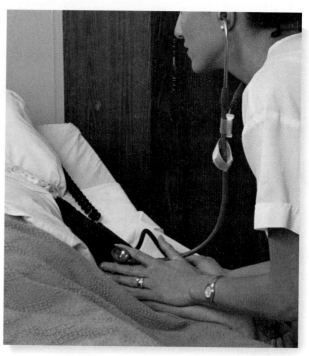

 Validate client's identity (check identaband and have client state name). **RATIONALE:** Client may say "Yes" if any name is asked. Identaband and client's stated name must correspond.

- Check for presence of allergy bracelet. **RATIONALE:** If client is allergic to the medication, physician should be notified and drug order clarified.
- Provide privacy.
- Inform client of drug name, purpose, and procedure for administration. **RATIONALE:** Clients have the right to this information as well as the right to refuse medication.

 Validate client's status (e.g., vital signs or other parameters affected by drug). **RATIONALE:** This action determines safety for drug administration.

SAFETY ALERT

- Always recheck a medication that the client has concern or doubt about.
- Do not leave medication at the client's bedside under the assumption that it will be taken.

SAFETY ALERT

- Medications that lower blood pressure should be held if client's systolic BP is less than 100 (or other parameter as directed).
- Medications that slow heart rate should be held if client's heart rate is less than 60.

SECTION TWO

ORAL MEDICATIONS

The oral route is most commonly used for drug administration. It is safe, convenient, and cost effective. In addition, the GI tract provides a large surface area for drug absorption. Some drugs, however, cannot be absorbed or are destroyed by enzymes or the acidity (low pH) of this environment, or are rendered unavailable to tissues by first passing through the liver (e.g., nitroglycerine). Either slow or accelerated gastric emptying will affect the drug absorption rate. Some medications are designed to be taken on an empty stomach, some to be taken with food.

Many of today's new medication delivery systems provide sustained drug delivery at a constant rate, decreasing the need for frequent dosing. Such slow-release tablets should not be crushed or capsules opened for ease of administration to clients who have difficulty swallowing or who have a feeding tube. Doing so could potentiate or obliterate the drug's action, resulting in a medication error with serious outcomes for the client. Check with the pharmacist before deciding to alter the form of any medication. Some medications can be substituted with a liquid form or a short-acting formulation that can safely be crushed for administration. Contact the prescribing physician for a substitute medication if formulation alternatives are unavailable or if the client is NPO, in which case another route must be used.

Most oral medications can be given through a nasogastric or gastrostomy tube if the nurse honors the General Precautions for Altering Drug Delivery (see Clinical Note on p. 428). If the medication is to be given before meals, a continuous feeding must be stopped temporarily for proper absorption. Each medication should be given separately, flushing before and after, necessitating careful recording of net fluid intake and adhering to any fluid restriction that may be imposed.

RATIONALE

- To provide the most common, easiest, and least expensive route of administering medications
- To provide sustained drug action and increased absorption time
- To provide oral liquid medication to client who has difficulty swallowing pills
- To provide oral medication mixed with food for client who is fluid restricted
- To provide oral medication via feeding tube
- To ensure that client receives medication

ASSESSMENT

- Check that client is not NPO for diagnostic or therapeutic purposes.
- Assess that client is alert, cooperative, and able to swallow.
- Check that medication is to be taken with food or on empty stomach.
- Assess that volume of liquid required to dilute medication is acceptable considering any fluid restriction.
- Check that medication's action will not be affected (potentiated or obliterated) if medication delivery is altered.
- Check vital signs, lab data, or other parameters affected by medication to be given.
- Make sure that medication and tube feeding scheduling allow for medication to be given on empty stomach (if indicated).

TABLETS AND CAPSULES

Equipment

- Pill from bottle or in unit dose packaging
- Paper soufflé cups
- Water or other liquid for swallowing medication

SKILL

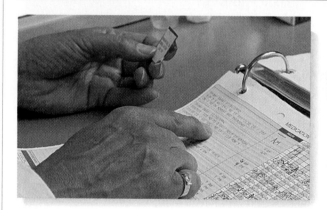

1 Leave tablet or capsule medication in unit dose packaging. **RATIONALE:** This maintains identity of drug. If medication is not taken, it can be returned to client's medication box.

- Dispense bottled tablet or capsule into bottle lid, then drop from lid into client's medication cup. **RATIONALE:** This action controls number of pills placed in cup.

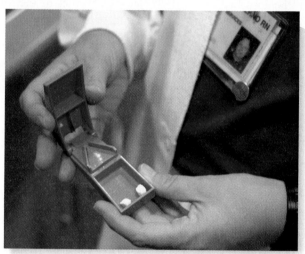

2 Open package to cut or break pill if partial dose is to be given.

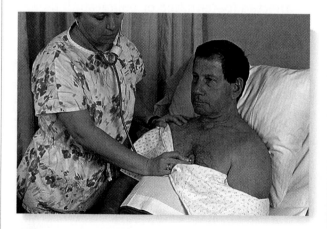

3 Place client in sitting position; assess vital signs if indicated. **RATIONALE:** Sitting position facilitates swallowing. Vital signs influence decision making about administering certain medications.

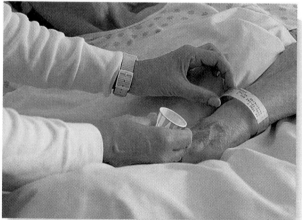

4 Open unit dose package, place pill in cup, and hand cup to client. Provide water or other liquid, making sure client swallows medication.

LIQUIDS

Equipment

- Liquid medication in bottle
- Calibrated cup

SKILL

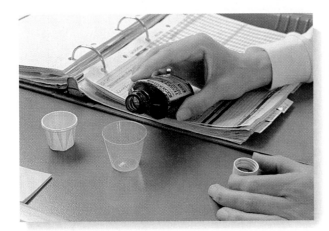

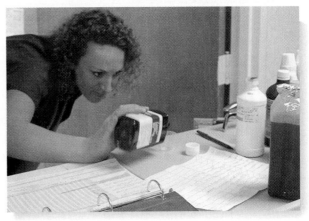

1 Shake bottle if indicated. **RATIONALE:** To suspend medication that has settled.

- Remove bottle lid and place upside down. **RATIONALE:** This prevents contamination of lid.

2 Hold calibrated medication cup at eye level, or place on firm surface with calibrations at eye level. **RATIONALE:** This facilitates accuracy of dose dispensed.

- Hold bottle so that label will not be soiled if medication drips onto bottle, and pour prescribed amount of medication into calibrated cup.
- Administer medication per skill for administering oral tablets or capsules.
- Provide water following medication, unless topical effect is intended (e.g., cough syrup).

CRUSHED OR ALTERED TABLETS AND CAPSULES

Equipment

- Pill from bottle or in unit dose packaging
- Pill crusher (pestle or other device)
- Soft food for administration

CLINICAL NOTE

GENERAL PRECAUTIONS FOR ALTERING DRUG DELIVERY

Safe Actions

- Chewable medications *can be* crushed safely.
- Powder from capsules *can be* mixed with food or liquid.
- Contents of liquid-filled capsules *can be* squeezed out through a hole punched with a large-gauge sterile needle or aspirated and then mixed with food or liquid, but should not be administered sublingually.
- Beads from opened capsules *can be* sprinkled over soft food, but should not be chewed.
- A sublingual formulation still *can be* given sublingually if the client is NPO.

Unsafe Actions

- *Do not* crush enteric-coated tablets. **RATIONALE:** Coatings are used to allow intestinal absorption of the drug, protect the medication from stomach acid, or protect the stomach from the medication.
- *Do not* crush long-acting tablets. **RATIONALE:** Sustained action over hours is the advantage of extended-release versions of drugs. Crushing could yield a toxic dose and eliminate the sustained action needed through the day.
- *Do not* crush contents of capsules (e.g., spansules) with beads or pellets. **RATIONALE:** These are intended for sustained-release action.
- *Do not* give sublingual formulations orally. **RATIONALE:** Ingredients may be inactivated by stomach acid.
- *Do not* crush sublingual formulations.
- *Do not* give oral medications sublingually. **RATIONALE:** This could yield a toxic dose since the medication would be absorbed directly into the bloodstream and skip the intended pass through the liver for early metabolism before entering the bloodstream.

SKILL

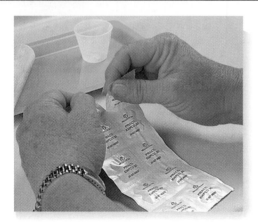

1 Leave pill in unit dose packaging and place on firm surface. **RATIONALE:** Labeled packaging maintains identity and prevents loss of medication. If client does not take medication, it can be returned to drawer.

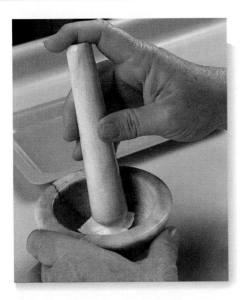

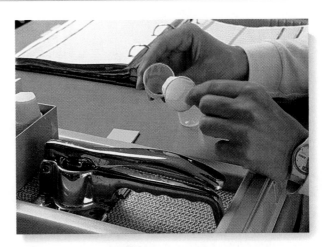

3 Alternatively, place pill between two soufflé cups. **RATIONALE:** The cups confine the medication.

2 Pound to crush pill with pestle or other tool, pulverizing thoroughly.

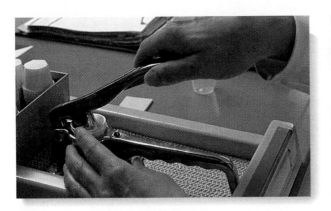

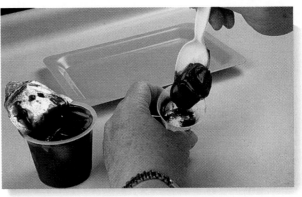

4 Crush "sandwiched" pill with pill crusher. Remove any uncrushed pill coating if medication is to be given per feeding tube. **RATIONALE:** To prevent tube clogging.

5 If giving orally, mix pulverized medication (or powder from opened capsule) carefully in small amount of soft food (pudding, jelly, applesauce). **RATIONALE:** For many clients with swallowing difficulty, soft food is easier to swallow than liquids.

6 Open capsule and sprinkle beads over soft food to administer. Warn client not to chew beads. **RATIONALE:** Beads are formulated for a sustained timed-release therapeutic effect.

- Ensure client has received all of medication.
- Offer liquid or food to cleanse palate.

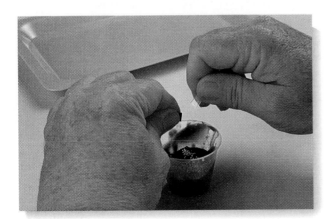

NASOGASTRIC AND ENTERAL TUBE MEDICATIONS

Equipment

- Appropriately prepared medication (use liquid medication when possible)
- Water for dilution and flushing
- 50-mL irrigating piston syringe
- Clean gloves

SKILL

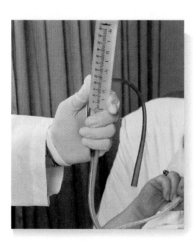

1 Stop tube feeding if medication is to be given on an empty stomach for absorption (e.g., before-meals [a.c.] medication). **RATIONALE:** Some medications are not absorbed if taken with food or other medications.

- Prepare each medication separately: Pulverize thoroughly or empty capsule of contents. **RATIONALE:** This maintains discrete identity of each medication. If, for some reason, a particular medication must be withheld, it can be identified.
- Dilute crushed tablet or powder from capsule in 30 mL warm water. **RATIONALE:** This facilitates tube administration.

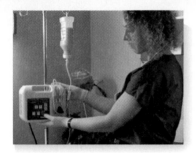

3 Administer each medication separately, allowing to flow through NG tube by gravity. **RATIONALE:** This allows identification of each medication given.

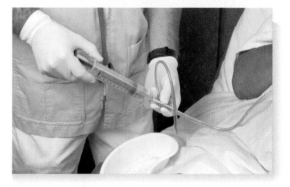

2 Disconnect NG tube from feeding tube, maintaining asepsis of connecting adapter.

- Check residual volume, return residual, and flush NG tube. **RATIONALE:** This validates gastric capacity for receiving medication and flush solution.

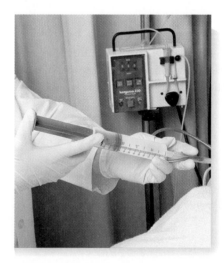

4 Flush tube with 15 to 30 mL water after each medication (monitor amount to record on intake and output [I&O] sheet). **RATIONALE:** Flushing reduces risk of tube clogging.

- Restart tube feeding at appropriate time.

CHARTING

- Date and time
- Medication and dosage
- Route of administration
- Rationale for PRN and STAT medications
- Client's pre- and postadministration assessment data (if indicated)

- Reason for client's refusal or nurse's decision not to administer medication
- Volume of liquid used for medication dilution and flushing (if I&O indicated)

SECTION THREE

TOPICAL MEDICATIONS

Topical agents are commonly used for a local effect. Dermal medications (lotions, creams) are applied to rashes, lesions, or burns of the skin for their local anti-inflammatory, anti-infective, or anesthetic effect. Inflamed, abraded, or denuded skin will absorb drugs readily, as will hydrated (as opposed to dry) skin.

Some medications are specifically formulated to be applied (via adhesive patch or disc) for slow absorption through the skin (transdermally) to gain access to the circulation for a systemic effect. Such systems allow drugs to be delivered at constant rates over days, months, or even years. The advantage is that much less drug is lost to metabolism in the GI tract or liver before it reaches the bloodstream.

Ophthalmic (eye) medications are administered for infections and inflammatory processes as well as for glaucoma and for diagnostic purposes. Topically applied eye medications are used most often for their local effects; unwanted systemic effects are possible, however, if the ophthalmic drops drain through the tear duct and enter the systemic circulation via nasal mucosal absorption. Such absorption is not subjected to hepatic first-pass metabolism.

Otic (ear) medications usually come in liquid form and are administered locally (topically) to treat conditions of the external ear. If the condition is not relieved by externally applied agents, systemic drugs may be necessary.

While most nasal drops are administered for a local effect (e.g., antihistamine), some applications are given for a systemic effect (e.g., antidiuretic hormone). Since nasal mucous membranes absorb drugs readily, an intended local effect sometimes may result in systemic toxicity. It is essential that the nurse understand the purpose of the drug being administered as well as the rationale for the particular drug delivery system.

RATIONALE

- To apply agent that stops, slows, or prevents growth of microorganisms
- To reduce inflammation/congestion or itching
- To provide local analgesia or anesthesia
- To provide appropriate surface for drug absorption
- To prevent or relieve anginal attacks
- To decrease intraocular pressure
- To prepare for diagnostic or therapeutic procedures

ASSESSMENT

- Assess that selected area for application (e.g., chest, buttocks, or extremity) is consistent with manufacturer's recommendation.
- Check that area for application is clean, dry, hairless, and intact.
- Assess status of area being treated (e.g., rash, character and amount of any drainage).
- Assess client's subjective rating of discomfort.
- Assess potential systemic effect if medication intended for topical effect is absorbed.

TRANSDERMAL MEDICATIONS

Equipment

- Medication tube or patch
- Premeasured paper for paste
- Clear plastic wrap, if indicated
- Tape (if indicated)
- Pen for labeling dressing or patch
- Clean gloves

Preparation

① Locate and remove previous medication patch prior to applying new dose. **RATIONALE:** This prevents inadvertent overdosage.

- Dispose of used patch paper in biohazard box. **RATIONALE:** This protects others from exposure to medication.
- Cleanse selected site if indicated. **RATIONALE:** To promote adherence and absorption.
- Clip hair if necessary, but do not shave. **RATIONALE:** Shaving can cause microabrasions that facilitate growth of microorganisms.

SKILL

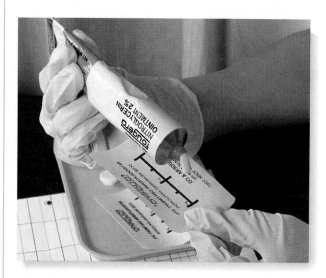

① Place prescribed medication directly on measuring paper (e.g., ½ to 1-in strip). **RATIONALE:** Gloves protect nurse's hand from absorbing medication.

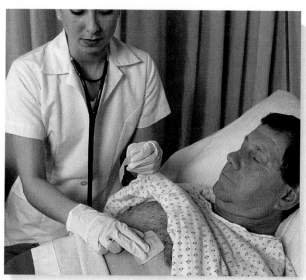

② Apply medicated paper to clean, dry, hairless, intact skin. (Manufacturer may specify site for application.) Alternate application sites with each dose of medication. **RATIONALE:** To prevent skin irritation.

- Use paper to spread medication paste over a 2-in area, and secure paper over medication with tape if necessary, or cover medication area with plastic wrap and tape. **RATIONALE:** To prevent loss of medication.

CLINICAL NOTE

Manufacturers' directions for application of transdermal agents differ significantly. Body temperature and blood flow to different regions influence the suggested application site. Always adhere to the manufacturer's specific guidelines and precautions when administering these systems.

Transdermal Patch

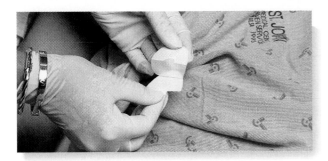

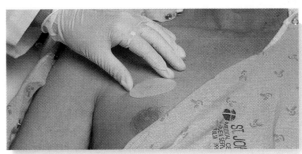

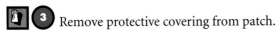 ③ Remove protective covering from patch.

④ Apply patch immediately after removing protective cover. Label patch with date, time, and your initials. **RATIONALE:** This documents drug application, and, since many patches are flesh colored, makes patch easy to find for removal before next application.

BEYOND THE SKILL

Dermal Medications

Equipment

- Medication container
- Gauze pads for cleansing
- Sterile tongue blade
- Appropriate dressing (if indicated)
- Pen for labeling dressing
- Clean gloves for intact skin
- Sterile gloves for lesions or burns

SAFETY ALERT

Wear sterile gloves when applying topical medication to open lesions such as burns.

1. Cleanse skin surface with soap and water unless contraindicated by client's condition. **RATIONALE:** This prepares site for drug absorption.
2. Dry thoroughly. **RATIONALE:** Wet skin enhances drug absorption and possible systemic effects. Systemic absorption of topical agents from open lesions can result in toxic effects.
3. Squeeze medication from tube, or, using tongue blade, take ointment/cream out of jar.
4. Using tongue blade, spread small, smooth, thin quantity of medication evenly over client's skin surface following direction of hair follicles; or, with gloved fingers, gently pat area to facilitate smooth application of ointment. **RATIONALE:** Softened medication applied with fingers ensures even distribution.

5. Protect skin surface with a sterile dressing, unless contraindicated. **RATIONALE:** Dressing ensures that medication does not rub off.
6. Label dressing with date, time, and your initials. **RATIONALE:** This documents application.

OPHTHALMIC DROPS

Equipment

- Prescribed ophthalmic (eye) drops (ocumeter)
- Cotton ball or tissues
- Clean gloves

Preparation

 Tilt client's head slightly backward. Give tissue to client for wiping off excess medication and ask client to look up. **RATIONALE:** The cornea is protected as client looks up.

- Uncap ocumeter and place cap on its side. **RATIONALE:** This prevents contamination of cap.

SKILL

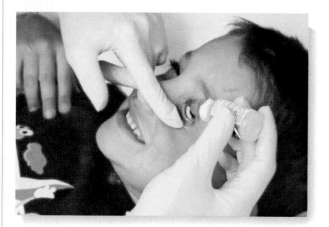

① Place ocumeter ½ to ¾ inch above eyeball with dominant hand. **RATIONALE:** This position reduces risk of dropper touching eyeball and causing injury.

- Stabilize hand holding ocumeter as necessary. Place nondominant hand on cheekbone and hand holding ocumeter on top. **RATIONALE:** This helps immobilize site.
- Expose lower conjunctival sac by pulling down on cheek. **RATIONALE:** To create a "cup" to receive drops.
- Without touching client's lids or lashes, drop prescribed number of drops into center of conjunctival sac. **RATIONALE:** Placing medication directly on cornea could cause injury to cornea.

SAFETY ALERT

When administering eyedrops, avoid potential unwanted systemic side effects by pressing the inner canthus for 2 min to prevent rapid drug absorption. Beta-adrenergic antagonists used to treat glaucoma can cause serious bradycardia if absorbed systemically.

OPHTHALMIC OINTMENTS

Equipment

- Prescribed ophthalmic ointment
- Tissues
- Clean gloves

SKILL

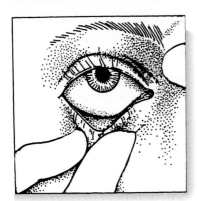

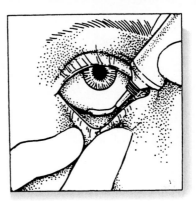

1 Expose lower conjunctival sac by pulling down on cheek. **RATIONALE:** This creates a trough for medication application.

2 Place tube tip ½ to ¾ inch above eyeball with dominant hand. Without touching client's lids or lashes, squeeze ribbon of ointment along the middle third of the inside edge of the lower lid. **RATIONALE:** This allows for twisting of tube to cut ointment ribbon.

- Ask client to close eyelids gently and move eyes. Very gently massage closed lid for client who cannot cooperate (e.g., comatose client). **RATIONALE:** This distributes medication over conjunctival surface.

OTIC MEDICATIONS

Equipment

- Prescribed otic (ear) drops
- Dropper

SKILL

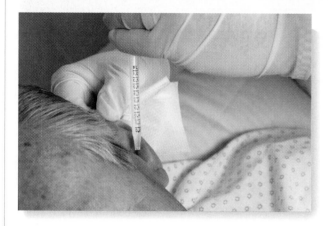

① Prepare client for instillation of ear medication by positioning on side, with ear to be treated uppermost, as follows:

- Warm medication bottle in your hand to body temperature. Fill medication dropper with prescribed amount of medication. **RATIONALE:** Instillation of cold medication can cause nausea or vertigo.

- Infant: Draw earlobe gently downward and backward. **RATIONALE:** This separates drum membrane from floor of cartilaginous canal.

- Adult: Lift auricle upward and backward. **RATIONALE:** This position straightens the ear canal.

- Instill medication drops, holding dropper slightly above ear. **RATIONALE:** This position protects dropper from contamination.

- Instruct client to remain on side for 5 to 10 min following instillation. **RATIONALE:** Prevents medication from escaping and facilitates distribution.

NASAL MEDICATIONS

Equipment

- Prescribed medication
- Dropper
- Tissue

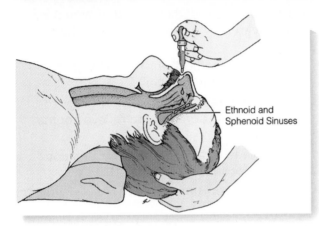

Ethnoid and
Sphenoid Sinuses

1 Fill dropper with prescribed amount of medication and instruct client to tilt head back. **RATIONALE:** Facilitates medication reaching sinuses.

- Place dropper just inside naris and instill correct medication dosage.
- Repeat skill in other naris.
- Wipe away any excess medication with tissue.
- Instruct client not to sneeze or blow nose and to keep head tilted back for 5 min. **RATIONALE:** This prevents medication from escaping.

- Date and time
- Medication and dosage
- Route of administration
- Rationale for PRN and STAT medication

- Client's pre- and postadministration assessment data (e.g., vital signs, client's description of discomfort, condition of site)

MUCOSAL MEDICATIONS

Mucosal medications may be administered for their local (topical) effect or for systemic (transmucosal) action. The mucosa of the lungs, mouth, nose, rectum, and vagina are readily available, and provide an abundance of blood vessels that promote direct entry of medications into the systemic circulation. Mucosal absorption helps ensure that the drug reaches the bloodstream before it is lost to metabolism in the GI tract or liver.

Sublingual (under the tongue) medications are absorbed rapidly and completely due to the vast network of capillaries in that area. This route is desirable for certain medications that are inactivated by first-pass metabolism when given orally (e.g., nitroglycerin).

Metered dose inhalers (MDIs) are designed to convert premeasured medication doses into mist for inhalation. This route is preferred for local treatment of a variety of pulmonary disorders and has the advantages of rapid onset of action, effectiveness of low doses, and fewer side effects compared with systemic administration. Bronchodilators and corticosteroids are frequently administered by this route. Some aerosolized drugs are being developed for the purpose of being absorbed transmucosally to achieve a systemic effect (e.g., insulin, morphine).

Nebulizers are frequently used for delivering bronchodilators to acutely ill clients who are confused, disoriented, extremely fatigued, very dyspneic, or unable to use an MDI. These units are less portable, more difficult to clean, and more expensive than MDIs. Drug delivery is slower and the dose delivered to the lungs is less predictable due to incomplete drug nebulization and dose loss to the environment during exhalation.

Suppositories are cone-shaped masses of solid medicated substance for introduction into the rectum or vagina either for a local or systemic effect. They are usually refrigerated and, when administered, melt at body temperature for slow absorption. Preferably these agents are administered at bedtime for retention and absorption.

The nurse must understand the rationale for both the drug being administered and the particular drug delivery system, as well as the desired therapeutic outcome for the individual client.

RATIONALE

- To provide sustained drug action over time
- To administer medications that would be inactivated by gastric secretions if taken orally
- To protect medications from first-pass metabolism by the liver
- To provide rapid absorption of drugs for immediate action (e.g., to relieve angina pectoris)
- To provide local therapy to airways and reduce systemic side effects
- To induce sputum production for diagnostic purposes
- To provide alternate route for medication administration when client is NPO (e.g., therapeutic procedure, diagnostic test, nausea, vomiting, comatose)
- To provide local anti-infective, anti-inflammatory, laxative, or contraceptive effects

ASSESSMENT

- Assess client symptoms substantiating need for emergency medication (e.g., vital signs, description of discomfort).
- Make sure client's blood pressure is 90 systolic or greater before administration (for nitroglycerine).
- Assess that client is able to cooperate with sublingual administration.
- Assess client's ability to activate MDI during inspiration.
- Check interval since client's last bowel movement (for administration of suppository).
- Assess character and amount of drainage or signs of inflammation in perineal area (before administering suppositories).

SUBLINGUAL MEDICATIONS

Equipment

- Prescribed tablet
- Stethoscope and sphygmomanometer (if indicated)

Preparation

1 Assess preadministration vital signs. Rapid-acting nitroglycerin, especially with repeated doses, can lower blood pressure due to its vasodilating effects.

SKILL

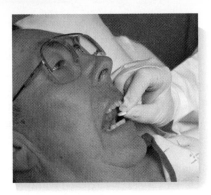

 1 Place or have client place medication under tongue. Explain that client should not swallow drug or eat, smoke, or drink until medication is completely absorbed. **RATIONALE:** The sublingual site is rich in capillaries for drug absorption. Eating, smoking, and drinking interfere with absorption.

- Evaluate client for desired drug action including relief of angina pectoris as well as possible side effects such as hypotension or headache.

SAFETY ALERT

Sublingual medications such as nitroglycerin can be administered to nonresponsive clients. These medications dissolve rapidly and quickly with minimal risk of aspiration.

METERED DOSE INHALER

Equipment

- Prescribed medication canister
- Metered dose inhaler (MDI) dispenser
- Tissues

SKILL

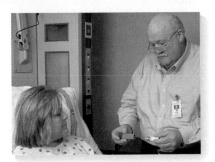

1 Insert medication canister (stem down) into longer part of metered dose dispenser.

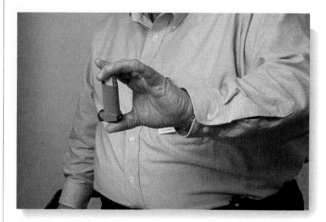

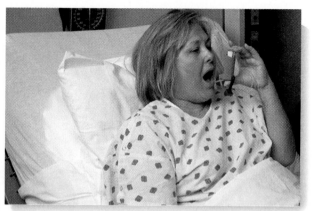

2 Hold canister upright and shake to mix medication with propellant before each MDI puff. **RATIONALE:** If propellant is not shaken, little or no medication will be delivered.

3 Instruct client to remove mouthpiece and hold inhaler 2 inches away from mouth (follow manufacturer's instruction). Client should be sitting or standing. **RATIONALE:** When inhaler is held in mouth, medication droplets are swallowed rather than mist being inhaled into airways.

- Instruct client to exhale through pursed lips. **RATIONALE:** This increases exhaled volume, allowing room for a greater inspiratory volume.
- Instruct client to depress inhalation device, releasing a puff of medication, while inhaling slowly (3 to 5 sec) and deeply through mouth. **RATIONALE:** With deep, slow inhalation, medication goes to lower respiratory tract.
- Instruct client to hold breath for 10 sec and slowly exhale through pursed lips. **RATIONALE:** Holding the breath allows time for the medication to be absorbed.
- Provide tissues. **RATIONALE:** Inhaled medication may stimulate coughing.

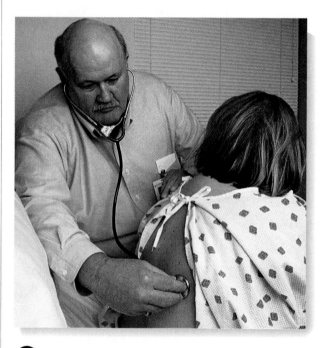

4 Assess client for subjective and objective improvement in breathing or possible adverse cardiac reaction to medication. **RATIONALE:** Bronchodilators can cause tachycardia or other dysrhythmias.

- Instruct client to wait 2 min between puffs if more than one puff is ordered and to shake canister before each puff. **RATIONALE:** Waiting between doses helps prevent paradoxical bronchospasm.
- Remove drug canister and clean mouthpiece daily, washing with soap and water and allowing to air dry. **RATIONALE:** To prevent microbial growth.

CLINICAL NOTE

- The size of the aerosol particle and the client's breathing pattern, age, and airway anatomy all influence the amount of inhaled drug that reaches the lung. Slow inspiratory flow rates and larger tidal volumes improve drug delivery to the lung. Holding inspiration for several seconds provides opportunity for deposition of inhaled drug.
- In contrast to liquid inhalers, dry powder inhalers are administered with the client's neck hyperextended. The client's lips are placed around the mouthpiece of the dispenser and inspiration is quick and deep.

MDI WITH SPACER

Equipment

- Prescribed medication canister
- Metered dose inhaler dispenser
- Spacer (aerosol chamber)
- Tissues

SKILL

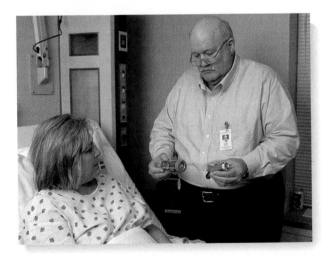

1 Assemble medication canister in MDI as in previous skill. Insert metered dose inhaler (MDI) mouthpiece into spacer.

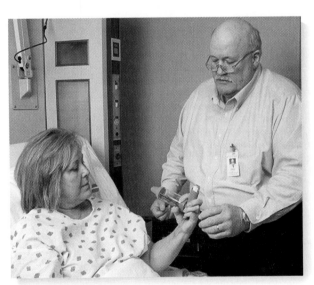

2 Holding upright, shake MDI and spacer unit. **RATIONALE:** Shaking mixes medication and propellant.

- Instruct client to exhale slowly through pursed lips. **RATIONALE:** This promotes a greater inspiratory volume.

CLINICAL NOTE

ASSESSING FLUID LEVEL IN MEDICATION CANISTER

Canister Level	Position in Water
Full	Sinks flat to bottom
Three-quarters full	Sinks to bottom; stands upright
Half full	Floats upright to top
One-quarter full	Floats to top at an angle
Empty	Floats flat to top

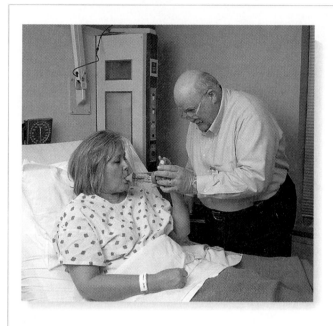

3 Remove mouthpiece cover from spacer.

- Instruct client to close lips around spacer mouthpiece.
- Activate MDI canister, pressing down with fingers to push it further into plastic adapter. **RATIONALE:** This releases metered dose of medication into spacer.
- After activation, instruct client to inhale slowly and deeply through mouth and hold breath 10 sec. **RATIONALE:** Spacer suspends medication momentarily, eliminating need for simultaneous activation of MDI on inhalation.
- Remove drug canister and clean mouthpiece and spacer daily, washing with soap and water and allowing to air dry. **RATIONALE:** This prevents microbial growth.

NEBULIZED AEROSOLS

Equipment

- Nebulizer aerosol (NPA) medication chamber
- T-piece, mouthpiece and corrugated tubing, or aerosol mask
- Air flow tubing
- Prescribed medication (e.g., bronchodilator)
- Prescribed diluent (normal saline)
- Wall or other source for compressed air or oxygen with flowmeter

SAFETY ALERT

Exhaled aerosols present a risk of second-hand exposure to airborne pathogens and medications. Gram-negative bacilli, particularly *Pseudomonas aeruginosa*, commonly contaminate arerosol solutions. One-way valves and filters in the expiratory limb of the nebulizer apparatus can reduce or eliminate this risk.

SKILL

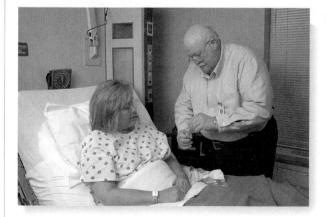

1 Dilute medication as ordered and place in nebulizer chamber.

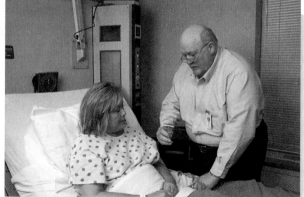

2 Keeping nebulizer vertical, connect top of nebulizer chamber to aerosol mask or to T-piece side arm.

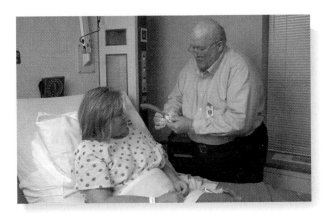

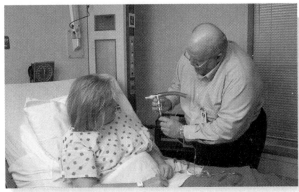

3 Attach corrugated tubing to one end of T-piece. Holding mouthpiece in its protective cover, attach mouthpiece to other end of T-piece.

4 Attach one end of air flow tubing to nozzle at side or bottom of nebulizer.

CLINICAL NOTE

If the client is receiving 3 L/min or less of oxygen therapy, deliver aerosolized medications with compressed air (yellow wall outlet). If the client is receiving 4 L/min or more of oxygen therapy, deliver the aerosol medication with the oxygen flowmeter (green wall outlet) set at 8 L/min.

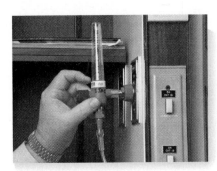

5 Attach other end of tubing to compressed air source. Turn on driving air or oxygen (8 L/min) source, and observe for mist generation.

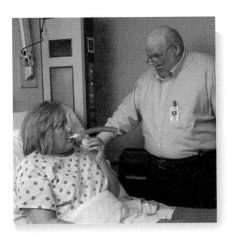

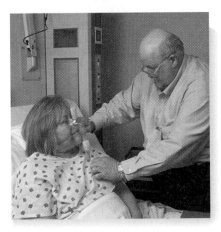

6 Instruct client to breathe normally in and out of mouthpiece or mask.

- Discontinue treatment when aerosol is no longer being produced.

- Turn power (air or oxygen flow) off, and unplug compressor (if used), or reset prescribed oxygen flow rate.

- Clean mouthpiece and place equipment in plastic bag at bedside. Rinse with sterile water every 24 hrs. Dispose of and replace components according to agency policy.

RECTAL SUPPOSITORIES

Equipment

- Prescribed suppository
- Water-soluble lubricant (K-Y Jelly)
- Paper towel
- Clean gloves

SKILL

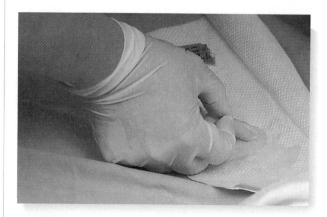

① Squeeze dollop of lubricant onto paper towel.
RATIONALE: Using lubricant or placing suppository in warm water to soften facilitates administration.

- Remove foil wrapper from suppository.
- Moisten suppository tip with warm water or lubricant.

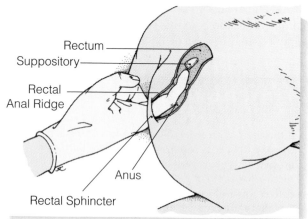

Rectum
Suppository
Rectal
Anal Ridge
Anus
Rectal Sphincter

② Place client in Sims' position (lying on left side with top leg flexed).

- Instruct client to bear down in order to identify anal opening and insert suppository into rectal canal beyond anal sphincter (approximately 4 cm).
RATIONALE: Prevents suppository from slipping out.
- Instruct client to lie quietly for 15 min.
RATIONALE: This promotes drug absorption.

VAGINAL SUPPOSITORIES

Equipment

- Prescribed suppository
- Vaginal suppository applicator (kept at client's bedside)

- Clean gloves

SKILL

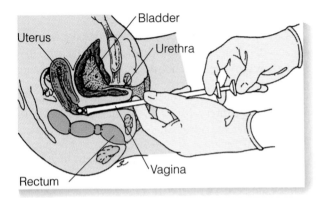

Uterus
Bladder
Urethra
Vagina
Rectum

1 Remove wrapper from suppository and insert into applicator. With client in dorsal recumbent or Sims' position, insert applicator with suppository into vaginal canal at least 2 in. **RATIONALE:** Prevents suppository from slipping out.

- Instruct client to lie quietly until suppository is absorbed. **RATIONALE:** This promotes medication retention and absorption.
- Wash applicator after use and store in protective wrap at client's bedside.

CHARTING

- Date and time
- Medication and dosage
- Route of administration
- Rationale for PRN and STAT medication

- Client's pre- and postadministration assessment data (e.g., client's subjective statements, vital signs, breath sounds, laxative results, condition of site)

CRITICAL THINKING FOCUS

SECTION ONE ▪ Medication Administration

Unexpected Outcomes

- Nurse is unsure of correct answer when calculating drug dose conversion.

- Medication is ordered by trade name and is dispensed in generic form.

- Medication dose on MAR is not consistent with medication dispensed.

- Narcotic count and sign-out sheets do not agree.

- Medication is scheduled on MAR to coincide with meals but it should be taken between meals.

- Medication slows client's heart rate to 56.

- Client states medication looks unfamiliar and asks why a new drug is being given.

Alternative Nursing Actions

- Request that another nurse check calculation or conversion.

- Validate discrepancy with pharmacology text or PDR or consult with pharmacist before administering.

- Validate medication with client's record, original source for medication order.

- Check medication sheets for narcotics signed out to specific clients. Check with another nurse who may have administered narcotics.

- Change MAR times to stagger meals, scheduling same hour intervals (e.g., q4h); next day's MAR should reflect your change.

- Hold medication and recheck vital signs in 30 min. Notify physician if vital signs continue to be unsafe for medication administration.

- Do not give medication (unless it *is* new). Recheck orders before giving, following steps for validation. Clients are usually familiar with their medications, and their questioning may prevent an error.

SECTION TWO ▪ Oral Medications

Unexpected Outcomes

- Client has difficulty swallowing medication and refuses to take orally.

- Client has an adverse reaction to medication.

Alternative Nursing Actions

- Contact pharmacist if in doubt about crushing tablet or opening capsule to administer.

- Stop or withhold medication. Notify physician at once; prepare to administer epinephrine to dilate bronchi and support blood pressure in case of anaphylaxis. If reaction is severe:
  —Keep client flat in bed with head slightly elevated.
  —Take vital signs every 10 to 15 min.
  —Assess for hypotension or respiratory distress.
  —Establish airway, if necessary.
  —Have emergency equipment available.
  —Provide psychologic support to client to alleviate fear.

- Record type and progression of reaction.

■ Client has difficulty swallowing tablet or capsule.	■ Follow steps of skill for crushed or altered tablets or capsules. If client is totally unable to swallow, do not attempt administering by mouth. Ask physician to order same or comparable medication by more appropriate route (e.g., parenteral, rectal).

SECTION THREE ■ Topical Medications

Unexpected Outcomes	**Alternative Nursing Actions**
■ Client has allergic reaction to topical medication.	■ Hold medication; notify physician. Continue to monitor client.
	■ Obtain order for antihistamine if necessary.
■ Transdermal patch does not stay on skin.	■ Cover with plastic wrap or tape in place.
■ Client develops severe bradycardia following administration of beta-adrenergic blocking agent (Timoptic) eyedrops for glaucoma.	■ While administering drops, press inner canthus to prevent medication drainage through tear duct and nasal mucosal absorption of the drug.
■ Client sustains injury shortly after initiation of miotic (pupil-constricting) eyedrops for glaucoma.	■ Inform client that pupil-constricting medications decrease the eyes' ability to accommodate to the dark. Discuss essentials of good lighting and other environmental safety measures.

SECTION FOUR ■ Mucosal Medications

Unexpected Outcomes	**Alternative Nursing Actions**
■ Client is unable to coordinate activation of MDI and inspiration.	■ Order spacer for easier use and more predictable drug delivery.
■ Client develops sore throat and signs of oral candidiasis from taking inhaled steroids.	■ Instruct client to rinse thoroughly after each treatment. Instruct client to clean inhalation equipment daily.
■ Client is unable to retain suppository.	■ Administer vaginal suppository at bedtime.
	■ Instruct client to maintain position for at least 15 min in order to allow absorption to occur.
■ Suppository is not retained.	■ Position client on abdomen, and hold buttocks together.
	■ Notify physician so that alternative route or a different medication can be tried.
	■ Instruct client to maintain appropriate position so that drug is absorbed.
	■ Ensure that suppository has been placed appropriately, 2 to 3 inches beyond internal anal sphincter. Run suppository under cold water to restore rigidity.

SELF-CHECK EVALUATION

PART 1 ▪ Matching Terms

Match the definition in column B with the correct term in column A.

Column A	Column B
a. a.a.	1. With
b. a.c.	2. Three times a day
c. b.i.d.	3. Drop(s)
d. c̄	4. After meals
e. p.c.	5. Of each
f. NPO	6. Twice a day
g. gtt	7. Before meals
h. PO	8. Nothing by mouth
i. t.i.d.	9. At bedtime
j. h.s.	10. By mouth

PART 2 ▪ Multiple Choice Questions

1. The least bioavailable route of medication administration is:

a. Transdermal.
b. Sublingual.
c. Inhaled.
d. Oral.

2. There are four biologic processes of drug utilization. The process in which the drug binds with plasma protein is:

a. Absorption.
b. Transportation.
c. Metabolism.
d. Excretion.

3. Most drugs are metabolized by the:

a. Kidney.
b. Plasma.
c. Liver.
d. Stomach.

4. Drugs are eliminated from the body by the process of:

a. Absorption.
b. Transportation.
c. Metabolism.
d. Excretion.

5. It is important to monitor for drug overdose in the elderly, even if the dosage is within the normal range, because:

a. Their digestive tracts function at a slower rate, and therefore the drug absorption rate is decreased.
b. They have more intracellular fluid than younger clients.
c. They have a lower percentage of fat than younger adults.
d. They often have a decreased serum albumin level.

6. For many medications, oral doses are much higher than parenteral doses because the drug is:

    a. Diluted by gastrointestinal secretions.
    b. Subjected to first-pass metabolism by the liver.
    c. Only partially absorbed in the gastrointestinal tract.
    d. Inactivated by gastric acid pH.

7. Free medication passes into its cellular site of action by:

    a. Unbinding from plasma protein.
    b. The process of osmosis.
    c. The process of active transport.
    d. Binding with plasma protein.

8. The purpose of computerized access systems of medication retrieval is to:

    a. Reduce the amount of time used in drug administration.
    b. Reduce the cost of medication administration.
    c. Control access to drugs and narcotics.
    d. Ensure the right client receives the right medication.

9. Safe measures for medication administration include:

    a. Validating an illegible order with another nurse.
    b. Validating illegible orders with the physician who wrote them.
    c. Crushing any oral medication for ease of administration.
    d. Discarding vaginal suppository applicators after use.

10. When a nurse inadvertently administers the wrong medication to a client:

    a. It is not necessary to record the medication administered unless adverse effects occur.
    b. It is not necessary to notify the client's physician unless adverse effects occur.
    c. It is not necessary to complete an unusual occurrence report unless adverse effects occur.
    d. Documentation, notification, and close monitoring of the client are essential.

11. When administering narcotics, the medication is signed out of the narcotic book:

    a. Before it is taken from the drawer.
    b. After it is taken out of the drawer.
    c. After it has been administered to the client.
    d. After any count discrepancies are corrected.

12. Which of the following actions is consistent with safe medication alteration?

    a. Sprinkling an opened capsule's beads onto food.
    b. Administering PO medication sublingually.
    c. Crushing an enteric-coated tablet for enteral tube administration.
    d. Crushing sublingual formulations.

13. Eardrops are administered to an adult by positioning the pinna:

    a. Up and back.
    b. Down and back.
    c. Up and forward.
    d. Down and forward.

14. Which of the following statements about MDI spacers is true?

    a. They eliminate the need for hand-mouth coordination.
    b. They decrease the amount of drug delivered.
    c. They are appropriate for adult use only.
    d. They reduce the risk of infection.

PART 3 ▪ Critical Thinking Application

Your client has recently suffered a stroke, which has caused him to have difficulty swallowing (dysphagia) and places him at risk for aspiration. When the previous shift nurse attempted to have him take his oral medications with water, he coughed and choked violently, so she discontinued efforts to complete his medication administration. One of this client's most important medications is Inderal LA 80 mg, a timed-release capsule, which is given once a day. This long-acting capsule cannot be opened and its contents emptied for convenient administration without interfering with the timed-release property of its formulation.

1. What types of consult would provide assistance in decision making about this client's swallowing problem and medication administration?
2. What actions would facilitate this client's swallowing and decrease the risk of aspiration?
3. What alternative method is there for administering the Inderal LA?
4. How will the nurse communicate adjustments in administration to the other staff members?

16

PARENTERAL MEDICATIONS

INTRODUCTION

Administration of medication by the parenteral route or injection exposes the body to two foreign objects: the hypodermic needle and the medication being injected. Parenteral administration requires sterile technique, proficiency, and precautions, and therefore, specialized training. Skills presented in this chapter cover the intradermal, subcutaneous, and intramuscular routes. Skillful preparation, accuracy in selection of the injection site, and precision in administration influence the effectiveness of the medication. Faulty technique and misdirected injection can hamper the medication's effectiveness and cause permanent injury to the client. Parenterally administered medications enter the bloodstream readily, have a more rapid onset of action when compared to the oral route, and have a potential for serious local or systemic complications.

The intradermal site is used to determine a client's immune response to a small quantity of injected antigen. Subcutaneous injections are administered into fatty tissue where there are few blood vessels, slowing absorption. The abdominal site offers the quickest absorption, followed by the arm, then the leg. Exercising an extremity will increase the rate of drug absorption. Since muscles are vascular, intramuscular injections are absorbed more rapidly. Intravenous medications are injected directly into the circulation, bypassing all barriers to absorption; therefore effects are immediate.

(continued on next page)

Parenteral medications come in vials, ampules, or cartridges. The medication vial label or ampule has a printed designation of acceptable sites for administration (e.g., IM, subq). Not all medications are appropriate for all injection routes. Some parenteral agents are prepared as powders that require a diluent for administration. The specific diluent indicated for a particular drug is directed on the medication insert or can be found in the *Physician's Desk Reference.*

PREPARATION PROTOCOL: FOR PARENTERAL MEDICATION SKILLS

Complete following steps before each skill.

1. Follow the skill for medication validation (see Chapter 15).
2. Wash hands.
3. Prepare medication according to skills for parenteral route.
4. Take medication to client's room; validate room, bed number, and client's identity (check identaband and have client state name).
5. Check for presence of allergy bracelet.
6. Provide privacy.
7. Inform client of drug name, purpose, and procedure for administration.
8. Assess vital signs or other parameters affected by drug to be given to determine safety for administration.
9. Place client in appropriate position for route of administration.
10. Don clean gloves.
11. Identify injection site, fully exposing it to locate pertinent landmarks (rotate among usable sites that are free of lesions, bruising, or induration).
12. Administer injection according to skill for specific site.

COMPLETION PROTOCOL: FOR PARENTERAL MEDICATION SKILLS

Make sure the following steps have been completed.

1. Quickly withdraw needle. Push safety device (safety glide) to retract needle. If using standard syringe and needle, do *not* recap.
2. Wipe injection site with alcohol swab.
3. Reposition client for comfort.
4. Dispose of needle-syringe unit in puncture-proof hazardous waste receptacle.
5. Remove and dispose of gloves, then wash hands.
6. Document medication on appropriate forms (medication administration record [MAR], client record).

INJECTION PREPARATION

Syringes and needles are available in a variety of sizes; appropriate equipment is selected depending on client factors, medication type, and the desired site of administration. Procedure for some medications (e.g., heparin, insulin) dictates that the nurse select a specific syringe (0.5- to 1-mL capacity). Some medications are prepared in prefilled cartridges that require the use of a special cartridge syringe for administration.

Needles vary in diameter (gauge): The larger the number, the smaller the gauge. Smaller-gauge needles are used for intradermal and subcutaneous injection of aqueous solutions, while larger gauges are used for more viscous medications. Needle lengths vary as well; longer ones are used for deep penetration to inject medication into muscle.

Nurses must be aware of potential danger to themselves when handling and disposing of biohazardous parenteral equipment, and should urge their employers to provide the safest possible equipment available. According to the Occupational Safety and Health Administration (OSHA), 800,000 health care workers are stuck by contaminated needles every year. Several states have passed legislation mandating the use of needles and other sharps with integrated safety features. A bill to protect health care workers was signed into law in November 2000. It will advocate that safe medical devices (retractable needles and devices that automatically cover the tips of used needles) be used in all health care settings.

RATIONALE

- To achieve rapid onset of drug action
- To ensure adequate drug absorption and predictable results
- To provide medication to clients who are NPO
- To prepare medication for injection using sterile technique

ASSESSMENT

- Check type and volume of medication ordered.
- Assess appropriate site for administering medication.
- Check that total volume to be administered is close to capacity of selected syringe.
- Check that needle length and gauge are appropriate for client's size and selected site for injection.

SAFETY ALERT

Parenteral equipment is most frequently associated with transmission of bloodborne pathogens. Protected needle systems should be used to protect against injury. In addition, all devices and equipment designed to prevent blood exposures must be monitored for continued safety.

WITHDRAWING MEDICATION FROM A VIAL

Equipment

- Medication in vial
- Syringe of closest capacity to hold medication
- Appropriate size needle

SAFETY ALERT

If multiple-use vials are opened, they should be marked with the date and time the container is entered. Consult the product label or package insert to determine if refrigeration is necessary. Unless contamination is suspected, the Centers for Disease Control (CDC) recommends that the vial be discarded either when empty or on the expiration date set by the manufacturer.

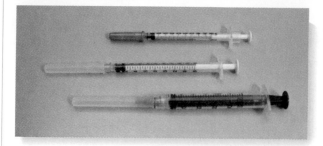

SKILL

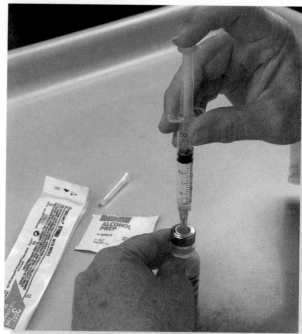

① Select appropriate syringe size: Capacity should closely accommodate volume to be administered. **RATIONALE:** This facilitates handling and accuracy in preparation.

- Assemble syringe and needle, maintaining sterility. **RATIONALE:** Infection/abscess may occur if equipment becomes contaminated.
- Remove vial cap and cleanse rubber top of vial with alcohol swab. **RATIONALE:** Manufacturer does not guarantee sterility of rubber top.
- Remove needle guard. Pull back on plunger of syringe to fill with an amount of air equal to amount of solution to be withdrawn. **RATIONALE:** Displacement of solution with air is necessary to prevent formation of a vacuum in the sealed vial.

② Insert needle into upright vial and inject air into vacant area of vial, keeping needle bevel above surface of medication. **RATIONALE:** If air is injected into the medication, bubbles may form, making drug withdrawal more difficult. Air creates positive pressure in the vial, allowing withdrawal of medication.

③ Invert vial and pull on plunger tip to extract desired amount of medication. Expel any air from syringe at this time, tapping side of syringe below air bubble. **RATIONALE:** Tapping below bubble makes it rise to needle hub area. Expelling air facilitates validation of dose withdrawn.

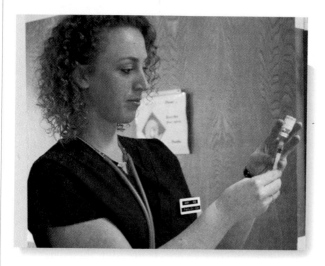

- Recheck amount of medication in syringe; turn vial upright and remove needle.
- Replace needle guard using the scoop method. **RATIONALE:** The scoop method is not necessary when recapping a sterile needle, but encourages development of a safe habit.
- Recheck medication label and dosage against medication record and any dose calculation. **RATIONALE:** This is another safety check.
- Dispose of or replace equipment appropriately. **RATIONALE:** Glass, needles, and syringes are disposed of in biohazard puncture-resistant containers to prevent injury.

WITHDRAWING MEDICATION FROM AN AMPULE

Equipment

- Medication in ampule
- Syringe of closest capacity to hold medication

SKILL

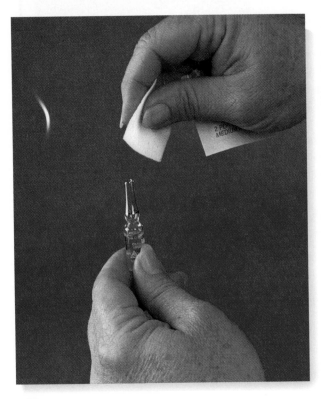

1 Tap stem of ampule, or, holding stem tip, briskly flick wrist to move all medication to ampule base.

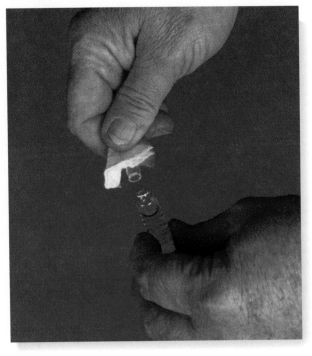

2 Using alcohol swab or dry gauze square, grasp and snap off stem of ampule, breaking away from you. **RATIONALE:** Directing movement of sharp object away from body prevents injury.

3 Remove syringe needle guard and insert needle into ampule without touching side of ampule neck. **RATIONALE:** Avoid touching sides to prevent contamination of needle.

- If needle is long enough, withdraw appropriate amount of medication. Tilt or invert ampule if needle is short. Then return ampule to upright position and remove syringe.

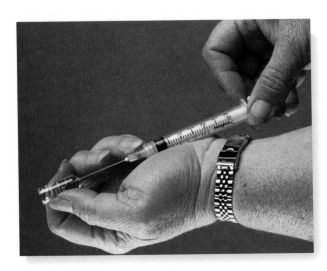

BEYOND THE SKILL

Preparing a Prefilled Cartridge Syringe

Equipment

- Prefilled medication cartridge-needle unit
- Cartridge syringe (e.g., Carpuject or Tubex)

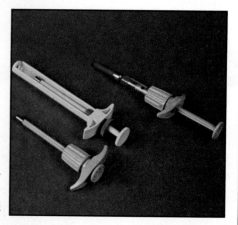

Skill

1. Insert prefilled medication cartridge-needle unit into cartridge syringe barrel, twisting syringe flange clockwise until it is secure. Screw plunger rod onto screw at bottom of medication cartridge. Remove needle guard and express air bubbles if indicated.

2. Check amount of solution in medication cartridge to determine if dosage is greater than required amount; if so, invert syringe and gently expel excess medication. Be especially careful to maintain sterility of needle. **RATIONALE:** If permanent needle is contaminated, cartridge becomes contaminated and must be discarded.

   - Replace needle guard using the one-hand scoop method.

MEDICATIONS COMBINED IN ONE SYRINGE

Equipment

- Vials of medications that are compatible when mixed together

- Syringe with capacity for total volume of the two medications
- Alcohol swabs

SKILL

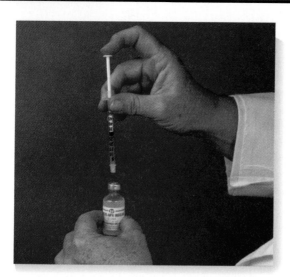

1 Follow skill for withdrawing medication from a vial, *with the following alterations:* (a) Swab top of first vial, (b) swab top of second vial. Inject displacement air into first vial.

CLINICAL NOTE

When combining medications in one syringe using vial and ampule, follow these steps:

■ Using syringe you will use for administration, follow skill for withdrawing medication from a vial (see page 453).

■ If using entire contents of ampule, use same syringe to withdraw ampule medication.

■ For partial dose of ampule contents, use unit dose syringe and follow skill for withdrawing medication from an ampule (see page 455). Drawing ampule medication into unit dose syringe ensures accuracy of dosage.

■ Remove needle from prepared syringe.

■ Pull air into syringe to accommodate medication from unit dose syringe.

■ Carefully insert needle of prepared unit dose syringe into needle hub of large syringe and inject medication into syringe.

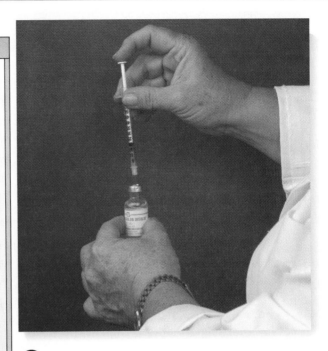

2 Inject displacement air into second vial (do not withdraw needle).

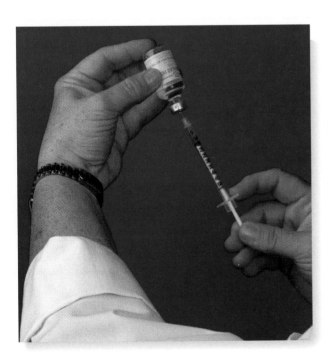

3 Withdraw desired amount of medication from second vial.

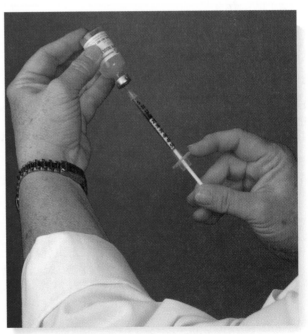

4 Carefully withdraw desired amount of medication from first vial.

SECTION TWO

INTRADERMAL INJECTIONS

The intradermal route, just under the top layers of the skin, is used to inject a very small (e.g., 0.1 mL) volume of a substance (antigen) to elicit a client's immune or sensitivity response. The inner aspect of the forearm is typically used for this type of testing. Alternate sites include the upper arm, upper chest, and shoulder blade areas. The client's reaction to the substance indicating immune or allergic response is monitored at the injection site (e.g., noting induration indicating immune response to tuberculin PPD).

Many agencies also use the intradermal route to administer a local anesthetic prior to a venipuncture procedure.

RATIONALE

- To determine cellular immune response to common antigens
- To diagnose exposure to the tuberculosis microorganism
- To detect possible carriers of tuberculosis
- To anesthetize site prior to venipuncture

ASSESSMENT

- Assess for previous exposure to tuberculosis, previous positive skin test, or previous BCG vaccination (PPD is contraindicated in these situations).
- Assess that site is free of dermatitis.
- Assess that skin is dry at planned injection site.
- Assess that client is not allergic to local anesthetic (e.g., lidocaine).

INTRADERMAL INJECTIONS

Equipment

- Unit dose (1 mL) tuberculin syringe with ¼-in to ⅝-in-long needle (small 25 to 27 gauge)
- Medication (e.g., 0.1 mL Purified Protein Derivative antigen)
- Alcohol swabs
- Dry gauze square
- Pen to mark injection site for identification
- Clean gloves

SAFETY ALERT

For tuberculin testing, instruct client to return and have the site checked by the health care provider in 48 to 72 hrs.

Preparation

✋ ① Select lesion-free injection site on hairless undersurface, upper third of forearm (for skin testing) or site selected for venipuncture. Use alcohol swab to cleanse area with circular motion, moving from inside outward, and allow alcohol to dry. **RATIONALE:** Cleanse from selected site outward to prevent contamination from periphery.

- Remove needle guard.
- Grasp client's outer forearm to gently pull skin tight on undersurface for skin testing.

SKILL

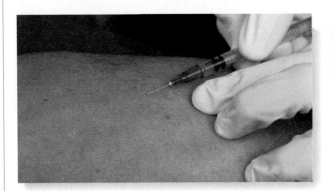

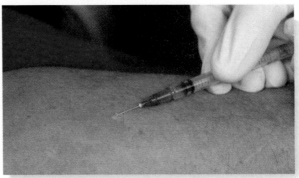

① Hold syringe almost parallel to skin and, with bevel facing up, insert needle tip (about ⅛ in). **RATIONALE:** Bevel up facilitates visualization of injected substance.

- Do *not* aspirate. **RATIONALE:** There is no risk of intravascular injection with correct intradermal technique.

② Slowly inject medication, observing for wheal (blister) formation and blanching at site. **RATIONALE:** Wheal formation indicates proper injection. If no wheal develops, injection was given too deeply.

- Withdraw needle at same angle as inserted. Do *not* recap.
- Pat site with dry gauze. Do *not* massage area. **RATIONALE:** Massage could disperse medication.

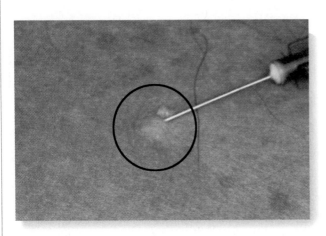

③ Use pen to mark injection site for future assessment; if more than one test is being performed, number injection site and record number and corresponding antigen in client's record.

CHARTING

- Date and time
- Medication and dosage
- Route of administration

- Site of administration
- Client teaching for follow-up evaluation of skin test

SECTION THREE

SUBCUTANEOUS INJECTIONS

Subcutaneous injections are administered into fatty tissue under the skin, where there are few blood vessels and nerves. This site can be used only for medications that are not irritating to tissue. Drug absorption is slower than when administered into muscle.

The most common sites used are the outer surface of the upper arm, the anterior thigh, and the abdomen (avoiding the area 1½ inches around umbilicus). Alternate sites include the ventrodorsal gluteal area and scapular areas of the upper back. Typically a small amount (less than 2 mL) of medication is injected.

RATIONALE

- To deliver a small volume of a nonirritating agent to be absorbed slowly
- To avoid hematoma formation

ASSESSMENT

- Check that the drug to be administered is nonirritating.
- Check that the volume of drug to be administered is less than 2 mL.
- Check results of laboratory tests (e.g., PTT or blood glucose) for specific medications.

SUBCUTANEOUS INJECTIONS

Equipment

- Syringe (3 mL) with ⅝-in needle (25 to 29 gauge)
- Medication vial or ampule
- Alcohol swabs
- Clean gloves

SAFETY ALERT

Irritating medications such as Vistaril must not be administered subcutaneously, as a sterile abscess or tissue necrosis may result. Such medications should be administered by another route.

SKILL

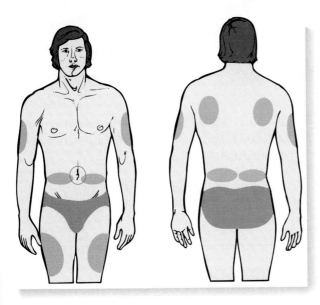

1 Select site for injection, alternating sites for each injection. **RATIONALE:** This prevents repeated trauma to tissue.

- Avoid area around umbilicus (inside red circle).

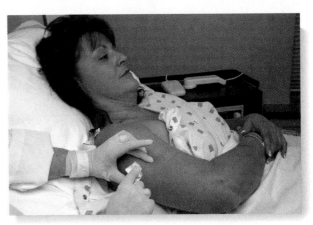

2 With selected site fully exposed, cleanse area with alcohol swab using circular motion moving from inside outward. Allow alcohol to dry. **RATIONALE:** This prevents alcohol from tracking into tissue with injection.

- Remove needle guard.

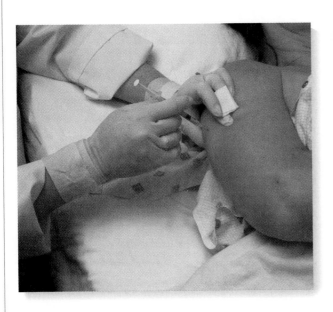

3 Use thumb and forefinger to gently grasp subcutaneous tissue ("pinch an inch") on posterior-lateral aspect, mid-upper arm (or other appropriate site). Holding syringe like a dart or between thumb and forefinger, insert needle at 45° or 90° angle. **RATIONALE:** Angle varies with amount of subcutaneous tissue, selected site, and needle length.

- Hold syringe barrel with dominant hand, and, with same hand, aspirate by pulling back on plunger. If no blood appears, administer injection. If blood appears, withdraw syringe, discard, and prepare new injection. **RATIONALE:** Blood indicates needle has entered a blood vessel. Injecting drug may be dangerous.

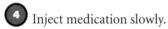

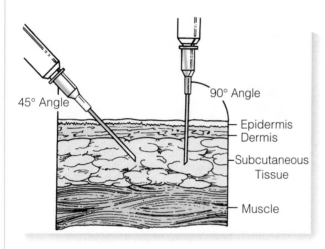

45° Angle

90° Angle

Epidermis
Dermis

Subcutaneous
Tissue

Muscle

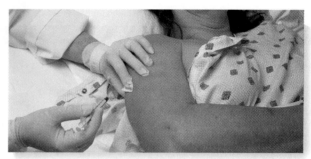

4 Inject medication slowly.

5 Wait 10 sec, then withdraw needle quickly. Do *not* recap. **RATIONALE:** Waiting before withdrawing needle prevents medication leakage.

■ Release tissue and gently massage injection site with alcohol swab. **RATIONALE:** Massaging area aids absorption.

HEPARIN INJECTIONS

Equipment

■ Unit dose syringe with small needle (25 to 29 gauge) or prefilled syringe
■ Heparin vial
■ Alcohol swabs
■ Clean gloves

SKILL

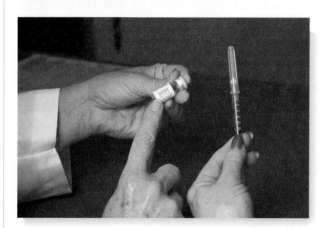

1 Double-check heparin vial label and prepared dose with another nurse before administration. **RATIONALE:** This safeguard helps prevent errors.

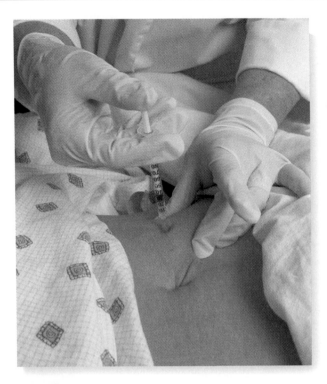

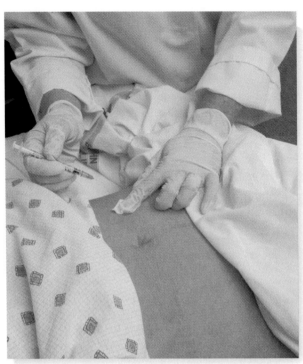

 2 Place client in supine position. **RATIONALE:** This facilitates site selection.

- Using abdomen or area above iliac crests, gently pinch up a fold of fat between thumb and finger. **RATIONALE:** Extremities must be avoided to prevent inadvertent intramuscular deposition of the drug and hematoma formation.
- Holding fat fold throughout injection, introduce full length of needle and inject heparin. Do not aspirate before injecting heparin. **RATIONALE:** To reduce risk of hematoma formation.

3 Quickly withdraw needle and hold alcohol swab to site, but *do not* massage area after withdrawing needle. **RATIONALE:** To prevent hematoma formation.

SAFETY ALERT

Do not aspirate or massage heparin or low-molecular-weight heparin (Lovenox) injections, as these actions may cause tissue damage and bruising.

INSULIN INJECTIONS

Equipment

- Insulin syringe that most closely accommodates prescribed number of units (50 or 100 U/mL capacity)
- Small gauge needle (25 to 29 gauge)

- Prescribed insulin(s) vial(s)
- Alcohol swabs
- Clean gloves

CLINICAL NOTE

- Insulin is administered to facilitate glucose transport into cells, where it is used as energy. Additional insulin is required by all clients with Type 1 diabetes and some clients with Type 2 diabetes. Since insulin lowers blood sugar, it is essential to obtain blood glucose levels before administration, and to monitor blood glucose levels periodically. A form of fast-acting carbohydrate should always be available to treat hypoglycemia.
- Many clients receive a mixed regimen of short-acting regular insulin (clear solution) and intermediate-acting insulin (cloudy solution). The cloudy solution bottle is rolled between the palms before preparation to achieve uniform suspension.
- When mixing two preparations of insulin, follow the skill for medications combined in one syringe (page 456). Draw up the regular insulin (clear solution), and then draw up the intermediate-acting insulin (cloudy solution). This prevents contamination of unused regular insulin with another insulin that can affect its action.

SKILL

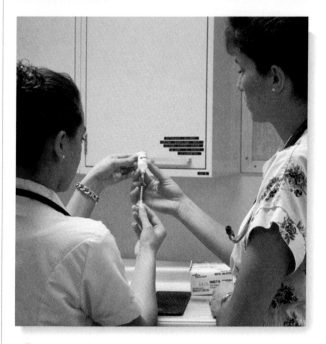

 SAFETY ALERT

In-use vials of insulin should not be refrigerated because cold insulin causes local irritation at the injection site. Open, unrefrigerated vials should be discarded after 1 month.

1 Validate type of insulin and prepared dosage with another nurse. **RATIONALE:** This safeguard helps prevent errors in preparation.

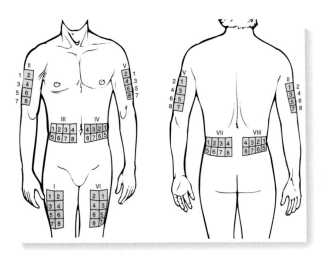

2 Avoid overuse of injection sites and dramatic changes in daily insulin absorption by selecting injection site spaced 1 inch from previous injection; systematically rotate within a body area before moving to another body part. **RATIONALE:** Tissue damage and erratic absorption occur with repeated use of same injection site.

- Inject insulin into abdominal area. **RATIONALE:** Absorption is quickest and most reliable in the abdomen, and this area is preferred for consistent control.

- Do not aspirate following injection or massage after withdrawing needle. **RATIONALE:** Massaging hastens drug absorption.

TABLE 16-1	INSULIN TYPES AND THERAPEUTIC ACTION				
Types	**Source**	**Onset**	**Peak**	**Duration**
Rapid-acting				
Humalog (Lispro)	Human	5–15 min	0.5–1.5 hrs	3–5 hrs
Short-acting				
Iletin IIR	Pork (purified)	0.5–1 hr	2–4 hrs	6–8 hrs
Novolin R	Human			
Humulin R	Human			
Velosulin BR	Human (buffered insulin for insulin pumps)			
Intermediate-acting				
Iletin II N	Pork (purified)	1–2 hrs	4–12 hrs	12–18 hrs
Humulin N	Human			
NPH*	Pork (purified)			
Novolin N	Human			
Mixtures of NPH/regular				
Humulin 70/30	Human (70% NPH, 30% regular)			
Novolin 70/30	Human (70% NPH, 30% regular)			
Humulin 50/50	Human (50% NPH, 50% regular)			
Iletin II L	Pork (purified)	2 hrs	8–12 hrs	12–16 hrs
Humulin L	Human			
Novolin L	Human			
Long-acting				
Humulin Ultralente	Human	8 hrs	18 hrs	24–36 hrs

*Neutral protamine Hagedorn.

Insulin is produced by two companies: Eli Lilly and Novo-Nordisk. These companies use different names for the same short-, intermediate-, or long-acting forms of insulin or their mixture. Different preparations of insulin have different onsets, peaks, and durations of action. The most typical concentration of insulin is 100 U/mL.

Human insulin is biologically engineered through the process of recombinant DNA technology.

FINGER-STICK BLOOD GLUCOSE TESTING

Equipment

- Penlet
- Automatic lancet
- Test strips
- Soap and water
- Tissue or sterile gauze squares
- Clean gloves

Preparation

1 Wash client's fingertip (side where lancet will puncture) or heel with soap and water. **RATIONALE:** Use soap and water if repeated sticks are done, as alcohol toughens skin and may alter reading. Warm water increases blood flow to area.

2 Instruct client to place arm at side of body for several seconds. **RATIONALE:** This engorges fingertips for ease in obtaining sample.

3 Take cover off Penlet and insert lancet, twisting into place. Replace cover of Penlet. Cock Penlet to pull lancet back into Penlet.

SKILL

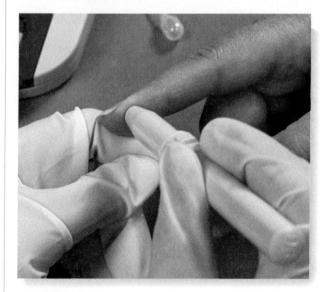

1 Place tip of sampling pen against side of finger. Activate to force lancet downward by pressing gently on activating button. Lancet punctures skin immediately. Use shallow skin penetration. **RATIONALE:** This causes less tissue damage.

- Gently massage base of finger, stroking toward puncture site. Do not squeeze or apply pressure to site. **RATIONALE:** Massaging increases blood flow to fingertip.
- Wait a few seconds to allow blood to collect at puncture site.

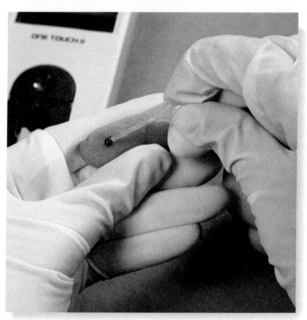

2 If using capillary suction bulb to obtain blood specimen, place tip of capillary bulb at base of blood drop. Fill tubing (not bulb) with blood.

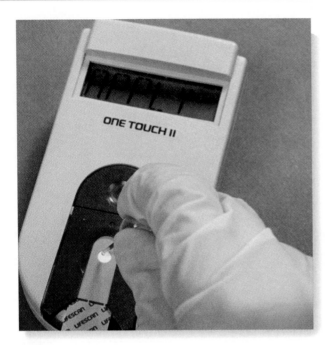

SAFETY ALERT

If the client is Type 1 insulin-dependent diabetic, test for ketonuria when blood glucose reading is over 250 mg/dL. Ketoacidosis should be reported and may require medical management.

3 Place large drop of blood onto test strip.

- Use a tissue to apply firm pressure for at least 10 seconds directly over puncture site to ensure thorough clotting. **RATIONALE:** Applying pressure to a wider area will create a bruise.
- Dispose of used equipment in biohazard container.

BEYOND THE SKILL

Use of Glucose Meters

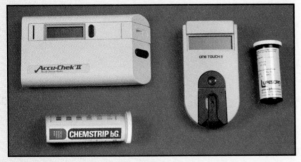

Many types of glucose meters are available today and may be used by clients for self-monitoring. General steps for their use include:

- Apply a drop of blood to a special reagent test strip.
- Allow the blood to stay on the strip for a specified amount of time.
- Place the strip in the glucose meter.
- Note the meter's digital readout of the blood glucose value.

- Date and time
- Medication and dosage
- Route of administration
- Site of administration

- Client's pre- and postadministration assessment data (e.g., blood sugar, pain rating)
- Rationale for PRN and STAT injections

SECTION FOUR

INTRAMUSCULAR INJECTIONS

Intramuscular injections are given deeply into muscle, which is rich with blood vessels, for rapid drug absorption. Intramuscular injections may be more painful than others because nerves are more plentiful in muscle. Because of the proximity of blood vessels and nerves, skillful technique and special precautions are necessary. Well-defined anatomic landmarks are used for individual injection site selection to avoid accidental intravascular deposition of drug and to prevent nerve injury.

Injection volume is usually limited to less than 4 mL for a large muscle. Needle length and gauge selection is based on the drug, the client's size, and the selected site for injection.

Muscles used for injection include the ventrogluteal, vastus lateralis, dorsogluteal, and deltoid.

- The ventrogluteal site is preferred for injection because of its relative lack of large nerves, blood vessels, and fat. It is suitable for most age groups.
- The vastus lateralis muscle of the thigh is thick and well developed in most adults and children and lacks major blood vessels and nerves. The injection site should be confined to the middle third of the muscle. This site is commonly used for pediatric clients.
- The dorsogluteal site is more difficult to locate and the least desirable of all intramuscular injection sites because major blood vessels and the sciatic nerve are located there. In addition, most people (especially women) have a thick layer of fat in this area, making true intramuscular injection less likely.
- The deltoid is a small muscle mass located in the upper arm near the shoulder, close to major vessels and the radial nerve. It is reserved for injecting a small volume (0.5 to 1 mL) of a nonirritating substance.

RATIONALE

- To deliver medication for rapid absorption into bloodstream
- To administer medications that are too irritating to be given subcutaneously (e.g., Vistaril)
- To provide medication to clients who are NPO, nauseated, or vomiting

ASSESSMENT

- Check type and volume of medication to be given.
- Assess client's size and age.
- Assess status of previous injection sites.
- Check any restriction imposed on client positioning.
- Assess relevant vital signs, laboratory data, or other parameters affected by drug to be given.
- Check that selected site is clearly visible for identification of landmarks and safety of administration.
- Check that selected site is free of local tissue damage.

INTRAMUSCULAR INJECTIONS

Equipment

- Medication vial or ampule
- Syringe (3 mL) with 1½-in needle (21 to 23 gauge)
- Alcohol swabs
- Clean gloves

SAFETY ALERT

Frequently, injections intended for muscle deposition are given into fat due to insufficient needle length. This is particularly true for injections given to women. Proper injection technique requires a sound knowledge of the anatomy involved.

SKILL

1 Fully expose area to select site for injection, alternating sites for each injection. **RATIONALE:** Facilitates visualization and palpation of landmarks.

- Cleanse area with alcohol swab using circular motion, moving from inside outward. Allow alcohol to dry. **RATIONALE:** Prevents tracking of alcohol into tissue.
- Remove needle guard.

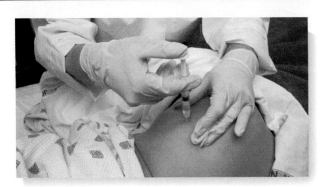

2 Use thumb and forefinger to spread skin taut, or grasp muscle in a small client to increase mass. **RATIONALE:** This will ensure needle placement in muscle belly.

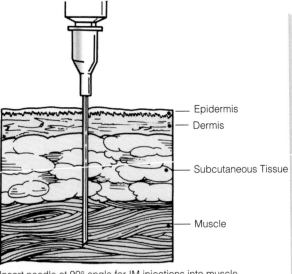

Insert needle at 90° angle for IM injections into muscle.

Epidermis
Dermis
Subcutaneous Tissue
Muscle

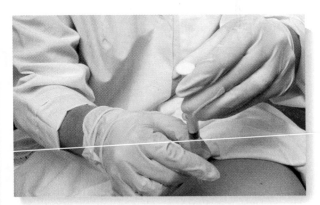

4 Pull back on plunger to aspirate for presence of blood. If blood returns, discard and prepare a new injection.

- Inject medication slowly.
- Withdraw needle at same angle as inserted. Retract needle if using safety syringe or do *not* recap needle.
- Press site with gauze.

3 Insert needle at 90° angle into muscle belly, using a quick darting motion. **RATIONALE:** This angle facilitates medication reaching muscle.

SKILL

Ventrogluteal Site

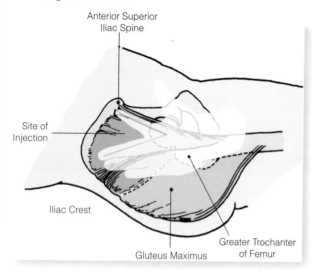

Anterior Superior
Iliac Spine

Site of
Injection

Iliac Crest

Gluteus Maximus

Greater Trochanter
of Femur

1 With client lying on side with upper leg flexed and rotated slightly forward, place your palm on client's greater trochanter and point your index finger to the anterior superior iliac spine. Use your right hand for client's left hip, and vice versa.

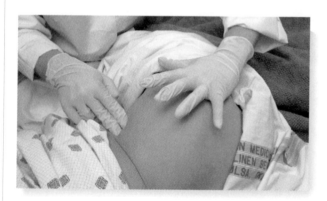

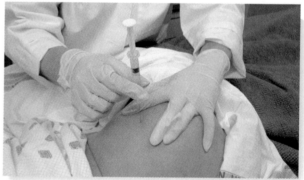

2 Spread your other three fingers posteriorly toward buttocks to create a V that confines the injection site.

3 Inject medication slowly at 90° angle within V area formed by fingers.

Vastus Lateralis Site

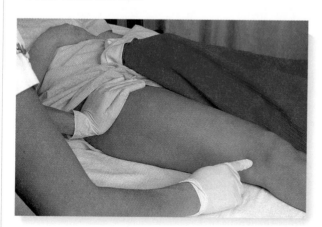

1 With client lying supine or in a sitting position, identify greater trochanter and lateral femoral condyle.

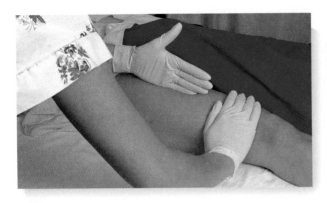

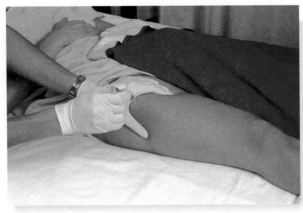

2 Select site bound by mid-anterior thigh on front of leg, mid-lateral thigh on side, and a hand's breadth below greater trochanter at proximal end and another hand's breadth above knee at distal end.

3 Inject medication slowly at a 90° angle into muscle.

Dorsogluteal Site

SAFETY ALERT

- Do not use the upper outer quadrant of the buttocks to identify the dorsogluteal injection site. The buttocks include fat tissue that extends well below the gluteal muscle and varies significantly among individuals. Intersecting vertical and horizontal lines on the buttocks can easily include the sciatic nerve and major blood vessels in the upper outer quadrant, possibly exposing them to serious and permanent injury if an injection is placed there.
- Chemical injury to the sciatic nerve can occur from the injection of irritating medications near the nerve. To avoid sciatic nerve injury, locate the dorsogluteal injection site above an imaginary line drawn between two bony landmarks: the greater trochanter and posterior superior iliac spine.

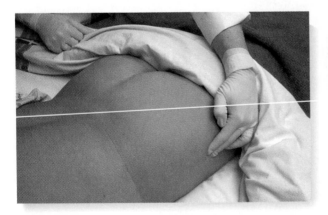

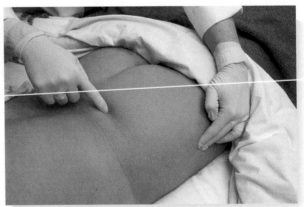

1 Assist client into prone (face-down) position with toes pointed inward; expose entire buttock area and locate client's greater trochanter. **RATIONALE:** Injection site must be clearly exposed to allow unobstructed view of area and identification of landmarks. Toes-inward position relaxes muscles and decreases pain on injection.

2 Locate posterior-superior spine of iliac crest (some clients have a dimple at this site). **RATIONALE:** This will help in location of correct injection site.

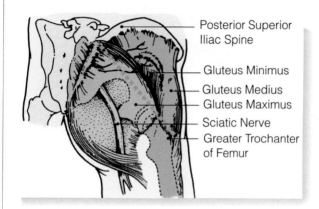

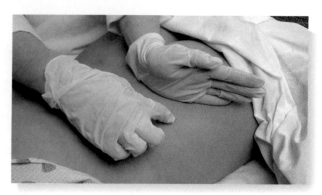

3 Review illustration of anatomy of dorsogluteal site as necessary.

4 Draw an imaginary line between the two bony landmarks (trochanter and posterior superior iliac spine).

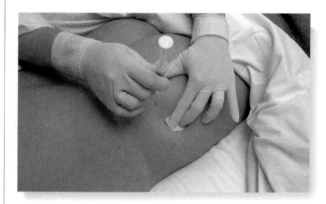

5 Inject medication slowly at 90° angle (perpendicular to flat surface on which client is lying) above and outside of imaginary diagonal line created by the bony landmarks.

Deltoid Site

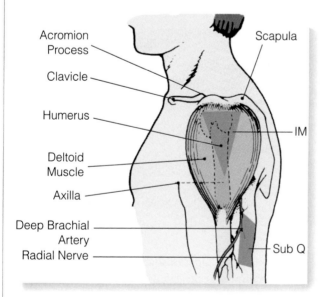

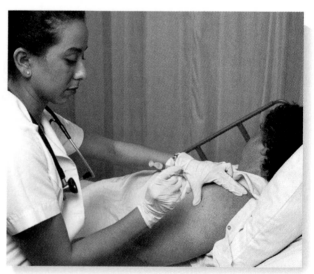

1 With client sitting, standing, or lying, locate deltoid site on outer lateral aspect of upper arm.

2 Inject medication within area two fingerbreadths below lower edge of acromion for top boundary, and opposite axilla for bottom boundary.

Z-TRACK INJECTIONS

Equipment

- Prepared medication in syringe
- Extra sterile 2-in needle (22 gauge)
- Alcohol swabs
- Clean gloves

Preparation

1 Follow the appropriate skill for injection preparation, with the following additions:

- After validating that correct medication dosage has been withdrawn, add 0.3 to 0.5 mL of air to syringe. **RATIONALE:** Air injection follows medication, clears needle, and prevents medication from leaking back into subcutaneous tissue after injection.
- Attach new 2-inch sterile needle to syringe. **RATIONALE:** A new needle prevents introduction of medication that could be irritating to tissue. A long needle allows medication to go deep into muscle.

SKILL

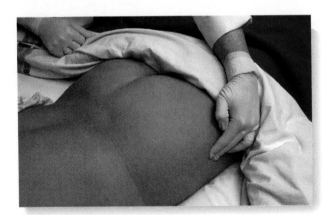

1 Assist client to lie in a prone position, if possible. **RATIONALE:** This position provides best perspective for identifying dorsogluteal landmarks (posterior superior iliac crest and greater trochanter).

- Cleanse injection site with alcohol.

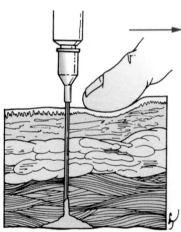

Z-Track Injection

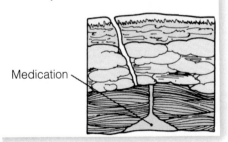

Medication

2 Pull skin 1½ in laterally away from injection site. **RATIONALE:** This tissue displacement creates a track that keeps medication from seeping back into subcutaneous tissue.

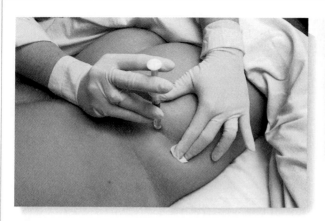

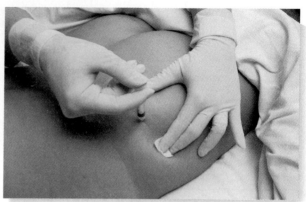

3 Maintaining displacement, insert needle at 90° angle.

- Aspirate by pulling back on plunger, checking to see if needle is in blood vessel. If blood is aspirated, needle is in a blood vessel; discard and prepare new injection. **RATIONALE:** Serious injury could occur if medication is injected intravenously. *Only medications specifically formulated and ordered for intravenous administration may be injected intravenously.*

4 Inject medication and air bubble slowly and wait 10 sec, keeping skin taut. **RATIONALE:** Permits muscle relaxation and absorption of medication.

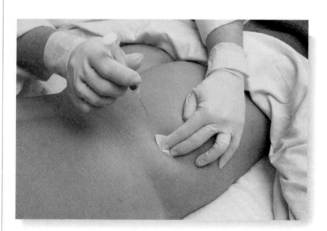

5 Withdraw needle and release retracted skin. **RATIONALE:** Lateral tissue displacement interrupts needle track and seals medication in muscle when tissue is released.

- Apply light pressure to site with alcohol pad. Do *not* massage. **RATIONALE:** Massage may disperse medication into subcutaneous tissue and cause tissue damage.

CHARTING

- Date and time
- Medication and dosage
- Route of administration
- Site of administration

- Client's pre- and postadministration assessment data (if indicated)
- Rationale for PRN and STAT injections

CRITICAL THINKING FOCUS

SECTION ONE ▪ Injection Preparation

Unexpected Outcomes

- Preoperative medications are not compatible in same syringe.

Alterative Nursing Actions

- Prepare separate injections for administration.

SECTION TWO ▪ Intradermal Injections

Unexpected Outcomes

- Client has anaphylactic allergic response to intra-dermally injected antigen.

Alternative Nursing Actions

- Maintain patent airway.
- Position client for optimal cerebral perfusion—trunk horizontal, legs elevated.
- Notify physician immediately.
- Have emergency equipment available and be prepared to carry out the following actions following physician's orders:

    -Administer oxygen at 6 L/min via nasal cannula.

    -Insert IV line for fluid resuscitation and drug delivery.

    -Administer epinephrine for bronchodilation.

    -Monitor client for response to treatment.

    -Monitor vital signs frequently until client's status stabilizes.

SECTION THREE ▪ Subcutaneous Injections

Unexpected Outcomes

- Ecchymosis (bruising) occurs following heparin injection.

Alternative Nursing Actions

- Rotate injection site.
- Do not inject medication into bruised area.
- Do not aspirate before injection or massage site following needle withdrawal.
- When forming fat pad in preparation for injection site, do not pinch tightly.
- Apply ice to area prior to injecting heparin.

SECTION FOUR ▪ Intramuscular Injections

Unexpected Outcomes

- Client complains of pain when injection is adminis-tered IM at dorsogluteal site.

Alternative Nursing Actions

- Use dorsogluteal site only when necessary.
- Obtain order for warm moist packs.
- Take greater care to identify anatomical landmarks.
- Place client in prone position (on abdomen) for injection.

- Irritating medication intended for intramuscular site is inadvertently administered subcutaneously.

- Use Z-track and added air bubble technique; inject into muscle at a 90° angle and wait 10 sec before withdrawing needle.
- Notify physician immediately and complete unusual occurrence report.
- An antidote may be necessary to reverse action of medication.
- Monitor client's response closely and report adverse findings immediately.

SELF-CHECK EVALUATION

PART 1 ▪ Matching Terms

Match the definition in column B with the correct term in column A.

Column A	Column B
_____ a. Ampule	1. Within a muscle
_____ b. Anticoagulant	2. Administration by injection
_____ c. Aspirate	3. Withdraw by negative pressure
_____ d. Cartridge	4. Within the upper layers of the skin
_____ e. Incompatibility	5. Area of hardness
_____ f. Induration	6. Single-dose drug-needle unit
_____ g. Intradermal	7. Glass container for injectable medication
_____ h. Intramuscular	8. Physical or chemical interaction when drugs are mixed
_____ i. Parenteral	9. Within the fat tissue under the skin
_____ j. Subcutaneous	10. Agent that slows the process of blood clotting

PART 2 ▪ Multiple Choice Questions

1. Which of the following needles should the nurse select when preparing to administer a pain medication subcutaneously to an obese client?

a. 27 gauge, ½ in.
b. 25 gauge, ⅝ in.
c. 22 gauge, 1 in.
d. 20 gauge, 1½ in.

2. Subcutaneous injections for pain are most commonly injected in which area?

a. Abdomen.
b. Buttocks.
c. Arm.
d. Lateral thigh.

3. The medication order is to give heparin 2000 U subcutaneously. The vial contains heparin 5000 U/mL. How many milliliters will you administer?

a. 0.2.
b. 0.4.
c. 0.6.
d. 0.8.

4. The nurse should not massage the site following heparin injection in order to:

    a. Maintain heparin in the subcutaneous tissue.
    b. Prevent rapid absorption of medication.
    c. Prevent tissue damage.
    d. Prevent discomfort.

5. Which of the following steps is correct when preparing to administer two types of insulin?

    a. Two separate syringes must be used.
    b. Air is placed in the regular insulin vial first.
    c. Air is placed in the intermediate-acting insulin vial first.
    d. The intermediate-acting insulin is drawn up first.

6. When administering Humulin insulin, the nurse expects its onset of action to be:

    a. 10 min.
    b. 30 min.
    c. 45 min.
    d. 1 hr.

7. The abdomen is the preferred site for insulin administration because:

    a. Absorption is slower than in the arms or thighs.
    b. Access to the site is easy.
    c. The injection is less painful.
    d. Absorption is the most consistent.

8. The nurse wears gloves when administering parenteral injections in order to:

    a. Protect against exposure to the medication.
    b. Reduce the risk of needle stick.
    c. Protect against exposure to blood.
    d. Maintain sterile technique.

9. Which of the following routes of injection has the most rapid absorption?

    a. Intradermal.
    b. Subcutaneous.
    c. Intramuscular.
    d. Intravenous.

10. Which of the following is the preferred site for intramuscular injection in adults?

    a. Dorsogluteal.
    b. Deltoid.
    c. Ventrogluteal.
    d. Vastus lateralis.

11. Which of the following needles should be used to administer an intramuscular injection to an obese client?

    a. 22 gauge, 1½ in.
    b. 20 gauge, 1 in.
    c. 18 gauge, 1½ in.
    d. 23 gauge, 1 in.

12. Which of the following statements is most correct regarding the Z-track technique of injection?

    a. Express all air from the needle and syringe before administration.
    b. Massage the skin following injection.
    c. Do not aspirate to check for needle placement.
    d. Wait 10 sec after injecting medication before removing the needle.

13. Landmarks for the ventrogluteal site include the:

    a. Anterior superior iliac spine and lateral femoral condyle.
    b. Anterior superior iliac spine and greater trochanter.
    c. Lateral femoral condyle and greater trochanter.
    d. Posterior superior iliac spine and greater trochanter.

14. Intradermal injections are administered to:

    a. Hasten medication absorption.
    b. Prevent hematoma formation.
    c. Determine a client's immune response.
    d. Avoid nerves and blood vessels.

PART 3 ▪ Critical Thinking Application

This is Nancy's third hospitalization for diabetic ketoacidosis this year. She has been an insulin-dependent diabetic for 5 years (since age 9). For several years Nancy has used two daily insulin injections, a combination of regular and NPH (intermediate-acting) insulin before breakfast and dinner.

 This year Nancy made the cheerleading A squad—quite an achievement and an honor that requires practice before and after school, enrollment in gymnastics class, and participation at evening and weekend games, some of which are out of town. In addition, Nancy must attend cheerleading camp this summer and is preparing for all-state competition trials.

 Nancy's diabetes is stabilized during hospitalization, but shortly before discharge she confides in you that she hates needles, the shots really hurt, and, in fact, she prepares the syringes and sometimes just throws them away. In addition, she has experienced low blood sugar on occasion while cheerleading and knows that something happens with her insulin "overreacting" at these times. It makes her uncoordinated and confused, but she just can't take time out to eat sugar. She's afraid of losing her position on the A squad that she worked so hard to achieve.

1. Select an appropriate nursing diagnosis for this scenario.
2. Based on this data, identify Nancy's psychosocial needs and developmental tasks at age 14.
3. Identify how insulin absorption and action are influenced by exercise and site of administration.
4. Suggest an alternative way for Nancy to maintain her insulin coverage without discomfort and erratic absorption rates.

17

INTRAVENOUS FLUIDS AND BLOOD

INTRODUCTION

The body's internal environment is made up of fluids (primarily water) and electrolytes (dissolved substances), which are constantly adjusting to maintain an environment that supports life-sustaining physiologic processes. Fifty to 70 percent of an average person's body weight is water. The obese and elderly have less body water, and infants, although they have the greatest percentage of body water, are unable to compensate readily for water losses. Physiologic factors place these clients at greater risk for fluid balance problems.

Most of our body water (66 percent) is located inside our cells. The remaining 34 percent is outside the cells: 75 percent of this extracellular fluid is interstitial (surrounding our cells), and the remaining 25 percent circulates as intravascular plasma within the vascular system. The intravascular fluid space is the smallest, yet the most critical for life support. Normally, the extracellular and intracellular spaces have equal osmotic pressure, or *osmolality* (about 290 mOsm), so fluid does not move between these two major compartments. In contrast, constant exchange of fluids occurs between the two extracellular (interstitial and intravascular) fluid compartments. The

(continued on next page)

movement of fluid between the two extracellular fluid compartments is controlled by two opposing forces: osmotic pressure of plasma proteins holding fluid within the vessels, and hydrostatic pressure in the arterioles forcing fluid into the tissue spaces. An increase in venous hydrostatic pressure, or a decrease in plasma proteins, will result in the retention of fluid in the interstitial space (edema).

Body water balance is dependent upon homeostatic physiologic responses to fluid gains (intake) and fluid losses (output). To balance a typical amount of fluid intake, the kidneys will produce 1 to 2 L of urine per day. An increased fluid intake, however, will result in an increased urine output, and vice versa. The major sources of intake and output are shown in Table 17-1.

TABLE 17-1	AVERAGE DAILY FLUID GAIN AND LOSS			
Intake (mL)		**Output (mL)**		
Oral intake (liquid and food)	2300	Urine	1500	
Cellular catabolism		Skin	600 (Insensible loss by evaporation)	
of proteins, carbohydrates, and fats	300	Lung	300 (Insensible loss by vapor)	
		Feces	200	
	2600		2600	

Urine production by the kidneys is influenced by two major hormones: antidiuretic hormone (ADH), secreted by the posterior pituitary gland, and aldosterone from the adrenal cortex. These regulatory hormones stimulate the kidneys to retain body fluid in response to any threat of fluid volume depletion or increased extracellular fluid osmolality (e.g., dehydration, hemorrhage, decreased cardiac output, or other stress states). ADH also stimulates thirst, which causes us to seek water. Elderly, infant, institutionalized, immobilized, or otherwise dependent clients are at risk for fluid volume deficit because of their depressed thirst response or inability to respond to the thirst drive.

When the kidneys sense a decreased cardiac output (e.g., hypovolemia or heart failure), they release renin. This enzyme activates angiotensin, which causes blood vessels to constrict in order to maintain blood pressure. It also stimulates the adrenal cortex to release aldosterone to maintain blood volume by decreasing the kidneys' production of urine. In order to clear the blood of the end products of cellular metabolism, however, the kidneys must produce a minimum of 500 to 600 mL of urine each day. When urine production falls below this minimum amount (a state of oliguria), nitrogenous wastes accumulate in the blood. This is reflected by a rise in serum BUN and creatinine, a condition called *azotemia*.

Body fluids contain dissolved electrolytes that influence not only fluid balance, but also vital cellular processes. The major intracellular electrolytes are potassium, magnesium, phosphate, and sulfate. Major extracellular electrolytes are sodium, chloride, and bicarbonate. As with body fluids, it is essential to maintain a balance of these important electrolytes by replacing what is lost on a daily basis. Stress, illness, and even medical management can influence gains and losses of these important elements.

TABLE 17-2	MAJOR ELECTROLYTES

Cations (+)		Anions (−)	
Na^+	Sodium	Cl^-	Chloride
K^+	Potassium	HCO_3^-	Bicarbonate
Ca^{2+}	Calcium	HPO_4^{2-}	Phosphate
Mg^{2+}	Magnesium		

Fluid and electrolyte balance can be threatened by any disruption of health. Therapeutic measures frequently necessitate peripheral or central intravenous infusion of fluids and electrolytes to cover daily insensible (nonmeasurable) losses and to dilute the end products of metabolism excreted by the kidneys. IV fluids are also administered to correct deficits (e.g., hemorrhage) or to compensate for ongoing abnormal fluid losses (e.g., gastric suction). In addition, when illness produces an intense requirement for nutrients (e.g., burn clients) or when the gastrointestinal tract is nonfunctioning (e.g., pancreatitis), infusion of parenteral nutrition is indicated.

The following skills are employed in caring for clients experiencing actual or potential disruptions of fluid and electrolyte balance necessitating intravenous therapy.

PREPARATION PROTOCOL: FOR INTRAVENOUS FLUIDS AND BLOOD SKILLS

Complete the following steps before each skill.

1. Verify fluid therapy or specimen to be obtained is consistent with physician's order in client's record.
2. Evaluate client's age and medical status.
3. Evaluate client's renal status and other pertinent lab data (e.g., electrolytes, CBC, serum glucose).
4. Prepare a time strip to coincide with fluid volume to be infused (do not use felt-tip pen).
5. Wash hands.
6. Inspect infusion product for expiration date, leaks, and signs of contamination.
7. Spike solution bag and prime tubing and filter, if used.
8. Program infusion parameters into pump delivery system.
9. Verify client's identity (check identaband and have client state name).

COMPLETION PROTOCOL: FOR INTRAVENOUS FLUIDS AND BLOOD SKILLS

Make sure the following steps have been completed.

1. Flush intermittent peripheral or central catheter infusion lock, or initiate infusion therapy at prescribed rate.
2. Dispose of equipment in puncture-resistant biohazard receptacle.
3. Remove and dispose of gloves.
4. Wash hands.
5. Document venipuncture, site condition and care, and infusion therapy on appropriate forms (medication administration record [MAR], client record, intake and output sheet, transfusion record).
6. Monitor infusion, IV site, and client response regularly.
7. Document discontinuation of IV therapy and removal of intact cannula on appropriate forms (MAR, client record, I&O sheet, transfusion record).

(continued on next page)

PREPARATION PROTOCOL: FOR INTRAVENOUS FLUIDS AND BLOOD SKILLS (CONT'D)

10. Provide privacy; explain procedure and purpose to client.
11. Position client for comfort and optimal visibility for skill performance.
12. Identify client's dominant hand and condition of veins.
13. Don clean gloves.
14. Access infusion site or validate patency of established site.

SECTION ONE

IV THERAPY PREPARATION

Intravenous (IV) therapy is a serious and complex responsibility that requires not only proficiency in performance, but also familiarity with the anatomy involved, ever mindful use of principles of asepsis, and expertise in prevention, identification, and management of complications that may occur with treatment. Many agencies utilize a certification process to validate the competency of nurses providing infusion therapy, and some states allow only registered nurses to provide this specialized care.

IV fluids are medications and require a physician's order. They are ordered to meet daily fluid and electrolyte requirements for the client who is NPO, to correct a fluid and electrolyte or blood deficit (e.g., due to vomiting or hemorrhage), or to replace abnormal ongoing losses due to NG suction or draining wounds. The type and amount of fluid administered will be based on these types of need as well as the client's age and general health status and the results of laboratory tests. Most clients receive crystalloid saline and/or glucose infusions, frequently with the addition of potassium, to cover electrolyte losses due to illness and stress.

Clients receiving IV fluids require physical assessment of fluid status, regular monitoring of response to IV therapy, and documentation of fluid intake and output (I&O) from all sources. Shift and 24-hr I&O totals are evaluated and the physician is notified of any unantici-

pated imbalance (e.g., urine output <30 mL/hr), as more intensive monitoring may be indicated.

RATIONALE

- To establish closed system for delivery of IV fluids
- To prevent air or particulate embolism
- To deliver IV fluids at consistent rate
- To provide continuous or intermittent IV fluid therapy

ASSESSMENT

- Follow physician order for type, rate, and duration of IV therapy.
- Check relevant laboratory data (e.g., electrolytes, BUN/creatinine, CBC).
- Assess expected outcomes of therapy (e.g., diuresis).
- Assess that fluid for infusion is clear and free of particulate matter.
- Make sure administration set is compatible with infusion delivery system (dedicated tubing may be required).

CLINICAL NOTE

Intravenous fluids are classified according to their tonicity (osmolality) in relation to normal blood plasma.

■ **Hypotonic fluids** have lower osmolality than plasma. They are administered to correct dehydration as they move from blood vessels into the cells.

—Examples are 0.45 percent NaCl, 0.2 percent NaCl, or 5 percent dextrose in water or combined with hypotonic saline.

—Excessive infusion can cause water intoxication or depletion of circulating volume.

■ **Isotonic fluids** have the same osmolality as plasma. They are administered to expand the intravascular space to correct hypovolemia as in shock.

—Examples are lactated Ringer's, 0.9 percent (normal) saline, and 5 percent dextrose in normal saline. One liter of normal saline (0.9 percent NaCl) meets the usual daily requirement for these electrolytes in an adult.

—Excessive infusion can cause circulatory overload and pulmonary edema.

■ **Hypertonic fluids** have greater osmolality than plasma, and are used primarily to pull fluid from cells and the interstitial space into the intravascular space to relieve edema. Hypertonic (>10 percent dextrose) parenteral nutrition solutions are irritating to peripheral veins and so must be infused into central veins, where blood flow is greater.

—Examples are >5 percent dextrose solutions, colloidal products such as dextran, and 3 percent saline (rarely used).

—Excessive infusion can cause cellular dehydration and circulatory overload or diuresis.

IV SYSTEM PREPARATION

Equipment

- IV fluid in bag
- Fluid infusion time strip (optional)
- Primary administration tubing set (compatible with infusion pump)
- Day or date identification sticker
- Needleless Luer Lock cannula for connecting IV tubing to client's IV site
- Add-on particulate filter (according to agency policy)
- Electronic infusion device or free pole for gravity infusion

Preparation

1 Remove outer wrap around IV bag (may be wet due to condensation).

- Inspect bag carefully for leaks by applying gentle pressure to bag. Hold bag up against both a dark and light background to examine for discoloration, cloudiness, or particulate matter. **RATIONALE:** Bag must be discarded if damaged or if there is any evidence of change that may indicate contamination.

SKILL

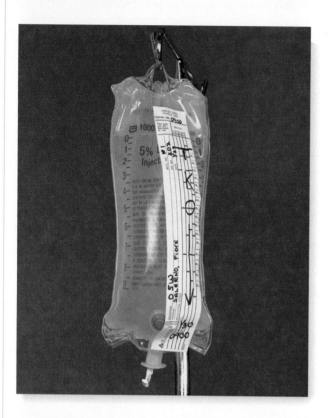

1 Affix time strip (optional) and suspend bag.

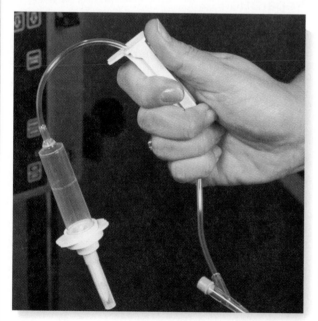

2 Close tubing regulator clamp.

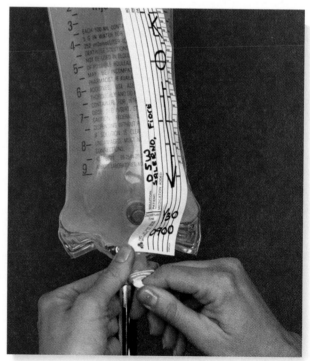

3 Remove plastic protectors from bag port and IV tubing spike.

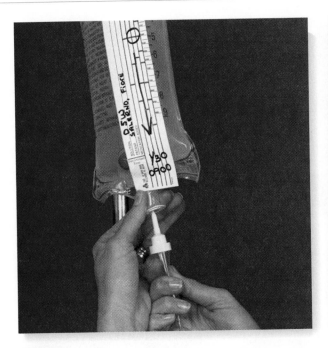

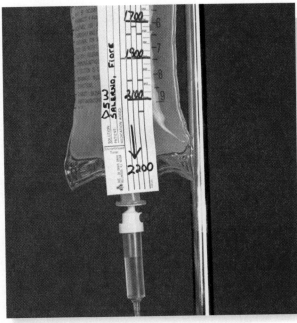

4 Squeeze drip chamber and insert tubing spike into bag port, holding port securely to prevent contamination. **RATIONALE:** Squeezing chamber during insertion prevents entry of air into bag.

5 Release pressure on drip chamber until chamber is partially full. **RATIONALE:** Drip chamber allows monitoring of fluid delivery.

- Attach add-on terminal filter (if indicated). **RATIONALE:** Filters may reduce risk of infection or particulate embolism.
- Remove protective cap at end of tubing; unclamp and purge tubing and filter of air.
- Invert and tap Y-injection sites to remove air as tubing primes. *Note:* Refer to administration set instructions for priming integral pump cassettes. **RATIONALE:** Removal of air prevents air embolism and promotes system function.

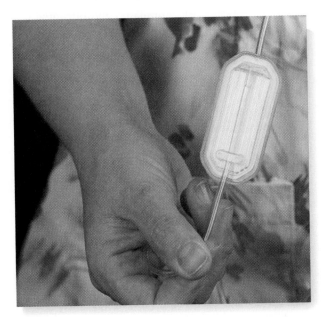

6 Hold filter pointing downward so proximal (closest to client) half of filter fills with fluid first, then invert to complete filter priming, tapping air out as filter primes.

 SAFETY ALERT

Add-on devices such as filters, cannula caps, injection ports, and needleless systems increase the risk of infection due to handling and the potential for separation. Preferably, these devices are an integral part of the administration set. If used, they should be changed along with administration set changes and should be discarded if their integrity is compromised.

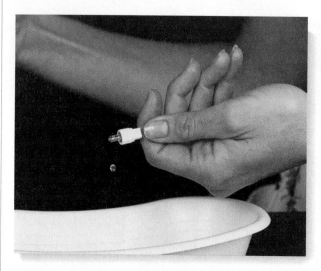

7 Hold tubing tip higher than tubing-dependent loop while priming. **RATIONALE:** Air rises and passes out as fluid primes tubing.

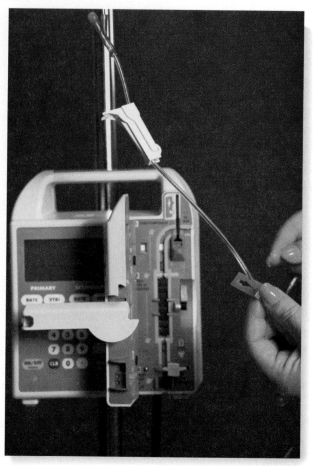

8 Close tubing clamp when priming is complete. Place needleless Luer Lock cannula on end of tubing. **RATIONALE:** This maintains sterility before infusion is established and attaches to resealable cap of IV cannula. Needleless connections protect against needle stick injury.

- Affix day-date identification sticker. **RATIONALE:** Duration of use can be identified.

- Load administration set into electronic pump according to manufacturer's instructions. **RATIONALE:** Most pumps require dedicated tubing and specific loading format.

CLINICAL NOTE

Some IV fluids are prepared in glass bottles. These require a steady source of air to maintain an infusion. These bottles may contain a tube through which air enters to allow fluid to leave the bottle. If a tube is not present, glass bottles require the use of vented tubing that incorporates an air side port just above the drip chamber. To assemble:

- Remove metal cap, metal disc, and rubber diaphragm from IV bottle. Listen for the inrush of air when the rubber diaphragm is removed. The inrush of air replaces the vacuum in the bottle. If inrush does not occur, discard the bottle.
- Place the bottle on a firm surface to spike.
- Proceed as in preparing to administer fluid from a plastic bag (step 4).

BEYOND THE SKILL

Infusion Regulation Devices

Various flow control devices are available to assist the nurse in the accurate delivery and monitoring of IV fluids. These utilize line power (AC) and have a backup battery feature allowing client mobility or transport. Such devices incorporate a message system that alarms the nurse about system problems and the need to troubleshoot various components of the system (e.g., occlusion or air in line).

- Controllers are pole-mounted electronic devices that are seldom used today, but may be necessary for backup equipment. They depend on gravity for flow; no pressure is added to maintain infusion or overcome resistance. Flow rate can be increased by raising the bag for greater gravity pressure. These devices regulate flow by counting drops, which are converted to milliliters per hour.

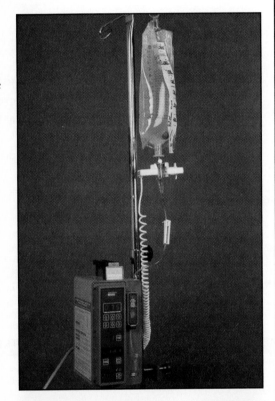

- In contrast to gravity flow devices, positive-pressure infusion pumps maintain preselected volume delivery by adding pressure to overcome resistance to fluid flow produced by the tubing diameter, filter, viscosity of infusing fluid, cannula, etc. Pumps usually require the use of specially designed administrations sets. When the system is working with normal resistance, delivery pressure is minimal. When resistance (5 psi over baseline) develops in the catheter or tubing, the pump adds pressure (within limits) to maintain infusion. Changes in resistance at the insertion site due to infiltration or thrombosis may not set off the system's alarm, and site problems could become serious. When the pump's maximum pressure limit is reached, an occlusion pressure alarm sounds. The nurse must become familiar with infusion devices by reading the manufacturer's literature and adhering to all instructions to ensure safe, efficient operation.

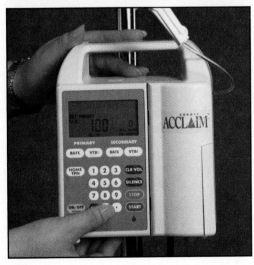

(continued on next page)

■ Simpler, but less precise or reliable, flow control can be achieved by using a tubing product that incorporates a dialed flow control mechanism for delivery of the prescribed milliliters of fluid per hour.

■ Alternatively, by calculating the drops per minute necessary to deliver the desired quantity of fluid per minute/hour, fluids can be administered by gravity and manual roller clamp adjustment without the use of mechanical devices. Refer to the administration set for its specific drops/mL.

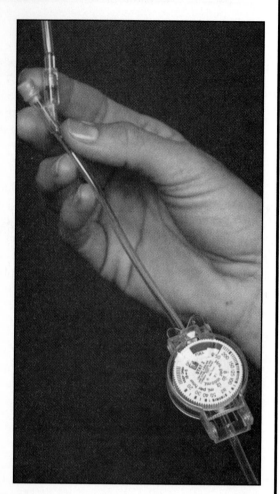

Three basic types of IV tubing include:

■ Tubing with drip factor of 10 to 15 drops/mL

■ Tubing with microdrip factor of 60 drops/mL

■ Y-tubing for blood transfusion with drip factor of 10 drops/mL

To calculate IV flow rate in drops per minute:

A. $\dfrac{\text{Total amount of solution in container}}{\text{Number of hours to run}} = \text{mL/hr}$

B. $\dfrac{\text{mL/hr} \times \text{drop factor}}{60 \text{ min}} = \text{gtts/min}$

SECTION TWO

IV FLUID ADMINISTRATION

Each state's Nurse Practice Act guides agency policies and procedures outlining the nurse's responsibilities in establishing and maintaining intravenous access and administering fluid and electrolyte solutions, blood components, and IV medications. In addition to Joint Commission on Accreditation of Healthcare Organizations (JCAHO) accreditation criteria and American Association of Blood Banks standards regarding administration of blood components, the Centers for Disease Control and Prevention and the Intravenous Nurses Society continually refine procedural guidelines and standards of practice for safe intravenous therapy.

Intravenous procedures require special precautions, conscientious adherence to principles of asepsis, proficient skill, and keen judgment. These therapies have evolved with such complexity that many agencies have established IV nursing therapy teams to focus solely on this area of care and serve as a resource to other personnel. You must become familiar with your particular agency's regulations and role parameters in order to avoid confusion about IV therapy.

The peripheral vasculature is convenient, easy to access, and most frequently selected for short-term IV therapy. Site selection is influenced by the client's medical condition, age, and current activity levels as well as the type and volume of fluid to be infused. Veins of the upper extremity are used, starting distally and moving proximally up the arm with subsequent sites.

All vascular access therapies place the client at risk for potentially life-threatening complications including phlebitis, thrombosis, infiltration of fluid, extravasation of medication, infection, and embolism. Careful client assessment, familiarity with equipment, and conscientious adherence to standards of care and agency-specific policies and procedures are essential for prevention or immediate intervention when therapy-related complications occur. IV therapies also place the nurse at high risk for exposure to bloodborne pathogens. The use of needles and sharps must be avoided whenever possible. Instead, select blood-drawing devices with integrated safety features designed to prevent injury, such as shielded retracting or self-blunting, and use resealable injection caps/ports and needleless or blunt cannula devices for connecting and accessing IV lines.

RATIONALE

- To establish vascular access for intermittent or continuous IV therapy
- To administer fluids and electrolytes
- To provide parenteral nutrition
- To transfuse blood or blood components
- To establish access for delivery of routine or emergency medications
- To obtain blood specimens for diagnostic purposes
- To stabilize catheter site to prevent phlebitis, infiltration, or dislodgement

ASSESSMENT

- Verify type, purpose, and duration of prescribed IV fluid therapy.
- Note client's age.
- Review client's medical and surgical history (mastectomy, dialysis fistula/shunt).
- Assess fluid intake and output trends.
- Review client allergies (e.g., iodine, shellfish).
- Verify client's identity (e.g., check identaband and have client state name).
- Assess client's understanding of procedure.
- Assess condition of client's veins.
- Check that peripheral IV access site (or central catheter) is intact and patent.

VENIPUNCTURE

Equipment

- Disposable tourniquet or blood pressure cuff
- Povidone-iodine wipe or alcohol (if client is allergic to iodine)
- Sterile winged needle (short tubing with terminal injection cap attached)
- Tuberculin syringe with 0.1 mL of 1 percent lidocaine without epinephrine (optional for over-the-needle application)
- Sterile over-the-needle catheter (for over-the-needle venipuncture)
- Alcohol swabs
- Sterile resealable injection cap
- Catheter extension tubing with resealable lock cap (for over-the-needle catheter)
- Sterile syringe with 1 mL normal saline solution and needleless cannula for priming
- Prepared IV administration setup (for infusion)
- Tape (½ in wide)
- Transparent semipermeable dressing or sterile 2 × 2 gauze
- Clean gloves
- Armboard, if indicated

Preparation

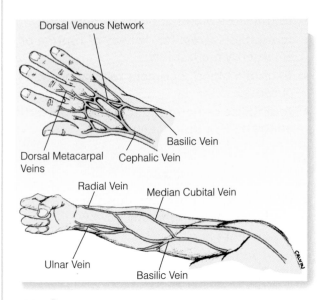

Dorsal Venous Network

Basilic Vein

Dorsal Metacarpal Veins   Cephalic Vein

Radial Vein   Median Cubital Vein

Ulnar Vein

Basilic Vein

 Select site for venipuncture. Inspect both arms, palpating and visualizing course of veins.

SAFETY ALERT

If gloves interfere with ability to palpate vein, don them just before venipuncture skill. Do not shave venipuncture site. Shaving can produce microabrasions that facilitate growth of organisms and development of infection. Hairy sites can be clipped with scissors.

SAFETY ALERT

In November 2000 the Needlestick Safety Prevention Act was passed. This bill amends the existing Bloodborne Pathogen Standard administered by the OSHA. It requires the use of safer devices to protect individuals in all states from sharps injuries.

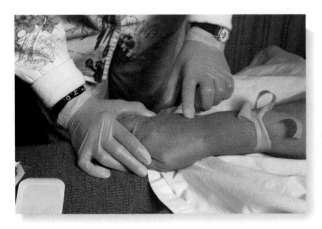

2 Identify superficial, easily palpated vein, large enough for needle insertion and advancement. Select area free of lesions and scars and away from joints. Use most distal site, reserving more proximal sites for future IV therapy. Reserve larger veins for hypertonic solutions, blood, and viscous fluids. *Note:* Select winged needle for children or elderly clients who have small or fragile veins. Avoid veins in arm with previous infiltration, on side of mastectomy, or with dialysis fistula/shunt. Avoid lower extremities.

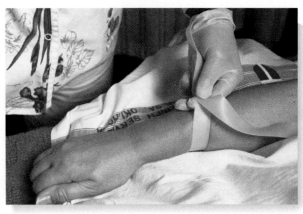

3 Apply tourniquet 6 inches above selected site or use blood pressure cuff. **RATIONALE:** To distend selected vein.

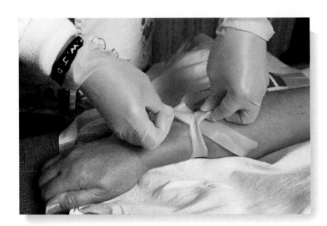

4 To apply tourniquet, overlap ends, lift and stretch, then tuck top end under bottom; keep ends pointing away from puncture site. **RATIONALE:** Tourniquet traps blood and engorges vein for better visibility.

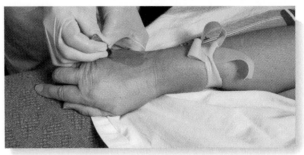

5 Prep site with povidone-iodine; if client is allergic, use alcohol. When alcohol is used, apply with friction for a minimum of 30 sec. Allow prep to dry completely for germicidal action to take place. **RATIONALE:** This creates an antibacterial barrier around the puncture site.

SKILL

Winged Needle

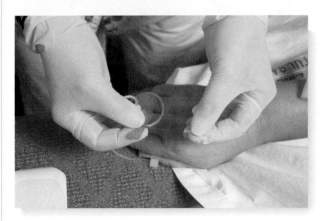

 1 Remove protective cap from winged needle.

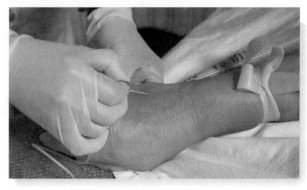

2 Anchor vein by placing thumb of nondominant hand below selected site and pull skin taut distally. **RATIONALE:** This secures vein and prevents rolling.

■ Using strict aseptic technique, hold needle (bevel up) with wings pinched together, and enter client's skin at a 15 to 30° angle. Enter skin next to or alongside vein. Flatten angle once needle is under skin and then enter vein from side; or, insert needle through skin below intended puncture site, then enter vein. **RATIONALE:** Inserting needle through skin and into small vein with one thrust will result in hematoma formation.

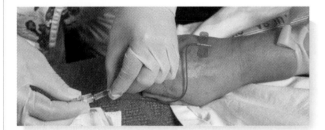

3 Carefully advance needle to wings; observe for flashback of blood in needle tubing. Affix sterile resealable injection cap to end of winged-needle tubing. **RATIONALE:** This is used for lock flushing or for connecting an infusion.

■ Release tourniquet. **RATIONALE:** To prevent hematoma formation.

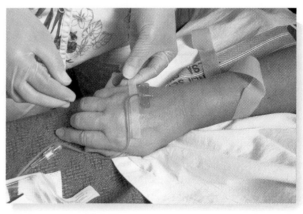

4 Secure needle with ½-inch tape; place with adhesive side up under tubing.

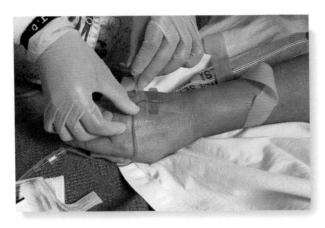

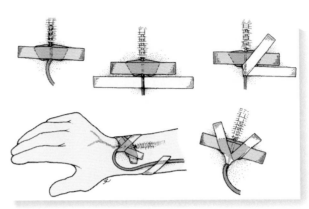

5 Fold tape ends over wings, making a V to secure. Avoid taping directly on insertion site. **RATIONALE:** Insertion site should be left uncovered for assessment and easy access.

6 Alternatively, use chevron (X) method. Place sticky side of tape under hub; cross ends of tape over to opposite side of needle, securing to skin; then apply another piece of tape across wings of chevron.

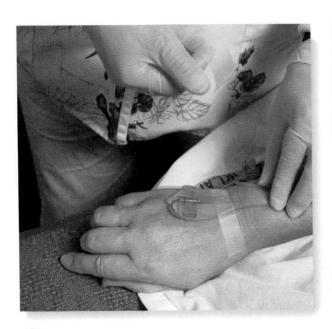

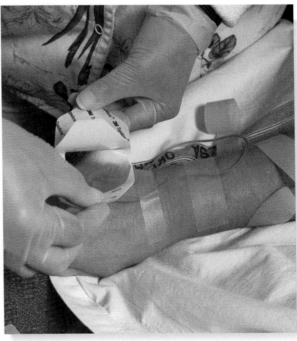

7 Loop and tape winged-needle tubing a short distance from insertion site. **RATIONALE:** This protects site from tension if tubing is inadvertently pulled.

8 Apply occlusive transparent dressing over infusion site.

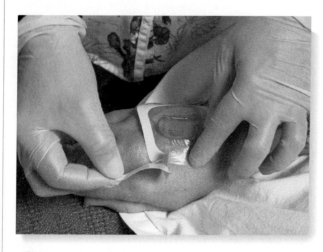

9 Smooth down dressing edges as frame is removed. Alternatively, apply sterile 2 × 2 gauze square and tape occlusively. **RATIONALE:** This stabilizes system.

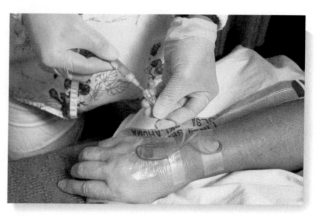

10 To lock, prep injection cap with alcohol swab and flush with 1 mL NS solution. Label dressing with date and initials. **RATIONALE:** Site should be rotated in 72 hrs.

■ Attach armboard if site is near area of flexion to ensure that circulation is not impaired and infusion site is visible. **RATIONALE:** To reduce risk of cannula displacement and injury.

Over-the-Needle Catheter

CLINICAL NOTE

SELECTING PERIPHERAL IV CATHETER GAUGE
Use the smallest-gauge and shortest catheter that accommodates the vein and allows optimal fluid flow.

24 gauge	For slow infusions in elderly clients or via small hand veins
22 gauge	For routine antibiotics and maintenance fluids via hand or arm veins
22 to 18 gauge	For fluids via forearm
20 gauge (or larger)	For blood components
18 gauge	For high-viscosity drugs
16 gauge	For administering large volumes of fluid rapidly via large veins

1 Administer intradermal local anesthetic at this time, if indicated. **RATIONALE:** To reduce discomfort of venipuncture.

Some agencies allow the intradermal injection of a local anesthetic (e.g., 0.1 mL of 1 percent lidocaine without epinephrine) to relieve the discomfort of venipuncture. Since this intervention carries the risk of anaphylaxis and vascular injury, routine use is not recommended. Analgesic creams are preferred. Refer to your agency's policies and procedures, and also see the skill for intradermal medications in Chapter 16.

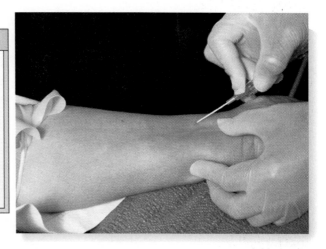

2 Hold and stabilize device, and insert needle at a 45° angle, either alongside vein or ½ inch distal to (below) selected puncture site.

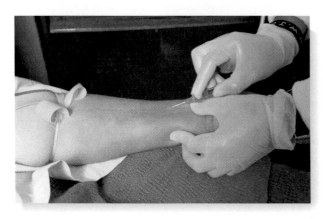

3 After bevel enters vein and blood flashes back, reduce angle and advance unit into vein lumen. Observe for backflow of blood in plastic hub. **RATIONALE:** This indicates you are in vein.

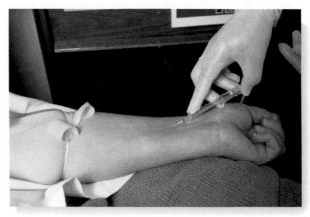

4 Hold needle and gently advance plastic catheter hub over needle and up vein to desired length. **RATIONALE:** This prevents inadvertent puncture of vein.

■ Alternatively, advance entire unit up vein to desired length and then remove needle/stylet.

5 Release tourniquet after accessing vein. **RATIONALE:** This prevents loss of blood due to tourniquet pressure.

■ Place protective gauze pad under hub, hold hub in place, and gently withdraw needle/stylet, leaving flexible catheter within vein.

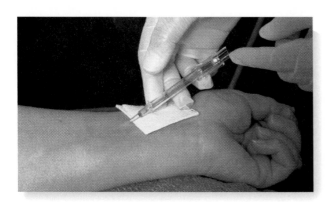

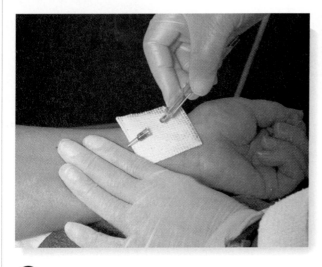

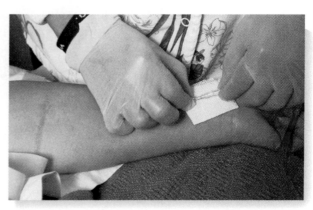

6 Apply pressure on vein proximal to catheter. **RATIONALE:** To prevent blood loss.

7 Affix resealable injection cap, primed extension tubing, or prepared administration set. **RATIONALE:** To maintain IV access for administration of fluids or medications.

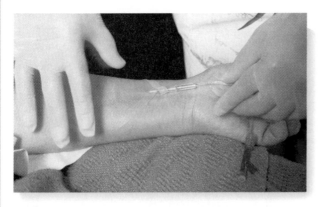

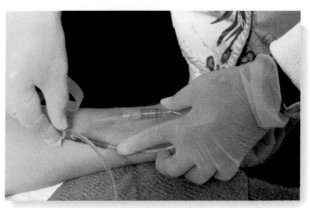

8 Secure cannula with tape, chevron fashion.

9 Loop and tape IV tubing close to site. **RATIONALE:** This reduces risk of tension at skin and cannula junction.

10 Apply transparent dressing over site and part of hub, then label with initials and date. **RATIONALE:** Transparent dressing allows visualization of cannula and skin junction.

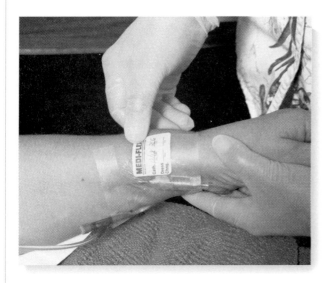

SAFETY ALERT

Edema at IV site may indicate infiltration of infusion. Monitor site closely; it may be necessary to change IV site.

BEYOND THE SKILL

IV Catheter Extension Tubing

A short extension tubing with a resealable injection cap attached to the IV cannula provides easy access for intermittent infusions and protects the IV site from manipulation trauma. It can be inserted directly into the IV cannula or connected into a resealable injection cap with a Luer Lock adapter. To assemble:

 1. Swab tubing's terminal injection cap and insert syringe cannula.

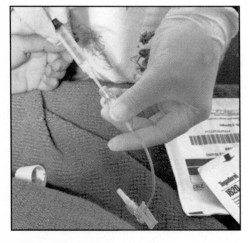

2. Remove protector at opposite end and prime extension tubing with 1 mL normal saline solution.

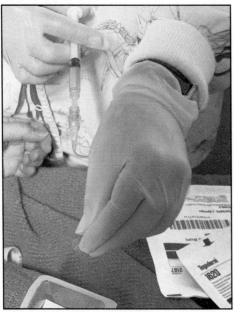

(continued on next page)

3. Add needleless cannula to tubing if attaching to a capped catheter. Swab client's established IV cannula resealable cap and connect extension tubing, or

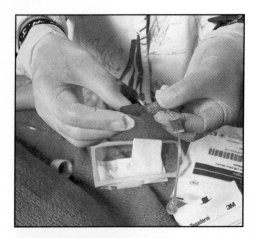

4. Insert primed extension tubing directly into client's IV catheter.
▪ Flush with 1 mL normal saline solution (optional).

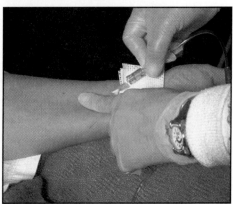

5. Dress site.

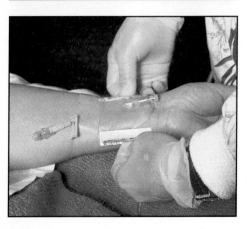

PERIPHERAL IV FLUID INFUSION

Equipment

- Prepared IV administration setup
- Alcohol swabs
- Infusion control device
- Clean gloves

SKILL

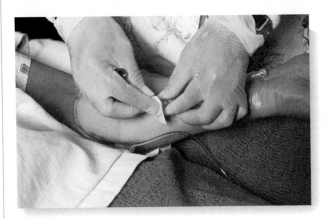

① Prep client's peripheral cannula (or extension tubing) injection cap with alcohol.

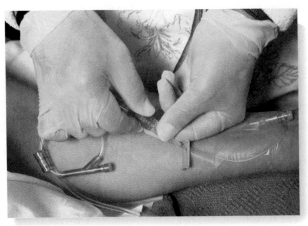

② Affix Luer Lock of primed IV administration set to peripheral cannula injection cap.

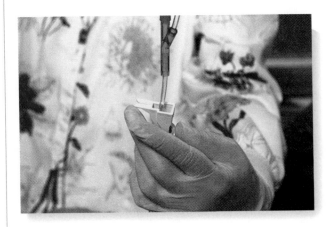

③ Open IV tubing clamp and observe drip chamber. **RATIONALE:** Fluid should flow easily and there should be no sudden swelling at IV site.

- If used, program infusion pump delivery parameters (e.g., delivery rate in milliliters per hour and volume to be infused) and initiate fluid infusion.

BEYOND THE SKILL

Intake and Output Measurement

Generally, daily intake and output measures, though not exactly equal, are within 200 mL of each other. To evaluate the client's fluid balance, record all measurable sources of fluid intake (such as fluids with and between meals, tube feedings, liquid medications, IV fluids, IV medications and flushes) and all measurable sources of fluid output (urine, emesis, diarrhea, drainage sites). Also, consider less obvious, nonmeasurable sources of fluid intake and loss such as food, increased metabolism (e.g., fever), rapid breathing, and perspiration. Since there are many sources of error in these types of recordings, compare total balances for several consecutive days and record the client's daily body weight for another helpful index of fluid balance. Deficits or excesses of fluid and electrolytes can be manipulated with replacement or other appropriate therapy.

| TABLE 17-3 | | INTAKE AND OUTPUT FLOW SHEET | | | | | | | | |

Date	Time	IV No.	IV Started	Description	IV Intake	Oral Intake Output	Urine	Other	N/G
1/9/02	9 A			Full liquid breakfast		620			
	9:45 A			Vomitus				400	
	10:30 A	#1	1000						
	12 N						450		
	2:30 P						400		
				7–3 total	500	620	850	400	100
	6:30 P	#2	1000						
	9 P						500		
				3–11 total	1000	npo	500		350
1/10/02	2:30 A	#3	1000		450				
	5 A						350		
				11–7 total	1000	npo	350		375
				24-hour total	2500	620	1700	400	825

DISCONTINUATION OF PERIPHERAL IV

Equipment

- Gauze square
- Tape
- Clean gloves

SKILL

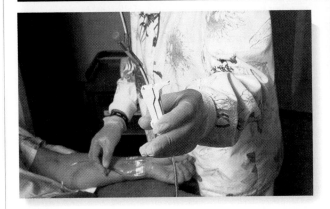

1 Turn off infusion (gloves are optional for steps 1 and 2).

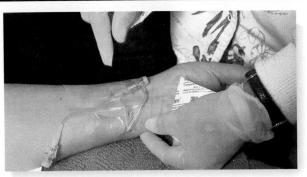

2 Loosen dressing and tape, peeling dressing edges back toward puncture site. **RATIONALE:** This minimizes trauma to puncture site.

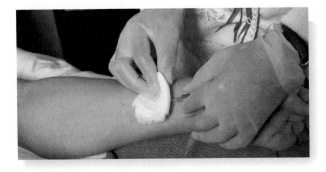

 3 Hold folded gauze to site while removing infusion catheter—do not use alcohol swab. **RATIONALE:** Alcohol causes site to bleed.

SAFETY ALERT

Reliable adhesion is important until time for removal. Remove dressings slowly and carefully, from edges toward the IV insertion site, peeling the tape or dressing parallel (not perpendicular) to the skin. Pulling the tape or dressing at a right angle can exert sufficient tension to tear fragile skin. An adhesive remover can be used when removal is anticipated to be difficult.

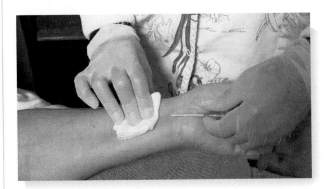

4 Apply pressure to gauze over puncture site.

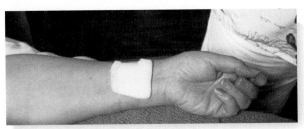

5 Tape gauze into place. Hold pressure for several minutes if client has been receiving antithrombotic or anticoagulant therapy. **RATIONALE:** This ensures hemostasis and prevents bleeding or hematoma formation.

PHLEBOTOMY

Equipment

- Vacutainer assembly with shielded or self-blunting needle
- Plastic vacuum blood collection tubes (appropriate for tests)
- Alcohol swabs
- Gauze squares or cotton balls
- Clean gloves
- Disposable tourniquet
- Tape

CLINICAL NOTE

Phlebotomy (obtaining a blood specimen from a peripheral vein) differs from venipuncture performed to initiate IV fluids. This skill is not legally restricted to certified personnel, but must be performed by competent personnel, since a very important part of accurate medical diagnosis and treatment involves clinical testing of the client's blood. Most agencies require didactic and supervised practicum training sessions followed by periodic evaluation to ensure that personnel are qualified to meet the laboratory's blood collection and processing standards.

SKILL

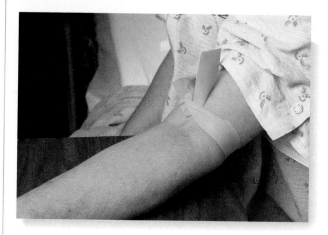

1 Apply tourniquet (or blood pressure cuff inflated to level between systolic and diastolic pressure) 4 to 6 inches above client's elbow; ask client to open and close fist. **RATIONALE:** This increases trapped blood and makes vein more easily palpable.

- Select puncture site free of IVs or fistula, and on opposite side from mastectomy; avoid scars, bruising, or edema. **RATIONALE:** IV fluids can contaminate specimen. Injury to an extremity with altered lymphatic function or life-sustaining access can cause serious complications and disability.
- Palpate antecubital (inner elbow) area with index finger to select best vein (medial is preferred)—vein will bounce back after being touched. **RATIONALE:** Index finger is most sensitive for locating vein.

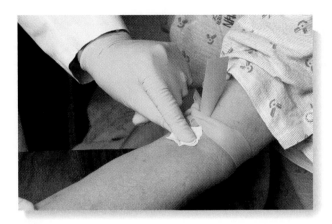

2 Cleanse area with alcohol swab, moving 2 inches outward in a circular motion, and allow to dry. **RATIONALE:** Moving away from intended site prevents moving microbes toward area. If puncture is performed before alcohol dries, specimen may hemolyze.

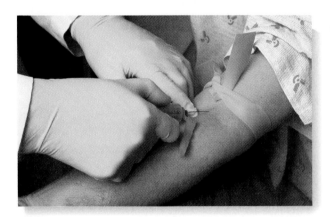

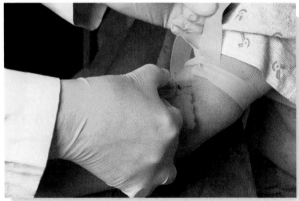

3 Clamp vein down by placing thumb or fingertip of nondominant hand below intended puncture site. Hold Vacutainer assembly between thumb and last three fingers of dominant hand, resting index finger on needle hub. With bevel up, insert needle at a 15 to 30° angle. **RATIONALE:** Steeper angle increases risk of passing through vein into deeper structures.

- Keeping client's arm in downward position and maintaining tube below puncture site, insert blood collection tube into holder and onto needle to guideline on needle holder. **RATIONALE:** This prevents backflow of blood from tube.

- As soon as needle is in vein, grasp flange of needle holder and push tube forward until butt end of needle punctures stopper, exposing full lumen of needle.

4 Have client relax fist, and release tourniquet. **RATIONALE:** Hemolysis occurs with prolonged tourniquet use. If needle is withdrawn before tourniquet is removed, hematoma will form.

- Fill tube until vacuum is exhausted and blood flow ceases, then remove tube from holder; if additional specimens are needed, insert next tube into holder and fill.

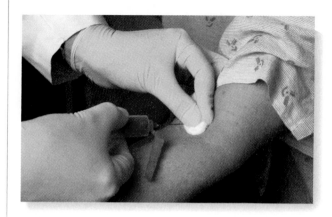

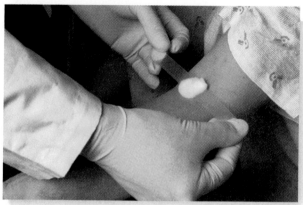

5 Place gauze square/cotton ball over puncture site and carefully remove needle.

6 Apply pressure to puncture site, then tape gauze/ cotton into place. Do not have client bend elbow. **RATIONALE:** Bending elbow causes hematoma formation.

- If tube contains an additive, gently invert tube 5 to 10 times. **RATIONALE:** To mix blood with additive.
- Once drawn, completely label tube of blood at client's bedside (with time, date, and your initials). **RATIONALE:** Delayed labeling increases risk of error and potential injury to client.

CHARTING

- Date, time, and site of catheter insertion
- Type and gauge of catheter placed
- Number of attempts at venipuncture
- Type of dressing applied
- Condition of IV site
- Flush solution and frequency of flushes
- Time of fluid initiation
- Type and amount of fluid initiated

- Infusion regulation device used
- Tubing changes
- Amount of fluid administered (include in I&O record)
- Client's response to therapy
- Time of discontinuation of IV site
- Purpose and dispensation of blood specimen drawn

CENTRAL VENOUS CATHETERS

Long-term intravenous therapy may require central venous access, especially when peripheral veins are no longer available or when irritating drugs or hypertonic fluids (e.g., parenteral nutrition) are infused. Central lines are especially useful for obtaining blood specimens from the neutropenic client. A variety of soft, pliable, single or multilumen central catheters may be inserted percutaneously (e.g., via subclavian vein) for use for up to 2 months. Longer-term catheters are surgically tunneled or implanted subcutaneously by a physician, while the peripherally inserted central catheter (PICC) can be advanced centrally via an arm vein by a specially educated, certified IV nurse. PICCs are less invasive and less expensive than other central catheters.

The central venous catheter extends into the superior vena cava. Because so much blood normally flows through this large vein, this placement minimizes vessel irritation and sclerosis due to infusion. For all centrally placed catheters, an x-ray is taken to verify the catheter's central position before infusion therapy is initiated.

In order to prevent air embolism, lumens must be clamped or the client must not inhale during tubing changes or any time a central venous catheter is open to the atmosphere (unless the catheter incorporates a Groshong valve). Since the PICC's exit site is below heart level, there is less risk of air embolism when the system is open to the atmosphere.

Patency of an unused central venous catheter is maintained by the regular instillation of a small volume of dilute heparin (100 U/mL) into each lumen. The Groshong valve is incorporated into a variety of long-term central venous catheters, including implanted ports and PICCs. This three-position valve allows forward flow infusion, but prevents backflow of blood unless negative pressure is applied. Catheters with Groshong valves require instillation of saline alone to maintain patency. There is no need for heparin flush, and external clamps are not used. Catheter insertion site protection and stabilization are accomplished by regular antimicrobial cleansing and sterile dressing changes. Gauze dressings are changed every 48 to 72 hrs, while a transparent dressing alone can be changed every 3 to 7 days.

RATIONALE

- To provide intermittent or continuous administration of fluids and electrolytes
- To provide parenteral nutrition
- To transfuse blood or blood components
- To administer routine or emergency medications
- To obtain blood specimens for diagnostic purposes
- To stabilize and protect catheter site to prevent contamination or dislodgement
- To provide ongoing visualization for evaluation of site

ASSESSMENT

- Check client's age and medical condition.
- Assess client allergies (e.g., iodine or shellfish).
- Review type, purpose, and duration of prescribed IV fluid therapy.
- Check type and frequency of dressing change.
- Assess type and amount of flush solution and required flush frequency.
- Verify client's identity (check identaband and have client state name).
- Assess client's understanding of procedure.

CENTRAL IV FLUID INFUSION

Equipment

- Primed IV administration set with needleless Luer Lock connector
- Infusion delivery pump
- Povidone-iodine swabs
- Syringe with 5 mL normal saline (for flush)
- Clean gloves

SKILL

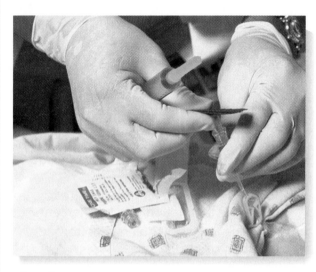

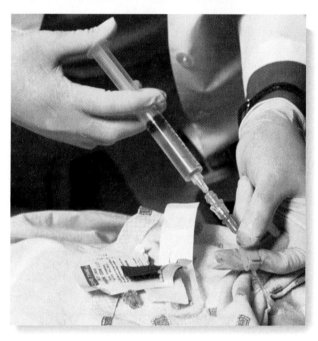

① Prep central lumen cap with povidone-iodine and allow to dry.

② Insert needleless cannula of saline flush syringe and unclamp lumen (clamp is not present on PICCs or catheters with Groshong valves).

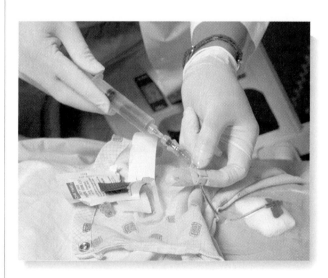

③ Begin flush; briefly aspirate for blood return. **RATIONALE:** To evaluate patency of system. *Note:* Dead-space air is frequently encountered on aspiration of central lines. To avoid reinjecting this air, hold syringe vertically, so the air rises to end of syringe barrel; continue flush, but do not inject air.

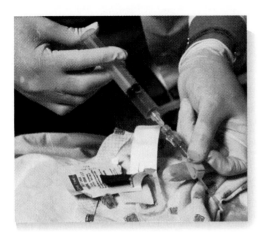

4 Instill syringe contents. **RATIONALE:** Flush clears lumen of inline dilute heparin.

- Near completion of injection, continue pressure on plunger as syringe is withdrawn to maintain positive pressure in line. Alternatively, clamp lumen before withdrawing syringe. **RATIONALE:** To prevent aspiration of blood into lumen.

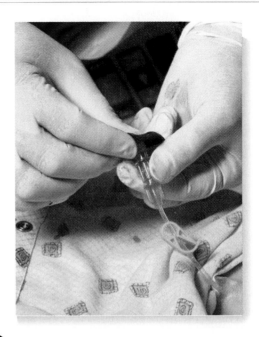

5 Prep cap again. **RATIONALE:** For asepsis.

SAFETY ALERT

For the PICC, flush with minimal force using a pulsating motion. This action creates turbulence for catheter cleansing.

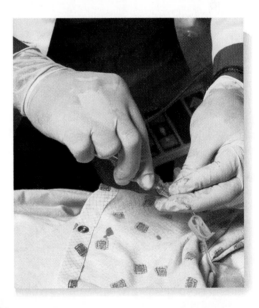

6 Access central line with IV tubing Luer Lock connector, unclamp lumen, then initiate IV infusion.

TABLE 17-4	CENTRAL VENOUS CATHETER MAINTENANCE		
CVC	**Flush Solution**	**Frequency**	
Percutaneous catheter, short-term	2 to 3 mL dilute heparin per lumen	q12hr to daily, and after each use	
Catheter with Groshong valve, long-term	5 mL normal saline ONLY	Weekly and after each use	
PICC without Groshong valve	5 mL dilute heparin per lumen	Weekly and after each use	
PICC with Groshong valve	5 mL normal saline ONLY	Weekly and after each use	

CENTRAL VENOUS CATHETER ACCESS CAP CHANGE

Equipment

- Povidone-iodine swabs
- Sterile resealable injection cap
- Syringe with 5 mL normal saline solution (for flush)
- Syringe with 2 to 3 mL dilute heparin (for maintenance if no Groshong valve present) OR new primed IV fluid administration set with needleless cannula
- Clean gloves

SAFETY ALERT

It is recommended that central venous catheter access caps be changed weekly.

SKILL

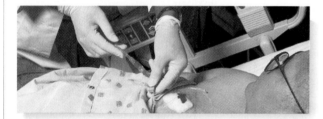

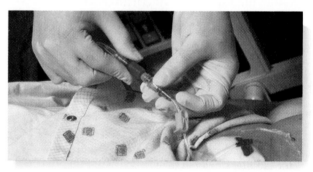

① Place client in supine position. Clamp catheter lumen using online slide or squeeze clamp. **RATIONALE:** Unless catheter incorporates Groshong valve, catheter must be clamped before cap removal to prevent air embolism during cap change. Alternatively, have client hum or perform Valsalva maneuver during cap change.

② Stop infusion and disconnect line from existing access cap.

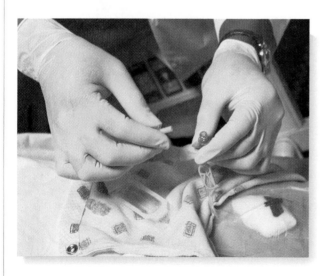

③ Using aseptic technique, remove existing cap and insert new one. Prep injection cap with povidone-iodine and flush catheter/lumen, or insert new primed tubing and initiate infusion.

CLINICAL NOTE

CENTRAL VENOUS CATHETER COMPLICATIONS

Signs and Symptoms	Possible Cause
Redness, swelling at site	Infiltration, hematoma, sepsis
Crepitus on chest	Subcutaneous emphysema that can lead to respiratory distress
Respiratory distress with recent central catheter placement	Pneumothorax
Arm, shoulder, or neck pain	Infiltration or thrombosis
Temperature elevation	Catheter-related infection

CENTRAL VENOUS CATHETER DRESSING

Equipment

- Povidone-iodine swabs
- Sterile 2 × 2 gauze pads (optional)
- Transparent semipermeable dressing
- Tape (½ in)
- Steri-Strips (for PICC)
- Receptacle for soiled dressing

- Clean gloves
- Sterile gloves
- Two masks (according to agency policy)
- Primed IV administration set with Luer Lock connector (if tubing change indicated)

Preparation

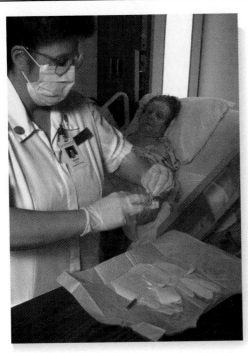

1 Set up needed sterile equipment before removing client's dressing (dressing changed q48 to 72 hrs). Don mask if client is neutropenic. **RATIONALE:** This reduces risk of infection.

2 Position client supine. **RATIONALE:** Supine or Trendelenburg (head down) positions reduce chance of air embolism if lumen cap is changed.

- Turn client's head away from insertion site and place mask on client's nose and mouth if necessary. **RATIONALE:** This reduces insertion site exposure to microorganisms.

SKILL

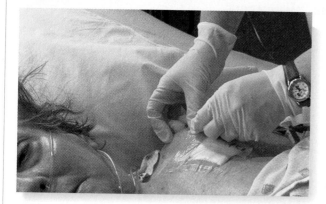

1 Carefully remove old dressing or tape without pulling on catheter. Remove edges toward insertion site. **RATIONALE:** This prevents stress on insertion site.

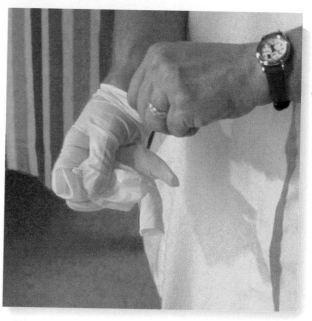

2 Remove gloves with soiled dressing inside and discard.

SAFETY ALERT

The use of scissors at or near any infusion site is prohibited.

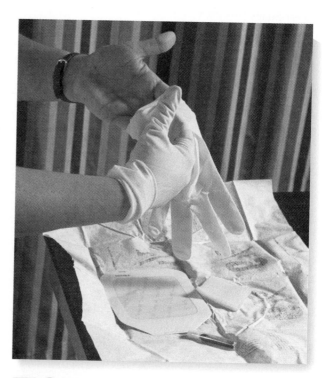

3 Don sterile gloves.

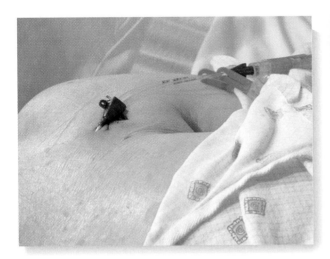

4 Inspect site for loose sutures; signs of infection, inflammation, or infiltration; and length of exposed catheter. **RATIONALE:** Abnormal findings must be reported and will guide decision making.

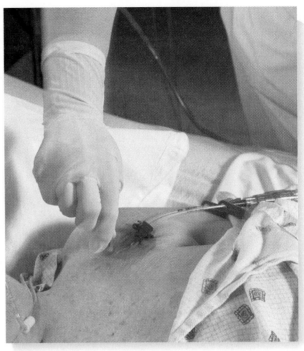

5 Cleanse insertion site, sutures, and catheter with iodine swabs, working from insertion site outward in circular motion. Repeat three times. **RATIONALE:** Most catheter infections are caused by normal flora on the skin.

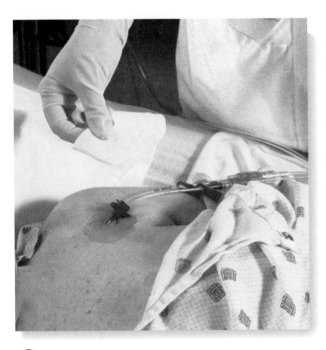

6 Place 2 × 2 gauze pad over insertion site (optional).

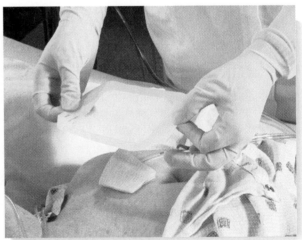

7 Cover with sterile transparent dressing, or use transparent dressing alone (according to agency policy). **RATIONALE:** Transparent dressings allow visualization of skin and cannula junction site.

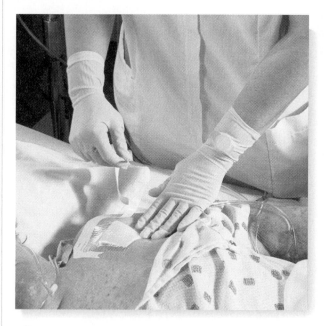

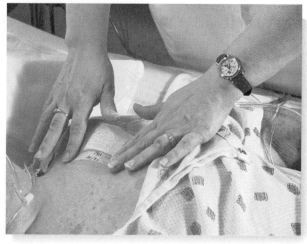

 Label dressing with date and your initials.

8 Smooth dressing edges as frame is removed.

Peripherally Inserted Central Catheter (PICC) Dressing

SAFETY ALERT

- Routine application of antimicrobial ointment to insertion sites should be avoided because it macerates the skin and promotes fungal growth.
- If gauze is used for central catheter dressing, it is covered occlusively with tape and all edges are secured (or covered with a transparent dressing). It is still considered a gauze dressing that retains moisture and may harbor bacteria. Gauze dressings should be changed every 48 hrs.
- Any dressing should be changed when it becomes damp, soiled, or loose. Diaphoretic clients may require more frequent dressing changes.

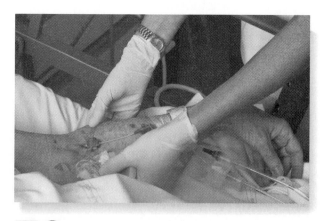

1 Very carefully remove old dressing and Steri-Strips from peripherally inserted central catheter (PICC) site. Note distance catheter extends from insertion site. **RATIONALE:** Catheter is secured by tape only and is not sutured in place. Length of catheter exposure should remain consistent.

- Discard old dressing and gloves.

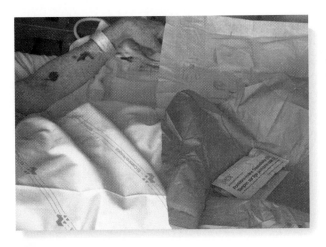

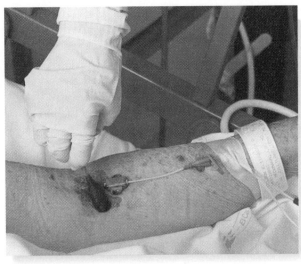

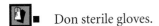

(2) Check site for bleeding or signs of phlebitis. **RATIO-NALE:** Bleeding may occur with arm use. Phlebitis is the most common complication.

 ■ Don sterile gloves.

(3) Clean skin and catheter junction site and exposed catheter with povidone-iodine swabs using circular movement from site outward, repeating three times. Allow to dry. Do not blow on arm or wave hand to hasten drying. **RATIONALE:** Antibacterial action does not take effect until solution is dry. Waving hand or blowing may contaminate site.

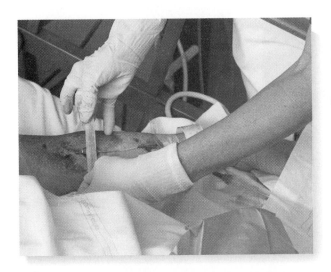

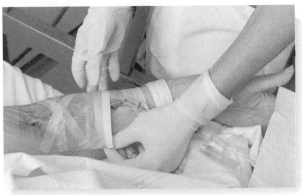

(5) Cover exit site with transparent sermipermeable dressing; label with date and your initials.

(4) Apply Steri-Strips to catheter exit site or hub to stabilize.

SAFETY ALERT

Avoid taking blood pressure in arm with PICC unless absolutely necessary. If necessary, take manually, NOT with automatic cuff, as they hyperinflate.

BLOOD SPECIMEN FROM A CENTRAL VENOUS CATHETER

Equipment

- Syringe (10 mL) with needleless cannula
- Syringe (10 mL) filled with sterile normal saline with needleless cannula
- Syringe (3 mL) filled with heparinized saline (100 U/mL heparin) with needleless cannula
- Povidone-iodine swabs
- Vacutainer tube holder and Vacutainer collection tubes
- Clean gloves

SAFETY ALERT

When obtaining a blood specimen from a central catheter that has multiple lumens, all infusions through the catheter must be stopped for 1 min prior to obtaining blood samples.

SKILL

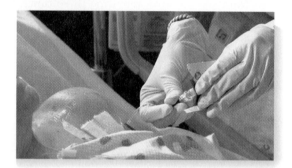

1 Unclamp most proximal lumen of multilumen catheter; swab cap and hub with povidone-iodine for 30 sec and allow to dry. **RATIONALE:** Proximal port specimen will not be contaminated if fluids are infusing distally.

CLINICAL NOTE

Newer catheter caps accept a syringe hub for administration of fluids or withdrawal of blood specimens, eliminating the need for either uncapping the catheter or using a needleless cannula.

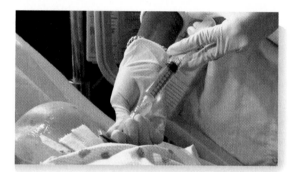

2 Insert needleless cannula of 10-mL syringe into cap and unclamp catheter.

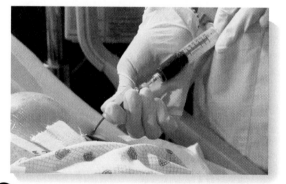

3 Slowly withdraw 5 mL of waste blood from catheter and clamp catheter. **RATIONALE:** Waste specimen should be equal to three times the dead-space volume of the catheter. This assures removal of flush solution from catheter before blood sample is obtained.

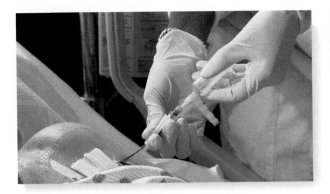

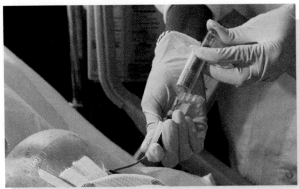

④ Swab cap again, then insert Vacutainer holder.

⑤ Insert collection tube to withdraw required amount of blood for laboratory tests. Fill tube until vacuum is exhausted and blood flow ceases.

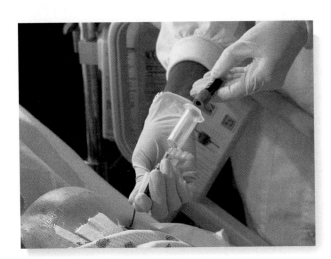

⑥ Remove tube from holder and insert next tube into holder to obtain additional samples if needed. **RATIONALE:** Each laboratory test requires a specific number of milliliters of blood. Check manual for specific tube and additives/preservatives needed for each test.

- Gently invert sample tubes 5 to 10 times. **RATIONALE:** This mixes blood with tube additive.

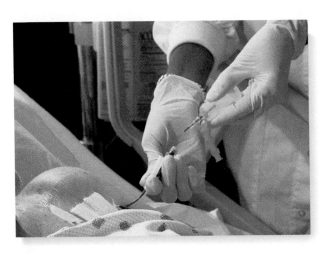

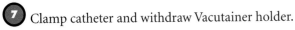

⑦ Clamp catheter and withdraw Vacutainer holder.

⑧ Swab cap.

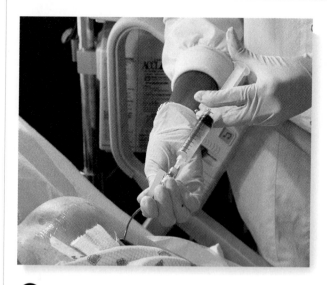

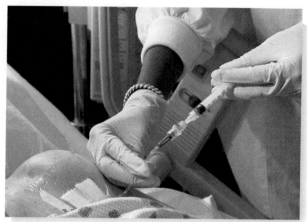

9 Insert 10-mL saline flush syringe; unclamp catheter, flush catheter, clamp, then remove syringe. **RATIONALE:** Flushing catheter reduces incidence of occlusion.

10 Swab cap again and insert 3-mL dilute heparin flush syringe; unclamp lumen, flush, clamp, then remove syringe, or maintain pressure on plunger and withdraw syringe while completing flush. **RATIONALE:** Dilute heparin maintains patency of central catheter. *Note:* Clamping lumen or maintaining positive pressure while removing syringe prevents creation of negative pressure and blood backflow into the catheter.

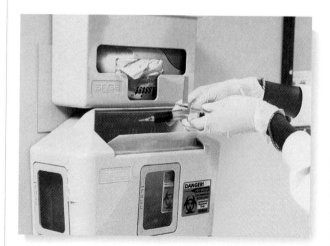

11 Discard waste syringe and used supplies in biohazard box.

CLINICAL NOTE

Vacuum tubes should not be used on central venous catheters (or PICCs) with Groshong valves. Specimens are obtained using a syringe with needleless cannula.

- Flush catheter with 20 mL of normal saline solution.
- Withdraw and discard 5 mL of blood in biohazard container. (Optimal amount of waste is three times the dead-space volume of the catheter).
- Using 10-mL syringes with needleless cannulas, withdraw required amount of blood for laboratory tests.
- Flush with 10 mL of normal saline solution, using pulsating motion.
- Carefully transfer blood from syringes into the appropriate laboratory specimen tube, supported in a laboratory basket. Do not hold the receiving tube in your hand.
- Gently invert specimen tube 5 to 10 times.

- Date and time of skill
- Type and amount of fluid administered (include in I&O record)
- Infusion regulation device used
- Condition of insertion site
- Dressing type and frequency of change

- Tubing and injection cap changes
- Flush solution, amount, and frequency
- Patency of lumens
- Client's response to therapy
- Purpose and dispensation of blood specimen drawn

SECTION FOUR

PARENTERAL NUTRITION

When clients are unable to maintain adequate nutrition, their body stores of carbohydrates, then fats, and finally plasma and tissue protein are metabolized for energy. Protein is essential for tissue growth and repair and the replacement of body cells. Since the body does not store protein beyond that needed, its use, unless it is replaced, can result in serious nutritional deficiency that increases the risk of morbidity and mortality.

While the gastrointestinal tract is the preferred route for nutrition since it is more physiologic, less expensive, and safer, introducing nutrients intravenously (parenteral nutrition) can maintain or restore a client's nutritional health. Bypassing the normal gastrointestinal system, this route provides a source of nitrogen for those with non-functional GI tracts or those with high caloric requirements (e.g., burn clients) or acute hypoalbuminemia.

Balanced blends of nutrients (carbohydrate, fats, and protein), including vitamins and minerals, can be administered peripherally using isotonic concentrations of glucose (less than 20 percent dextrose). Peripheral formulations are incomplete and therefore insufficient for nutritionally depleted clients, and therapy is limited to less than 3 weeks. In contrast, hypertonic preparations, used to achieve tissue synthesis, repair, and growth, are nutritionally complete (total parenteral nutrition), but irritating due to their osmolality, and must be administered through a central, high-flow vein. Rapid dilution of these preparations decreases the risk of phlebitis, clot formation, and hemolysis. These preparations are useful for long-term therapy. Administration may be continuous or cyclic.

Parenteral nutrition requires special handling and management, presents greater risk for metabolic and catheter-related complications, and is the most expensive method of feeding.

RATIONALE

- To provide dextrose as source of carbohydrate to spare body protein
- To provide amino acids as source of protein to maintain or restore nitrogen balance for tissue growth and repair
- To provide lipids as source of calories and essential fatty acids
- To provide vitamins, minerals, and essential trace elements
- To meet fluid and electrolyte needs

ASSESSMENT

- Check client's height and weight and skin fold and mid-arm circumference measurements.
- Review client's dietary and health history.
- Review laboratory tests (electrolytes, lymphocyte count, serum protein and albumin, total iron binding capacity).
- Assess client's daily fluid balance.

- Check that established IV site (peripheral or central) is patent and free of signs of infection.
- Ensure that client's blood glucose level is checked every 8 hrs and remains within normal limits.
- Check that liver function tests are normal.
- Make sure parenteral formulation is refrigerated (4°C) until used.

- Make sure IV tubing and filter are changed every 24 hrs.
- Check vital signs (necessary for baseline, as reaction can occur with lipid emulsion infusion).
- Assess central infusion as indicated (based on osmolarity of admixture).

PARENTERAL NUTRITION AND LIPID INFUSION

Equipment

- Parenteral nutrition formula in bag or bottle mixed within last 24 hrs (or refrigerated)
- IV lipid solution
- Nonphthalate tubing infusion set for lipids
- IV tubing with needleless cannula
- Air-eliminating filter (0.22 μm) for *nonlipid* admixtures
- Air-eliminating filter (1.2 μm) for *lipid-containing* admixtures
- Infusion pump(s)
- Povidone-iodine swabs
- Glucometer
- Clean gloves

SAFETY ALERT

- Hyperglycemia (due to high concentration of glucose) is the most common complication of parenteral nutrition. Exogenous regular insulin remains stable, and may be added by the pharmacist to the parenteral admixture to promote glucose control.
- Since parenteral nutrition induces increased production of endogenous insulin, abrupt discontinuation can precipitate postinfusion hypoglycemia. Therapy must be weaned gradually.

Preparation

1 Examine bottle or bag for separation of emulsion, fat globules, or froth. **RATIONALE:** Do not use if these are present; contamination may have occurred.

2 Swab bottle stopper (if indicated); connect tubing with filter to solution bottle/bag, and prime tubing. **RATIONALE:** This purges system of air.

SKILL

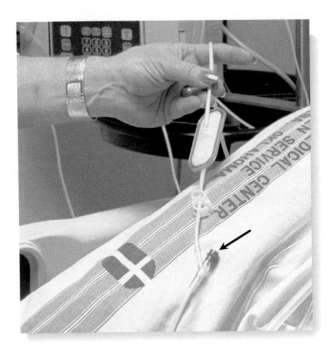

2 If piggybacking lipids into parenteral solution tubing, use port closest to client, below tubing filter. Infuse fat emulsion initially at 1 mL/min for adults. **RATIONALE:** This limits volume infused if side effects occur.

- Monitor vital signs every 10 min, observing for side effects during first 30 min of infusion. **RATIONALE:** If allergic reaction occurs, infusion should be stopped and physician notified.

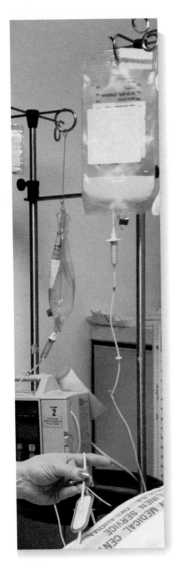

1 Prep client's central lumen cap IV site with povidone-iodine, insert tubing cannula, and initiate infusion using infusion pump. Discard any partially used bottles/bags, and use a new administration set with each unit (unless additional units are administered consecutively, in which case administration set should be changed every 24 hrs). **RATIONALE:** The dextrose and protein content of the solution creates greater potential for microbial growth; frequent set changes are required.

CLINICAL NOTE

Since lipid particles are so large, inline filters are not used when parenteral fat emulsions are infused separately. Total nutrient admixtures contain dextrose, amino acids, and lipids in one container, eliminating the need for separate lipid infusions. Use a 1.2-μm filter for these all-in-one solutions.

- Time and date of infusion
- Parenteral nutrition product administered
- Amount and rate of infusion (include on I&O sheet)
- Location and status of infusion site

- Daily weight
- Client's response (e.g., finger stick blood sugars) and nursing intervention

SECTION FIVE

BLOOD TRANSFUSION

Few conditions require transfusion of whole blood; instead, for economical and practical purposes, separate components (packed RBCs, platelets, fresh frozen plasma) are administered to correct specific deficiencies such as anemia and bleeding disorders. Because these are physiologic rather than pharmacologic substances, they require special processing, storage, and handling. Blood is typed using the ABO and Rh antigens systems for compatible cross matching with the recipient's blood. Platelet concentrates do not require cross matching, and type O (Rh negative) blood (universal donor) can be administered to recipients having any blood type.

The Food and Drug Administration (FDA) and the American Association of Blood Banks establish standards of performance for the provision of safe transfusion. Blood donors are screened, and their blood is tested for antibodies to transmittable viruses (e.g., HIV, hepatitis B and C). While the risk of contracting an infection is small, many clients planning elective surgery choose to donate their own (autologous) blood preoperatively to minimize the risk of infection and transfusion reaction. The same testing is required on autologous as on donated blood. In some cases, the client may arrange for designated or directed donation from friends or relatives. This has not been demonstrated to be safer than receiving blood donated by volunteers, and since 48 to 72 hrs are required for processing, directed donations are not suitable for emergency use.

RATIONALE

- To restore or expand circulating volume
- To improve oxygen-carrying capacity of blood
- To treat bleeding or clotting disorders
- To treat deficiencies of specific component in the client's blood (e.g., albumin)

ASSESSMENT

- Assess client's CBC (hemoglobin, hematocrit, platelets, etc.).
- Review client's history of previous reaction to blood transfusion.
- Make sure client has signed consent for blood transfusion.
- Ensure that IV site is patent with large-gauge cannula.
- Check that the number and blood type on unit match client's blood ID bracelet name, type and number, and compatibility report (confirm with another nurse).
- Make sure blood was released by blood bank no longer than 20 min ago.
- Check that blood unit date has not expired.
- Check that blood bag is free of bubbles, cloudiness, dark color, or sediment.
- Assess that client's temperature is normal and documented prior to blood transfusion.
- Make sure infusion pump is suitable for blood (older peristaltic types may cause hemolysis).

BLOOD TRANSFUSION

Equipment

- Blood unit (packed RBCs)—must be hung within 20 to 30 min after leaving blood bank refrigerator
- Bag (250 mL) of 0.9 percent saline for line flush (no substitute)
- Y-set blood tubing with filter and needleless cannula (*Note:* Tubing must be compatible with infusion device if used)
- Antimicrobial swabs
- Infusion pump (suitable for blood transfusion)
- Clean gloves
- Protective garb, if indicated (gown, goggles, mask)

SAFETY ALERT

Blood is stored in the blood bank at 1 to 6°C and, once dispensed, must be hung within 20 to 30 min. Routine transfusions should not be warmed. If warming is required, as in massive transfusions, a blood warming device is used. Blood should NEVER be warmed in hot water or a microwave. Once blood is warmed, it must be used or disposed of, as it cannot be returned to the blood bank. Hemolysis of blood occurs at temperatures above 104°F.

SKILL

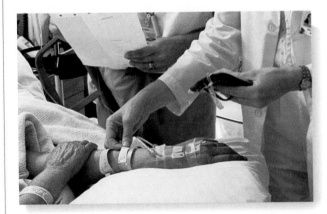

1 With another nurse, verify each unit (according to agency policy) with client's name and medical record number, blood group/Rh, and blood bank ID number, and sign confirmation of this verification on transfusion tag.

- According to agency policy, record vital signs prior to transfusion and periodically throughout, along with client assessment for any signs of transfusion reaction or fluid volume overload (e.g., cardiac client).

- Close all clamps on Y-set tubing.
- Aseptically spike bag of normal saline with one arm of Y-tubing. **RATIONALE:** Normal saline alone is used with blood. Dextrose causes cellular changes.
- Open clamps on both arms of Y-tubing to flush.
- Close clamp on free arm of Y-set (blood side).
- Open clamp of main line below tubing filter, prime tubing, then close clamp. **RATIONALE:** Tubing must be purged of air.
- Agitate blood unit bag gently. **RATIONALE:** This mixes blood cells with anticoagulant additive in bag.
- Expose port of blood unit bag; remove protective cover from free arm of Y-tubing, spike bag, and hang unit.
- Prep client's injection port and insert tubing cannula. Open clamp on Y-arm to blood unit and close clamp on Y-arm to normal saline. Load tubing into infusion pump if used. **RATIONALE:** Pump helps regulate transfusion rate.

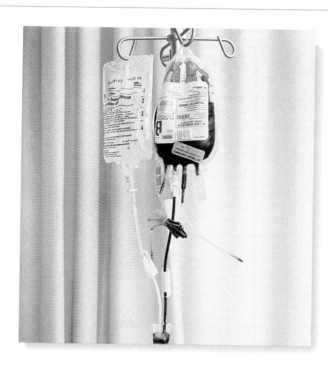

2 Open main line clamp and start transfusion, administering slowly (25 to 50 mL) for first 15 min (rate 100 mL/hr), then increase flow rate. **RATIONALE:** Slow administration limits amount infused and allows time to observe for adverse reactions. Most reactions occur in the first 15 min.

- Monitor vital signs 15 min after starting transfusion and periodically throughout transfusion; record on transfusion tag record. **RATIONALE:** Pretransfusion temperature provides baseline measure. A 1°C rise in temperature is a sign of transfusion reaction.

SAFETY ALERT

Most clients can tolerate a flow rate of 1 unit of packed cells in 1½ to 2 hrs. If client cannot tolerate completion of unit within 4 hrs, unit may be divided by the blood bank for two transfusion sessions.

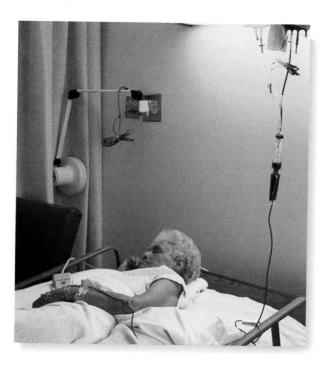

3 Observe client closely for adverse signs: chilling, backache, headache, nausea or vomiting, tachycardia, tachypnea, respiratory distress, rash, itching, hypotension. **RATIONALE:** Adverse signs necessitate immediate discontinuation of transfusion.

- Agitate blood bag each time client is checked.
- When transfusion is complete, flush tubing with normal saline.
- Use new administration set for each subsequent unit transfused.

TABLE 17-5	TRANSFUSION REACTIONS

Type	Clinical Manifestations	Nursing Interventions
Bacterial	Sudden increase in temperature Hypotension Dry, flushed skin Abdominal pain Headache Lumbar pain Sudden chill	Stop transfusion immediately and remove blood tubing. Maintain IV site; change tubing and start infusion of normal saline. Observe for shock. Monitor vital signs every 15 minutes. Insert Foley catheter and monitor urine output hourly. Notify physician and obtain order for antibiotic and steroids/shock management. Draw blood cultures before antibiotic administration. Send remaining blood and tubing to laboratory for culture and sensitivity.
Allergic	Mild: urticaria and hives, pruritus Severe: respiratory distress, wheezing Anaphylactic: shock, loss of consciousness	Stop transfusion immediately if symptoms are severe—immediate resuscitation may be necessary. Monitor vital signs for possible anaphylactic shock. If symptoms are mild, slow down transfusion and notify physician. Monitor for signs of progressive allergic reaction as transfusion continues.
Hemolytic	Severe pain in kidney region and chest Pain at needle insertion site Fever (may reach 105°F), chills, flushing Dyspnea and cyanosis Oozing of blood at IV site Headache Hypotension Hematuria	Stop transfusion immediately and remove blood tubing. Start normal saline infusion at keep-open rate with new IV tubing. Obtain vital signs. Notify Blood Bank STAT. Administer oxygen. Notify physician. Obtain orders for IV volume expansion and diuretic or vasopressor to dilate renal blood vessels to prevent acute renal tubular necrosis. Complete transfusion reaction form. Send two blood samples (from different sites), urine specimen, remaining blood and tubing, and transfusion record to laboratory. Monitor vital signs every 15 minutes for shock. Monitor urine output hourly for possible acute renal failure.

CHARTING

- Type and amount of blood administered
- Amount of normal saline infused
- Time transfusion began and ended
- Vital signs before transfusion, 15, 30, and 60 min after transfusion begins, then hourly until transfusion is completed
- Client's response to therapy
- Any unusual clinical manifestations; any nursing interventions

CRITICAL THINKING FOCUS

SECTION ONE ▪ IV Therapy Preparation

Unexpected Outcomes

- One manufacturer's product color coding does not coincide with those you have relied on in the past.

- A particular product is unreliable; staff reports chronic defects (e.g., confusing labels, leakage, separation, malfunction, expired product, contamination).

Alternative Nursing Actions

- Never rely upon color coding for identifying product. Color coding systems are not standardized. To prevent errors, read labels carefully.

- Report product defects to head nurse or supervisor so information can be relayed to appropriate department or agency (e.g., pharmacy, infection control, risk management).

SECTION TWO ▪ IV Fluid Administration

Unexpected Outcomes

- Venipuncture to initiate IV therapy is unsuccessful.

- Vein rolls and is difficult to enter.

- Vein is fragile and balloons around needle on entry.

- Phlebotomy for peripheral blood specimen is unsuccessful.

Alternative Nursing Actions

- Remove needle and dress site.
- Select another site more proximal in vein or use other extremity.
- Have client hang arm below heart level to promote venous filling.
- Apply warm packs to promote venodilation.
- Reposition tourniquet for sufficient vein engorgement.
- Push blood in vein up toward tourniquet to distend vein.
- Alter needle entry angle.
- Avoid the one-step entry method since this frequently results in through-and-through vein puncture.
- After two failed attempts, seek a more experienced person to perform venipuncture.

- Apply traction with thumb and index finger to stabilize skin and vein; maintain traction until venipuncture is complete.
- Select smaller-gauge catheter.
- Advance catheter slowly.

- Release tourniquet as soon as vein entry is evident.
- Distend vein using blood pressure cuff rather than tourniquet.
- Avoid use of tourniquet if veins are very fragile or if client is taking an anticoagulant.
- Enter vein with needle bevel down.

- Loosen tourniquet, as it may be too tight for venous flow.

■ Change position of needle: advance or withdraw slightly, but do not probe.

■ Try another Vacutainer tube; the one in use may have lost its vacuum.

■ Client develops pain and redness along vein site (phlebitis).

■ Discontinue infusion and remove catheter.
■ Apply warm compresses.
■ Start IV at another site.
■ Select large vein when administering irritating agents.
■ Anchor cannula to prevent motion in vein.

■ Infusion flow rate is sluggish.

■ Compare extremity against other extremity to rule out infiltration.
■ Try to aspirate, but do not irrigate cannula; there may be a clot at the end of cannula that could be flushed into the bloodstream.
■ Elevate bag for greater pressure if gravity infusion method is being used.
■ Reposition extremity to relieve positional obstruction (e.g., bent elbow, arm rotation).

■ Infusion site becomes pale, cool, and swollen (infiltration).

■ Do not rely on backflash of blood to determine that cannula is in vein.
■ Remove IV tubing from pump and maintain keep-open rate; lower fluid bag below IV site. If blood returns, needle is in vein, but fluid may be leaking into tissue if bevel has pierced vein wall.
■ Place tourniquet proximal to infusion site tightly enough to restrict venous blood flow. Set IV to slow rate and remove tubing from infusion pump. If infusion continues to drip, fluid is infiltrating into surrounding tissue.
■ Discontinue infusion, elevate extremity, and restart IV at another site.
■ Apply warm compresses to encourage vein dilation and absorption of infiltrated fluid.
■ Notify physician if solution contains potassium or other irritating component (e.g., 10 percent dextrose).

SECTION THREE ■ Central Venous Catheters

Unexpected Outcomes

■ Central venous catheter insertion site becomes inflamed.

Alternative Nursing Actions

■ Notify physician immediately so catheter can be discontinued if catheter-related sepsis is suspected. Antibiotic therapy may be indicated.
■ Cut tip of catheter off with sterile scissors and place in sterile container. Send to laboratory for culture and sensitivity for specific causative organism.
■ Cleanse insertion site with povidone-iodine and apply sterile dressing.

- Blood specimen cannot be aspirated even though solution flows through central venous catheter.

- Use less negative pressure on syringe when aspirating blood. Tip of catheter may be sucking against wall of vessel.
- Have client perform Valsalva maneuver to change intrathoracic pressure.
- Have client raise arms above head or change position. This can alter position of catheter.
- Change client's position.

- Air enters vascular system because central catheter is open to atmosphere; client experiences chest pain, shortness of breath, or coughing (air embolism).

- IMMEDIATELY clamp catheter (use rubber band if Groshong valve is present).
- Turn client to left side with head lower than rest of body (Trendelenburg position) to trap air in right heart.
- Notify physician STAT.
- Administer 100 percent oxygen per order.

SECTION FOUR ▪ Parenteral Nutrition

Unexpected Outcomes

- Client develops hyperglycemia.

Alternative Nursing Actions

- Monitor blood glucose levels every 4 to 6 hrs.
- Limit dextrose to less than 25 percent if possible.
- Request order for admixture of insulin to parenteral formula.
- Maintain blood glucose <200 mg/dL.
- Discuss addition of lipids as calorie source.
- Discuss need for sliding-scale insulin therapy with physician.

- Client develops hypoglycemia.

- Gradually decrease infusion when discontinuing parenteral nutrition.
- Assess blood glucose 1 hr after discontinuing parenteral nutrition.
- Infuse 10 percent dextrose in water (50 percent dextrose may be needed).

- Infusion is sluggish.

- Assess filter; plugged filter is the most common cause of infusion failure. Change filter and tubing.
- Check finger stick blood sugar.
- Observe for signs of hypoglycemia (weakness, trembling, sweating, hunger) caused by decrease in dextrose delivery.

- Electrolyte deficiencies occur.

- Limit initial parenteral nutrition to 1000 kcal/24 hrs and increase gradually.
- Provide electrolyte replacement.
- Continue to monitor electrolyes as they move intracellularly with parenteral nutrition.

SECTION FIVE ▪ Blood Transfusion

Unexpected Outcomes	Alternative Nursing Actions

Unexpected Outcomes

- Cardiac client becomes short of breath due to fluid overload during transfusion of packed RBCs.

Alternative Nursing Actions

- Reduce infusion rate.
- Place client in sitting position with feet dependent.
- Request blood bank to split packed RBC unit for two sessions of transfusion.
- Discuss with physician option of administering IV diuretic as prophylaxis.
- Discuss with physician option of CVP monitoring during transfusion.

Unexpected Outcomes

- Transfusion reaction occurs (fever/chill, urticaria, shortness of breath, back pain).

Alternative Nursing Actions

- Stop transfusion, remove administration tubing, and flush cannula cap to keep vein access, or use new IV tubing and infuse normal saline at keep-open rate.
- Check transfusion reaction form for appropriate nursing intervention per agency.
- Complete all relevant nursing actions.

Unexpected Outcomes

- Client develops only mild itching (allergic reaction) during transfusion.

Alternative Nursing Actions

- Slow down transfusion, and notify physician for orders.
- Assess client frequently during transfusion.
- Notify blood bank.
- Complete report of transfusion reaction.
- Note symptoms and interventions in client's record.

Unexpected Outcomes

- Transfusion flow is sluggish.

Alternative Nursing Actions

- Check client's IV site.
- Gently agitate blood bag to mix blood cells with anticoagulant.
- Raise blood bag higher on IV pole.
- Squeeze flexible tubing to promote blood flow.
- Adjust clamp on tubing. As blood passes over filter, more blood microaggregates clog filter and slow drip rate.
- Replace IV tubing.
- Utilize an infusion pump, especially if administering blood through a small catheter or lock.
- Apply warm pack to infusion site, as cold blood may induce venospasm.

Unexpected Outcomes

- Blood has been infusing for 4 hrs.

Alternative Nursing Actions

- Discontinue blood bag and discard or send to blood bank (according to agency policy).
- Flush peripheral cap or maintain IV with normal saline solution or ordered IV fluid.
- Monitor vital signs for complications.

SELF-CHECK EVALUATION

PART 1 ▪ Matching Items

Match the definition in column B with the correct term in column A.

Column A

_____ a. Infiltration
_____ b. Phlebitis
_____ c. Oliguria
_____ d. Hypotonic
_____ e. Osmolality
_____ f. Hydrostatic pressure
_____ g. Venipuncture
_____ h. Groshong valve
_____ i. Valsalva maneuver
_____ j. Phlebotomy

Column B

1. Obtaining a blood specimen from a vein
2. Pulling pressure of plasma proteins that maintains intravascular volume
3. Tension exerted on a vessel wall
4. Having lower osmolality than plasma
5. Establishment of an opening into a vein
6. Exhalation against a closed glottis
7. Urine production of less than 500 mL/day
8. Movement of IV fluid into the interstitial space
9. Inflammation of a vein
10. Remains closed; opens forward to positive pressure, opens backward to negative pressure

PART 2 ▪ Multiple Choice Questions

1. A winged-needle IV system is preferred for:
   a. Long-term IV use.
   b. Hypertonic fluid infusion.
   c. Transfusion of blood.
   d. Temporary infusion.

2. The most important factor to consider when selecting a vein for initiating IV therapy is that the vein site should:
   a. Be large and deep.
   b. Allow client mobility.
   c. Be most distal in the arm.
   d. Be located in a lower extremity.

3. The purpose of injecting an intradermal anesthetic before venipuncture is to:
   a. Dilate the vein.
   b. Decrease the discomfort of venipuncture.
   c. Decrease the discomfort of infusion.
   d. Prevent venospasm.

4. The administration of a hypotonic IV solution will result in:
   a. Expansion of intravascular fluid.
   b. Expansion of intracellular fluid.
   c. Contraction of intracellular fluid.
   d. Equilibration of intravascular and intracellular fluids.

5. The administration of a hypertonic IV solution will result in:

    a. Extracellular fluid expansion.
    b. Intracellular fluid expansion.
    c. Extracellular fluid contraction.
    d. Equilibration of extracellular and intracellular fluid.

6. Central venous catheters place the client at increased risk for:

    a. Phlebitis.
    b. Infiltration.
    c. Sepsis.
    d. Air embolism.

7. In order to prevent air embolism when a central venous catheter is open to the atmosphere, the nurse should:

    a. Have the client exhale.
    b. Have the client inhale.
    c. Unclamp the catheter lumen.
    d. Place the client in a Fowler's position.

8. The unique feature of the peripherally inserted central catheter (PICC) is that it:

    a. Is tunneled subcutaneously.
    b. Requires no maintenance flushing.
    c. Requires no dressing.
    d. Can be inserted by a specialized nurse.

9. Care for the client with a PICC with Groshong valve includes:

    a. Daily dressing changes.
    b. Weekly maintenance with heparin injection.
    c. Pulsating irrigation technique.
    d. Forceful irrigation technique.

10. Of the following blood specimens, the one that should not be collected with a Vacutainer is a specimen from a:

    a. Peripheral vein.
    b. PICC with Groshong valve.
    c. Percutaneously inserted central catheter.
    d. Client with bleeding tendencies.

11. The client who wishes to receive blood donated by a family member should be informed that:

    a. There is decreased risk of disease transmission.
    b. Typing and cross matching of the donated blood is not necessary.
    c. The donated blood is no safer than random donor blood.
    d. There will be no delay in availability of the donated blood.

12. When administering blood, the tubing is primed with:

    a. Normal saline.
    b. 5% D/W.
    c. 5% D/LR.
    d. 10% D/W.

13. A blood transfusion should be started at a rate of:

    a. 5 mL/hr.
    b. 10 mL/hr.
    c. 50 mL/hr.
    d. 100 mL/hr.

14. When suspecting a possible transfusion reaction, the nurse should first:
   a. Notify the physician for emergency orders.
   b. Obtain a urine specimen and notify the blood bank.
   c. Discontinue the transfusion and tubing.
   d. Switch the infusion to the priming normal saline.

PART 3 ▪ Critical Thinking Application

Mrs. Owens, a 34-year-old client with morbid obesity, has been admitted to your unit following exploratory abdominal surgery for lysis of adhesions. She has a nasogastric tube for decompression and is receiving intravenous fluids (half saline with dextrose and potassium chloride) at a rate of 125 mL/hr. On postoperative admission assessment, you note that her arms and legs are edematous, though she is grossly overweight and differentiation between edema and obesity is often difficult. Her IV is infusing without a problem (drip rate is maintained and pump alarms are not sounding occlusion), but her arm appears swollen and is cool to the touch.

1. Evaluating the IV, what are the implications of a swollen arm that feels cool to the touch when no pump alarm is sounding?

2. Based on this data, what are indications of infiltration?

3. What assessment techniques would assist the nurse in validating proper IV infusion?

18

INTRAVENOUS MEDICATIONS

INTRODUCTION

The advent of intravenous (IV) maintenance devices has led to ever increasing utilization of the intravenous route for continuous or intermittent delivery of medications. The intravenous route provides immediate and total drug absorption into the venous circulation, with almost instantaneous distribution of a high concentration of drug to tissues and prompt physiologic results; therefore it is ideal for achieving and maintaining predictable drug levels for desired therapeutic effects. It is especially useful for administering irritating agents when properly diluted, and for emergency situations when immediate effects are desired.

While the intravenous route is more comfortable for the client than are other parenteral routes, it is the most hazardous. Many incompatibilities exist among medications and IV solutions. Adverse or toxic responses are more likely to occur (especially with rapid injection) and must be recognized immediately so that remedial actions can be initiated. Safe administration requires strict adherence to pharmacologic guidelines, diligent attention to the Five Rights of Medication Administration (see Chapter 15), and vigilant client monitoring.

(continued on next page)

As with all medications, a physician prescribes the IV drug and IV solution as a signed written order in the client's chart. The order includes the medication and its dosage, route, and frequency of administration. Before giving medication intravenously, the nurse first must validate that this skill falls within the scope of nursing practice and must adhere to agency restrictions regarding professional qualifications and the handling of particular medications.

The nurse must consider the combined directives in the preparation protocols for medication administration (see Chapter 15), parenteral medications (see Chapter 16), and intravenous fluids and blood (see Chapter 17), as well as the following guidelines for the preparation of IV medications.

PREPARATION PROTOCOL: FOR INTRAVENOUS MEDICATIONS SKILLS

Complete the following steps before each skill.

1. Verify that medication is consistent with physician's order in client's record.
2. Evaluate pertinent lab or other client data relevant to drug being administered (e.g., serum drug levels, vital signs, ECG, concomitant medications).
3. Validate that medication is appropriate for intravenous use.
4. Carefully note medication manufacturer's guidelines for IV infusion or injection.
5. Determine compatibility of medication with all components of current infusion system.
6. Inspect medication for expiration date, discoloration, and cloudiness.
7. Wash hands.
8. Prepare medication according to manufacturer's instructions (dilution is frequently required).
9. Prepare medication label and attach it to container if indicated, adding date, time, and signature.
10. Verify client's identity (check identaband and allergy bracelet and have client state name).
11. Provide privacy; explain procedure and purpose to client.
12. Position client for comfort and optimal visibility for skill performance.
13. Verify patency of established IV site.
14. Program pump/delivery system infusion parameters (if indicated).
15. Don clean gloves.

COMPLETION PROTOCOL: FOR INTRAVENOUS MEDICATIONS SKILLS

Make sure the following steps have been completed.

1. Flush intermittent peripheral or central catheter infusion lock using positive-pressure technique.
2. Dispose of equipment in puncture-resistant biohazard receptacle.
3. Remove and dispose of gloves.
4. Wash hands.
5. Document IV medication, dose, and time of administration on appropriate forms (e.g., medication administration record [MAR], chart, intake and output sheet).
6. Monitor and document client's response to therapy (e.g., vital signs, pain rating), and intervene accordingly.

I V   M E D I C A T I O N S

Intravenous (IV) medications are administered through an established intermittent or continuous peripheral or central intravenous system by a variety of mechanical and manual techniques. Since IV systems are closed systems and must be maintained as such, tubing injection ports or locks must be disinfected just before entry for medication administration. For safety and accuracy, timed drug delivery (e.g., piggyback) should be regulated by an infusion control device. While pumps are an adjunct to this aspect of nursing care, they do not relieve the nurse of responsibility for monitoring and ensuring safe administration of intravenous medications.

Methods of IV Medication Delivery

Three methods are used to administer medication through an established intravenous system:

- **Continuous infusion** of medication, accomplished by admixing medication with a large volume of infusate to be infused slowly over a period of time (e.g., heparin drip). These solutions are usually prepared by the pharmacist.
- **Intermittent infusion** of medication (e.g., antibiotics) diluted in a volume of diluent into an established primary line by piggyback (secondary) or volume control device.
- **Injection** of medication directly into an IV system by IV push, slowly over a designated time period (e.g., Lasix), or rapidly by IV bolus into a primary infusion via tubing port or through an existing peripheral or central catheter cap or lock.

Delivering medication intravenously is a very serious nursing responsibility. The nurse must be familiar with the intended as well as possible adverse effects of the medication and must adhere to all protocols for safe administration. Once in the circulation a drug cannot be retrieved, and client responses may be grave. There is no margin of error.

RATIONALE

- To administer medication when traditional routes are inadequate or inappropriate
- To administer medications that irritate or are destroyed by the gastrointestinal system
- To administer medications for immediate drug action
- To achieve high drug concentration
- To maintain constant blood levels of medication

ASSESSMENT

- Check that drug is indicated for intravenous injection or infusion.
- Review special precautions or contraindications referred to in drug manufacturer's guidelines.
- Review guidelines for medication preparation and storage.
- Assess type of administration set, solution, and infusion control device in use.
- Know compatibility and stability of medication with primary infusing solution and all components of infusion system.
- Review type and amount diluent to be used.
- Check time interval over which drug is to be administered.
- Check availability of specific drug antidotes (e.g., naloxone) and emergency supplies.
- Assess that existing infusion site is patent and free of signs of infiltration, phlebitis, or infection.
- Assess client's understanding of rationale for therapy.
- Establish baseline vital signs for evaluating response to patient-controlled infusion of opioid.

SAFETY ALERT

- All precautions mandated in the preparation protocols for Chapters 15, 16, and 17 also apply to the following skills for administration of IV medications.
- Not all parenteral medications are intended for intravenous use. Refer to an IV medication text when in doubt.

IV PIGGYBACK (SECONDARY) MEDICATION

Equipment

- Pharmacy-prepared medication bag with label, including name of medication, date, time, expiration date, rate for infusion, and client's name.
- Secondary administration set (short tubing and needleless cannula)
- Established compatible primary infusion
- Extension hook to lower primary infusion (if indicated)
- Alcohol swab

SKILL

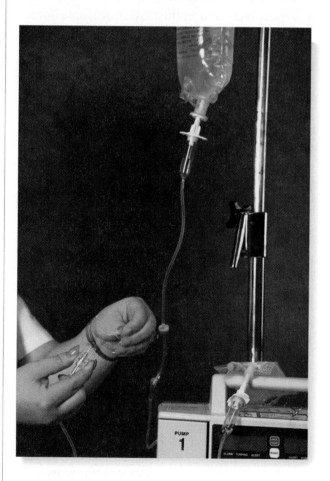

1 Clamp secondary administration set short tubing and spike medication bag. **RATIONALE:** Clamping tubing prevents loss of medication.

- Swab injection port of primary tubing (above infusion pump, or on loaded tubing cassette), remove protector, and insert needleless cannula of secondary piggyback tubing. **RATIONALE:** This establishes communication between medication and primary tubing.

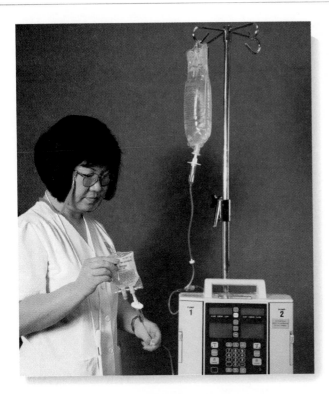

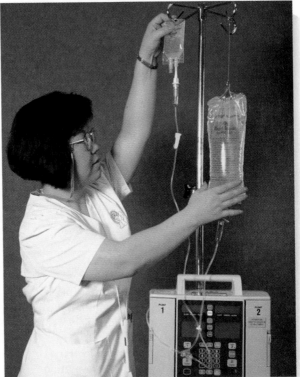

2 Momentarily lower secondary bag below primary bag, open clamp on secondary tubing, allowing primary solution to flow retrograde into secondary bag tubing (back-priming) until drip chamber is one-third full; then reclamp secondary tubing or hang piggyback (secondary) medication bag on IV pole and back-prime secondary tubing using infusion pump back-prime control (if present). **RATIONALE:** Retrograde priming prevents loss of medication and environmental exposure of drug.

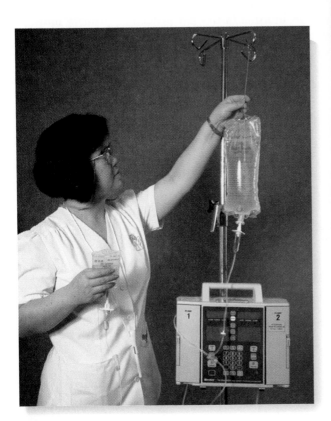

3 Lower primary bag using extension hook.

4 Hang secondary bag on IV pole. **RATIONALE:** Primary solution ceases flow because of increased hydrostatic pressure in higher secondary bag. *Note:* Some infusion pumps control secondary infusions without necessitating bag height differentials.

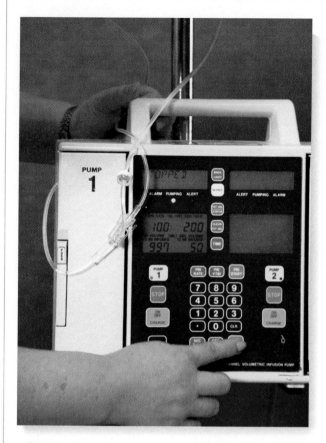

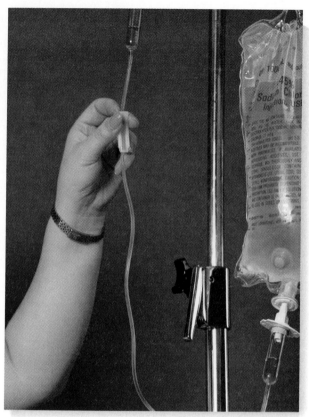

5 Program secondary settings of infusion pump, if used (volume and rate to be infused).

6 Unclamp secondary tubing and initiate secondary infusion to run independently; primary infusion will resume at its preset rate when secondary volume has been infused.

SAFETY ALERT

To check for extravasation of medication, place a tourniquet proximal to peripheral infusion site tight enough to restrict venous blood flow. Set tubing roller clamp to keep-open (or slow) rate, and remove tubing from infusion pump. If the infusion continues to drip, fluid is extravasating into the surrounding tissue.

IV MEDICATION USING VOLUME CONTROL SET

Equipment

- Primary IV solution compatible with drug to be infused
- Calibrated volume control set (e.g., Volu-Trole)
- Extension tubing with Luer Lock connector (if necessary)

- Prescribed medication prepared in syringe with needleless cannula
- Alcohol swab
- Label with medication, date, time, and nurse's initials

SKILL

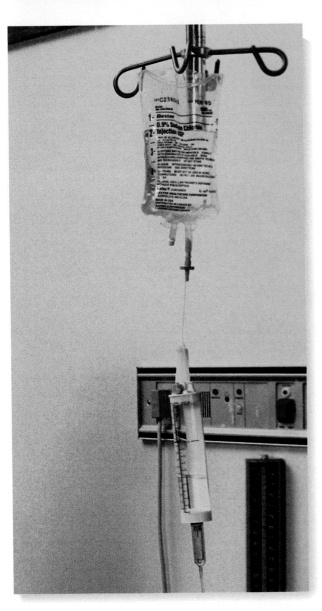

1 Add extension tubing to volume control set (if necessary). Close both clamps on volume control set tubing (above and below volume chamber). Open chamber's air vent by turning clamp located on top of volume chamber. **RATIONALE:** This allows air displacement by fluid.

- Spike IV bag with volume control set tubing and hang.
- Open upper clamp on control set tubing and fill chamber with IV solution so chamber is one-third full, then close upper clamp. Open lower clamp, squeeze drip chamber underneath volume set to fill half-full, prime tubing, then close clamp. Attach tubing to client's IV site cannula and initiate slow flush infusion.

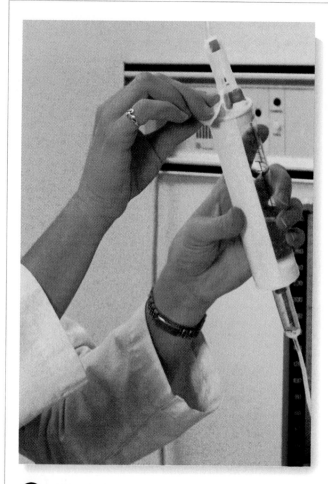

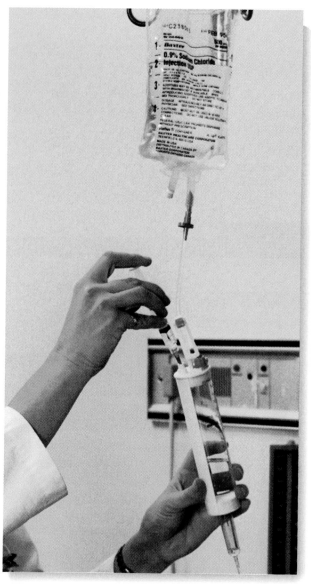

2 Swab injection port located on top of volume chamber with antimicrobial swab. **RATIONALE:** This action prevents contamination before injection of medication.

3 Inject prepared medication into chamber and agitate gently to mix medication with solution in chamber. Dilute medication (per order or PDR instructions) if necessary by opening upper clamp and adding additional fluid from IV bag (e.g., 500 mg medication in 50 mL solution).

- Open clamp on volume control set and adjust drip rate as prescribed for medication administration (e.g., number of gtts per minute).

- Affix medication label on volume control set (medication, dosage, and time medication infusion began). **RATIONALE:** Label alerts others to medication being delivered.

BEYOND THE SKILL

Adding Medication to IV Fluid

The addition (admixture) of medication to an IV solution for continuous administration is usually performed by the agency pharmacist according to standards established by the American Society of Health System Pharmacists (ASHP) and Occupational Safety and Health Administration (OSHA). Special precautions for this procedure include preparation in a laminar airflow environment (clean air center), strict adherence to requirements of asepsis, safety regarding components' stability and compatibility, proper dilution of agents, and control of extraneous particle addition to the admixture. Only under unusual circumstances will the nurse be called upon to compound a medication with parenteral solution. Refer to agency policy and approved list of medications allowed for admixture.

For admixture:

- Prepare prescribed medication in syringe according to insert or PDR.
- Prep injection port of compatible IV solution bag.
- Inject medication into bag, maintaining aseptic technique.
- Squeeze injection port to clear it of medication.
- Gently agitate bag to thoroughly mix IV solution and medication.
- Hold bag against both dark and light backgrounds to inspect for any precipitate.
- Affix medication label to IV bag (include medication, dosage, date, time, and initials).
- Insert IV tubing into bag and proceed with appropriate rate of administration as ordered.

After adding an administration set, the admixed solution must be infused or discarded within 24 hrs.

IV MEDICATION BY INJECTION (IV PUSH)

Equipment

- Syringe with medication, properly diluted, if indicated (*Note:* Medication and its diluent must be compatible with primary infusion solution)
- Two syringes (1 mL normal saline solution each) with needleless cannulas, for pre- and postmedication flush of the peripheral lock
- Two syringes (5 mL normal saline solution each) for central line pre- and postmedication flush
- One syringe (2 mL dilute heparin, 100 U/mL) for central line terminal flush, if indicated
- Antimicrobial swabs (povidone-iodine for central venous catheter lumen)
- Clean gloves
- Watch with second hand

SAFETY ALERT

Always use needleless products when accessing IV ports. If you must use a needle for injection into IV systems, select one no longer than 1 inch and no smaller (finer caliber) than 25 gauge so that the needle will not break and enter the system.

SKILL

IV Push into Peripheral Lock

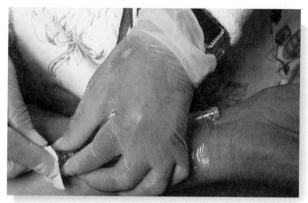

1 Prep resealable peripheral lock. Unclamp short catheter extension tubing of peripheral lock (if present) and inject saline (briefly aspirate to check for patency, then flush), noting swelling at insertion site. **RATIONALE:** Presence of blood and absence of swelling at catheter insertion site indicate that needle and infusion are probably in vein and not in surrounding tissue.

- Insert medication syringe cannula into lock injection port.

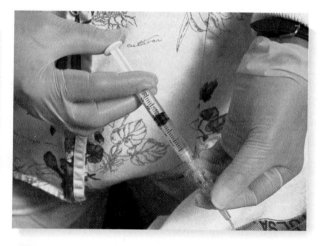

2 Note watch second hand; inject medication in allotments, timing administration rate (e.g., 0.1 mL q15sec) according to drug manufacturer's instruction (see medication insert or PDR). **RATIONALE:** Slow injection into client's circulation allows time for medication to be buffered and diluted, preventing "speed shock." It also allows observation of client's response.

- Prep lock again and flush system with 1 mL normal saline solution.

CLINICAL NOTE

Use positive-pressure technique when removing the flush syringe from a peripheral or central lumen cap. Clamp the lumen before removing the cannula (if present) or withdraw the syringe as you complete the saline or dilute heparin flush in order to prevent negative-pressure aspiration of blood into lock or catheter.

IV Push into Central Venous Catheter

SAFETY ALERT

For central venous catheter (SASH technique):

- Always use povidone-iodine to prep central venous catheter lumen ports.
- Central catheters with Groshong valves do not require lumen clamps or heparin maintenance.

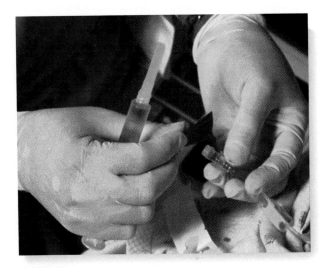

 1 Prep central lumen cap with povidone-iodine. **RATIONALE:** To prevent entry of microorganisms into the circulation.

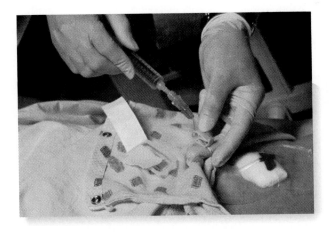

2 Use SASH (saline, administration, saline, heparin) technique.

- S = Unclamp lumen, insert cannula of 5-mL syringe of saline, briefly aspirate, then flush. **RATIONALE:** Presence of blood indicates that lumen is patent.
- A = Prep cap and administer medication as in previous skill.
- S = Prep cap and flush lumen with 5 mL saline.
- H = Follow with injection of 2 mL dilute heparin, using positive-pressure technique. Reclamp lumen. **RATIONALE:** To maintain lumen patency.

CLINICAL NOTE

Before administering any medication through an existing infusion, the nurse must validate intravenous line placement. Blood flashback is not a reliable indicator. To validate peripheral access, place a tourniquet proximal to the primary infusion; slow the infusion drip rate and remove tubing from infusion pump. Make sure the infusion slows or stops before injecting the IV medication.

To administer IV medication into an existing infusion:

- Insert medication syringe into lowest injection port (nearest client) of tubing.
- Temporarily clamp primary tubing with nondominant hand because this prevents retrograde injection of medication. This action is not necessary if pump is used to deliver primary infusion.
- Inject medication in evenly spaced increments (e.g., 0.2 mL at a time), then allow primary solution to flush increment toward client; repeat process until completed. This flushing of small increments prevents inadvertent delivery of a discrete mass as a bolus.

SAFETY ALERT

In contrast to IV push, an IV bolus of a drug is rapidly injected in order to achieve an immediate desired drug level, usually for emergency situations. Toxic levels of drug can result in speed shock and cardiac arrest. Emergency equipment and antidotes must be readily available. Always refer to the pharmaceutical company's instruction for IV drug injection before administering.

CHARTING

- Date and time of administration
- Dosage and dilution of medication
- Method of IV drug administration (e.g., IVPB, IVP)
- Rate of continuous infusion
- Pre- and postmedication flush solution (e.g., normal saline) if indicated for compatibility and for maintaining patency of site

- IV site status
- Pre- and postmedication client responses (e.g., vital signs, client's pain rating, location and character of pain)

SECTION TWO

PATIENT-CONTROLLED ANALGESIA

The experience of pain is a mixture of physical sensation, physiologic changes, and psychosocial factors. The pain source may be mechanical, chemical, thermal, electric, or ischemic. Sensory nerve endings in the periphery (nociceptors) receive the stimulus and send messages to the spinal cord. Nonopioid analgesics interrupt these pain impulses.

In the spinal cord, the messages are relayed along sensory pathways that ascend to the thalamus. Here, the autonomic nervous system is activated. Sensations then travel to the parietal lobe of the cerebral cortex where they are interpreted, the person becomes aware, and almost instantaneously responses are activated.

The client's interpretation of pain is influenced by

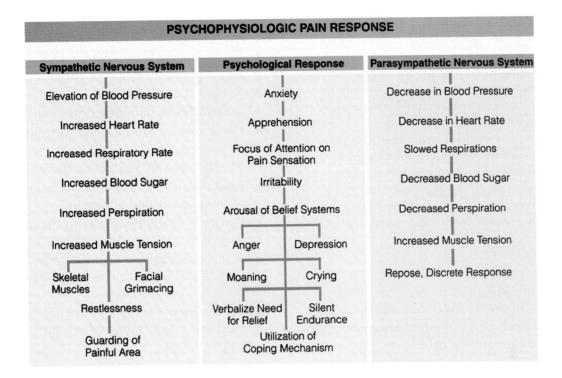

PSYCHOPHYSIOLOGIC PAIN RESPONSE

Sympathetic Nervous System	Psychological Response	Parasympathetic Nervous System
Elevation of Blood Pressure	Anxiety	Decrease in Blood Pressure
Increased Heart Rate	Apprehension	Decrease in Heart Rate
Increased Respiratory Rate	Focus of Attention on Pain Sensation	Slowed Respirations
Increased Blood Sugar	Irritability	Decreased Blood Sugar
Increased Perspiration	Arousal of Belief Systems	Decreased Perspiration
Increased Muscle Tension	Anger / Depression	Increased Muscle Tension
Skeletal Muscles / Facial Grimacing	Moaning / Crying	Repose, Discrete Response
Restlessness	Verbalize Need for Relief / Silent Endurance	
Guarding of Painful Area	Utilization of Coping Mechanism	

culture, previous experiences with pain, beliefs about self, interpretation of the future, present environment, and others in that environment. Finally, intensity of pain is influenced by what the sensation means to the client, as well as the client's level of anxiety, degree of fatigue, and number of other environmental stressors.

Acute physical pain due to illness, injury, or surgery, while it is temporary and subsides with time, arouses autonomic nervous system and psychological responses that can have a negative effect on recovery, causing serious complications such as hypoventilation and atelectasis, delayed mobility, deep vein thrombosis, and paralytic ileus. Pain interferes with the work necessary to prevent such complications; timely and adequate pain management facilitates recovery. Chronic pain, such as that experienced with cancer, is prolonged (defined as lasting more than 6 mo) and persists at a static or increasing level of intensity. It serves no purpose, and depletes the person's emotional and cognitive energies and quality of life.

Opioid analgesics interfere with the brain's perception of pain, as well as spinal cord transmission of painful stimuli to the brain. Thus, these drugs may be helpful in the management of both acute and chronic pain because they make the intensity of the pain manageable even while the client is still aware of the pain.

The promotion of comfort and alleviation of pain is one of the most important goals of nursing care. Indeed, in most cases, the nurse has the power to relieve pain or to withhold pain relief. Unfortunately, studies reveal that not only is pain underreported, but also, commonly, analgesics are underutilized and pain is inadequately treated in all settings. These studies have also given us new awareness of the pain phenomenon and effective options for its management. When pain relief is delayed, the client requires larger doses of medication than would have been necessary had intervention been started earlier. The client is also at greater risk for adverse events as a consequence of requiring higher doses.

Margo McCaffery has defined pain as "whatever the patient experiencing pain says it is, existing whenever he says it does." Since pain is a subjective experience, the nurse is totally dependent upon the client to describe the sensation of pain, to identify its location, and to know how much analgesia is required to relieve it. It follows that clients can best monitor and meet their own pain management needs.

Patient-controlled analgesia (PCA) is one of the most successful methods of pain relief because it permits the client to control the delivery of an analgesic and maintain therapeutic blood levels of the drug. This method also reduces time-consuming nursing activities. Clients do not over-medicate, but in fact use less medication with PCA, enjoy quicker recovery, and experience fewer complications. When clients are in control of their symptoms, or their lives with persistent symptoms, they are freed to improve their quality of life through achieving other goals.

PCA uses an electronically controlled programmable infusion syringe-pump system that is piggybacked into an established IV line. After a loading dose for effective analgesia and safe client response is determined, the PCA is programmed to deliver an analgesic (usually an opioid) at a continuous basal rate, independent of the primary infusion. Built-in features allow client-initiated boluses of pain medication to be delivered independently or in addition to a basal analgesic infusion. Safety features include a security mechanism that prohibits tampering with programmed pump controls. Finally, the PCA pump records the number of times the bolus button is activated, and the cumulative dose of medication delivered.

As with other parenteral medications, the physician orders the predetermined analgesic maintenance basal dose, initiated bolus doses, and a set lockout interval of 5 to 10 min during which the PCA pump cannot be activated. This allows time for an administered dose to have its effect and prevents inadvertent overdosage due to boluses.

RATIONALE

- To promote client's autonomy in pain control
- To avoid drug peaks and troughs associated with other parenteral routes of administration
- To keep narcotic within therapeutic levels
- To shorten postoperative recovery period and prevent complications of immobility
- To improve quality of life and decrease client's anxiety around pain control issues

ASSESSMENT

- Assess client's candidacy for PCA use.
- Assess client's medical or surgical condition.
- Review client allergies.
- Assess client's pain description and rating.
- Check and record baseline vital signs.
- Review client's experience with and effectiveness of adjunctive therapies.
- Assess client's ability to self-administer patient-controlled analgesia.
- Ensure availability of specific drug antidotes (e.g., naloxone) and emergency supplies.
- Assess existing infusion site status (should be patent and free of signs of infiltration, phlebitis, or infection).
- Make sure primary maintenance infusion solution is compatible with medication to be administered.

CLINICAL NOTE

There are several tools for assessing the degree of pain a client is experiencing. Help the client select an appropriate tool; then, whichever scale is chosen, maintain its use throughout the course of pain control.

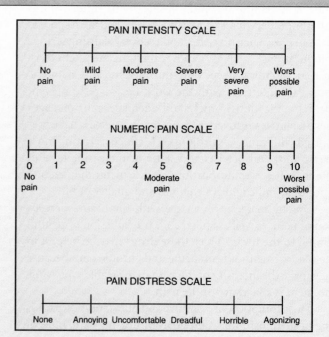

Examples of pain scales. Acute Pain Management: *Operative or medical procedures and trauma.* US Department of Health and Human Services, Public Health Service, pp. 116–117.

PCA

Equipment

- Prepared primary infusion set with delivery pump
- PCA infuser pump (refer to manufacturer's instructions)
- Prescribed medication cartridge or vial and injector (usually morphine, 30-mL injector, 1- or 5-mg/mL concentration, or Demerol, 30-mL injector, 10-mg/mL concentration)
- PCA administration tubing
- Extension set with Luer Lock adapter

SAFETY ALERT

If vial or injector is cracked and unusable, discard contents according to agency protocol in the presence of another licensed nurse and sign off on narcotic record. Dispose of vial/injector in bio-hazard sharps container. Replace with new vial.

Preparation

1 Prepare client by explaining rationale and specific functions of PCA.

2 Assemble prescribed PCA medication cartridge following instructions on vial carton.

- Snap caps from injector (plunger with long needle) and vial.

SKILL

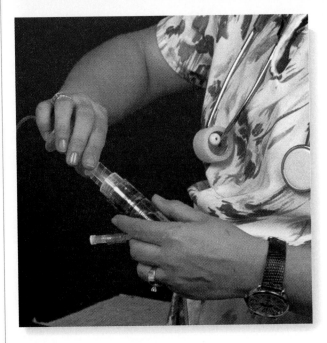

1 Connect plunger to cartridge by twisting them together.

- Remove air from vial by pushing on plunger.
- Secure back-check valve on cartridge/injector and tighten PCA set to back-check valve before proceeding. **RATIONALE:** Back-check valve must be attached to prevent accidental overdosage due to cracked or malpositioned PCA vial injector.

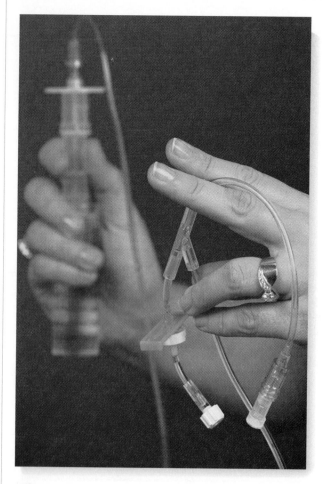

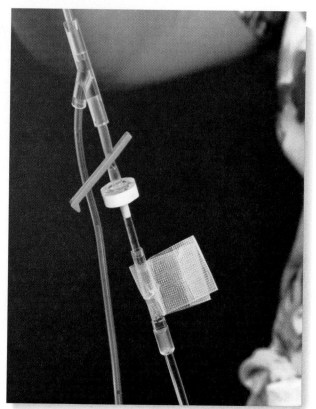

② Prime PCA tubing with medication only to the Y, then clamp tubing. **RATIONALE:** Overdose could occur if entire tubing is primed with medication.

③ Attach primary maintenance IV securely to unprimed Y-arm of PCA tubing. **RATIONALE:** To establish primary infusion.

- Clamp PCA tubing and prime short arm and lower tubing of PCA set with maintenance IV solution. **RATIONALE:** This clears air from remainder of tubing.
- Unlock and open door of PCA pump. Activate drive release mechanism by pinching spring-loaded lever and move drive assembly to uppermost position.

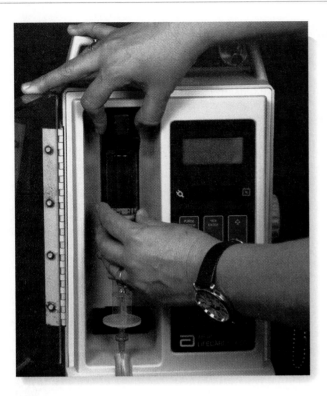

4 Load vial/injector into holder by moving drive assembly downward (position so vial calibrations are visible). Clamp securely, listening for a click. **RATIONALE:** Click indicates that vial/injector is properly inserted and locked into position.

- Rotate vial/injector to inspect for leakage or cracks. **RATIONALE:** Improper loading may cause vial/injector to crack. Vial/injector may not leak until delivery pressure is applied. Cracked vial/injector may cause overdelivery of medication to client.

PATIENT CONTROLLED ANALGESIA (PCA)—USING THE PCA INFUSION PUMP

DATE:	TIME:	DRUG ALLERGIES:

A. DRUG/CONCENTRATION: **Check One**
  Morphine = 1 mg/mL .... ☐
  Meperidine = 10 mg/mL.. ☐
  Other _____ _____ = mg/mL .... ☐

B. PCA/BASAL (Patient Controlled with Background Continuous Infusion)
  Please specify doses in mL rather than mg when ordering.

  1. Specify DOSE (patient controlled): _____ mL
     Pump range is 0.1–9.9 mL
     Suggested dose: Morphine   0.5–1.5 mL (0.5–1.5 mg)
                       Meperidine 0.5–1.0mL (5–10mg)

  2. Specify DELAY (PCA dose lockout interval): _____ min
     Pump range is 3–60 min
     Suggested interval: 10–15 min

  3. Specify BASAL RATE (continuous infusion): _____ mL/hr
     Pump range is 0.0–10.0 mL/hr
     Suggested continuous rate: Morphine   1.0–2.5 mL/hr (1.0–2.5 mg/hr)
                                Meperidine 1.0–1.5 mL/hr (10–15 mg/hr)

  4. Specify 1 HOUR LIMIT (maximum combined PCA + basal rate): _____ mL
     Pump range is 1.0–30 mL
     Suggested limit: Morphine   5–10 mL/hr (5–10 mg)
                  Meperidine 4.0–5.5 mL/hr (40–50 mg)

  5. Specify BOLUS dose (initial loading dose) if desired: _____ mL
     Specify if bolus dose may be repeated and frequency/interval:
     _____

     Pump range is 0.0–9.9 mL
     Suggested bolus dose: Morphine   3–5 mL (3–5 mg)
                     Meperidine 2.0–2.5 mL (20–25 mg)

C. Additional PCA orders: _____
_____

D. If patient persistently complains of inadequate analgesia, notify Physician.

  Physician's Signature: _____

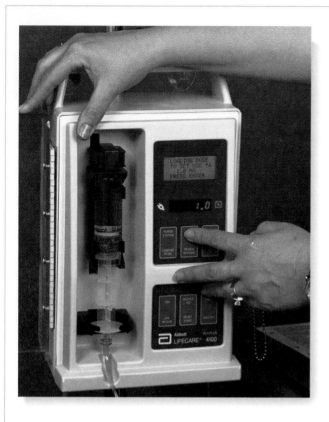

5 Following prescribed parameters, input and validate drug and dose by responding to PCA screen (e.g., "Drug—morphine 1 mg? Yes or No."). Then, follow pump commands to program prescribed dosing:

- Calculate number of milliliters needed for correct milligram dose.
- Set loading dose (e.g., morphine sulfate 2 mg), bolus dose (e.g., 0.5 mg), and basal rate (e.g., 2 mg per hour).
- Set prescribed lockout interval (period during which PCA infuser cannot be activated; e.g., 10 min).
- Set prescribed hourly limit of medication client can receive.
- Connect terminal Luer Lock of tubing to client's IV cannula and initiate primary infusion. Check that tubing clamps are open.

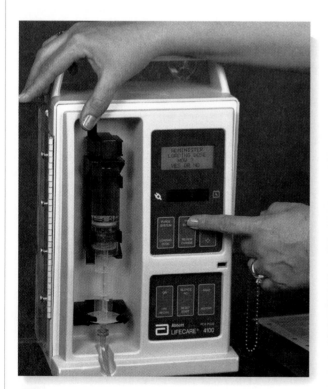

6 Press and release LOADING DOSE to administer. **RATIONALE:** Loading dose is first dose given to client, initiating pain management.

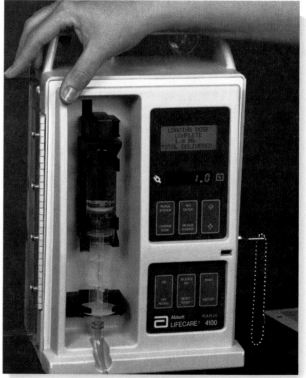

7 Check that display screen shows loading dose volume delivered. Monitor client's response after loading dose.

SAFETY ALERT

If it is necessary to administer any medication that is incompatible with the PCA infusion, you must establish a second IV site.

SEDATION SCALE

1. Client is awake and alert, initiates conversation.
2. Client is occasionally drowsy, but responsive.
3. Client is drowsy, but arousable. May drift off to sleep after being aroused.
4. Client shows minimal or no response to stimulus.

Note: This scale is an example of a sedation assessment that may be used in your facility.

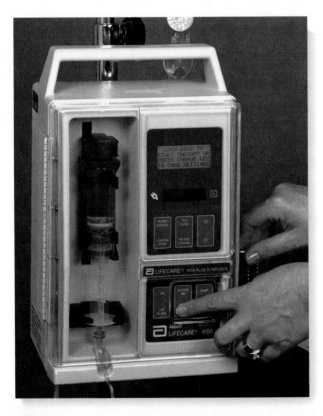

8 Review commands you have programmed, and reset if necessary. (*Note:* Have another nurse double-check your entries.)

- Close and lock security door to initiate client control. Remove key and place with narcotic keys or follow agency protocol. **RATIONALE:** Door must be locked to read READY message. This indicates infuser is now in client control mode and first dose is available to client.

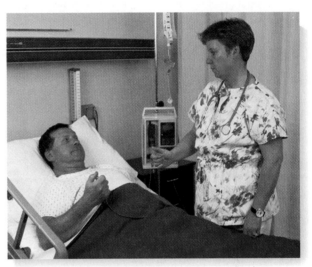

9 Hand control button to client, and review PCA instructions with client. **RATIONALE:** This provides opportunity for clarification if necessary. Remind client that nobody else should activate pump and to inform nurse if there is need for assistance, if pump alarms, or if pain is unrelieved.

- Monitor client's pain and sedation ratings regularly as directed:
  —If sedation level is 2, record VS, pain rating, and sedation level qh × 4, then q4h.
  —For escalation therapy, record VS, pain rating, and sedation level qh × 2, then q4h.
  —For respiratory rate <10, stop pump and notify physician; also check VS and pulse oximetry.
  —For respiratory rate <8, stop pump, give naloxone as prescribed, and notify physician.

CLINICAL NOTE

- The incorporation of noninvasive and nonpharmacologic approaches to pain management can help to reduce the client's perception of and reaction to pain, and to enhance the analgesic effect of medication and the health status of the client. Options may include the use of deep breathing, visualization, and imagery, and physical agents such as electric stimulators, massage-vibration or biofeedback techniques, and various adjunct therapies such as cold or heat.

- The body also has biochemical pathways (endorphins, catecholamines, and cortisol) that act as psychophysiologic linkages to produce a therapeutic placebo response. Various types of emotional and cognitive behavioral interaction between caregiver and client (or client and self) can invoke potentially powerful and independent effects, positive or negative (nocebo effect), through this placebo response. While there is no complete explanation for this neuroanatomic/biochemical response, studies suggest that it is mediated by endogenous endorphins.

- Other inexpensive, notably nontoxic, and ethically sound therapeutic strategies include:
  - Rituals that convey meaning and bring comfort through their simple predictability (e.g., taking vital signs, a special greeting, or wearing a particular uniform)
  - Interest in the whole person and interacting over time
  - Caring, sensitivity, and empathy
  - Being viewed as reliable and trustworthy
  - Engaging the client in decision making
  - Adapting to the client's needs, values, and life goals

CHARTING

- Cartridge medication/concentration (e.g., morphine 1 mg/mL)
- Medication, date, time, and amount of loading dose
- PCA basal (continuous) infusion dose
- PCA bolus dose and lockout interval
- Total dose given over 8-hr period (Press CLEAR VOLUME to read)
- Client's pain rating and other response, including vital signs as directed

CRITICAL THINKING FOCUS

SECTION ONE ■ IV Medications

Unexpected Outcomes

- Extravasation of medication occurs.

Alternative Nursing Actions

- Discontinue infusion; attempt to aspirate drug.
- Apply ice compress to area.
- Research medication; some agents have specific antidotes for extravasation injury.
- Notify physician.
- Administer irritating or vesicant medications through a central venous catheter.

- Piggyback (secondary) bag does not infuse adequately.

- Check that primary IV bag is lower than secondary bag (if infusion device requires).
- Ensure that cannula is positioned properly in primary injection port and secondary bag is sufficiently spiked.

- Solution in primary IV tubing is incompatible with medication to be administered via secondary piggyback.

- Prior to administering medication, flush primary tubing with solution compatible with medication (e.g., normal saline, 5 percent D/W).
- Piggyback separate compatible flush fluid and run during drug administration (e.g., IV push).

- Solution infuses sluggishly through peripheral lock.

- Check extremity for swelling or pain due to possible extravasation.
- Gently turn lock to establish flow.
- Reposition client's extremity.
- Initiate new IV site.

SECTION TWO ▪ Patient-Controlled Analgesia

Unexpected Outcomes

- Client experiences inadequate pain control when using bolus method PCA.

Alternative Nursing Actions

- Consider combining on-demand bolus with continuous basal infusion of analgesic.
- Add continuous basal infusion to on-demand bolus of medication only at night to maintain blood level of medication during sleep.
- Incorporate nonpharmacologic physical approaches to pain management (transcutaneous electrical nerve stimulation [TENS], heat or cold, biofeedback), change client's position, provide backrub.
- Add cognitive or behavioral methods of pain control (relaxation, imagery, deep breathing).

- Client experiences breakthrough pain when using continuous infusion PCA for chronic pain control.

- Discuss need to increase dose of opioid as tolerance develops.
- Administer additional prescribed PRN opioid or nonopioid medication for breakthrough pain.

- Client develops side effects from opioid analgesic (bradypnea, hypotension, nausea and vomiting, dizziness).

- Monitor client's response to therapy closely and regularly.
- Report client's response to physician so adjustment can be made.
- Withhold one or two doses until side effects resolve.
- Have client call for assistance to ambulate.
- Consider using bolus-only method of PCA.
- Consider alternative analgesic medication.

- Client fears addiction with PCA.

- Explore client's interpretation of addiction, and clarify misunderstandings.
- Assure client that effective pain management carries negligible (less than 1 percent) risk of addiction.

- Client is not self-medicating with PCA.

- Inform client that pain control is more effective and less medicine is needed when therapeutic serum level is consistently maintained.
- Emphasize degree of pain control client can achieve with PCA.
- Review and demonstrate PCA, then supervise client's use with appropriate feedback.
- Inform client that goal is to prevent recurrent pain rather than subdue it.
- Inform client that PCA is most effective when client administers bolus every 5 to 10 min.

- Elderly client utilizing PCA develops post-operative delirium.

- Suggest substitution of another opioid in place of meperidine hydrochloride (Demerol) if being infused.
- Suggest discontinuation of basal rate infusion and use bolus dosing only.

SELF-CHECK EVALUATION

PART 1 ▪ Matching Items

Match the definition in column B with the correct term in column A.

Column A	Column B
_____ a. Endorphin	1. Foreign substance carried in the blood stream that can impede or obstruct circulation
_____ b. Infiltration	
_____ c. Compatibility	2. Capable of being mixed and administered without undergoing undesirable chemical or physical change or loss of effectiveness
_____ d. Extravasation	
_____ e. Basal	3. Endogenous morphinelike peptide
_____ f. Embolism	4. Rapid injection of a drug intravenously for peak drug level and immediate effect
_____ g. Bolus	
_____ h. Analgesia	5. Compulsive need to use a drug
_____ i. Radiopaque	6. Unable to be penetrated by x-rays
_____ j. Drug addiction	7. Inadvertent administration of vesicant solution or medication into surrounding tissue
	8. Continuous maintenance infusion
	9. Absence of sensibility to pain
	10. Inadvertent administration of a nonvesicant solution into surrounding tissue

PART 2 ▪ Multiple Choice Questions

1. Admixture of medication to an IV solution should be performed:
   a. 24 hrs before administration.
   b. Wearing a mask.
   c. Immediately before administration.
   d. By a pharmacist.

2. Back-flushing a secondary set for medication administration is preferred because:

   a. It protects the environment.
   b. It transfers air into the medication bag.
   c. Asepsis is guaranteed.
   d. It is done at the bedside.

3. When administering an IV medication that is incompatible with the primary infusion, the nurse must:

   a. Clamp and flush the primary tubing and administer the medication.
   b. Disconnect the primary infusion and administer the medication through the cannula site.
   c. Request that the physician order another primary infusion.
   d. Inject the medication into another vein.

4. If an irritating medication inadvertently extravasates into the surrounding tissue, the nurse should:

   a. Apply a warm, moist pack.
   b. Elevate the extremity.
   c. Apply a tourniquet.
   d. Apply an ice pack.

5. If it is necessary to use a needle to inject a medication through a resealable access cap, which of the following needles should the nurse select?

   a. 27 gauge, ½ in.
   b. 22 gauge, 1½ in.
   c. 20 gauge, 1 in.
   d. 18 gauge, 1 in.

6. The distinguishing feature of a bolus injection is that it is:

   a. Never diluted.
   b. Given rapidly.
   c. Administered only by a physician.
   d. Administered by piggyback.

7. The last step in administering a medication per central catheter with Groshong valve is to:

   a. Swab the cap with povidone-iodine.
   b. Flush the catheter with dilute heparin.
   c. Flush the catheter with saline.
   d. Clamp the catheter.

8. Which of the following best describes using the positive-pressure technique of syringe withdrawal?

   a. The flush syringe is withdrawn while pressure is still being applied to the plunger.
   b. The medication syringe is withdrawn with 0.2 mL remaining.
   c. The client exhales while the medication syringe is removed from the catheter cap.
   d. The client exhales while the flush syringe is removed from the catheter cap.

9. When administering a piggyback (secondary) medication, the bag is hung above the primary infusion because:

   a. Medications have higher specific gravity than primary solutions.
   b. Gravity will cause the higher bag to infuse first.
   c. It is more visible for the nurse to monitor.
   d. If the secondary bag hung below the primary bag, the medication will flow into the primary bag.

10. Which of the following statements is true of opioid analgesics?

  a. They cause periods of apnea.
  b. They decrease the tidal volume of breathing.
  c. They decrease the depth but increase the rate of breathing.
  d. They decrease the rate but increase the depth of breathing.

11. The most appropriate candidate for PCA use is:

  a. A toddler, but with parents present.
  b. A nonresponsive client with head injury.
  c. An elderly client with Alzheimer's disease.
  d. A postoperative alert client.

12. Clients who use patient-controlled analgesia usually:

  a. Require less pain medication.
  b. Have slower postoperative recovery.
  c. Require supplemental pain medication.
  d. Experience more respiratory depression.

13. If the PCA client's respiratory rate is depressed (rate of 10), the nurse should:

  a. Administer naloxone (Narcan) 0.2 mg IV.
  b. Discontinue the PCA.
  c. Obtain pulse oximetry.
  d. Obtain other vital signs (P, BP).

14. Nurses can evoke a placebo response in the client by:

  a. Administering a sugar pill.
  b. Telling the client to "be strong."
  c. Showing a caring attitude.
  d. Encouraging diversional activity.

PART 3 ▪ Critical Thinking Application

The client assigned to you has a diagnosis of advanced Alzheimer's disease and prostate cancer with metastasis to the bone. He is 75 years old, and recently has been hospitalized for palliative care. You know he is in pain, but he is unable to relate the degree of pain clearly to the staff or his family.

1. What methods are used to assess pain?

2. What method of pain assessment applies to this client?

3. What is unique about pain assessment in this case?

4. How can the nurse plan care and intervene to promote comfort in this client?

Gastrointestinal Therapy and Nutritional Support

19

GASTROINTESTINAL THERAPY

INTRODUCTION

Disturbances of fluid and electrolyte balance are commonly associated with gastro-intestinal dysfunction. The gastrointestinal tract digests ingested foods and transports nutrients across its mucosa into the bloodstream. Physical and mechanical processes of digestion begin in the mouth, where carbohydrates are broken down by mastication and alkaline salivary secretions. Swallowing is a complex, continuous three-stage process involving six cranial nerves and over 30 different muscles. Since the pharynx provides entrance to the esophagus as well as the trachea, precise coordination of structures must occur during this phase to ensure airway protection and prevent aspiration of contents into the airway. The entrance to the stomach is guarded by the lower esophageal sphincter.

The average meal remains for 3 hrs in the stomach, where digestion continues. The stomach's secretions of hydrochloric acid and pepsin break down proteins, while the acid pH environment helps protect against ingested pathogens. Vomiting, or suction decompression of acid gastric contents, primarily HCl, Na, and K, can lead to fluid and electrolyte imbalance with metabolic alkalosis, exhibited by high bicarbonate and elevated

(continued on next page)

pH on arterial blood gases. Since H_2 receptor antagonists (e.g., cimetidine) make gastric secretions less acid, their administration reduces the risk of metabolic alkalosis and electrolyte disturbance in clients who require gastric secretion suction or decompression.

The stomach's mechanical processes occur with intervals of peristalsis and relaxation of the pyloric sphincter as gastric content (chyme) moves into the small intestine (duodenum). Digestive processes continue within the sections of the small intestine (duodenum, jejunum, ileum) as enzymes break down protein to amino acids, fats to glycerol and fatty acids, and carbohydrates to monosaccharides. Here most nutrients and water are absorbed into the circulation and several important vitamins (e.g., B_{12}, riboflavin, thiamin) are formed. While 7 to 10 L of electrolyte-rich secretions mix with the chyme, only 600 to 800 mL enter the large intestine. Secretions of the small intestine have an alkaline pH, with less bactericidal effect, making this environment more vulnerable to bacterial invasion. Alkaline intestinal fluid loss, which may be due to diarrhea or intestinal decompression, can lead to fluid and electrolyte imbalance with metabolic acidosis exhibited by low bicarbonate and low pH on ABGs.

The ileocecal valve separates the small intestine from the large intestine. In the large intestine, fluids and electrolytes continue to be absorbed to solidify the stool, and mucus is secreted to lubricate the waste as it moves toward the rectum for storage and final elimination after a water loss of approximately 200 mL.

In summary, the role of the gastrointestinal tract is to dilute, digest, transport, and absorb nutrients and secretions. When gastrointestinal pathology disrupts this process, intestinal obstruction develops. Cessation of peristalsis (ileus) due to neurogenic impairment or traumatic stress, abdominal pathology, electrolyte imbalance (hypokalemia), or bowel manipulation during surgery results in alteration of both movement and absorption, which allows secretions and gas to accumulate in the system. Progressive accumulation of gases and fluid distends the bowel and compresses bowel wall capillaries. This inhibits the bowel's capacity for absorption. It also makes the bowel permeable, which causes transudation of intravascular plasma fluid into the bowel. This transudation further increases bowel contents and compression of bowel wall capillaries. As a result, intestinal fluid and bacteria may enter the peritoneal cavity, resulting in peritonitis, and the resulting toxins may enter the circulation, leading to septic shock. Transudation of fluid from the intravascular space can also result in hypovolemic shock and hemoconcentration leading to vascular clotting.

Decompression through intubation to remove fluids and gas may be necessary to prevent or correct fluid and electrolyte imbalances and infection due to temporary dysfunction of the gastrointestinal tract. This also alleviates discomfort, nausea, and vomiting and reduces the possibility of aspiration. A partial obstruction or temporary cessation of gastrointestinal function may be entirely managed with this intervention.

Intubation may also be used in the care of clients with gastrointestinal hemorrhage. Gastric bleeding creates a protein load that is digested and absorbed. Clients with impaired liver function are most likely to experience a GI bleed, but are unable to process a protein load normally. For these clients, the digestion of blood causes a precipitous rise in ammonia that can lead to metabolic encephalopathy with altered neurologic function, resulting in somnolence, loss of coordination, and coma. Intubation allows gastric lavage or washing, which not only removes blood to prevent metabolic encephalopathy but also allows estimation of acute blood loss in these cases.

PREPARATION PROTOCOL: FOR GASTROINTESTINAL THERAPY SKILLS

Complete the following steps before each skill.

1. Validate physician's written order for nasogastric (NG) tube insertion, decompression or lavage, or aspirated specimen testing.
2. Evaluate client's medical or surgical status.
3. Wash hands.
4. Verify client's identity; check identaband and have client state name.
5. Provide privacy; explain procedure and purpose to client.
6. Elevate client's position and bed height to appropriate level.
7. Optimize lighting for performance of skill.
8. Don clean gloves.

COMPLETION PROTOCOL: FOR GASTROINTESTINAL THERAPY SKILLS

Make sure the following steps have been completed.

1. Following intubation, initiate decompression suction or drainage as ordered.
2. Maintain client's position of elevation to reduce risk of pulmonary aspiration.
3. Monitor character of aspirated secretions.
4. Irrigate tube to validate and maintain patency q4hrs or as needed.
5. Remove and dispose of gloves.
6. Wash hands.
7. Monitor client's intake and output balance.
8. Monitor client's relevant lab data, including electrolytes, Hgb & Hct, and clotting factors.
9. Label specimen and send to laboratory for analysis if indicated.
10. Monitor character and amount of net lavaged gastric content and assess client's vital signs frequently.
11. Discard disposable equipment in biohazard waste receptacle.
12. Monitor enterostomy site for signs of leakage or irritation.
13. Monitor decompression (suction or drainage) device for proper functioning.
14. Return reusable equipment to appropriate area for disinfection and storage.
15. Provide regular nasal and oral hygiene for the enterally intubated (NPO) client.
16. Maintain IV fluid replacement therapy.

GASTROINTESTINAL TUBE THERAPY

Enteral tubes may be placed into various levels of the gastrointestinal tract (stomach, duodenum, or jejunum) for purposes of removing secretions (i.e., decompression). Tubes may be placed nasoenterally for short-term therapy or may require direct surgical placement for prolonged decompression. Clients undergoing gastrointestinal surgery, those with abdominal pathology (e.g., pancreatitis, mechanical obstruction), or those in whom surgery necessitates manipulation of gastrointestinal organs resulting in temporary obstruction due to cessation of peristalsis (ileus) require decompression.

The client experiencing bowel obstruction usually complains of constant severe abdominal pain and abdominal distention with nausea and vomiting, especially when the small intestine is involved. Initial abdominal assessment reveals hyperactive bowel sounds; as peristalsis slows, the sounds become high-pitched "tinkling," similar to the sound of water plunking into a bucket, then cease. Symptoms of dehydration and hypovolemic shock develop late in the obstructive process unless intubation with decompression and IV fluid supplementation are initiated.

Gastric bleeding creates an irritant that usually triggers vomiting, which may aggravate the bleeding. Emesis may be bright red (hematemesis) or have a "coffee-ground" appearance due to partial digestion. Gastric lavage or washing is used to remove irritating or toxic substances (e.g., blood or ingested poisons) from the stomach, preventing their digestion and absorption. This is usually accomplished using an irrigating syringe or gravity drainage.

Short, large, rigid nasogastric (NG) tubes have been used for years to remove fluids and gas that accumulate due to gastrointestinal obstruction. A life-threatening hazard of inserting any tube through the nose and advancing it into the stomach is inadvertent placement into the client's airway. Validation of tube placement is accomplished using a variety of techniques. Additionally, one must appreciate the anatomic invasion of intubation. Esophageal sphincters are rendered incompetent with nasoenteral tube placement, placing clients at risk for aspiration of gastric secretions into the respiratory tract.

Decompression is accomplished using a continuous or intermittent negative-pressure suction device while the client is kept NPO and given IV fluids. Since gastrointestinal secretions are isotonic with extracellular fluid, a guideline for fluid replacement is administration of a volume of normal saline or one-half normal saline with KCl equivalent to the previous day's drained secretions.

A unique feature of the intestinal tract is that it derives its nutrition directly rather than from the bloodstream. Thus, early ambulation, termination of decompression, and resumption of feeding into the GI tract are recommended. These interventions also help prevent fluid and electrolyte disturbances that may occur with prolonged decompression, NPO status, and IV fluid therapy. The nurse assesses for the return of gastrointestinal function as evidenced by the client's passage of flatus and the return of bowel sounds. Ongoing assessments include the client's tolerance of diet progression and elimination pattern.

RATIONALE

- To provide a means for gastrointestinal decompression for obstructive disease or surgical wound healing
- To provide a means for temporary postoperative decompression until normal gastrointestinal motility is restored
- To obtain gastric content samples for analysis (e.g., pH, occult blood, culture)
- To lavage the stomach to remove blood or toxic ingested substances
- To monitor the quantity of gastrointestinal bleeding

ASSESSMENT

- Verify that physician has written orders for type and purpose of tube to be inserted.
- Verify that order specifies suction or gravity drainage for decompression.
- Utilize a variety of validation techniques to determine that tube is patent and in desired position.
- Monitor quantity and character of aspirated secretions.
- Assess that tube remains patent by regular flushing.
- Assess client's abdomen (e.g., not distended, soft, presence/absence of bowel sounds) and subjective complaints.
- Monitor client's elimination pattern and character of stool.

- Monitor client's vital signs, intake and output (I&O), and relevant laboratory data (e.g., electrolytes, H&H, clotting factors).

- Monitor ongoing IV fluid replacement therapy.

LARGE-BORE NASOGASTRIC TUBE INSERTION

Equipment

- Nasogastric (NG) tube (e.g., Levin, Salem)
- Irrigating syringe (50 mL) with catheter tip
- Water-soluble lubricant (e.g., K-Y jelly)
- Towel
- Tissues
- Emesis basin
- Stethoscope
- Glass of water with straw
- Clean gloves
- Penlight or flashlight
- Tape

- Safety pin or rubber band to secure tube to client's gown
- pH chemstrip (if available)

SAFETY ALERT

Never insert or withdraw a nasogastric tube if the client is recovering from gastric surgery. Notify the surgeon if the tube is inadvertently dislodged.

SKILL

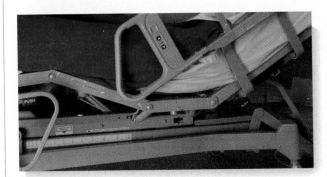

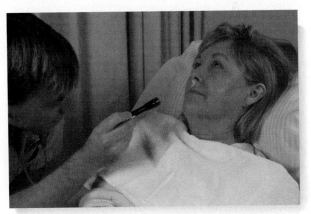

1 Elevate head of bed (HOB) to 45° angle. Check elevation gauge on bed frame under mattress. **RATIONALE:** Head elevation promotes safety during tube insertion.

- Place towel over client's chest and emesis basin within reach. Agree upon a signal client can use to stop you momentarily. **RATIONALE:** Client may experience discomfort or may gag or vomit during tube insertion.

2 Inspect client's nose to select naris that has better airflow; ask client about deviated septum and previous injury or surgery, and check ability to breathe through both nares by occluding one at a time.

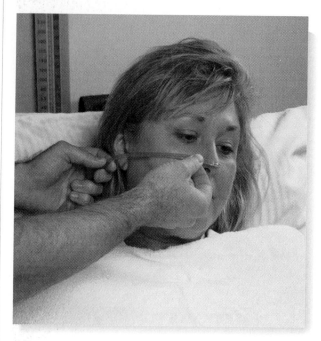

3 To determine length of tube to be inserted, use tube to measure from tip of client's nose to earlobe.

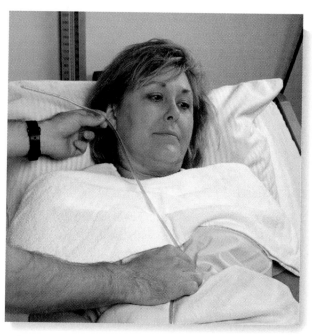

4 To this measurement, add length from earlobe to xiphoid process of sternum plus 6 in. Mark determined distance on tube with tape or pen. **RATIONALE:** This length should be sufficient to advance tube into client's stomach.

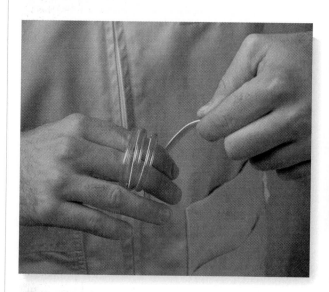

5 Coil end of tube over your fingers. **RATIONALE:** Coiling softens tube and facilitates insertion through client's nares.

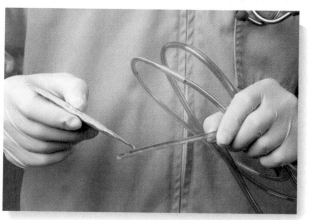

6 Lubricate the first 3 to 4 in of tube with water-soluble lubricant. **RATIONALE:** This facilitates advancement through nasal passage; if tube lubricated with oil-based lubricant is inadvertently passed into client's respiratory tract, complications could occur.

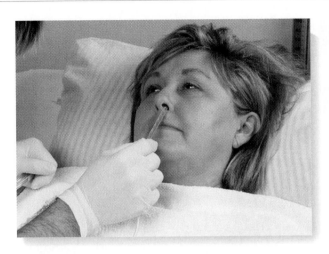

7 With client's head upright or slightly extended, carefully insert tube into client's nostril, aim it toward client's ear and downward, and gently advance it toward client's nasopharynx. **RATIONALE:** Turning and directing tube help it conform to anatomic passageways. When tube reaches nasopharynx, resistance will be felt.

SAFETY ALERT

Coughing and choking are normal responses for some clients; however, choking and coughing plus cyanosis or inability to speak indicate that the client is experiencing respiratory distress and that the tube may be in the airway.

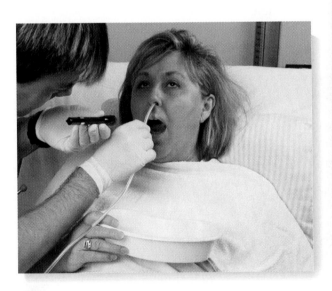

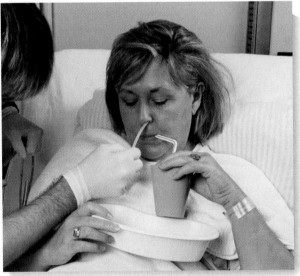

8 Have client open mouth and check with penlight to visualize tube. **RATIONALE:** To verify that tube is at back of throat and not coiled up in mouth.

- Once tube is advanced toward back of throat, have client flex head forward, then rotate tube 180° inward toward client's other nostril. **RATIONALE:** This helps direct tube past nasopharynx.

9 Ask client to dry-swallow or to sip water several times while advancing tube until tape mark is reached. If client gags, briefly stop tube advancement. **RATIONALE:** Swallowing opens upper esophageal sphincter and allows tube to enter esophagus.

- Aspirate 20 to 30 mL of air into syringe; attach syringe to free end of nasogastric tube to check for tube position. **RATIONALE:** Tube must be placed in client's alimentary canal, not respiratory tract.

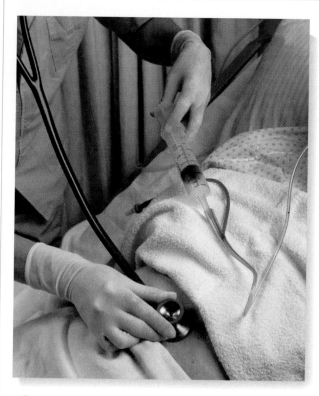

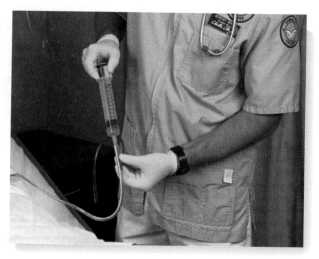

11 Keeping syringe attached, pull back on plunger to aspirate gastric contents; check for color and pH of contents (according to agency policy). **RATIONALE:** Since secretions may be obtained from tube inadvertently placed in client's airways or pleural space, pH testing of aspirated secretions helps determine where tube has been placed (see Beyond the Skill, "Nasogastric Tube Placement").

■ Use pen to mark tube near client's naris for future monitoring of tube placement and possible migration.

10 Place stethoscope over client's epigastric region, then inject air and listen for swooshing sound. **RATIONALE:** This indicates that tube has probably reached stomach.

 SAFETY ALERT

It is possible to hear the swoosh of air sounds when the tube has inadvertently been advanced into the lung or pleural space; therefore, the auscultatory method is unreliable as a sole measure for determining tube placement.

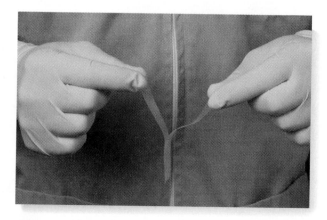

12 Make "pair of pants" of tape by using 2- to 3-inch piece of tape and splitting it half-way up the middle.

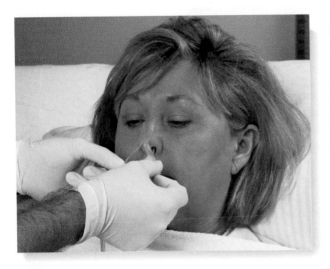

13 Place "body" part of "pants" tape on client's nose.

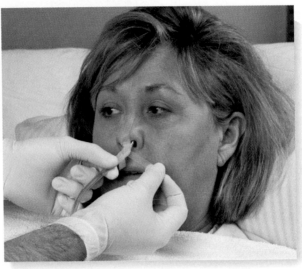

14 Wrap tape "legs" around NG tube. **RATIONALE:** To stabilize tube.

- Or use attachment device. **RATIONALE:** This reduces tissue trauma due to tube movement and helps prevent tube displacement.

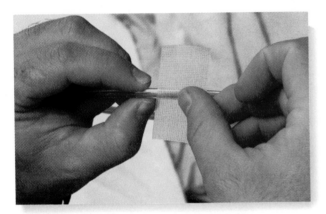

15 Loop piece of tape or rubber band around tube to pin it to client's gown.

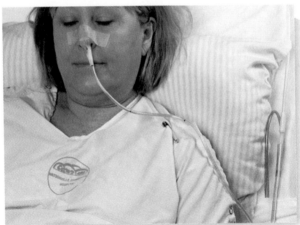

16 Pin tape or rubber band to client's gown to secure tube above client's stomach. **RATIONALE:** If tube is pulled, tension will be placed at pinned site rather than client's naris. Securing tube above stomach helps prevent leakage due to siphoning.

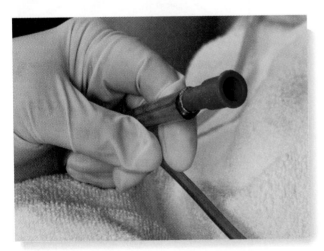

17 Plug end of tube, or connect end of tube to intermittent/continuous suction device for decompression.

BEYOND THE SKILL

Nasogastric Tube Placement

The pH and color of tube aspirate may be used to test nasogastric (NG) tube placement and to evaluate certain disease conditions. A low pH (<5) is a strong indicator that the tube is in the stomach, but pH measurement is unreliable for clients receiving medications that alter gastric pH or those with esophageal reflux of gastric contents. A higher than expected pH may be due to blood in the sample or reflux of intestinal bile. Gastric secretions are normally greenish to tan or off-white, or may be bloody or contain some mucus. In contrast, respiratory secretions are clear to light yellow with considerable mucus, and duodenal samples are deep golden yellow. A coffee-ground appearance of gastric secretions may represent digested blood, while a bright red color may indicate active bleeding or perhaps the ingestion of red food such as gelatin. In these cases, the hemo (Gastroccult) test may be used to validate suspicion of blood in the aspirate.

Skill

1. To test for presence of blood in aspirate, flush tube with 20 mL air, then aspirate 5 to 10 mL of gastric secretions.

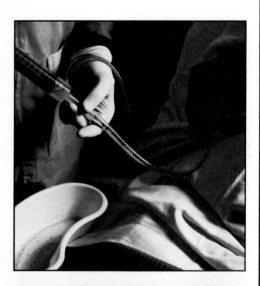

2. Dip pH test paper into 5 mL of tube aspirate.

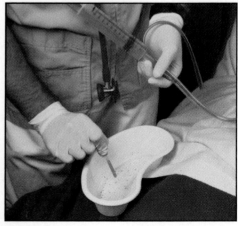

(continued on next page)

3. Alternate method: Place sample on Gastroccult card. Read pH within 30 sec by comparing color of paper with pH color guide. Gastric contents have pH of usually 0 to 4. Intestinal secretions have pH of 6 or more. If NG tube is in airway, pH will be 7 or more, but may be lower if client has aspirated gastric contents.

- When testing aspirate pH, one must determine if client is receiving an H_2 blocking agent, proton pump inhibitor, antacid, or other medication that increases gastric pH. The sustained effects of these medications alter gastric specimen pH, thus affecting ability to determine tube's location.

- Also, nurse must wait for at least 1 hr after administering any type of medication or feeding before obtaining gastric specimen for analysis.

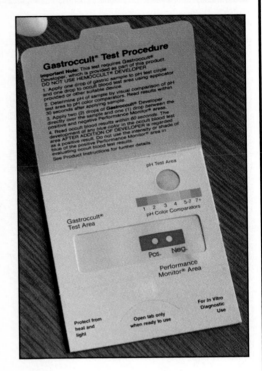

4. X-ray determination of tube placement remains the gold standard, and is mandatory if secretions cannot be obtained for testing.

ENTERAL DECOMPRESSION

Equipment

- Suction source with tubing, generally a wall unit or electrically operated suction machine, or bedside drainage bag for enterostomy tube gravity drainage
- Spindle (tapered) adapter to connect client tube to decompression (suction) tubing
- Towel
- Irrigating syringe (50 mL) with catheter tip
- Container of sterile normal saline solution
- Clean gloves
- Provisions for oral hygiene

SAFETY ALERT

Clients who are unable to ingest food or take fluids by mouth should receive regular oral and nasal hygiene to keep mucous membranes moist and to help prevent infection of the parotid glands. Oral hygiene also reduces the risk of aspiration pneumonia, as it decreases the number of pathogens in oropharyngeal secretions. Chewing gum or sucking on sugar-free candy also helps stimulate salivation, but excessive use can stimulate gastric secretions and electrolyte imbalance.

SKILL

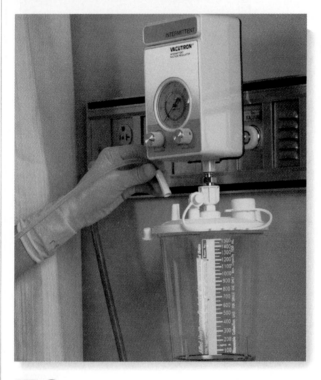

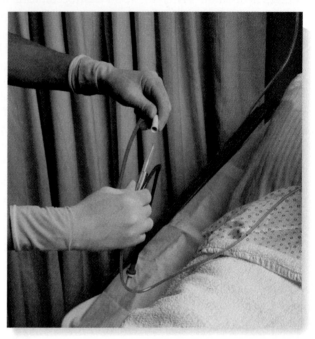

① Use tapered adapter to connect Levin tube to suction source extension tubing. Set on intermittent low suction (40 mm Hg) for decompression. **RATIONALE:** Intermittent suction allows gastric tube to release suction on stomach wall, reducing risk of mucosal erosion.

② Alternate method: Connect Salem sump tube with blue pigtail to continuous low suction (40 mm Hg) for decompression. **RATIONALE:** Continuous suction can be used because air vent lumen prevents excessive pressures from developing in stomach.

- For intermittent suction, set Gomco machine on HIGH (120 mm Hg) or wall source on LOW (40 mm Hg) suction.

- Or connect surgically placed intestinal enterostomy tube to bedside gravity drainage bag tubing. Note that contents flow into suction receptacle or gravity drainage bag.

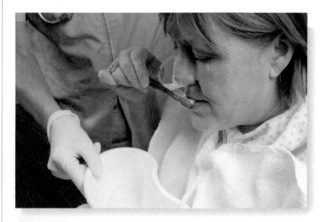

③ Provide regular oral and nasal hygiene. **RATIONALE:** To keep mucous membranes moist for client comfort and to prevent complications.

BEYOND THE SKILL

Salem Sump Tube Maintenance

The Salem sump tube has a double lumen specifically designed to reduce gastric irritation. One lumen has a terminal blue pigtail that provides an opening to the atmosphere to keep excess pressures from building up in the stomach. This port serves as an escape hatch for positive air pressure due to air swallowing, and, by allowing atmospheric pressure to enter the stomach, reduces negative suction pressure at the tube's tip, thus keeping the tip away from the stomach lining. Occasionally gastric contents siphon into the air vent tubing, necessitating tube clearance to restore proper functioning.

Skill

1. To prevent gastric fluid backup (siphoning) into blue lumen air vent, keep pigtail secured above level of client's stomach.

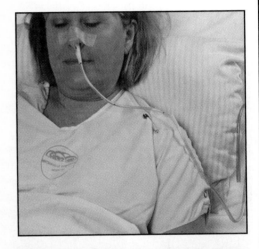

2. Or insert antireflux valve plug, blue side into blue pigtail. This one-way valve allows air to enter tube, yet prevents leakage of gastric secretions.

   ■ To cap tube, disconnect from suction source tubing and insert white tip of antireflux valve into sump tube lumen.

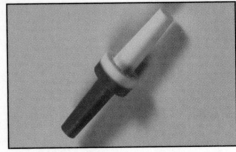

3. Should fluid siphon into vent tubing, clear it by instilling 20 to 30 mL of normal saline followed by 20 to 30 mL of air, then reinsert the antireflux plug if used. **RATIONALE:** This reestablishes air buffer between valve and stomach.

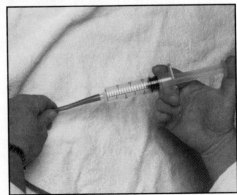

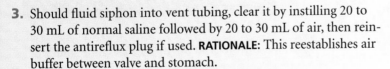

NASOGASTRIC TUBE IRRIGATION

Equipment

- Towel
- Stethoscope
- 50-mL irrigating syringe
- Container of sterile normal saline solution
- Clean gloves

SAFETY ALERT

- If water rather than normal saline is used to irrigate enteral decompression tubes, the production of gastric secretions will increase and increasing amounts of electrolytes will be washed out. Similarly, if the client is NPO but ingests ice chips ad lib, electrolyte imbalance due to washout can occur, causing metabolic alkalosis.
- Limit the use of ice chips by substituting chips made from an electrolyte solution, and provide oral hygiene to keep the client's mucous membranes moist for comfort.
- If the client is receiving adequate parenteral hydration (IV fluids), excessive thirst should not be experienced.

SKILL

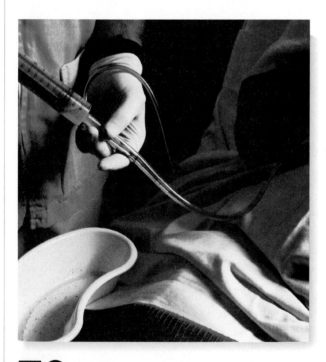

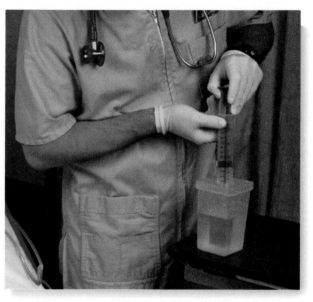

2 Draw up 20 to 30 mL of normal saline solution.

1 Place towel underneath tube to protect bed linens. Disconnect tube from suction. Determine tube placement by auscultation and aspiration of secretions as in previous skill. **RATIONALE:** To protect against inadvertent administration of irrigating solution into client's airway.

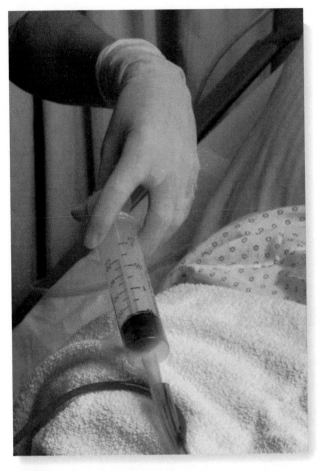

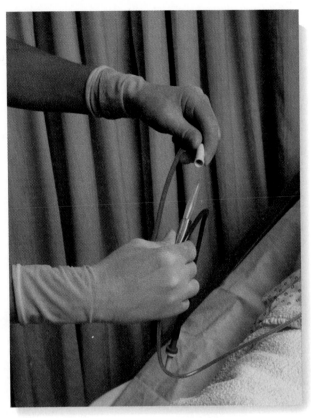

3 Gently instill normal saline into NG tube or remove syringe plunger, pour normal saline solution into syringe barrel, and allow solution to flow in by gravity.

4 Reconnect tube to suction, or reclamp tube if suction is not used. Record instilled amount on client's I&O record. **RATIONALE:** To help monitor client's fluid balance.

CLINICAL NOTE

GASTRIC LAVAGE
Gastric lavage or washing is usually performed as an emergency measure to remove a toxic or irritating substance from the stomach, thus preventing its absorption.

■ Monitoring I&O volumes carefully, instill 30 mL normal saline solution, then aspirate gastric contents (some authorities recommend water for lavage since it breaks up clots more easily than saline solution, is less expensive, and is easily available).

■ Note character and quantity of aspirated or drained contents.

■ Subtract total instilled volume from total aspirated volume to determine volume of gastric contents removed.

■ Continue repeating process until return is clear, or as ordered.

■ Record vital signs frequently and monitor client's response closely.

NASOENTERIC TUBE REMOVAL

Equipment

- Towel
- Stethoscope
- Irrigating syringe (50 mL)
- Container of sterile normal saline solution
- Tissues, paper towel
- Clean gloves

SAFETY ALERT

When assessing for the return of bowel sounds, use the diaphragm of the stethoscope to auscultate at each of the four quadrants. Be advised that it may require a 2-min assessment at each site to detect sounds. For a quick assessment, auscultate to the right of the umbilicus. Since bowel sounds are transferred throughout the abdomen, this site alone is an alternative to assessing all four sites.

S K I L L

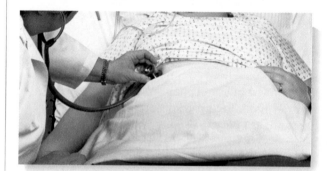

1 Assess client for return of bowel sounds. **RATIONALE:** Presence of bowel sounds indicates return of peristalsis and should be established before decompression tube or intestinal feeding tube is removed.

- Prepare client for tube removal by explaining that it may cause some nasal discomfort, coughing, sneezing, or gagging.
- Provide tissues and place towel or paper towels over client's chest.

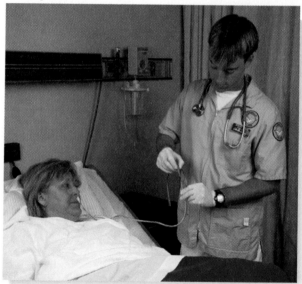

2 Flush tube with 20 mL normal saline. **RATIONALE:** To clear tube so that gastric contents do not inadvertently drain into esophagus on tube removal.

- Follow flush with bolus of air. **RATIONALE:** To free tube from stomach lining.
- Plug tube or clamp it by folding it over in your gloved hand.

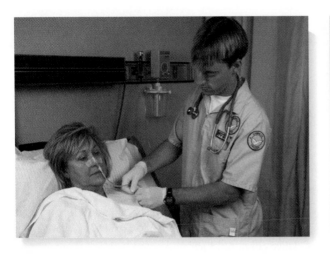

3 Unpin tube from client's gown.

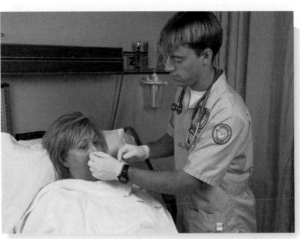

4 Loosen tape that secures tube.

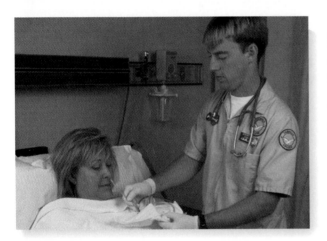

5 Pinch tube close to nostril; have client take deep breath and hold it while you withdraw tube. **RATIONALE:** Holding breath closes glottis and helps prevent aspiration.

- Wrap tube in towel. **RATIONALE:** To remove tube from client's view.

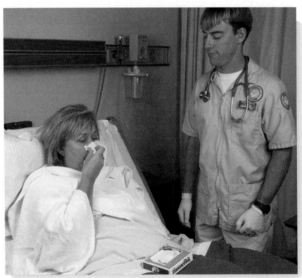

6 Offer oral and nasal hygiene.

CHARTING

- Date, time, and skill performed
- Type and size of tube inserted
- Client's intake and output; quantity, color, and character of secretions aspirated
- Frequency of tube irrigation and solution used
- Enterostomy tube site status
- Net volume of secretions obtained with gastric lavage
- Purpose and dispensation of sample aspirated secretions
- Abdominal assessment findings (i.e., bowel sounds, distention, subjective complaints)
- Provision of nasal and oral hygiene
- Time of nasoenteral tube removal
- Client's response to decompression interventions

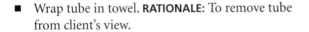
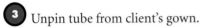

CRITICAL THINKING FOCUS

SECTION ONE ▪ Gastrointestinal Tube Therapies

Unexpected Outcomes

- Nasogastric tube is difficult to advance.

- Client coughs, is unable to speak, and becomes cyanotic during tube insertion.

- Salem sump pigtail tube leaks gastric contents.

Alternative Nursing Actions

- Select more patent nostril: Have client compress each naris and breathe in to determine which nostril is more patent.
- Relubricate tube and try again.
- Stiffen tube by cooling in iced water and lubricate first 3 to 4 in of tube to advance to posterior nasopharynx.
- Have client hold ice chips in mouth for a few minutes to numb nasal passage and suppress gag reflex.

- Immediately remove tube, as signs indicate tube is being advanced into client's airway.

- Flush with normal saline, then with air to clear.
- Keep blue pigtail at level above client's stomach.
- Insert antireflux valve plug.

SELF-CHECK EVALUATION

PART 1 ▪ Matching Terms

Match the definition in column B with the correct term in column A.

Column A	Column B
_____ a. Lavage	1. Second part of the small intestine; beginning of the lower gastrointestinal tract
_____ b. Decompression	
_____ c. Jejunostomy	2. Surgical opening into the stomach
_____ d. Gastrostomy	3. State of excessive alkalinity of body fluids due to accumulation of bicarbonate or loss of acid, which may result in increased pH of the blood (alkalemia)
_____ e. Alkalosis	
_____ f. Salem sump	
_____ g. Sphincter	
_____ h. Acidosis	4. Removal of pressure due to accumulation of gas or fluid
_____ i. Jejunum	5. Surgical opening into the jejunum
_____ j. Levin	6. Irrigating or washing out content of an organ
	7. State of excessive acidity of body fluids following the accumulation of acids or the loss of bicarbonate that may result in a decrease in pH of the blood (acidemia)
	8. Circular muscle constricting an opening
	9. Short single-lumen tube used for gastric decompression with low intermittent suction
	10. Short double-lumen tube used for gastric decompression with continuous suction

PART 2 ▪ Multiple Choice Questions

1. Nasogastric tubes are placed in clients with intestinal obstruction in order to:

a. Provide nutrition.
b. Monitor gastric secretion pH.
c. Provide decompression.
d. Monitor the amount of gastric secretions.

2. The major reason for establishing nasogastric suction in clients with liver dysfunction who are experiencing gastric bleeding is to:

a. Relieve pain and nausea.
b. Prevent vomiting and aspiration.
c. Prevent digestion and absorption of blood.
d. Decrease peristalsis and prevent diarrhea.

3. Which of the following describes the appropriate method for measuring tube length for nasogastric insertion? Measure from:

a. Nose to ear to xiphoid process plus 6 in.
b. Nose to ear to xiphoid process plus 10 in.
c. Ear to nose to xiphoid process.
d. Ear to nose, back to ear, and then to chin.

4. The client is asked to swallow during enteral tube insertion because swallowing:

a. Prevents tube advancement into the airway.
b. Opens the upper gastroesophageal sphincter.
c. Helps to lubricate the tube.
d. Distracts the client's attention from the procedure.

5. Indications that an enteral tube may have been inadvertently placed in the airway include:

a. Cyanosis and high-pH aspirate.
b. Cyanosis and low-pH aspirate.
c. Coughing and sneezing.
d. Dark yellow mucoid aspirate.

6. The least reliable method of determining gastric tube placement is:

a. Aspiration of gastric contents.
b. Auscultation of instilled air.
c. X-ray determination.
d. Measurement of aspirant pH.

7. The presence of old blood in gastric secretions is indicated by:

a. Presence of bright red blood.
b. pH less than 3.
c. Black, tarry appearance.
d. Coffee-ground appearance.

8. Respiratory secretions usually have the following characteristics:

a. pH greater than 7 and clear color.
b. pH less than 7 and dark gold color.
c. pH greater than 4 and greenish color.
d. pH less than 3 and mucoid appearance.

9. Intestinal secretions are usually decompressed using:

   a. NG tube and low intermittent suction.
   b. NG tube and gravity drainage.
   c. Jejunostomy tube and gravity drainage.
   d. Jejunostomy tube and intermittent suction.

10. The nasogastric decompression tube is taped to the client's gown above the level of the stomach in order to:

   a. Prevent siphoning of gastric contents.
   b. Prevent ulceration of the nares.
   c. Slow gastric emptying.
   d. Allow visibility of the tube.

11. Regular oral hygiene is indicated for the client who is NPO because it:

   a. Decreases thirst.
   b. Helps prevent respiratory infection.
   c. Helps prevent parotitis.
   d. All of the above.

12. For enteral tube removal, the client is asked to hold the breath in order to:

   a. Prevent aspiration of secretions during tube removal.
   b. Prevent bradycardia due to vagal stimulation.
   c. Open the glottis to facilitate tube removal.
   d. Open the upper esophagogastric sphincter.

13. The Salem sump tube pigtail functions to:

   a. Provide a port for gastric lavage.
   b. Provide an air vent to reduce intragastric pressures.
   c. Provide a port for the administration of medications.
   d. Prevent siphoning of gastric contents onto linens.

14. Decompression of gastric secretions can lead to metabolic alkalosis unless the client's intravenous fluid provides adequate:

   a. Potassium chloride supplementation.
   b. Hydrochloric acid supplementation.
   c. Sodium bicarbonate supplementation.
   d. Sodium chloride supplementation.

PART 3 ▪ Critical Thinking Application

Mrs. Ramsey, age 62, has been admitted to the hospital with complaints of painful abdominal distention and signs of dehydration after 2 days of vomiting. She is diagnosed with small bowel obstruction due to adhesions (scar tissue) from a remote abdominal hysterectomy.

1. What are the pathophysiologic effects of intestinal obstruction?
2. What potential fluid and electrolyte problems occur with small bowel obstruction?
3. How does the loss of gastric secretions differ from the loss of intestinal secretions?
4. What are the body's normal compensatory mechanisms for acid-base imbalances due to loss of gastrointestinal fluids?
5. What interventions help to correct these imbalances?

20

NUTRITIONAL SUPPORT

INTRODUCTION

Food is an undeniable necessity for the maintenance of life, and, as a symbol, equally important to our psychological health. Properly balanced nutrition helps to promote health and prevent illness. It is essential to the normal metabolic processes of growth, development, and healing. The recommended dietary allowance (RDA) is the most widely accepted standard for levels of nutrient sufficiency. As with any balance, excesses or deficiencies in RDAs can have general and long-lasting effects on our lives.

We can meet essential nutrient recommendations by following the guidelines shown in the Food Guide Pyramid published by the U.S. Department of Agriculture. The pyramid specifies five major food groups as well as the number of daily servings that fulfill each category and provide the necessary carbohydrates, fats, proteins, vitamins, and minerals. Recommendations are easy to follow because we can select from a variety of choices within each major group. Selections should be relatively low in fat, salt, and simple sugars. In addition, food intake needs to be balanced with regular physical activity so that we maintain an ideal body weight and avoid obesity, which is associated with increased morbidity and mortality. The body mass index

(continued on next page)

ESSENTIAL BODY NUTRIENTS

Carbohydrates

- Monosaccharides—glucose, fructose, galactose
- Disaccharides—sucrose, lactose, maltose
- Polysaccharides—starch, dextrin, glycogen, cellulose, hemicellulose

Fats

- Linoleic acid, linolenic acid, arachidonic acid

Protein

- Amino acids—phenylalanine, lysine, isoleucine, leucine, methionine, valine, tryptophan, threonine

Vitamins

- Fat soluble—vitamins A, D, E, and K
- Water soluble—vitamins B_1, B_2, B_6, B_{12}, niacin, pantothenic acid, folacin, biotin, choline, meso-inositol, para-aminobenzoic acid, vitamin C

Minerals

- Major elements—calcium, chloride, iron, magnesium, phosphorus, potassium, sodium, sulfur

Water

- Trace elements

(weight in kilograms divided by height in meters squared) should be kept within the range of 20 to 26.

Carbohydrates include simple sugars, complex sugars (starches), and cellulose. These nutrients are converted by the body into glucose to provide fuel for energy. Some of the glucose is stored in the liver as glycogen, which can be converted back to glucose as needed by the body. One gram of carbohydrate provides 4 kilocalories. The U.S. Senate's Select Committee on Nutrition and Human Needs recommends that 55 to 60 percent of our calories come from complex carbohydrates.

Fats or lipids are a more concentrated source for energy; each gram provides 9 kilocalories. They also carry fat-soluble vitamins (A, D, E, and K). Fats should make up no more than 25 to 30 percent of our daily caloric intake. Saturated fats should not exceed 10 percent of calories, and cholesterol should be limited to less than 300 mg daily. To reduce fat intake, we should limit meat, fish, and poultry to a cooked weight of 3 to 6 ounces daily. High-fat diets increase the risk of atherosclerotic cardiovascular disease and cancer.

Proteins are complex organic compounds that contain amino acids, which are critical to all aspects of growth and development of body tissues and the production of hormones and enzymes. Proteins become a source of energy only when the body's intake of carbohydrate or fat is insufficient. Proteins are broken down into 22 amino acids through the digestive process. Amino acids are used for tissue synthesis, and all but eight are produced by the body; these eight must be obtained from the diet. If a particular food con-

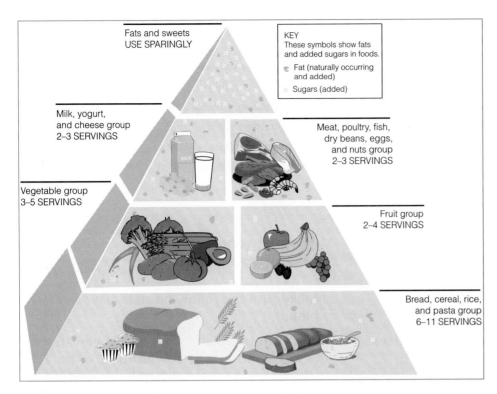

● **FIGURE 20-1** *USDA Food Guide Pyramid. Source: U.S. Department of Agriculture/U.S. Department of Health and Human Services, Washington, D.C.*

tains all eight amino acids, it is called a complete protein. Most meat and dairy products are complete proteins, while most vegetables and fruits are incomplete because they lack one or more essential amino acids. Several incomplete foods (for example beans and rice) can be combined to provide a complete protein. Each gram of protein provides 4 kilo-calories. Optimal daily intake of protein is 0.8 g per kilogram of body weight.

Vitamins and minerals are also essential to nutritional health. The RDA standard provides guidelines for fat- and water-soluble vitamins and minerals that can be met by ingesting a variety of common foods. Dietary supplements in excess of the RDA, such

NUTRIENT REQUIREMENTS FOR HEALING

- Total calories per day—2800 for tissue repair; 6000 for extensive repair
- Protein—40 to 50 g/day average person; 50 to 75 g/day in postoperative period; 100 to 200 g/day if needed for new tissue synthesis
- Carbohydrates—55 to 60 percent of calories, sufficient in quantity to meet calorie needs and allow protein to be used for tissue repair
- Fat—25 to 30 percent; not excessive, as that leads to poor tissue healing and susceptibility to infection
- Vitamins—vitamin C, up to 1 g/day for tissue repair; vitamin B, increased above normal for stress management; vitamin A, adjuncts autoimmune system; vitamin E, increases O_2 to tissues
- Minerals—zinc, aids tissue repair; selenium, aids cell repair; calcium/magnesium, relaxes nerves and maintains electric stimulation

as multivitamins, are not harmful. Excessive levels of certain vitamins and minerals, however, can have toxic systemic effects.

Nutrient guidelines for healthy people may not meet the needs of clients whose nutritional status is altered by illness, particularly conditions that affect oral intake or nutrient digestion, absorption, and utilization. Indeed, a degree of malnutrition is present in as many as 50 percent of hospitalized clients. Forced enteral nutrition support (tube feeding) may be prescribed to correct nutrient deficiencies, especially when acute illness compounds nutrient demands and high levels of protein and calories are required.

PREPARATION PROTOCOL: FOR NUTRITIONAL SUPPORT SKILLS

Complete the following steps before each skill.

1. Evaluate client's medical or surgical and nutritional status.
2. Wash hands.
3. Prepare enteral nutrition system according to manufacturer's instructions.
4. Label enteral nutrition system components with preparation time and date.
5. Verify client's identity; check identaband and have client state name.
6. Provide privacy; explain procedure and purpose to client.
7. Elevate client's position and bed height to appropriate level.
8. Optimize lighting for skill performance.
9. Don clean gloves.
10. Perform enteral intubation or validate tube patency and position for delivery of enteral nutrition.
11. Assess client's abdomen for bowel sounds, distention, and gastric residual volume before administering gastric bolus or continuous feeding.
12. Flush system before and after any feeding with 20 to 30 mL water.

COMPLETION PROTOCOL: FOR NUTRITIONAL SUPPORT SKILLS

Make sure the following steps have been completed.

1. Maintain client's position of elevation for continuous enteral nutrition, or for 2 hrs following intermittent bolus feeding.
2. Program infusion pump parameters for continuous enteral feeding as ordered.
3. Flush continuous feeding system every 4 hrs with 20 to 30 mL water.
4. Discard disposable equipment in biohazard waste receptacle.
5. Remove and dispose of gloves.
6. Wash hands.
7. Label, date, and refrigerate any unused feeding formula.
8. Discard any unused opened refrigerated formula after 24 hrs.
9. Change enteral nutrition delivery system daily, including reservoir, tubing, and syringe.
10. Monitor and document client's response to therapy (e.g., gastric residuals, signs of aspiration, tolerance to feeding, abdominal assessment, elimination pattern, intake and output [I&O], weight).
11. Monitor enterostomy site for signs of leakage or irritation.
12. Monitor pump infusion equipment for proper functioning.
13. Return reusable equipment to appropriate area for disinfection and storage.
14. Provide regular nasal and oral hygiene for the enterally intubated (NPO) client.

SECTION ONE

SMALL-BORE NASOENTERAL FEEDING

Many types of tubes are available for enteral feeding. They vary in length and lumen size (6 to 18 French) depending upon their intended placement (e.g., stomach, duodenum, jejunum). There are advantages and disadvantages to each type of tube used, position in the gastrointestinal tract, and method of enteral nutrition administration.

Large-bore tubes are inserted nasogastrically for short-term enteral nutrition (less than 30 days). Gastric feedings through large-bore tubes may be delivered through a syringe, by gravity, or utilizing an infusion pump. The physician's order specifies the frequency of feedings: intermittently (4 to 6 times daily), cyclically (over 12 hrs), or continuously (over 24 hrs).

Long, soft, pliable small-bore tubes made of silastic or polyurethane may be placed nasogastrically or nasointestinally (advanced beyond the pylorus). Nasally inserted small-bore tubes are more comfortable for the client, but such feeding requires continuous infusion using a pump and continuous client positioning with the head of the bed elevated. Enteral feeding into the small intestine is associated with greater risk of infection due to the alkaline environment. Closed formula systems and the use of feeding tubes with separate flush or medication ports help reduce the risk of enteritis caused by contamination when breaking and entering the system.

Inserting any tube nasoenterally is associated with the life-threatening hazard of inadvertent advancement and subsequent feeding into the respiratory tract, especially in clients with delayed gastric emptying. Tube misplacement, or displacement after insertion, can cause other serious complications such as pneumothorax and pleural effusion. Unfortunately, validation of small-bore tube placement is difficult compared to that for large-bore tubes because aspiration to obtain gastrointestinal contents frequently causes a small, flexible tube to collapse. Research studies suggest that while a variety of techniques are used to determine feeding tube placement, traditional methods are inadequate for all types of enteral intubation. X-ray validation continues to be the gold standard for determination of enteral tube placement and is mandatory before any feeding is initiated through a small-bore tube.

Tubes for long-term feeding (e.g., over 30 days) are placed surgically through the abdominal wall directly into the stomach (gastrostomy) or into the small intestine (jejunostomy). The PEG or PEJ tube is inserted endo-scopically from the inside out. Directly placed tubes are secured by a stabilizing bar (bumper), a large, mushroom-shaped tip, or a balloon inflated with water similar to the balloon on a Foley catheter.

For clients with a history of gastric reflux or aspiration pneumonia related to tube feeding, a small-bore jejunostomy tube is preferred. Jejunostomy tubes may be placed surgically or by laparoscopy. Special dual-purpose tubes (e.g., Moss tubes) allow gastric decompression and simultaneous administration of intestinal feeding. These tubes are often inserted during surgery so that enteral feeding can be initiated in the early postoperative period while the client is NPO. Intestinal feeding requires continuous pump infusion.

RATIONALE

- To provide a means for intermittent nutritional feeding into the stomach
- To provide a means for continuous nutritional feeding into the small intestine
- To provide a means for medication administration (see Chapter 15)

ASSESSMENT

- Verify that physician has written an order for type of nasoenteral tube to be inserted.
- Verify that order specifies desired placement of tube (e.g., gastric, intestinal).
- Verify that physician's order specifies type, amount, and frequency of enteral feeding.
- Validate client's identity; check room number and identaband and have client state name.
- Auscultate to ensure client has bowel sounds.
- Assess that client's nasal passage is patent to allow tube insertion.
- Determine if client is able to swallow to assist in tube advancement.
- Verify that tube is placed in desired location by using several validation techniques.

SMALL-BORE FEEDING TUBE INSERTION

Equipment

- Radiopaque nasointestinal small-bore tube (Keofeed, Dobbhoff) with stylet and tungsten-weighted tip
- Water-soluble lubricant (e.g., K-Y jelly)
- Towel
- Tissues
- Emesis basin
- Stethoscope
- Glass of water with straw
- Clean gloves
- Penlight or flashlight

SAFETY ALERT

Do not remove stylet until tube placement is confirmed to be where intended. Once removed, wire stylet cannot be replaced to facilitate tube repositioning without risk of tube damage and injury to client.

- Tape
- pH chemstrip (if available)
- Pen with indelible ink for marking tube
- Normal saline solution
- Syringe (60 mL or size manufacturer recommends)

SKILL

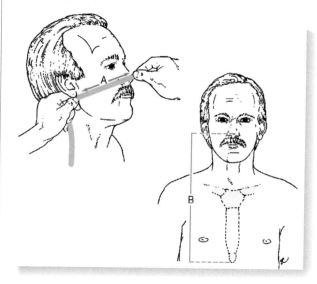

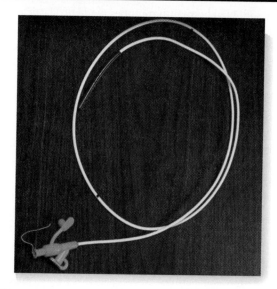

1 Determine length of tube insertion by measuring from tip of client's nose to earlobe, then to xiphoid process, then adding 10 inches. **RATIONALE:** Small bowel placement requires at least 40 inches of tubing. This additional measurement allows tube to migrate into small intestine.

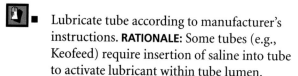 - Lubricate tube according to manufacturer's instructions. **RATIONALE:** Some tubes (e.g., Keofeed) require insertion of saline into tube to activate lubricant within tube lumen.

2 Check that guide wire (stylet) does not protrude through holes in feeding tube. Reposition guide if necessary. **RATIONALE:** To prevent trauma to mucosa.

- Proceed with steps for inserting nasogastric tube (see Chapter 19).
- Using syringe size that manufacturer recommends, flush tube with 30 mL air, then aspirate contents. Repeat steps if necessary to obtain specimen. **RATIONALE:** Small-capacity syringes exert excessive pressure that may collapse tube and prevent successful aspiration. Repeated attempts at insufflation and aspiration are frequently necessary to obtain return.

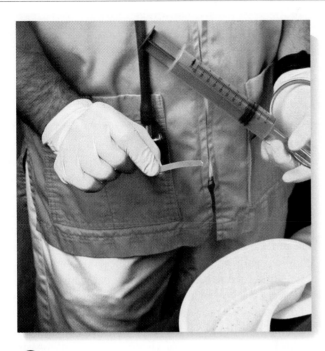

Since both intestinal and respiratory secretions have pH values higher than those of gastric secretions, identifying the position of a nasally placed tube based on secretion pH alone is only moderately helpful. Recent research indicates that a combination of pH level (>5) and bilirubin value (>5) can be used to correctly identify intestinal placement of the tube in 75 percent of cases.

③ Test aspirated secretions for pH (see Chapter 19). **RATIONALE:** pH helps determine tube's location. As tube advances into intestine, secretions will have higher pH than gastric secretions and color will be golden yellow.

- If tube has incremental measures, note and document measurement where tube enters nose. If there are no incremental markings, mark tube with indelible ink.

- Do not initiate feeding until tube placement is confirmed by plain film abdominal x-ray (KUB). **RATIONALE:** X-ray remains gold standard for determination of tube position.

CLINICAL NOTE

In order to encourage the tube to migrate into the duodenum, have the client assume a right-side-lying position for 1 to 2 hrs to allow natural digestive reflexes to expel the tube from the stomach.

- The intestinal tube's tungsten-weighted tip assists it to move through the pylorus and into the duodenum within 24 hrs.
- The client must be fasting during this period of time.
- If necessary, the physician may prescribe a prokinetic medication such as metoclopramide to induce transpyloric passage of the tube.

CHARTING

- Date and time
- Type and size of tube inserted
- Techniques used to validate tube placement

- Nature and amount of aspirated secretions
- X-ray determination of tube position (if indicated)

SECTION TWO

ENTERAL FEEDING

Well-nourished clients can tolerate a short period of caloric balance deficit, which may occur during brief illness or surgery. The body's fat stores provide calories during such periods. However, negative nitrogen balance, as seen with reduced serum albumin or reduced prealbumin, indicates that the client has already lost structural and functional proteins. Enteral nutrition (tube feeding) is prescribed for clients in negative nitrogen balance who are unable (e.g., due to dysphagia) or unwilling to eat, or who need a supplement to ingested food. Clients in catabolic states with intensive caloric requirements (e.g., burn or trauma clients) are also candidates for enteral feeding. Enteral feeding is preferred over parenteral intravenous nutrition (TPN) for the client who does not respond to simple oral food supplements. Unless an elemental formula is administered directly into the jejunum, the client's gastrointestinal tract must be functioning and without obstruction below the site of formula delivery.

The enteral route is safer, less expensive, and associated with fewer problems related to metabolism and sepsis than the parenteral route. Also, using the enteral route helps to maintain GI function and speeds regeneration of the small intestine, which receives its nutrition directly from food rather than from the bloodstream. Enteral nutrition preserves production of humoral antibodies, reduces bacterial overgrowth in the gut, and helps to maintain the gut's protective mucosal barrier by preventing translocation of bacteria and endotoxin from the gut, which may become a source of sepsis in the client. Since the small intestine is less affected than the stomach and colon by surgical ileus, postoperative feeding into the small intestine is feasible while the client is NPO.

Enteral formulas are available in powder form that must be reconstituted or in ready-to-use liquids. Depending on the client's needs, the formulas contain all or just one of the following: protein, carbohydrates, fat, electrolytes, vitamins, and minerals. Isotonic formulas are most commonly used, but special formulations are sometimes necessary. Modified enteral diets are available for clients with specific nutritional requirements: lactose-free or lactose-containing, fiber-containing, elemental (predigested), or modular formulations that provide additional macronutrient components (e.g., lipid, carbohydrate, or protein). Specialized formulas are also available for clients with trauma, pulmonary disease, renal failure, diabetes, liver failure, or immune deficiency.

Potential complications from enteral feeding include gastric hypomotility, altered drug absorption, and altered metabolism. Feeding directly into the small bowel must be continuous because osmotic loads cannot be buffered there as effectively as in the stomach. Rapid bolus feeding pulls fluid from the circulatory system into the gut to dilute the load and results in a temporary hypovolemic reaction. This dumping syndrome may cause diarrhea, cramping, weakness, lightheadedness, diaphoresis, and palpitations.

Mechanical problems due to tube obstruction or dislodgment are common, but the most serious complication of enteral feeding is tracheobronchial aspiration. This occurs in over one-third of clients receiving nasogastric feedings. It is more likely to occur in those with swallowing disorders, gastric paresis, altered gag reflex, or decreased level of consciousness.

Tubes placed through the nose alter the normal protective function of the upper and lower esophageal sphincters. While gastric placement is thought to pose the greatest risk for aspiration, tubes placed distal to the pylorus in the proximal small intestine (duodenum) have been associated with reflux into the stomach. Tubes placed into the jejunum, beyond the ligament of Treitz, should theoretically be associated with less risk of reflux. Still, aspiration is possible with continuous feedings delivered into the jejunum. Clearly, studies show that there is no reduced incidence of aspiration of tube feeding associated with feeding into any particular area of the gastrointestinal tract. Feeding aspiration may be silent or can cause gagging, fever, tachycardia, tachypnea, and respiratory distress. To determine if there is formula aspiration, the solution may be tinted blue. Alternatively, pulmonary secretions can be tested for the presence of glucose, but if secretions contain blood, this test may yield a false positive result.

RATIONALE

- To provide nutrients to clients who are unable to ingest normally (e.g., clients who are comatose or who have obstructive lesions)
- To provide nutrition for clients with severe protein or protein and calorie malnutrition
- To provide nutrition for catabolic clients with high metabolic requirements
- To provide individualized dietary supplementation for clients with specific diseases

- To promote healing of enterocutaneous fistulas by direct mucosal feeding
- To speed small bowel recovery following resection surgery
- To maintain fluid and electrolyte balance

ASSESSMENT

- Verify that physician has written specific order for nutritional product, method, amount, and frequency of administration.
- Review client's medical status and allergies.
- Auscultate client's abdomen to ensure presence of bowel sounds unless elemental formula is being administered into small intestine.

- Aspirate residual before each gastric feeding to ensure feeding rate is tolerated.
- Monitor frequency and consistency of client's stool.
- Monitor for development of ileus, abdominal distention, nausea or vomiting, or tube exit site complications.
- Monitor client's daily weight, fluid intake and output, and other signs of fluid volume excess or deficit.
- Monitor client's electrolyte status (e.g., Na, K, Cl, HCO_3).
- Monitor client's pre- and posttherapy nutritional status (e.g., BUN, creatinine, height and weight, serum albumin, blood sugar).

TABLE 20-1	COMPARISON OF ENTERAL TUBE FEEDING METHODS	
	Advantages	**Disadvantages**
Nasogastric	■ Easily placed. ■ Intermittent feeding is possible, so client is less confined. ■ Large-volume feeding may be delivered less often. ■ Tube placement does not require x-ray confirmation. ■ Acid environment may reduce infection. ■ Less risk of dumping syndrome. ■ Uses normal gastric emptying, preventing intestinal overload. ■ Less expensive; no feeding pump required.	■ Impairs competence of lower esophageal sphincter and swallowing of saliva. ■ Limited to 4 wk use. ■ Gastric retention, reflux, and aspiration are possible. ■ Large tube is uncomfortable and visible to others. ■ Naris ulceration may occur. ■ Tube becomes stiff or brittle over time. ■ Allows regurgitation by interfering with normal upper and lower esophageal sphincter function. ■ Gastric ulceration or fistulae may occur.
Gastrostomy or PEG	■ Long-term use is possible. ■ Allows intermittent feeding. ■ Normal gastric emptying occurs. ■ Tube is not visible to others. ■ Medication administration is easier. ■ Less risk of infection. ■ Client can ambulate. ■ Esophageal irritation is avoided.	■ Requires surgical placement with sedation or local anesthetic. ■ Requires local skin care. ■ May ulcerate gastric mucosa.

TABLE 20-1	COMPARISON OF ENTERAL TUBE FEEDING METHODS (CONT'D)

	Advantages	**Disadvantages**
Nasointestinal	■ Smaller tube is more comfortable. ■ Less risk of reflux and aspiration.	■ Requires x-ray confirmation. ■ Tube is more difficult to place. ■ Client is still at risk for aspirating naso-pharyngeal and gastric contents. ■ Elevated position must be maintained. ■ Constant infusion used; intermittent feeding not recommended because of osmotic response of small intestine. ■ Cramping, vomiting, distention, and diarrhea more common. ■ Requires pump; more expensive. ■ Tube can displace back into stomach (with constant infusion, this increases risk of aspiration). ■ Medication administration is difficult (liquid form preferred). ■ Greater risk of infection due to alkaline environment. ■ Limited to 4 wk use.
Jejunostomy	■ Tube position is guaranteed. ■ Tube is not visible to others. ■ Possibly less risk of reflux and aspiration.	■ Requires general anesthesia for placement. ■ Continuous infusion is required. ■ Local skin care is required. ■ Cramping, vomiting, distention, and diarrhea are more common. ■ Other disadvantages associated with nasointestinal feeding.

INTERMITTENT OR BOLUS GASTRIC TUBE FEEDING

Equipment

- Alcohol swabs
- Prescribed nutritional formula/product
- Calibrated container for measuring formula
- Irrigating syringe (50 mL) with catheter tip for bolus NG feeding

SAFETY ALERT

- Discard unused formula after 24 hrs.
- Change formula delivery syringe daily.

- Calibrated container of water for flushing
- Clean gloves

Preparation

1 Swab unopened formula container top with alcohol.

2 Date and refrigerate opened formula can.

3 Warm refrigerated formula to room temperature by placing container with desired amount of formula in basin of hot water.

4 Elevate head of bed to a 30° angle or higher.

5 Assess that NG or gastrostomy tube has not migrated.

SKILL

Intermittent Large-Bore Nasogastric Tube Feeding

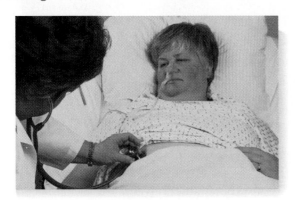

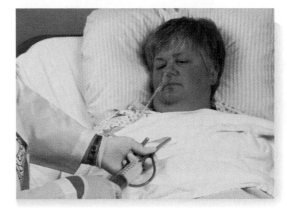

1 Assess client's abdomen and verify presence of bowel sounds. **RATIONALE:** Absence of bowel sounds indicates lack of peristalsis; gastric feeding should not be given in this case.

■ Determine position of NG tube using sounds with stethoscope, aspiration of gastric contents, and x-ray determination as previously described (see Chapter 19).

2 Aspirate gastric contents to determine residual volume. **RATIONALE:** If residual volume is greater than one-half of volume previously delivered, hold feeding and recheck in 1 hr.

■ Return aspirated contents to stomach. **RATIONALE:** Secretions contain electrolytes; their return helps prevent electrolyte imbalance.

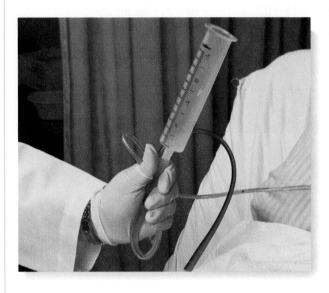

3 Remove plunger from syringe and attach empty syringe barrel to NG tube.

- Holding syringe no higher than 18 in above client's stomach, administer 30 mL water to flush and test tubing; clamp tubing by folding before syringe empties. **RATIONALE:** To prevent administering air into client's stomach.

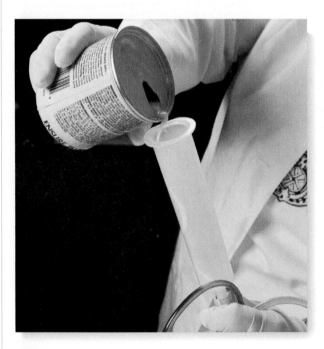

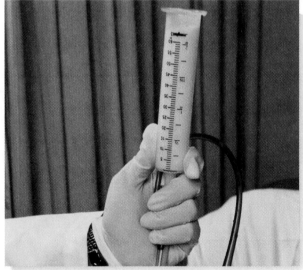

5 Clamp tubing before syringe empties or continuously fill syringe before it completely empties. **RATIONALE:** If syringe empties and tubing fills with air, additional formula will move this air into client's stomach and increase risk of vomiting.

4 Pour feeding product into syringe barrel and allow to flow slowly by gravity (over 15 min). **RATIONALE:** Forced delivery increases risk of cramping, nausea, or vomiting.

- Flush tubing with 30 mL water and clamp.

SAFETY ALERT

Gastric ileus or delayed emptying may result in retention of forced feedings and may impose a serious risk for aspiration and death, especially when feedings are continuous. To reduce the risk of aspiration:

- Aspirate gastric contents (NG tube) to determine retention before administering any intermittent feeding.
- For intermittent feedings, residual volume should not be greater than one-half the amount of previously delivered feeding.
- Regularly analyze residuals with continuously infused feeding to evaluate whether retained amount is significant; for instance, if formula is infusing at 100 mL/h and aspirated volume is greater than 100 mL, stomach is not emptying as fast as feeding is being infused.
- Keep head of bed elevated at all times for continuous feeding and for 2 hrs following intermittent (bolus) feeding.
- Report delayed gastric emptying to physician for possible pharmacologic management.

Intermittent Gastrostomy Tube Feeding

SAFETY ALERT

Assess for migration or change in length of exposed gastrostomy tube (usually ½ inch exposed) because change in exposed tube length may indicate tube displacement.

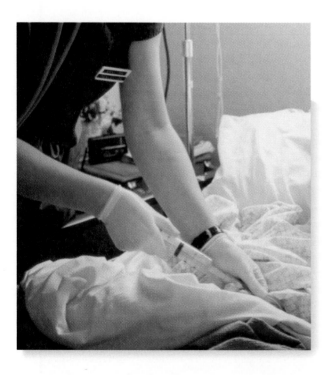

1 Aspirate gastric contents to determine residual volume as in previous skill. **RATIONALE:** Increased residuals may indicate that delayed emptying is occurring or that gastrostomy tube's internal stabilizer has migrated and is obstructing pyloric outlet. If residual secretions are unobtainable, tube may be displaced between stomach and abdominal wall, in which case administration of feeding could result in peritonitis.

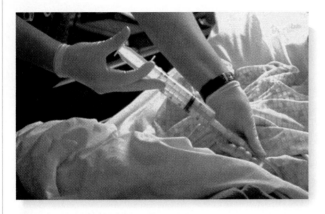

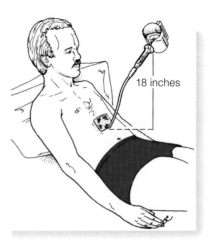

18 inches

2 Return aspirated contents to stomach. **RATIO-NALE:** To prevent electrolyte imbalance.

3 Slowly administer tube feeding through syringe barrel by gravity, following steps in previous skill.

BEYOND THE SKILL

Gastrostomy or PEG Tube Site Care

The PEG has two crossbar bumpers (stabilizers). One is on the tube inside the stomach; the other is on the tube externally where it exits the abdominal wall.

- The external bumper should be rotated 90° daily.
- Prepared split dressings or special dressing holders are used to secure PEG tubes.
- Dressings should be changed when they become wet, or daily.
- Dressings are placed over, not under, the external bar; dressings placed under the external bar can cause erosion of gastric tissue or abscess of the abdominal wall due to pressure on the internal bar within the stomach.
- The site should be assessed for signs of tube migration, dislodgment, infection, or skin problems.
- In special cases, a barrier dressing or paste may be required to protect the skin from GI fluid irritation; however, the use of an occlusive dressing is associated with greater risk for fungal infection.

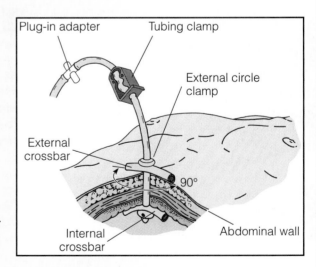

CONTINUOUS SMALL-BORE ENTERAL TUBE FEEDING

Equipment

- Prescribed formula in closed ready-to-infuse system (preferred)
- Formula reservoir or bag (if necessary)
- Infusion pump (not to exceed 40 psi)
- Administration tubing that is compatible with pump
- Label for client's name, date, and formula (if necessary)
- Sterile normal saline solution for flushing
- Sterile syringe for flushing (60 mL or size manufacturer recommends)

SAFETY ALERT

- Do not allow gastric formula to hang for over 8 hrs.
- Change formula reservoir and administration set daily.
- Discard closed formula system after 24 hrs.

SKILL

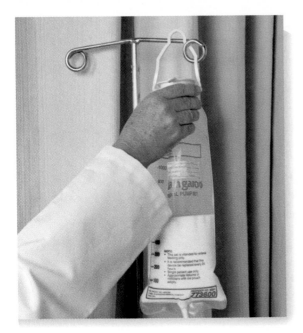

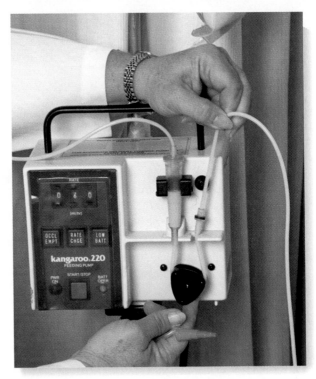

1 If using reservoir or bag for continuous intestinal feeding, fill with enough formula to limit hang time to 4 hrs. **RATIONALE:** To reduce risk of infection since intestine is a less protected alkaline environment.

- Initiate feeding with isotonic (300 mOsmol) or slightly hypotonic formula. **RATIONALE:** To prevent cramping and diarrhea.
- Connect administration tubing to formula reservoir (container or bag) and prime tubing per manufacturer's instructions.

2 Thread tubing through pump per manufacturer's instructions. Pump must not exceed 40 psi. **RATIONALE:** Excessive pressures can cause tube rupture.

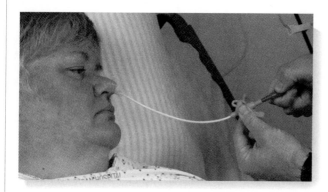

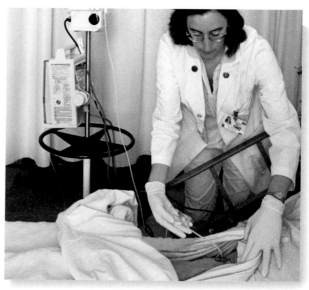

 ③ Connect feeding tube to client's small-bore nasoenteric tube.

④ Alternate method: Connect to client's small-bore jejunostomy tube.

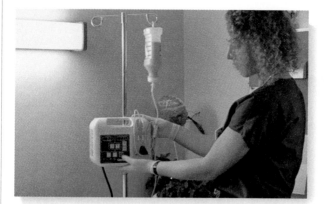

⑤ Start feeding at slow constant infusion rate (25 to 50 mL/hr). **RATIONALE:** To allow time to assess client's tolerance for feeding.

- If client tolerates feeding, increase rate in 8 to 24 hrs (increase by 25 to 50 mL/hr). **RATIONALE:** Incremental increases may be better tolerated (maximum rate is usually 100 to 150 mL/hr).

- Keep head of bed elevated at 30° angle all the time during constant infusion. **RATIONALE:** To reduce risk of aspiration.

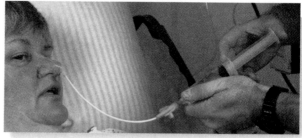

⑥ Flush continuous infusion tubing every 4 hrs with 30 mL normal saline or warm water. **RATIONALE:** To help prevent clogging.

- For closed system, inject into side port and use sterile syringe each time tube is flushed. **RATIONALE:** To reduce risk of system contamination.

SAFETY ALERT

- Tinting of the formula may enhance detection of aspiration, but should be used cautiously, especially in seriously ill clients. Instances of death have been associated with systemic absorption of blue dye (client's skin and internal organs become blue). It is thought that dye translocates by inhibiting the normal protective barrier processes of the gastrointestinal tract.

- Large containers of blue dye have been found to be contaminated. If dye must be added to the client's formula, a single dose unit (blue dye FD&C#1, FDA approved) should be used. Do not open any closed system (e.g., ready-to-hang formula container) to add dye.

CHARTING

- Date and time
- Quantity and character of residual volumes obtained
- Type and rate of feeding administered
- Type of infusion pump used
- Client's elevated positioning post bolus feeding
- Client's continuous elevated positioning for continuous feeding

- Client's response to feedings
- Frequency of tube irrigation; type and volume of solution used
- Abdominal assessment findings
- Assessment characteristics of tube insertion site
- Type and frequency of tube site dressing changes
- Frequency and type of oral hygiene provided

CRITICAL THINKING FOCUS

SECTION ONE ▪ Small-Bore Nasoenteral Feeding

Unexpected Outcomes	Alternative Nursing Actions
Tube is difficult to advance.	Have client hold ice chips in mouth for a few minutes to numb nasal passage and suppress gag reflex.
X-ray shows nasointestinal tube remains in stomach.	Position client on right side (1 to 2 hrs) to promote tube movement to distal antrum.
	Report to physician; metoclopramide injection may be required to facilitate tube movement.
	Do not initiate forced feeding until x-ray confirms tube is in duodenum.
Client coughs, is unable to speak, and becomes cyanotic during tube insertion.	Remove tube, as these signs indicate tube is being advanced into client's airway.

SECTION TWO ▪ Enteral Feeding

Unexpected Outcomes	Alternative Nursing Actions
Tube is obstructed and cannot be irrigated or pump's occlusion alarms sound repeatedly.	Check that tube is not kinked or twisted.
	Establish regular flushing schedule using 30 mL warm normal saline or water q4hr.
	Avoid use of acidic or carbonated flush solutions as they may precipitate protein.
	Flush small-bore tubes every 4 hrs or more frequently to prevent clogging.
	If possible, obtain liquid form of medications delivered by tube.

- Thoroughly dissolve or crush pills to be administered per tube, administer each pill separately, and flush with 10 mL of water or normal saline before and after each medication.
- Utilize special clog zapper system, which includes small-bore tubing applicator, syringe, and clog-zapping solution.

- Gastrostomy or PEG tube site leaks formula and accumulates crusty drainage.

- Rotate external bar daily; if it cannot be rotated freely, notify physician.
- Make sure daily dressing is placed over, not under, external stabilizing bar to prevent tension on internal bumper and erosion of gastric tissue.
- Cleanse exit site daily with soap and water and allow to dry before dressing.
- Report purulent drainage, redness, or tenderness to physician.

- Client develops diarrhea when feeding is started.

- Consult dietitian about osmolarity of formula.
- Slow formula feeding rate.
- Avoid addition of blue dye to formula.

- Client receiving enteral feeding develops diarrhea due to system contamination.

- Use careful handwashing when setting up or opening system or adding formula.
- Check expiration date on formula.
- If adding dye to formula, only use individual single dose of food dye FD&C #1. Large dye containers may be source of formula contamination.
- Do not open closed systems to add dye. Do not allow gastric formula to hang over 8 hrs (4 hrs for intestinal formula); discard closed formula system after 24 hrs.
- Change formula reservoir, administration set, or delivery syringe daily.
- Store unopened formula containers in cool, dry place.
- Date and refrigerate opened cans and discard after 24 hrs.
- Discard unused reconstituted (powder) formula after 24 hrs.
- If possible, use stopcock rather than disconnecting tube system to aspirate or deliver fluids.
- Consult with dietician or physician about use of prefilled ready-to-hang formula as closed system.
- Flush reservoir with sterile water before refilling with formula.

- Client receiving enteral nutrition develops intractable diarrhea, vomiting, and silent bowel.

- Discontinue all feeding and notify physician and other members of nutrition team.

- Gastric residual is greater than 50 percent of amount administered in previous feeding.

- Withhold feeding temporarily and recheck. Formula may be too concentrated; faster emptying occurs if feeding has same osmotic pressure. Report increasing residuals to the physician.

SELF-CHECK EVALUATION

PART 1 ▪ Matching Terms

Match the definition in column B with the correct term in column A.

Column A

_____ a. Ileus
_____ b. Paresis
_____ c. Aspiration
_____ d. Anabolism
_____ e. Jejunostomy
_____ f. Naso-
_____ g. Enteral
_____ h. PEG
_____ i. Catabolism
_____ j. Dysphagia

Column B

1. Destructive phase of metabolism; breakdown of complex substances into simple ones for the release of energy
2. Surgical opening into the jejunum of the small intestine
3. Constructive phase of metabolism resulting in cellular repair and growth
4. Intestinal paralysis due to obstruction or muscle paralysis secondary to chemical or mechanical stimuli
5. Partial or incomplete paralysis
6. Inhalation of blood or fluid due to dysfunction of the pharyngeal stage of swallowing
7. Alteration in the ability to swallow
8. By means of the gastrointestinal tract
9. Through the nose
10. Endoscopically placed gastric tube

PART 2 ▪ Multiple Choice Questions

1. Which of the following statements is true regarding enteral nutrition?

a. It is more expensive, but safer than parenteral nutrition.
b. It protects the integrity of the GI tract.
c. It is less convenient than parenteral nutrition.
d. It cannot provide total nutritional support.

2. Which of the following clients would be a candidate for enteral feeding?

a. A client with an obstructing esophageal lesion.
b. A client with an absorptive disorder (e.g., Crohn's disease).
c. A client requiring decompression management.
d. A client experiencing acute GI bleeding.

3. The most natural way to deliver enteral nutrition is:

a. Per jejunostomy tube.
b. Per gastrostomy tube.
c. Parenterally.
d. Nasointestinally.

4. The desired placement for tube delivery of enteral nutrition for the client at high risk for aspiration is:

a. Nasogastric tube.
b. Nasointestinal tube.
c. Jejunostomy.
d. Gastrostomy.

5. The most accurate method of determining enteral tube placement is:

   a. Auscultation of injected air.
   b. Testing the pH of aspirated secretions.
   c. Checking the color of aspirated secretions.
   d. X-ray.

6. The most common nosocomial cause of diarrhea in tube-fed clients is:

   a. Hyperosmolar formula.
   b. Fast feeding administration rate.
   c. System contamination.
   d. Overdilution of formula.

7. A gastric feeding should be withheld if the residual volume is:

   a. 50 mL.
   b. 100 mL.
   c. The same as the previous residual.
   d. 50 percent of the volume previously delivered.

8. Before administering an intermittent bolus feeding (200 mL) per nasogastric tube, the nurse aspirates 90 mL of residual gastric contents. The nurse should:

   a. Notify the physician.
   b. Hold the feeding and recheck residual in 1 hr.
   c. Reinsert the aspirate and administer the feeding.
   d. Discard the aspirate and administer the feeding.

9. Following administration of a tube feeding, the client should remain in the following position:

   a. Head of bed elevated 30°.
   b. Supine, lying on the right side.
   c. Supine, lying on the left side.
   d. Position of the client's choice.

10. It is essential to check the residual before administering a nasogastric feeding because greater than expected residual volume may indicate that:

   a. The formula is stimulating hypersecretion of gastric juices.
   b. The enteral product is too dilute.
   c. Gastric ileus may be present.
   d. The nasogastric tube may be obstructing the pyloric outlet.

11. The most serious complication associated with gastrostomy tubes is:

   a. Skin irritation due to leakage.
   b. Tube misplacement into the abdominal cavity.
   c. Tube obstruction.
   d. Dumping syndrome.

12. Which of the following must be obtained before continuous enteral feeding by small-bore tube is begun?

   a. Validation that aspirated contents have pH >6.
   b. Validation that aspirated contents have pH <6.
   c. Confirmation of tube position by x-ray.
   d. Client's height, weight, and nutritional status.

13. The greatest advantage of using nasointestinal tubes for enteral nutrition is:

    a. Risk for infection is lower.
    b. Risk of aspiration is lower.
    c. Intermittent feeding is possible.
    d. Long-term use is possible.

14. The use of blue dye to color enteral formula is associated with:

    a. Decreased risk of feeding aspiration.
    b. Increased risk of formula contamination.
    c. Improved visualization on validation x-rays.
    d. Reduced risk of bacterial translocation and sepsis.

PART 3 ▪ Critical Thinking Application

Mr. Bradley has been diagnosed with cancer of the liver. He is admitted to the hospital with brain metastases. He complains of no appetite, refuses most meals, and becomes significantly malnourished with drastic weight loss. Impairment of his hepatic and neurologic status has caused intermittent periods of nonresponsiveness and inability to eat. Mr. Bradley's family is asking about alternative nutrition options, and the physician requests that the family make decisions about treatment options.

    1. If nutritional support is indicated, what are the processes normally followed?
    2. Who has the primary decision-making power about medical treatments such as nutritional support?
    3. Do health care providers have an obligation to provide extraordinary care?
    4. Once artificial feeding is initiated, can health care providers discontinue it?
    5. In what ways can health care providers offer symbolically significant care?

21

URINARY

ELIMINATION

INTRODUCTION

The primary structures of the urinary system are the kidneys, ureters, bladder, and urethra. Each kidney produces urine, which is carried to the bladder by the ureter. Peristaltic waves, pressure, and gravity propel urine through the ureters so that it can be discharged into the bladder.

The bladder serves as a reservoir for urine until the urge to void takes place. When the act of micturition or urination occurs, urine passes through two sphincters and is transported from the bladder to the external environment by the urethra.

The anatomic position of the bladder and the structure of the urethra differ in males and females. In both sexes the bladder is posterior to the symphysis pubis. In females, however, the bladder is anterior to the vagina and the neck of the uterus. In males, the bladder is anterior to the rectum. The urethra of the female is about 1.5 in (4 cm) long; in the male it is about 8 in (20 cm) long.

(continued on next page)

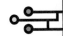

The urethra, bladder, ureters, and kidney pelves are lined with a continuous layer of mucous membrane. Because there is no break in the continuity of the lining, bacteria introduced into the normally sterile system can spread rapidly throughout the tract. When the bladder is empty, the lining falls into folds that provide pockets where bacteria can multiply. Since the membrane is highly vascular, bacteria can easily enter the bloodstream and septicemia can result.

PREPARATION PROTOCOL: FOR URINARY ELIMINATION SKILLS

Complete the following steps before each skill.

1. Check physician's order and client plan of care.
2. Gather equipment.
3. Check client's identaband.
4. Explain purpose of procedure to client.
5. Instruct client/family as indicated.
6. Wash hands.
7. Put on gloves when collecting output.

COMPLETION PROTOCOL: FOR URINARY ELIMINATION SKILLS

Make sure the following steps have been completed.

1. Measure output findings and document on I&O record.
2. Discard disposable equipment and trays.
3. Remove gloves and discard appropriately.
4. Position client for comfort.
5. Wash hands.
6. Report any abnormal or unusual findings.

SECTION ONE

INTAKE AND OUTPUT

One of the most important tasks a nurse performs on a daily basis is the accurate documentation of the client's I&O findings. Most clients require I&O monitoring following surgical intervention, major trauma, or systemic dysfunction.

The accurate measurement of intake and output provides the following vital information regarding the client:

- Estimate of fluid and electrolyte status
- Estimate of function of cardiac and renal systems
- Guide to replacement of intravenous fluids when client is NPO
- Guide to replacement of intravenous fluids when client has abnormal losses or fluid shifts
- Estimate of progress of client with drainage following medical interventions
- Estimate of effects of cardiotonic and diuretic medications

I&O should be a nursing order if indicated by the client's condition and/or medication profile and not ordered by the physician.

RATIONALE

- To measure and record I&O, providing vital information for physician and nurse
- To accurately measure all forms of fluid intake and output, including urine, gastric, and drains
- To identify alteration in fluid status of client and design appropriate action plan

ASSESSMENT

- Assess client's plan of care to see if intake and output is ordered.
- Assess client's plan of care and progress to determine if intake and output is necessary if not included in physician's orders.
- Assess client's ability to assist in keeping an I&O record.
- Identify all potential sources of output (urine, drainage from tubes, liquid stools, vomiting, wound drainage not collected in drainage tubes).

- Observe color, clarity, and odor of urine.
- Identify all agency forms where recording of intake and output must occur on your assigned shift.
- Assess for signs of dehydration, overhydration, and weight change (most accurate assessment of fluid balance).

MEASURE AND RECORD INTAKE

Equipment

- Glass or cup
- I&O bedside form with fluid conversion

- I&O chart record
- Graduate for measurement of urine and other output

SKILL

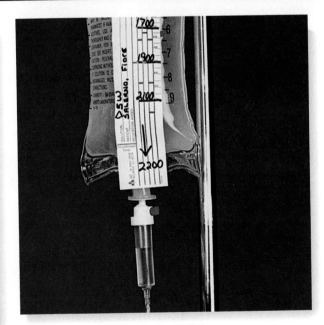

2 Record time, amount, and type of IV fluids in appropriate space on bedside form.

1 Measure all fluids taken orally according to agency values.

- Record time, amount, and type of oral fluids in appropriate space on bedside form.

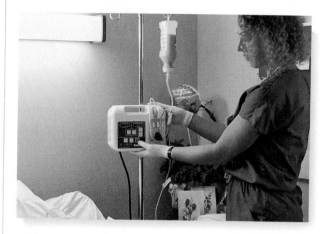

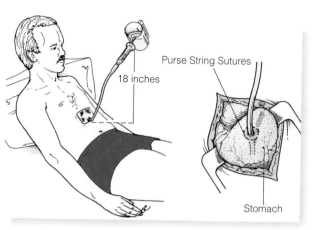

18 inches

Purse String Sutures

Stomach

3 Record time, amount, and type of continuous NG tube, G tube, or J tube feedings and medications on bedside form.

4 Record time, amount, and type of intermittent NG tube, G tube, or J tube feedings and medications on bedside form.

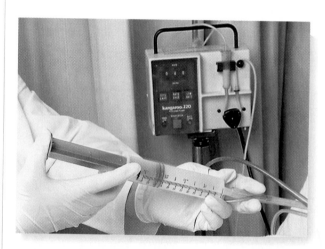

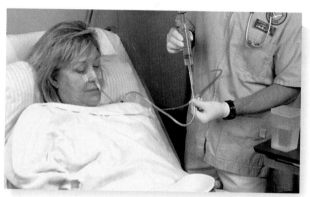

6 Record time, amount, and type of fluids instilled for flushing tube used for intermittent feedings on bedside form.

5 Record time, amount, and type of fluids instilled for flushing continuous feeding tube on bedside form.

SAFETY ALERT

Remember to include intermittent IV medications as fluid intake. (Medications given by infusion pump or piggyback are usually dissolved in 10 to 100 mL of compatible fluid.) This adds up to an appreciable amount when a client receives multiple IV medications.

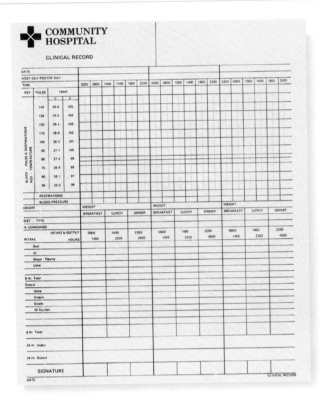

7 Accurately calculate 8-hr totals of each type of intake from bedside form.

- Transfer to graphic sheet on client's chart (appropriate columns on 24-hrs I&O record).

MEASURE AND RECORD OUTPUT

Equipment

- Bedpan or urinal
- Graduate for measurement of output
- Calibrated drainage bag
- Clean gloves
- I&O chart record

SKILL

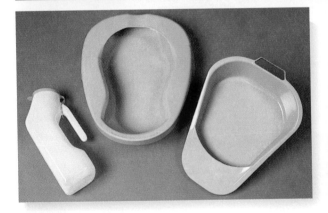

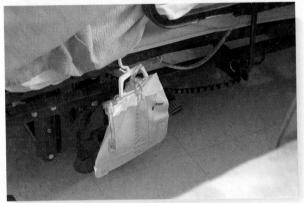

1 Offer bedpan or urinal as appropriate.

- Run warm water over bedpan and dry.
- Pad bedpan if necessary for very thin clients.

2 Use calibrated drainage bag to monitor urinary output.

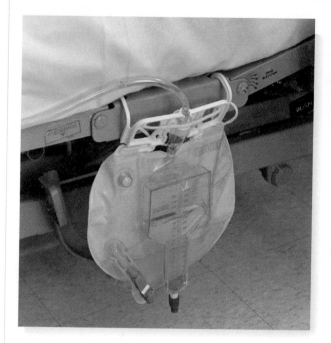

3 Use Foley drainage bag with hourly urinometer if close monitoring is required.

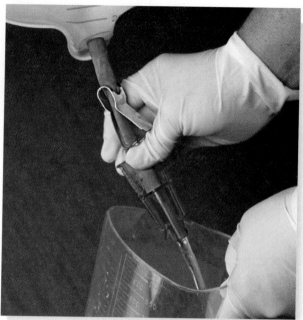

4 Empty urinal, bedpan, or Foley drainage bag into graduate or commode "hat" and note amount of urine.

- For most accurate record, empty urine into graduate. **RATIONALE:** Measurement from Foley drainage bag or hat is only approximate.
- Note color and odor of urine.

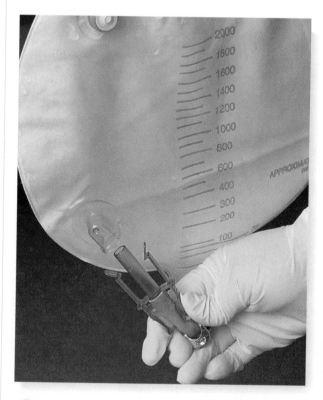

5 Be sure to clamp and replace drainage spout securely. **RATIONALE:** If drainage spout is not replaced securely, urine will drain onto floor, resulting in inaccurate urinary output measurement and safety hazard created by wet floor.

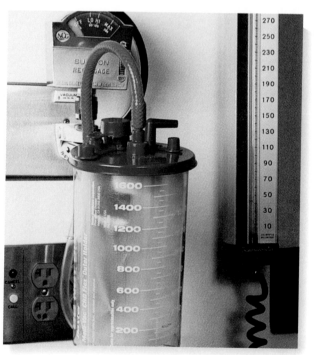

6 Document amount of drainage in NG suction and mark on suction container.

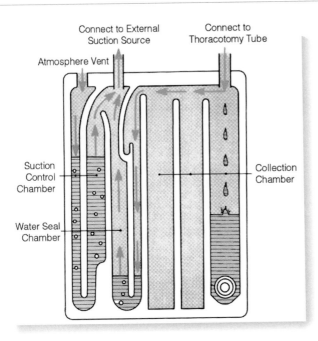

Connect to External Suction Source
Connect to Thoracotomy Tube
Atmosphere Vent
Suction Control Chamber
Water Seal Chamber
Collection Chamber

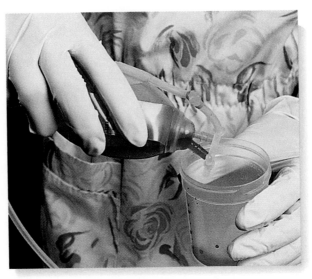

8 Empty wound drainage collection system (either Jackson-Pratt or Hemovac) containers into graduate or calibrated specimen container and record amount of drainage.

7 Note amount of drainage in collection chamber of chest tube drainage system and mark on container.

SAFETY ALERT

Be sure to reconnect and resume wound drainage systems according to manufacturer directions after measuring output. Otherwise, suction will not operate effectively, and drainage will collect in the client, delaying wound healing and increasing the risk of infection.

BEDSIDE INTAKE AND OUTPUT RECORD

Name _____   Date _____

Room # _____

	Intake			Output		
	Oral	IV		Urine	Emesis	Drainage
7 am – 3 pm			7 am – 3 pm			
Total			Total			
3 pm – 11 pm			3 pm – 11 pm			
Total			Total			
11 pm – 7 am			11 pm – 7 am			
Total			Total			
24hr Total			24hr Total			

Measurements

Glass 240cc   Ice Cream 100cc
Cup 150cc   Jello 100cc
Bowl 150cc   Ice Chips 5cc/Cube
Juice Glass 100cc
Coffee Pot 240cc

9 Record time and amount of all output on bedside I&O record.

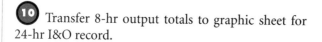

10 Transfer 8-hr output totals to graphic sheet for 24-hr I&O record.

- Complete 24-hr output record by adding all three output totals together; place totals on graphic sheet (if task for your shift).

CHARTING

- Time and amount of all oral fluid intake
- Eight-hour total of all IV and enteral fluids
- 24-hr total of all fluid intake
- Time and amount of all urinary output

- Time and amount of all drainage (e.g., NG or T tube)
- 8-hr total of all fluid output
- 24-hr total of all fluid output

SECTION TWO

URINE STUDIES

Nursing responsibilities include collecting and performing tests on urine specimens. Most urine specimens are collected as clean-catch or midstream samples. Single urine specimens are obtained through random sampling. The majority of urine tests are completed in the laboratory. A common urine test performed in the nursing unit is checking the specific gravity of a urine specimen. Urine glucose is sometimes tested in the nursing unit using a dip strip. Urinary ketone bodies are also checked with the dip Keto-Diastix strip.

RATIONALE

- To determine if urine studies are time dependent
- To determine if first voided specimens are to be discarded
- To provide baseline data for further evaluation
- To determine presence of bacteria or hemoglobin in urine
- To assist in determining fluid balance of client

ASSESSMENT

- Assess client's ability to void when specimens are needed.
- Assess color and odor of urine: Unusual color can indicate concentration and hydration status, presence of blood or urobilinogen, or side effects of medications.
- Assess for cloudiness and unusual odor of urine that can indicate early signs of infection.
- Determine approximate time when testing should be done.
- Review diagnostic tests and drugs that interfere with test results and alert appropriate health team members.

OBTAIN URINE SPECIMEN USING BEDPAN

Equipment

- Bedpan
- Clean gloves
- Toilet tissue
- Absorbent pad (if indicated)

SKILL

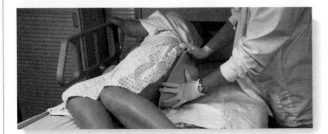

1 Place client on side.

- Place absorbent pad under client's hips.
- Slip warmed bedpan under client's hips, with large end of bedpan at hip level.

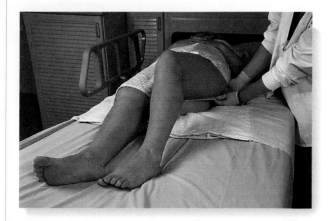

2 Roll client back onto bedpan.

- Raise head of bed for client comfort.
- Remove pan after client has voided.
- Assist client to wipe as necessary.
- Reposition client for comfort.

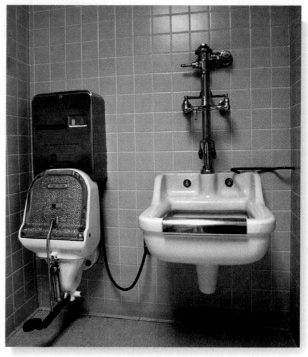

3 Clean bedpan and return to appropriate storage area.

CLINICAL NOTE

To use a urinal, place the base of the urinal flat on the bed between the client's thighs. Place the penis into the urinal and instruct the client to begin to urinate into the container. It is easier for the client to use the urinal if he can sit on the edge of the bed. Instruct the client to lower the urinal below the level of the bed and place it between his thighs. He can then urinate directly into the container.

OBTAIN URINE SPECIMEN USING COMMODE

Equipment

- Commode with locking wheels or rubber-tipped legs
- Toilet tissue
- Nurse's call bell
- Bath blanket
- Slippers
- Clean gloves

SKILL

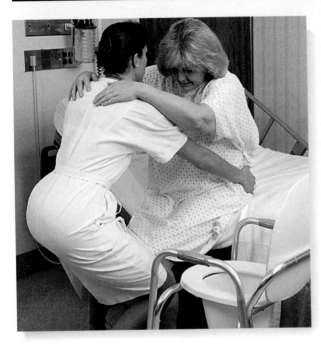

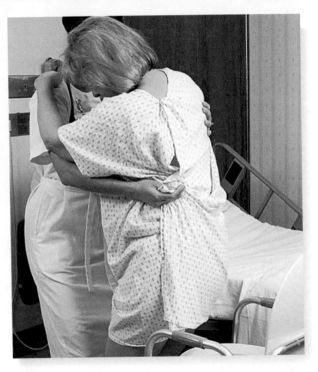

1 Place commode at foot of bed. Be sure to lock wheels.

- Place slippers on client.
- Instruct client to grasp your shoulders.
- Place your hands securely around client.
- Pivot client in front of commode.

2 Lower client onto commode, using correct body mechanics; ensure client is securely positioned on commode.

- Ensure nurse's call bell is close to client.
- Cover client with bath blanket for warmth and privacy.
- Assist client to wipe self after voiding.
- Assist client back to bed.
- Empty commode pan, clean, and replace in commode. Remember to document I&O if needed.

MEASURE SPECIFIC GRAVITY

Equipment

- Clean gloves
- Urinometer
- Cylinder
- Urine specimen

SKILL

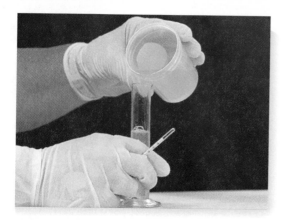

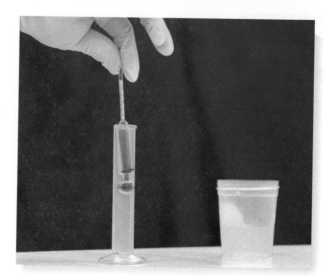

① Take urinometer and cylinder to client's room.

- Fill cylinder with 20 to 30 mL of urine (approximately three-fourths full).
- Place cylinder on flat surface.

② Place urinometer into cylinder and spin with your fingers so urinometer floats freely and does not touch side of cylinder. **RATIONALE:** If urinometer stays against side of cylinder, false reading occurs.

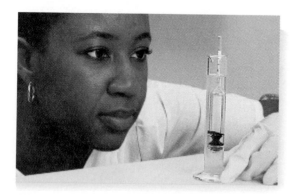

③ Take reading just before spinning stops by checking curved portion of urine level on scale of urinometer. Normal specific gravity is 1.003 to 1.030. Urinometer scale is 1.000 to 1.060.

- Empty and wash cylinder.
- Rinse urinometer with cool water. **RATIONALE:** Cool water prevents urinary proteins from coagulating and adhering to side of cylinder.

CLINICAL NOTE

To determine urinary glucose using test tape, follow these steps:

- Have client void, or collect specimen from closed system.
- Pour small amount of urine into specimen container.
- Dip test strip into urine.
- Compare color change with color chart on test strip container after waiting prescribed length of time identified on container. Results are read as a percent (1/10% to 2%) or as a one plus (+ or +1) to a four plus (++++ or 4+).

DETERMINE URINARY KETONE BODIES

Equipment

- Container with urine specimen
- Clean gloves
- Keto-Diastix strips or Acetest tablets

SKILL

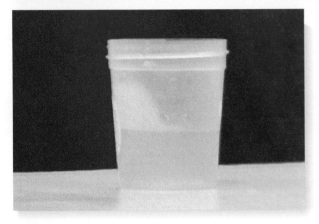

1 Collect urine specimen.

- Pour small amount of urine into specimen container.

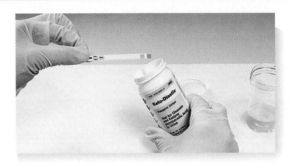

2 Remove Keto-Diastix strip from sealed bottle.

- Dip Keto-Diastix strip into urine.

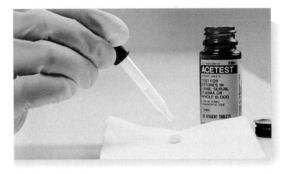

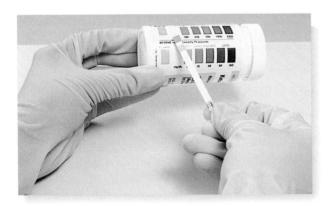

3 Compare results on strip with color chart on bottle.

- Discuss results with client. **RATIONALE:** Reinforces client teaching and participation in plan of care.

4 Alternate method: Use Acetest tablets to measure urinary ketone bodies. Obtain second voided urine specimen. **RATIONALE:** Second voided specimen is more accurate measure of present condition of client.

- Place Acetest tablet on piece of paper towel. **RATIONALE:** White towel reflects color and maintains clean area for tablet.
- Place one or two drops of urine on Acetest tablet. Wait 1 min.
- Compare color of tablet with chart colors. Dark purple indicates positive results. (Results range from negative to positive to strongly positive).

CHARTING

- Amount, color, appearance, and odor of urine
- Techniques effective in stimulating voiding
- Results of specific gravity reading
- Results of Keto-Diastix test
- Nursing interventions completed as result of test findings
- Difficulty obtaining specimen (if appropriate)
- Method of obtaining specimen
- Results of Acetest tablet test
- Physician notified, if appropriate

SECTION THREE

CATHETERIZATION

Catheterization of the urinary bladder involves inserting a small sterile tube through the urethra into the bladder, allowing urine to drain. Nurses are involved in assessing the need for this procedure, securing the physician's order, performing the procedure while maintaining sterility of all equipment and specimens, and reassessing the client's condition following the procedure. There are three types of urinary catheters: two that enter the bladder through the urethra and one that is inserted by a physician just above the symphysis pubis. Of the two that enter the bladder through the urethra, one is called a straight catheter and is intended to be inserted and removed after the bladder is drained or a specimen is obtained. The second type of catheter is one that enters the bladder through the urethra and is intended to remain in the bladder for an extended period of time. This catheter includes an inflatable balloon that holds the catheter in place and is called a retention or indwelling catheter. The catheter that is inserted above the symphysis pubis is called a suprapubic catheter. Nurses are responsible for maintaining the functioning of suprapubic catheters following insertion.

RATIONALE

- To determine need for intermittent catheterization
- To promote urinary elimination
- To determine emptying ability of bladder after voiding
- To completely assess abdominal and pelvic pain
- To prevent or relieve bladder distention
- To obtain sterile urine specimen
- To prevent urinary tract infections through catheter care

ASSESSMENT

- Assess client's bladder for distention.
- Identify purpose of catheterization.
- Check physician's orders for type of catheterization procedure.
- Assess client's ability to cooperate with positioning for procedure.
- Assess urinary meatus and catheter for exudate, edema, inflammation, and general cleanliness.
- Assess need for perineal care before catheterization procedure.

DRAPE CLIENT

Equipment

- Bath blanket

SKILL

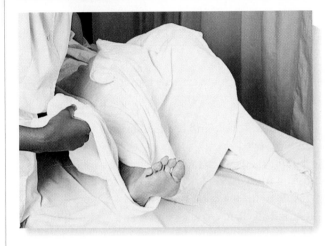

1 Bring bath blanket to bedside and raise bed to HIGH position; lower side rail nearest you.

- Place bath blanket over female client's top linen so one corner of blanket is pointed toward client's head to form diamond shape over client.
- Instruct client to hold onto bath blanket. Fanfold top linen to foot of bed or place it on chair.
- Ask client to flex knees and keep them spread apart with feet firmly placed on bed.
- Wrap lateral corners of the bath blanket around client's feet in spiral fashion until they are completely covered.

SAFETY ALERT

Take care to drape client properly, wrapping ends of bath blanket securely around legs and feet. Unsecured ends of blanket can become loose and contaminate sterile field during procedure.

CLINICAL NOTE

Drape a male client by placing bath blanket or towel over chest and fanfolding linen down to cover lower extremities.

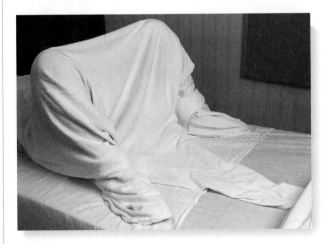

2 Place lower corner of bath blanket between knees toward foot of bed covering perineum.

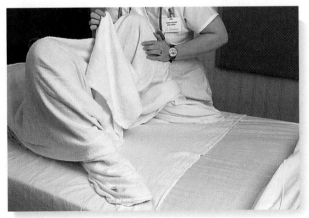

3 Fold lower corner of bath blanket back over abdomen when ready to begin catheterization procedure. **RATIONALE:** Draping provides additional warmth and prevents unnecessary exposure of perineum prior to procedure being performed.

CATHETERIZATION

Equipment

- Appropriate catheter tray
- Bath blanket
- Washcloth (optional)
- Towel (optional)
- Soap (optional)
- Basin with warm water (optional)
- Additional light source (if needed)
- Clean gloves

Preparation

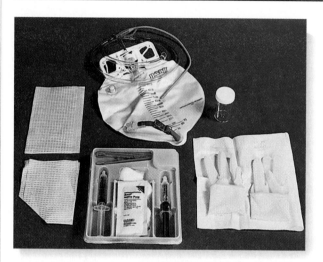

1 Gather appropriate catheterization tray and take to bedside.

- Check light source and bring additional light source if needed.
- Remind clients to maintain position as directed during procedure—knees flexed for females, legs separated for males.
- Remind all clients to keep hands away from sterile field during preparation and procedure.
- Position bed in HIGH position; lower side rail nearest you.

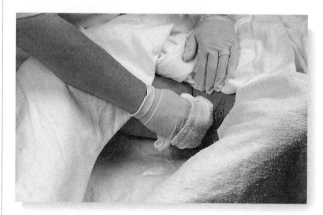

2 Visualize meatus in female clients and prepare to wash area.

- Withdraw foreskin from uncircumcised males and wash penis.
- Dry perineum thoroughly and cover genital area for privacy.
- Ensure client safety by raising side rail while away from bedside.
- Discard towels and water and replace basin.

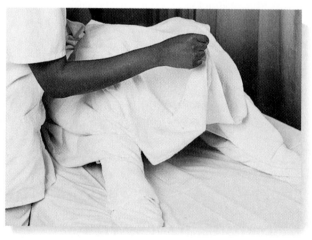

3 Drape client according to protocol.

STRAIGHT CATHETER (FEMALE)

SKILL

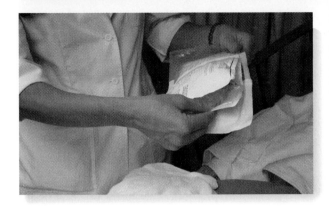

① Follow steps for preparation and draping client.

- Open sterile package by tearing package on lined edge of plastic wrap.

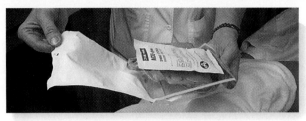

② Open and remove inner sterile package.

- Place plastic wrap at foot of bed for waste disposal.
- Place catheter tray between client's legs. Instruct client to flex knees.
- Remove sterile absorbent pad and place with absorbent side up under client's buttocks. Ask client to raise buttocks, if able, to facilitate placement.

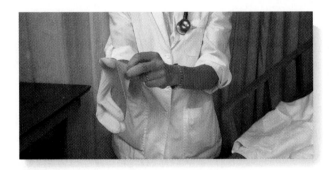

③ Don sterile gloves.

- Remove contents from tray and arrange conveniently on sterile field or place tray close to sterile field.

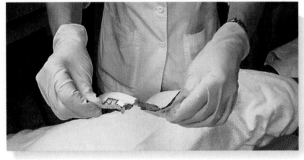

④ Open package of antiseptic solution and pour over cotton balls.

- If tray contains Betadine swabs, open package of swabs and place upright in tray.

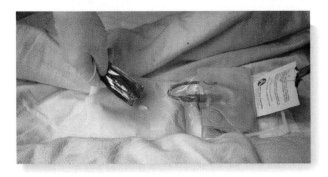

⑤ Open package of lubricant and squeeze onto sterile field.

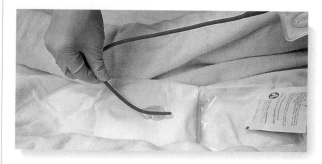

6 Pick up catheter tip and lubricate generously.

- Place catheter back on tray or leave catheter sitting on sterile field in lubricant.
- If specimen is required, uncap specimen container.
- Position urine collection receptacle close to client.

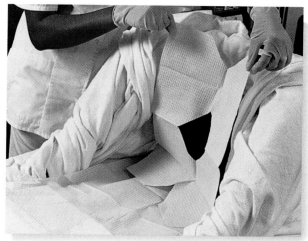

7 Place fenestrated drape over perineum, exposing meatus.

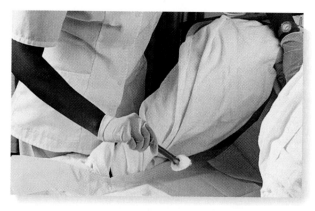

8 Cleanse client's meatus.

- Separate labia minora with your nondominant hand.
- Use forceps to pick up absorbent ball that has been saturated with antiseptic solution with your dominant hand (or pick up saturated Betadine swab).

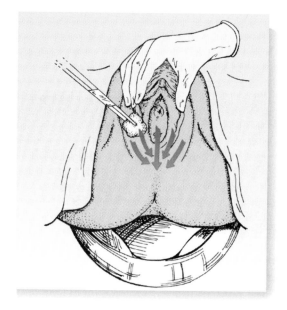

9 Use one downward stroke of forceps or swab to cleanse meatus. **RATIONALE:** Using one downward stroke, clean from least contaminated area to most contaminated area.

- Discard absorbent ball or swab in plastic cover at foot of bed. **RATIONALE:** Using new cotton ball or swab with each downward stroke prevents transfer of microorganisms.
- Repeat previous two steps at least three or four times. **RATIONALE:** This prevents contamination of urinary meatus.
- Discard forceps in plastic bag at foot of bed.

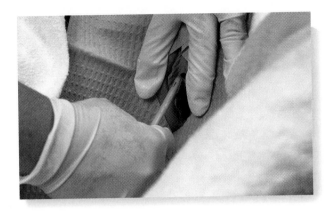

10 Pick up sterile lubricated catheter with sterile gloved hand, keeping drainage end in collection container, and insert 2 to 3 inches or until urine begins to flow.

- Move hand holding labia open to hold catheter in place.
- Place sterile specimen container under drainage end of catheter if specimen is needed and fill container with approximately 30 mL of urine.
- Replace catheter drainage end in collection container and allow urine to flow until it ceases.
- Pinch catheter closed when urine ceases to flow, and remove gently and slowly.

STRAIGHT CATHETER (MALE)

SKILL

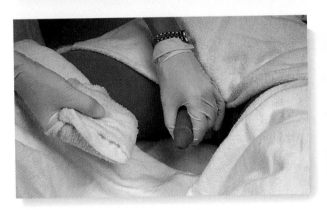

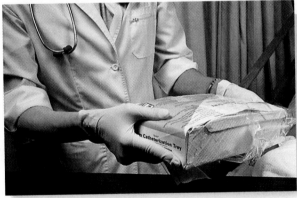

1 Follow steps for preparation.

- Place client in supine position with knees slightly apart. **RATIONALE:** This position relaxes abdominal and perineal muscles.
- Drape client by placing bath blanket over chest area; fanfold top linen down to cover lower extremities, exposing genital area.
- Wash genital area as directed in preparation. Hold penis, exposing meatus, and cleanse tip of penis using circular motion.
- Remove gloves, wash hands, and prepare for catheterization.

2 Open sterile package on lined edge of plastic wrap.

- Place plastic wrap at foot of bed for waste disposal.
- Place catheter tray between client's legs or on thighs if client is able to cooperate. If not, place catheter tray at client's side near the thigh.

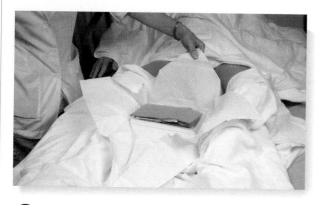

3 Open outer wrap away from sterile package with last turn toward penis.

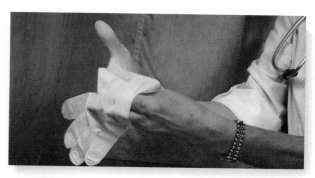

4 Don sterile gloves.

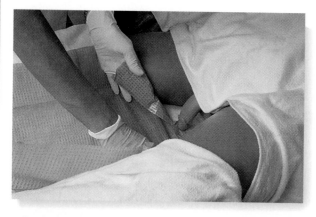

5 Place absorbent pad over thighs and under penis with absorbent side up.

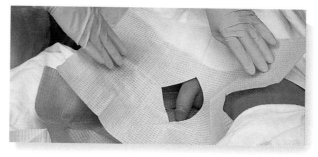

6 Place fenestrated drape over penis.

- Open antiseptic package and pour solution over cotton balls, or open Betadine swabs.
- Uncap syringe filled with lubricant or open lubricant package and squeeze lubricant onto sterile field. Syringe may be filled with lubricant from package if using alternative method.

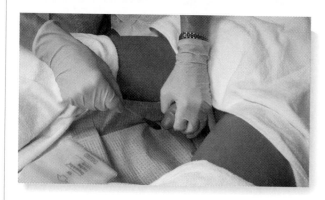

7 Hold penis upright in nondominant hand. **RATIONALE:** Holding sides of penis prevents closing of urethra.

- With dominant hand, use forceps to pick up saturated cotton ball or use Betadine swab to cleanse meatus.
- Cleanse meatus using one circular stroke with cotton ball or swab. Discard cotton ball or swab into plastic bag at foot of bed.
- Repeat cleansing motion around tip of penis. Cleanse three times, using new cotton ball or swab each time.
- Continue to hold penis with your nondominant hand.
- Discard forceps into plastic bag.

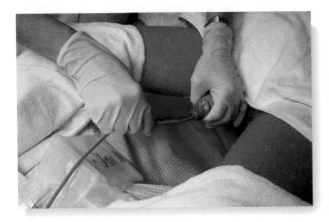

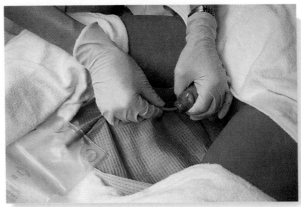

8 Place end of catheter in specimen container or urine collection container. (Newer systems have plastic container connected to catheter). **RATIONALE:** This allows specimen to be collected or urine to drain into container without urine leaking over sterile field.

- Lubricate tip of catheter 3 to 4 inches down with generous amount of lubricant.
- Pick up catheter with sterile gloved hand about 3 to 4 inches from lubricated tip of catheter.
- Lift penis to 90° angle (perpendicular to body) and exert slight traction by pulling upward. **RATIONALE:** This movement straightens urethra for easier insertion of catheter.
- Alternate method: Insert tip of lubricant syringe slightly into urethral opening and instill lubricant directly into urethra. If catheter tray does not have syringe, place sterile syringe on tray before gloving. **RATIONALE:** Inserting lubricant syringe directly into urethral opening prevents injury to lining of urethra. Because only tip of catheter is lubricated, lubricant may not get past urethral opening.

9 Insert catheter about 8 inches until urine begins to flow.

- If catheter meets resistance at sphincter, decrease angle of penis to 45°, twist catheter, and ask client to take a deep breath. **RATIONALE:** Taking a deep breath helps relax external sphincter. If persistent resistance is felt and catheter is unable to be inserted without difficulty, remove catheter and notify physician.
- Obtain urine sample if needed. Place 30 mL of urine in specimen container.
- Pinch tubing and transfer end of catheter into collection container.
- Allow urine to drain into collection container until flow stops.
- Remove catheter from container; place lid on specimen bottle.
- Discard tray.

RETENTION CATHETER (FEMALE)

Equipment

- Same as in "Drape Client" and "Straight Catheter (Female)" skills
- Disposable catheter kit with appropriate size catheter (size 8 to 10 for child, size 14 to 18 for adult female, size 18 to 20 for adult male)
- Closed drainage set
- Tape

SKILL

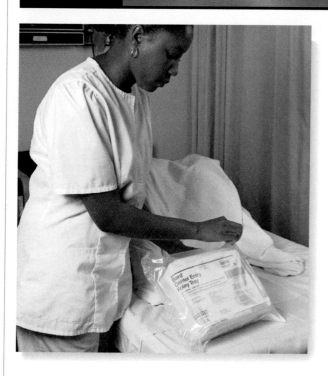

1 Follow steps for preparation.

- Remove contents from tray.
- Place plastic bag at foot of bed for waste disposal.
- Place catheter tray between client's legs.

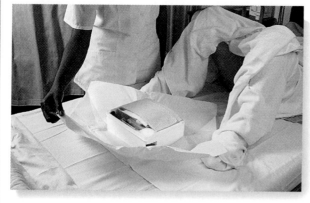

2 Fold back corner of bath blanket to expose perineum.

- Open white outer wrap away from package.
- Bring white wrap under client's buttocks.

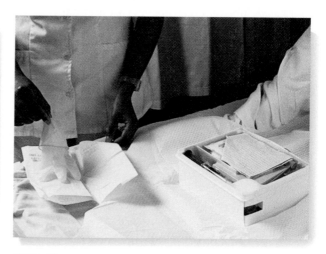

3 Don sterile gloves.

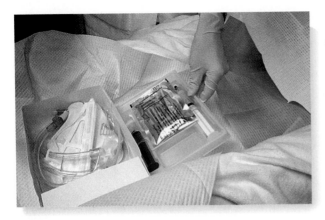

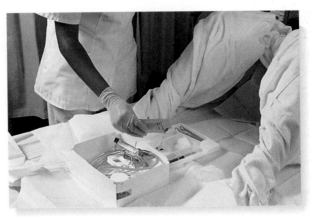

4 Separate layers of catheter tray and view contents.

- Place portion of tray with catheter and drainage bag at back portion of sterile field.

5 Tear package of antiseptic solution open and pour solution completely over cotton balls, or open package of Betadine swabs.

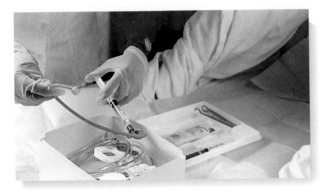

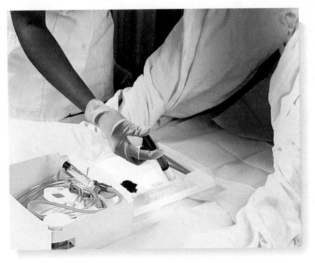

6 Test catheter balloon.

- Remove rubber protector from syringe filled with sterile water.
- Insert tip of prefilled syringe into catheter side arm to inflate balloon.
- Ensure that at least 10 mL sterile water is in syringe, as balloon usually holds more than 5 mL of water. **RATIONALE:** Catheter can be expelled if balloon is not inflated with appropriate amount of water.
- Omit pretesting steps for catheters with prefilled balloons. **RATIONALE:** Once prefilled balloons are opened and fluid is forced into balloon at tip of catheter, fluid cannot be aspirated back into syringe.
- Inflate balloon with 10 mL sterile water and check for leaks.
- After testing balloon, withdraw solution back into syringe. You may leave syringe attached to side arm of catheter.

7 Uncap syringe filled with lubricant, or open package filled with sterile lubricant and squeeze onto catheter tray.

- Remove catheter from sterile covering.

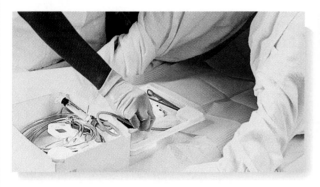

8 Generously lubricate catheter tip. Leave sterile catheter lying in lubricant while you prepare for insertion. **RATIONALE:** Lubricating catheter prevents friction and trauma to meatus and urethra.

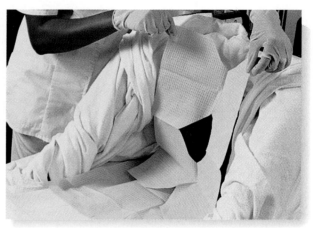

9 Position fenestrated drape over client.

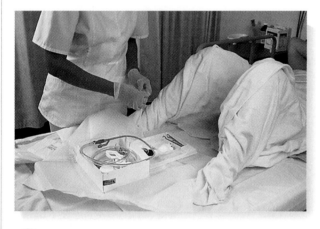

10 Position equipment prior to cleansing and insertion.

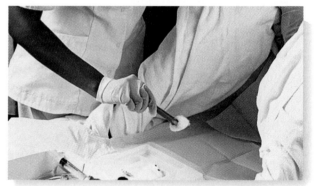

11 Cleanse client's meatus as in previous skill.

- Continue to hold labia apart until you insert catheter.
- Discard contaminated forceps in plastic bag at foot of bed when completed.

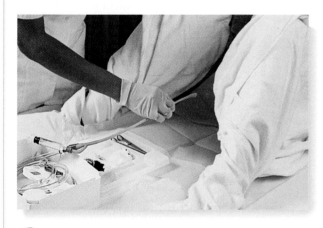

12 Grasp catheter approximately 2 inches from tip and move toward client's meatus.

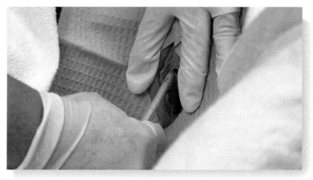

13 Insert catheter 2 to 3 inches into meatus or until urine starts to flow. Guide catheter gently 1 to 2 inches beyond point at which urine starts to flow. **RATIONALE:** Inserting catheter further into bladder ensures that it is beyond neck of bladder.

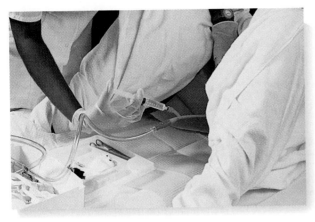

CLINICAL NOTE

- If catheter has a prefilled balloon at the drainage end, inflate the retention balloon by releasing the clamp on the prefilled balloon port.
- Retract the catheter until you feel resistance. **RATIONALE:** This indicates correct position of the catheter.

14 Move hand, separating labia, to hold catheter in place.

- Inject entire contents of prefilled syringe into side arm of catheter used for balloon inflation. Do not use excessive force to insert syringe into inflation lumen. **RATIONALE:** Valve stem may be pushed too far into valve.

SAFETY ALERT

If client complains of pain on installation of water, immediately aspirate the sterile water. **RATIONALE:** The catheter is probably in the urethra rather than the bladder.

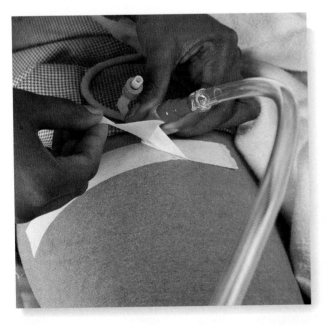

15 Tape catheter to inside or top of leg with 1-in non-allergenic tape, or use catheter holder if available (follow manufacturer's directions).

- Place one piece of tape on client's leg.
- Take second piece of tape and encircle catheter, leaving two "tails" on tape.
- Secure tails from tape on catheter to tape on client's leg. **RATIONALE:** To prevent pulling on catheter.

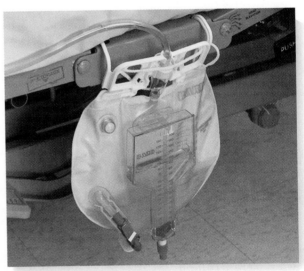

16 Attach drainage bag to bed frame (not side rails).

- Discard used supplies.
- Remove and discard gloves and wash hands.

RETENTION CATHETER (MALE)

Equipment

- Same as for "Retention Catheter (Female)" skill

SKILL

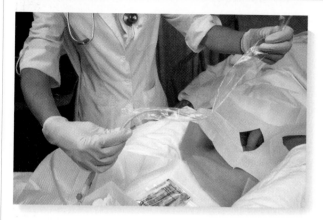

1 Follow steps outlined in skills for preparation and draping client.

- Don sterile gloves.
- Separate the two containers.
- Place container with cotton balls or Betadine swabs and lubricant toward client.
- Place container with catheter and urine bag toward foot of bed (next to first container).
- Place fenestrated drape over penis.
- Remove outer covering from catheter.

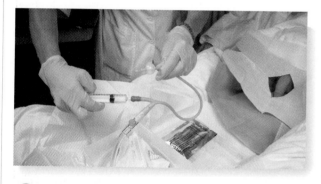

2 Test catheter balloon as described in "Retention Catheter (Female)" skill.

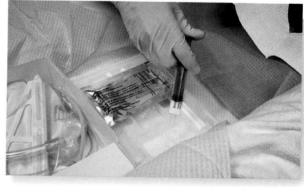

3 Squeeze lubricant onto sterile tray.

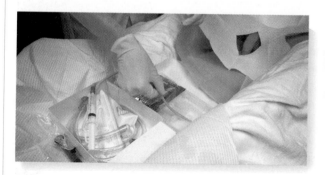

4 Lubricate catheter generously about 3 to 4 inches down and leave catheter in lubricant until ready to insert, or leave lubricant in syringe to insert lubricant directly into urethra.

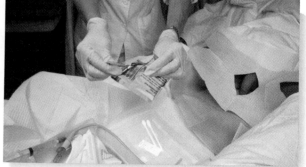

5 Open antiseptic solution container and saturate cotton balls with solution, or open package containing Betadine swabs.

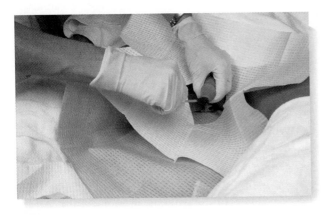

With your dominant hand, use forceps to pick up cotton ball with antiseptic solution, or pick up Betadine swab.

■ Cleanse meatus first with one circular stroke, using forceps with cotton ball or Betadine swab.

■ Discard swab or cotton ball into plastic bag at foot of bed.

■ Repeat circular cleansing motion around tip of penis. Cleanse three times, using new cotton ball or Betadine swab each time. **RATIONALE:** Using circular motion around tip of penis prevents bacteria from entering urinary meatus.

■ Continue to hold penis with nondominant hand.

■ Discard forceps into plastic bag as appropriate.

6 Hold penis upright with your nondominant hand. Hold sides of penis to prevent closing of urethra.

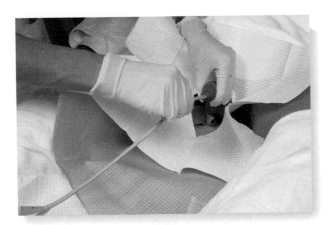

7 Pick up catheter with sterile hand 3 to 4 inches from tip of catheter.

■ Lift penis to 90° angle (perpendicular to the body) and exert slight traction by pulling upward. **RATIONALE:** This movement straightens urethra for easier insertion of catheter.

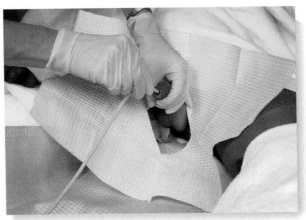

8 Insert catheter about 8 inches until urine begins to flow.

■ If resistance is met at sphincter, twist catheter and ask client to take a deep breath. **RATIONALE:** Taking a deep breath helps relax external sphincter. If persistent resistance is felt and catheter is unable to be inserted without difficulty, remove catheter and notify physician.

■ Guide catheter gently and slowly 1 to 2 inches beyond point at which urine begins to flow. **RATIONALE:** Insertion of catheter further into bladder ensures that it is beyond neck of bladder.

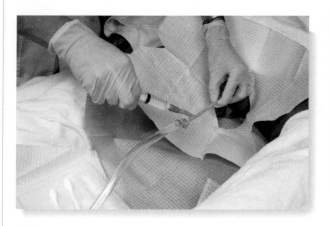

CLINICAL NOTE

- If catheter has a prefilled balloon at the drainage end of the catheter, inflate the retention balloon by releasing the clamp on the prefilled balloon.
- While maintaining pressure on the syringe plunger, retract the catheter until you feel resistance.

9 Change position of nondominant hand to hold catheter in place.

- Inject entire contents of prefilled syringe into side arm of catheter used for balloon inflation.

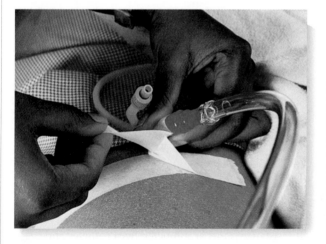

10 Tape catheter to side of leg using nonallergenic tape or tape catheter to abdomen with 1-inch tape. **RATIONALE:** This prevents pressure on penoscrotal angle.

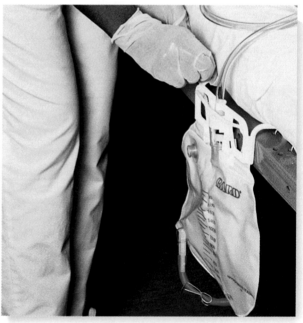

11 Attach drainage bag to bed frame (not side rails).

REMOVE RETENTION CATHETER

Equipment

- 10-mL syringe
- Paper towel
- Catheter clamp

- Soap, water, towels
- Clean gloves

SKILL

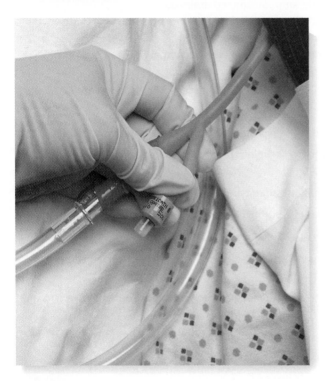

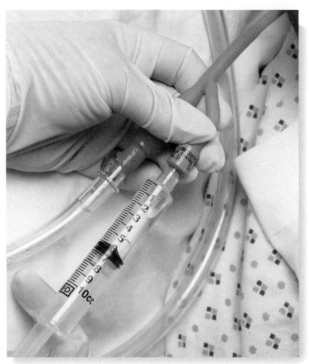

1 Clamp catheter and remove tape that attaches catheter to client's leg.

- Insert empty 10-mL syringe into balloon port of catheter. Do not cut catheter. **RATIONALE:** Balloon may not deflate completely when cut.

2 Withdraw fluid from balloon (usually 5 to 10 mL in balloon).

- Pull gently on catheter to ensure that balloon is deflated before attempting to remove. **RATIONALE:** Damage to urethra can occur if balloon is not completely deflated.
- Hold paper towel under catheter with your nondominant hand.
- If resistance is not met, pinch catheter with fingers to clamp and slowly withdraw catheter, allowing it to fall onto paper towel.
- Disconnect catheter bag from bed frame.

CLINICAL NOTE

COMPLICATIONS ASSOCIATED WITH LONG-TERM INDWELLING CATHETERS

Several complications are associated with long-term indwelling catheter placement, and therefore this procedure is to be avoided as much as possible. Alternative methods of urinary drainage for clients with incontinence include the use of protective undergarments, condom catheters in males, and intermittent self-catheteritization for clients who are able to do so.

Complications	Interventions
■ Urinary tract infection	■ Follow sterile technique for catheterization procedures.
	■ Provide meticulous catheter care.
	■ Provide meticulous perineal care following defecation.
	■ Ensure adequate fluid intake.
	■ Assess frequently for unobstructed drainage.
	■ Assess frequently for characteristics of urine output (color, clarity, amount, presence of sediment, odor).
	■ Assess client frequently for early signs of urinary tract infection, with appropriate reporting and follow through.
	■ Replace indwelling catheter at least every 2 wk.
■ Catheter leaks	■ Ensure patency of catheter.
■ Pain	■ Ensure catheter balloon is inflated in bladder and not in urethra.
■ Bladder spasms	■ Ensure that catheter is draining properly and is not plugged with sediment or blood.
■ Urethral sphincter damage	■ Report abnormal assessment and obtain appropriate medical order.
■ Urethritis	■ Use sterile technique during catheter care.
■ Epididymitis	■ Monitor and treat early signs of UTIs.
■ Prostatitis	■ Properly tape catheters in all clients to prevent tension and chronic irritation.
■ Scrotal abscess	■ Tape catheter to abdomen in males to prevent pressure on penoscrotal angle.
■ Prostatic abscess	■ Monitor for signs of infection following incision.
■ Urinary stones	■ Ensure adequate fluid intake.
	■ Take precautionary measures to prevent urinary stasis.
	■ Identify early signs of UTIs.

CHARTING

- Type of catheterization
- Amount, color, and odor of urine obtained
- Size of catheter used
- Client's tolerance of procedure
- Specimen sent to lab (if ordered)
- Catheter care provided
- Condition of urinary meatus and perineum
- Catheter removed
- Voiding: time and amount of urine voided after catheter removal
- Intake and output

SECTION FOUR

EXTERNAL CATHETERS

When the primary reason for use of a catheter is incontinence, the external catheter is used for male clients. The use of the condom catheter minimizes the risk of complications that frequently occur with long-term use of indwelling catheters. Leg bags are used as an alternate method for collecting urinary drainage. Frequently the nurse will need to attach either an indwelling catheter or a condom catheter to a continuous drainage collection system or to a leg bag, depending on the client and the situation. The following situations may occur that will necessitate this procedure:

- On initial insertion or changing of an indwelling catheter, original tubing attached to drainage collection system by manufacturer is defective or becomes contaminated during procedure.
- Client is ambulatory or upright during the day, and a continuous drainage system is inappropriate for client's activities.
- Client is being discharged with an indwelling catheter or condom catheter in place. (Be sure to send a large collection system home with client as well).

Teach the client or caregiver how to change the collection system from leg bag to large collection system for continuous drainage at night.

RATIONALE

- To provide a means for dealing with incontinence in male clients
- To prevent urinary tract infections in clients who are at risk but require a method of urine collection to maintain continence
- To collect urine for specimens
- To prevent skin irritation due to urinary incontinence

ASSESSMENT

- Assess genital area for signs of irritation and edema during use of condom catheter.
- Assess client's activity level to determine when leg bag or continuous drainage system is necessary.
- Determine ability of client/caregiver to learn how to change from leg bag to continuous drainage system using aseptic technique.

CONDOM CATHETER

Equipment

- Condom sheath
- Urine collection system

- Clean gloves

SKILL

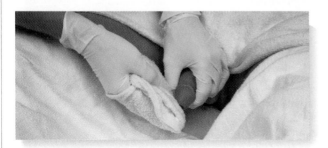

1 Wash, rinse, and dry penis thoroughly. **RATIONALE:** External catheter needs to be placed on clean, dry skin for secure fit.

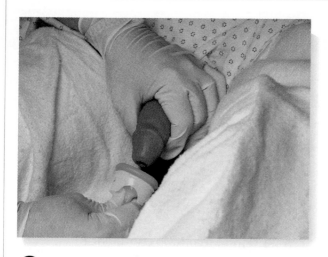

2 Pinch catheter closed and place tip of penis into catheter and against fingertips of nondominant hand. Hold plastic collar in place.

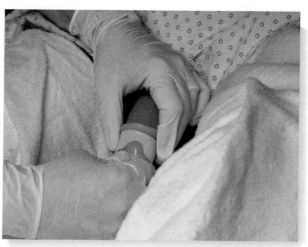

3 While holding catheter in place, unroll catheter, with nondominant hand, up shaft of penis. Do not allow catheter to wrinkle. **RATIONALE:** Wrinkles allow urine to collect in pockets, which can lead to skin irritation.

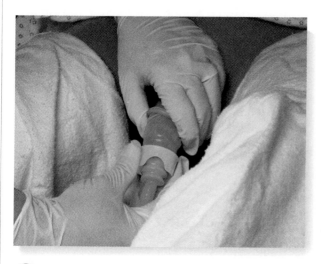

4 Remove and discard plastic collar.

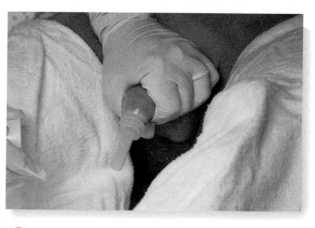

5 Squeeze catheter to adhere sheath to skin.

6 Attach external catheter to leg bag.

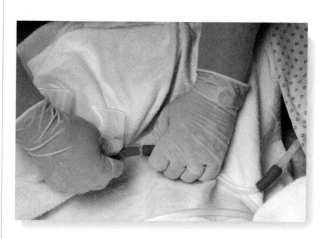

ATTACH LEG BAG TO CATHETER

Equipment

- Leg bag
- Alcohol wipes
- Clean gloves

SKILL

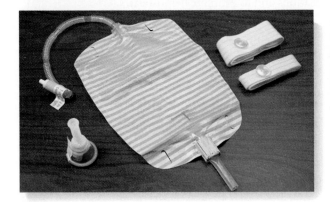

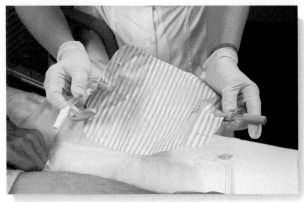

1 Gather leg bag and alcohol wipe.

- Disconnect drainage tubing from indwelling or condom catheter.
- Wipe leg bag and catheter connectors with alcohol (unless sterile package was just opened; then wipe exposed connector with alcohol).

2 Connect longer tip of leg bag or drainage tubing to catheter.

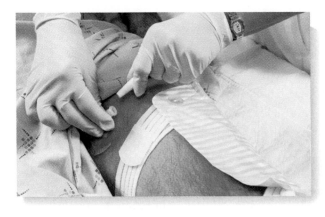

3 Connect leg bag to catheter.

- Secure leg bag to lower leg by placing strap through bag and around leg.
- Secure strap by placing button through opening of strap.
- When removing leg bag and replacing continuous gravity drainage system, reverse process, taking care to wipe all connections with alcohol before switching tubing.

CHARTING

- Condom catheter applied
- Size of catheter used
- Condition of genital area
- Type of protective coating applied to skin

- Whether catheter is connected to leg bag or continuous drainage system
- Amount, color, and odor of urine
- Client's tolerance of procedure

CATHETER AND BLADDER IRRIGATION AND INSTILLATION

The flow rate of urine drained from the bladder of a client with an indwelling catheter is usually sufficient to cleanse the lumen and promote patency of the catheter and tubing. However, where there is significant sediment or bloody drainage, indwelling catheters can become plugged with debris and will not flow properly. Nurses are instructed to irrigate the catheter either through the port on the drainage tube or by opening the closed system. When possible, it is preferable to maintain the patency of the system and irrigate the catheter through the closed system. This method of irrigation decreases the chance of contamination and thus reduces urinary infections. Following surgery on the bladder or prostate, significant bleeding and clotting can be expected. In these situations, the risk of the catheter becoming plugged is prevented by the use of a triple-lumen Foley catheter (the third lumen is for irrigation) and continuous bladder irrigations. Continuous bladder irrigations rinse clots and debris from the bladder. This rinsing prevents bladder spasms and excess bleeding. Postoperative bradycardia can also be prevented by eliminating clots and bladder spasms. Continuous bladder irrigation is also used to instill medications and to promote hemostasis.

RATIONALE

- To remove blood clots following prostatic surgery
- To instill medications into client's bladder
- To ensure patency of drainage system
- To relieve bladder spasms

ASSESSMENT

- Assess for distended bladder.
- Assess for bladder discomfort.
- Note rate of urine flow from bladder.
- Determine presence of active bleeding or clot formation.

IRRIGATE CATHETER BY OPENING A CLOSED SYSTEM

Equipment

- Sterile irrigation set (new one for each irrigation)
- Clean gloves
- Sterile gloves
- Sterile normal saline irrigant (or solution as ordered)
- Catch basin
- Antiseptic swab
- Absorbent pad

SKILL

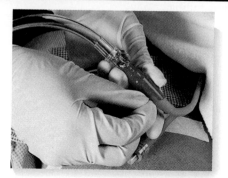

1 Expose catheter connection by removing plastic covering.

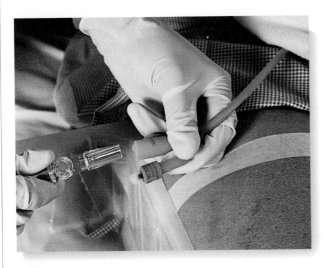

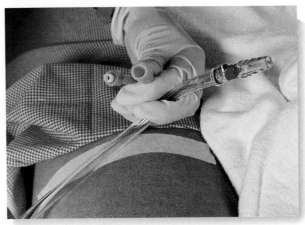

2 Disconnect catheter from drainage tube.

- Place sterile protective cap over end of drainage tube. **RATIONALE:** This will prevent contamination of tip of tubing.
- Coil tubing on bed.
- Place end of catheter over edge of catch basin. **RATIONALE:** If end of catheter touches linens, underpad, exposed skin surfaces, or drainage tube, it will be considered contaminated.
- Remove clean gloves and don sterile gloves.

3 Alternate method: Disconnect catheter from drainage tube and hold end of collection tubing in nondominant hand.

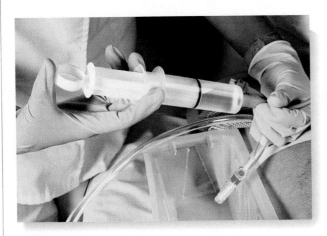

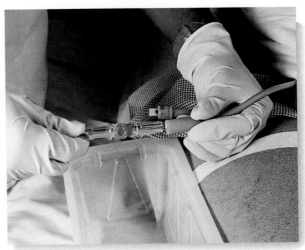

4 Instill 30 to 50 mL of irrigant into catheter with gentle but firm pressure.

- Remove syringe and allow solution to drain.
- Lower catch basin to facilitate solution to return by gravity.
- Continue to irrigate client's bladder until fluid returns are clear and clots are removed.
- Remove protective top from drainage tube and wipe with antiseptic swab or alcohol sponge.

5 Wipe end of catheter with antiseptic swab or alcohol sponge.

- Reconnect catheter to drainage tube.

CLINICAL NOTE

After catheter instillation or irrigation, follow these steps:

- Ensure a straight line from tubing to drainage bag.
- Curl excess tubing loosely on bed.
- Secure tubing to bottom linen.
- Tape catheter to client's inner thigh using a commercially available catheter holder, or tape catheter to abdomen in a male.
- Measure solution in catch basin.

SAFETY ALERT

If the amount of solution in catch basin is less than the amount of solution instilled, subtract the amount from the output on the bedside I&O record. If the amount of the solution in the catch basin is more than the amount of solution instilled, add the amount to the output on the bedside I&O record. This discrepancy may occur as a result of retained irrigating solution that is not immediately expelled.

IRRIGATE CATHETER THROUGH A CLOSED SYSTEM

Equipment

- 21- or 25-gauge, 1-in needle
- 30-mL syringe
- Catheter clamp
- Sterile gloves
- Sterile irrigation set
- Catch basin
- Antiseptic swab
- Clean gloves

SKILL

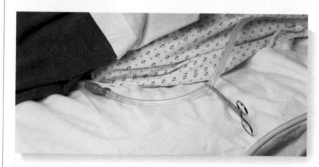

1 Fill syringe with irrigation solution.

- Clamp tubing just distal to injection port.

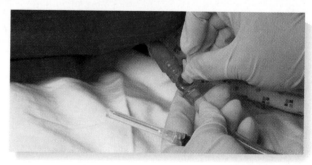

2 Swab injection port of catheter with alcohol swab or Betadine solution.

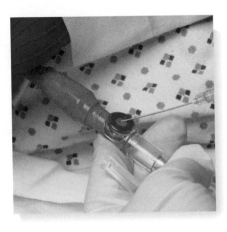

3 Insert needle into injection port.

- Inject slowly into injection port. **RATIONALE:** To prevent back-pressure in urinary drainage system.
- Remove syringe and needle from injection port.
- Unclamp drainage tube and lower catheter. **RATIONALE:** This facilitates drainage.
- Repeat irrigation steps until return is free of clots and debris.
- Measure output and record appropriate amount on bedside I&O record.

MAINTAIN CONTINUOUS BLADDER IRRIGATIONS

Equipment

- Irrigating solution and container
- Tubing
- IV pole

- Alcohol or Betadine swab
- Clean gloves

SKILL

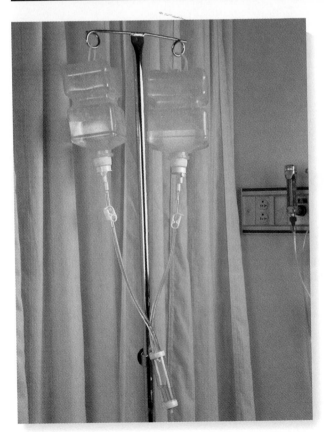

1 Obtain irrigation fluid from pharmacy or central supply and label with client's name, date, room number, type of solution, and additives if not prelabeled.

- Hang irrigation solution container on IV pole 24 to 36 in above bladder.
- Spike irrigation port of solution container and prime tubing.
- Fill drip chamber by pinching fluid chamber until half full.
- Remove protective cover from end of tubing using aseptic technique.
- Open roller clamp and allow irrigation solution to run through tubing until air is expelled. **RATIONALE:** This prevents air from entering bladder and causing discomfort.
- Close roller clamp.

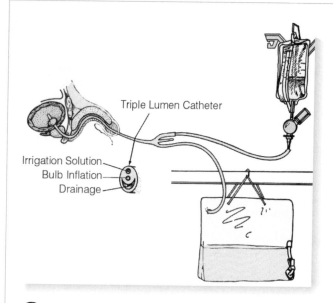

Triple Lumen Catheter

Irrigation Solution
Bulb Inflation
Drainage

With clear drainage, drip rate should be approximately 40 to 60 drops/min. When drainage is bright red or contains blood clots, the drip rate needs to be increased. **RATIONALE:** An increased drip rate will clear drainage and flush out clots, reducing the risk of bladder spasms and excessive bleeding.

- Change irrigation solution bottles and tubing using aseptic technique. Tubing should be changed a minimum of every 24 hrs.
- Monitor urine output at least every hour to observe patency of system.
- Empty drainage bag at least every 4 hrs.
- Subtract amount of irrigant infused from total output to obtain urine output.

2 Connect tubing to third lumen using aseptic technique.

- Remove gloves and discard.
- Adjust drip rate of solution by adjusting clamp on tubing to deliver prescribed hourly rate of irrigant.

INSTILL MEDICATION INTO BLADDER

Equipment

- Irrigation set
- 30-mL syringe and 21- to 25-gauge 1-in needle
- Alcohol or Betadine swab

- Irrigating solution
- Catheter clamp
- Clean gloves

SKILL

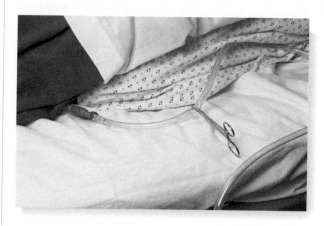

1 Draw up medication to be instilled into appropriately sized syringe using 21- to 25-gauge 1-in needle.

- Clamp drainage tube prior to instilling medication so that medication will be retained in client's bladder.
- Scrub port site on catheter tubing with alcohol or Betadine solution.

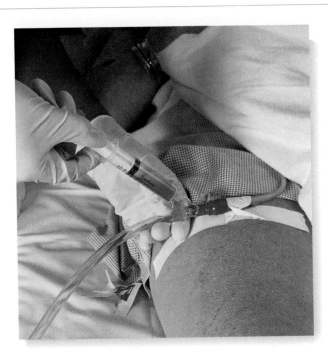

2 Insert needle at 90° angle into injection port.

- Instill medication slowly.
- Withdraw needle and cleanse port site with alcohol swab or Betadine swab.
- Remove gloves and wash hands.
- Keep tubing clamped for 15 to 20 min and observe for bladder distention or spasms.
- Unclamp tubing after 15 to 20 min.
- Subtract volume of medication instilled on bedside I&O records.
- Document medication on medication administration record.

CHARTING

- Type and amount of solution administered for irrigation
- Type and amount of medication administered
- Rate of administration of irrigating solution
- Description of urinary output, including color and presence of clots
- Discomfort, cramping, or pain
- Amount of actual urine output (minus irrigating solution)
- Signs or symptoms indicative of potential infection

SPECIMEN COLLECTION FROM A CLOSED SYSTEM

Specimens are frequently obtained from clients with indwelling catheters. The most common laboratory specimen is obtained to determine the presence of microorganisms. Sterile technique must be maintained throughout the skill to ensure accurate results.

RATIONALE

- To determine specific microorganism(s) causing urinary tract infection
- To obtain specimen for use in diagnostic urinary workup

ASSESSMENT

- Assess type of specimen required (sterile or clean).
- Check closed drainage system to determine if system has port for obtaining specimens or if catheter material has self-sealing protection.
- Identify amount of urine required for specimen.

SPECIMEN COLLECTION

Equipment

- Catheter clamp
- Syringe with 21- to 25-gauge 1-in needle
- Sterile specimen container
- Antimicrobial or alcohol swab
- Clean gloves

SKILL

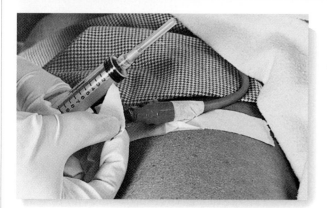

1 Clamp catheter tubing for 15 min. **RATIONALE:** Ensures adequate amount of time for collection of urine for specimen.

- Wipe aspiration port of drainage tube with antimicrobial or alcohol swab.

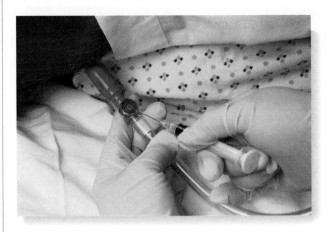

2 Insert needle into aspiration port at 30 to 45° angle. **RATIONALE:** Facilitates sealing of rubber in port following removal of needle.

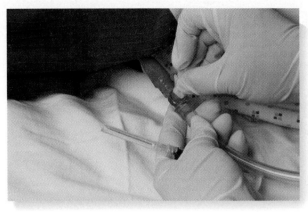

3 Allow urine to accumulate in tubing (2 mL is sufficient for specimen).

- Aspirate urine sample by gently pulling back on syringe plunger and then removing needle.
- Wipe aspiration port with antimicrobial or alcohol swab.
- Remove clamp.
- Empty syringe into sterile urine container (specimen may be taken to lab in syringe).
- Label container and take to lab within 15 min. If unable to do so within this time frame, refrigerate specimen in appropriate refrigerator.

CHARTING

- Type of specimen obtained
- Mode of obtaining specimen from port
- Color, consistency, and odor of urine

- Time of urine collection
- Time specimen sent to laboratory

CRITICAL THINKING FOCUS

SECTION ONE ▪ Intake and Output

Unexpected Outcomes

■ Fluid balance is not correct as stated on I&O record.

Alternative Nursing Actions

■ Report to charge nurse so she or he can determine if all nurses are keeping accurate records.
■ Check if client or family can help with keeping I&O record.
■ Check addition on I&O record to see if error was made.

■ Client does not maintain intake of at least 1500 mL.

■ Ensure that diagnosis allows 1500-mL intake.
■ Check if client is able to drink fluids without assistance.
■ Ensure that adequate fluids are available for client.
■ Determine client's preference for fluid (i.e., juice, jello, etc.).

■ Client voids in toilet when on I&O monitoring.

■ Document on I&O sheet, "voided in toilet."
■ Provide additional verbal instructions indicating all urine must be saved.
■ Place sign above toilet indicating, "All urine must be saved."

SECTION TWO ▪ Urine Studies

Unexpected Outcomes

■ Strips or tablets are discolored or moist.

Alternative Nursing Actions

■ Sensitivity is lost. Strips or tablets need to be disposed of and new ones used.
■ Keep new strips or tablets away from moisture by storing them in tightly covered container (original bottle for tablets, baby food jar for strips).
■ Always check tablet before using to ensure accurate results.

SECTION THREE ▪ Catheterization

Unexpected Outcomes

■ Catheter is inserted into vagina of female client.

Alternative Nursing Actions

■ Leave catheter in place and follow these actions:
—Reposition fingers to assist in visualizing urethral meatus.
—Have someone obtain new catheter and new gloves. You may need whole new kit if contamination of sterile field has occurred.
—Locate client's urinary meatus before inserting catheter and repeat procedure.

- Catheter is contaminated when insertion is attempted.

  - Obtain new catheter and repeat catheterization.
  - If sterile field has been contaminated, obtain new catheter kit and repeat procedure.

- Catheter cannot be inserted in female client.

  - Repeat procedure, following these actions:
    —Ask client to hold legs apart or ask for assistance from another health team member so you have better access to urethral meatus.
    —Before cleansing client, identify area of urethral meatus. Meatus may be in unusual anatomic location.
    —When cleansing with antiseptic solution, observe urethral opening for movement when pressure is applied to meatus.
    —Repeat catheterization procedure using new catheter kit and new gloves, or new catheter if kit has not been contaminated.

- Catheter cannot be inserted in male client.

  - Obtain new catheter kit and follow these actions:
    —Hold penis perpendicular to client's body.
    —Insert catheter while applying slight traction by gently pulling upward on shaft of penis.
    —If you encounter resistance, rotate catheter, increase traction, and change angle of penis slightly.
    —When urine begins to flow, lower penis.

- Urine appears to be leaking around catheter.

  - Catheter may not be inserted above sphincter, but rather in urethral channel. It may be necessary to insert new catheter.
  - Check amount of fluid in catheter balloon. If balloon is underinflated, leakage may occur.
  - Fill balloon to 10 mL with sterile water. Bacteriostatic water and sodium chloride contain substances that affect integrity of balloon.

- Urine exceeds 1000 mL with catheterization.

  - If Foley catheter is inserted, clamp catheter for 20 to 30 min and then unclamp.
  - If bladder appears grossly distended when palpitated, insert Foley catheter instead of straight catheter.
    —If urine exceeds 1000 mL, inflate balloon and clamp for 30 min.
    —Open clamp and drain remaining urine, then deflate balloon.
    —Remove catheter after urine flow ceases or notify physician of results and ask if Foley should be left in place.

- Catheter comes out with balloon still inflated.

  - Assess client for signs of urethral trauma (e.g., bleeding, pain).
  - Obtain new catheter and repeat catheterization procedure, making sure that balloon is inflated with at least 10 mL of water.

- Monitor urine output for bleeding.
- Notify physician to determine if Foley with 30-mL balloon should be inserted.

SECTION FOUR ▪ External Catheters

| **Unexpected Outcomes** | **Alternative Nursing Actions** |

Unexpected Outcomes

- Incontinence continues with use of wrinkle-free condom catheter.

- Penis becomes reddened and excoriated.

Alternative Nursing Actions

- Use smaller condom to provide wrinkle-free application.

- Remove condom catheter as much as possible to allow air to reach penile shaft.
- Notify physician for topical medication order.
- Diaper client and change frequently.
- Keep condom off penis until area is healed.
- Wash perineal area frequently.

SECTION FIVE ▪ Catheter and Bladder Irrigation and Instillation

Unexpected Outcomes

- Irrigation flow is not infusing at prescribed rate.

- Irrigation solution is not returned because of obstruction in system.

Alternative Nursing Actions

- May need to raise or lower IV stand with attached irrigation bag to assist in regulating flow using gravity.
- Move flow adjuster clamp to new site on tubing if flow is slower than ordered. (Tubing may be collapsed due to constant pressure from clamp.)
- If infusion rate slows, may indicate clots are blocking flow. Irrigate catheter following physician's orders.

- Follow these steps to obtain irrigation solution:
  —Aspirate solution from catheter, using moderate pull-back pressure.
  —If irrigant does not return, palpate client's bladder and instill 30 to 50 mL of irrigating solution to agitate and clear any clots.
  —If irrigant does not return, reconnect urinary system and observe for 30 min. Bladder spasms can block flow of urine through system.
  —If irrigant does not return, cleanse client's urinary meatus and catheter tubing with povidone-iodine (Betadine) solution. Gently insert Foley catheter further into client's bladder. If lumen opening of catheter is against wall of bladder, flow of urine will be obstructed.
  —If irrigant still does not return after the preceding procedures are performed, notify physician for further orders.

- Client's pain and anxiety cause "clamping down" and create obstruction in opening of catheter; thus irrigation solution is not returned.

- Help client practice relaxation techniques.
- Place warm towel over client's abdomen to ease bladder spasms.
- Reposition client to reduce pressure on catheter.
- If client is unable to expel irrigant, administer medications to relieve client's pain or bladder spasms.

- Client experiences excessive bladder spasms.

- Notify physician of bladder spasms to obtain order to place heating pad on client's abdomen.
- Follow physician's order and administer urinary antispasmodic.

- Bright red drainage continues even when solution flow rate is increased.

- Notify physician.
- Continue to infuse solution at rapid rate to cleanse client's bladder until you obtain physician's orders.
- Assess client for signs of anemia or significant blood loss. Take vital signs, observe capillary filling pressure, and observe mucous membranes for signs of anemia.

SECTION SIX ▪ Collecting Specimens

Unexpected Outcomes

- Insufficient amount of urine is available when specimen collection is attempted.

- Signs and symptoms of urinary tract infection occur.

- Bacteremia develops secondary to urinary tract infection.

Alternative Nursing Actions

- Clamp catheter tubing for 30 min.
- Reposition client.
- Check for kinking of catheter.

- Notify physician of client's signs and symptoms.
- Make sure there are no kinks in urinary system tubing and that system is not clamped off. This ensures that urine drains into catheter bag and does not stagnate in bladder.
- Give ordered antibiotics on correct time schedule.
- Do not interrupt closed urinary drainage system.

- Administer antibiotics as ordered.
- Encourage client to force fluids to flush out bladder.
- Use cranberry juice or other acid-producing (noncitric) juices.
- Obtain frequent vital signs and assessment data.
- Observe color and clarity of urine for further infectious problems.

SELF-CHECK EVALUATION

PART 1 ▪ Matching Terms

Match the definition in column B with the correct term in column A.

Column A

_____ a. Catheter
_____ b. Catheterization
_____ c. Distention
_____ d. Dysuria
_____ e. Excoriation
_____ f. Foley catheter
_____ g. Ketonuria
_____ h. Patency
_____ i. Sediment
_____ j. Specific gravity

Column B

1. Presence of protein in the urine
2. Breakdown of the epidermis
3. Insertion of a sterile tube into the bladder for removal of fluids or instillation of medications
4. Type of catheter inserted into the bladder for continuous urinary drainage
5. Weight of a substance compared with an equal volume of water
6. Stretching out or inflating of an organ with fluid or gas
7. Difficult or painful urination—an early sign of UTI
8. Substance settling at the bottom of a liquid
9. State of being freely open
10. Sterile tube inserted into a body cavity or vessel

PART 2 ▪ Multiple Choice Questions

1. Which one of the following actions is effective in safely stimulating voiding in the client who is having difficulty?

a. Putting spirits of ammonia on a cotton ball in the bedpan.
b. Placing the client in a bath of cool water.
c. Placing a hot washcloth on the client's abdomen.
d. Ambulating the client to stimulate peristalsis.

2. Which of the following statements about urine specific gravity is correct?

a. The normal range of urine specific gravity is 1.003 to 1.030.
b. The reading is taken at the fluid level on the side of the cylinder.
c. The reading is taken when the urinometer is stationary for 1 min.
d. The urinometer is spun without touching the side of the cylinder before the reading is taken.

3. In catheterizing a female client, which of the following steps should be completed after placing the absorbent pad under the client?

a. Place the outer white wrap under the client's buttocks.
b. Put on sterile gloves.
c. Open the sterile catheter package.
d. Pour antiseptic solution over cotton balls, or open sterile swabs.

4. If urine is not flowing after a catheter is inserted in a female client, the nurse should:

a. Insert the catheter a little further and wait a few seconds for urine to flow before reassessing placement.
b. Obtain a new, larger catheter and insert it.
c. Reassess; if catheter is in vagina, remove it and reinsert into meatus.
d. Remove catheter, check meatus, and reinsert catheter.

5. When urine begins to flow through the catheter, the next step in the procedure is to:

   a. Connect the catheter to the drainage tubing.
   b. Inflate the catheter balloon with sterile water.
   c. Place the catheter tip into the specimen container.
   d. Place the catheter tip into the collection receptacle.

6. Which one of the following nursing actions is important in addition to strict handwashing and gloving to reduce the risk of infection for clients with indwelling catheters?

   a. Antibiotic therapy.
   b. Aseptic catheter care on a daily basis.
   c. Emptying the collection bag every 2 hrs.
   d. Making sure there are dependent loops in the drainage tubing.

7. If urine test sticks or test tape become wet or discolored, the nurse should:

   a. Put them in the sun to dry out and then use them.
   b. Use them anyway; moisture will not affect the results.
   c. Discard them, obtain a new supply, and store in a dry place.
   d. Send the urine to the lab to be tested accurately.

8. Draping the female client for catheterization is done in a way that provides for warmth and privacy of the client and:

   a. Protects the sterility of the field during the procedure.
   b. Provides a clean place to put sterile equipment during the procedure.
   c. Protects the bed from spillage during the procedure.
   d. Covers the client's face so that she is not embarrassed by the procedure.

9. Which one of the following rationales is the most important reason to assess the client's ability to maintain positioning and remain still during a catheterization?

   a. Movement will cause pain for the client.
   b. Client movement may hinder your ability to locate the meatus.
   c. Client movement may compromise the sterility of the catheter.
   d. Client movement may increase the nurse's nervousness about the procedure.

10. After the catheter is in place and urine begins to flow, the nurse changes the position of the nondominant hand from separating the labia to holding the catheter until the:

   a. First 100 mL of urine have been removed.
   b. Client is able to hold the catheter in place.
   c. Catheter is taped to the client's leg.
   d. Balloon is inflated to hold the catheter in place.

11. When inserting an indwelling catheter in a male client, the penis should be held at a _____ degree angle to the body to straighten the urethra and facilitate insertion of the catheter.

   a. 30°.
   b. 45°.
   c. 90°.
   d. 120°.

12. Which of the following rationales explains why taping a long-term indwelling catheter to the abdomen of the male client is recommended? A catheter taped to the abdomen:

   a. Is easier to conceal and provides more privacy for the client.
   b. Decreases pressure on the penoscrotal angle.
   c. Prevents kinking of the drainage tubing.
   d. Is more convenient for the nurse.

13. When collecting a sterile specimen from an indwelling catheter, the nurse:

    a. Removes the required amount from the drainage bag.

    b. Clamps the catheter for 2 hrs prior to obtaining the specimen.

    c. Removes the required amount from the balloon port with a needleless syringe.

    d. Removes the required amount with a syringe from the port on the tubing.

14. Which of the following is the most important rationale for checking the glans of the client 30 min following application of a condom catheter?

    a. Client may have removed the condom catheter.

    b. Catheter may be interfering with circulation and output.

    c. Catheter may be leaking.

    d. It provides psychological support of the client.

15. Bladder distention due to obstruction by blood, sediment, or other debris can lead to serious complications in the client with compromised cardiac function due to a:

    a. Urinary tract infection.

    b. Sympathetic nervous system response.

    c. Vagal response.

    d. Hemorrhage.

PART 3 ▪ Critical Thinking Application

Mrs. Christofferson, a 64-year-old woman, is a first-day postoperative client. She had a bowel resection yesterday. The physician ordered her Foley catheter discontinued at 8 A.M. today. His additional order is to check for residual urine after her first voiding.

1. The client has not voided since the Foley catheter was removed 2 hrs earlier. What is your priority nursing intervention?

2. The client voids 600 mL of urine 6 hrs after removal of the Foley catheter. What is your priority intervention at this time?

3. Checking for residual urine, you obtain 120 mL of urine. What is your next intervention? What alternative action might you take if you suspect the client may exceed the normal amount of residual urine?

22

BOWEL ELIMINATION

INTRODUCTION

The organs and structures of the bowel elimination system are the mouth, esophagus, stomach, small intestine, and large intestine. The first three organs are involved in the upper gastrointestinal system, which functions to ingest, prepare, and begin the process of digestion. The small and large intestine are the organs of the lower gastrointestinal system and are the organs specifically involved with the process of elimination.

Many conditions affect the body's ability to effectively eliminate waste through normal defecation. Alterations in bowel motility can result from changes in the autonomic system, side effects of medications, congenital or acquired diseases, or intestinal muscle weakness. An obstruction in either the small or large intestine can affect normal bowel elimination, with the severity of symptoms depending upon the size and location of the obstruction. A third condition affecting normal elimination of waste through the bowel involves the circulatory system. Any alteration of the arterial blood supply, from complete obstruction of flow to partial occlusion due to atherosclerosis, inhibits bowel function to a greater or lesser degree. Lastly, there are several surgically induced alterations in bowel structure that affect elimination patterns. The colostomy,

(continued on next page)

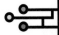

an artificially created opening from the colon to the abdominal surface, is used for the purpose of elimination of waste products. A colostomy can be temporary or permanent. A temporary colostomy is usually created as a result of severe bowel irritation, trauma, or occlusion. A permanent colostomy is primarily performed as a result of a cancerous tumor. An ileostomy is a permanent surgical intervention in which an artificially created opening is made from the ileum to the abdominal surface. It is usually necessitated as a result of Crohn's disease or ulcerative colitis.

Nurses are involved in assisting clients to maintain elimination patterns that promote health and well-being. The following skills relate to evacuation of the lower bowel and maintaining the function of altered structures in elimination.

PREPARATION PROTOCOL: FOR BOWEL ELIMINATION

Complete the following steps before each skill.

1. Check physician's orders and client plan of care.
2. Gather equipment.
3. Check client's identaband.
4. Explain purpose and procedure to client.
5. Instruct client/family as indicated.
6. Provide privacy.
7. Wash hands.
8. Put on clean gloves.
9. Place client in position that best facilitates procedure.
10. Place bed protector under client.
11. Allow client to assist, if appropriate.

COMPLETION PROTOCOL: FOR BOWEL ELIMINATION

Make sure the following steps have been completed.

1. Remove equipment; clean and store if not disposable.
2. Discard disposable equipment.
3. Assist client to position of comfort.
4. Remove soiled gloves and wash hands.
5. Record results of procedure in nurses' notes and graphic record, as appropriate.
6. Report any abnormal or ineffective results and obtain further orders, if appropriate.

SECTION ONE

RECTAL TUBE

One of the hazards of immobility and a frequent postoperative occurrence is the collection of gas in the client's bowel that he or she is unable to expel as flatulence. This situation is caused by hypomotility of the bowel due to decreased peristalsis. It can lead to significant abdominal distention and can be extremely uncomfortable for the client. A more serious complication results when the collected gas expands to such an extent that it interferes with diaphragmatic muscle contraction, compromising respiratory expansion and causing dyspnea. In this situation, or when hypermotile conditions cause persistent diarrhea, the nurse may insert a rectal tube to promote the removal of flatus or to collect loose stool.

RATIONALE

- To promote removal of flatulence following abdominal surgery or for clients who have swallowed excessive amounts of air
- To stimulate expulsion of flatus in lower digestive tract
- To prevent abdominal distention that can result in diaphragmatic muscle contractions and cause dyspnea
- To manage continual diarrhea

ASSESSMENT

- Assess client's complaints of pain, distention, or diarrhea.
- Assess bowel sounds.
- Note quality and depth of respirations.
- Note quality and rate of pulse.
- Gently palpate client's abdomen.
- Measure abdominal girth.
- Note presence or absence of hemorrhoids.
- Assess condition of perianal skin.

Equipment

- Rectal tube: size 22 to 30 straight (French) for adults size 12 to 18 (French) for children
- Small plastic bag or stool specimen container
- Hypoallergenic paper tape
- Water-soluble lubricant
- Bed protector
- Clean gloves

SKILL

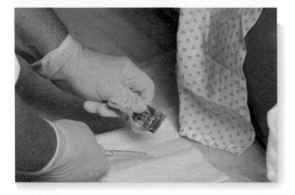

1 Place client on left side in a recumbent position and drape. **RATIONALE:** This position facilitates insertion of tube following normal curve of rectum and sigmoid colon.

- Tape plastic bag around distal end of rectal tube or insert tube into stool specimen container.
- Vent upper side of plastic bag to prevent inflation.
- Lubricate proximal end of rectal tube with water-soluble lubricant.

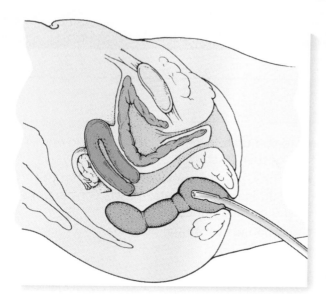

2 Gently separate buttocks and ask client to take deep breath. **RATIONALE:** Taking deep breath relaxes anal sphincter and prevents tissue trauma during tube insertion.

- Gently insert tube into client's rectum, past external and internal anal sphincters (4 to 6 inches in adults).
- Gently tape tube in place with hypoallergenic tape.
- Leave tube in place no longer than 20 min. **RATIONALE:** Prolonged stimulation of anal sphincter may result in loss of neuromuscular response. Prolonged presence of catheter may cause pressure necrosis of mucosal surface.
- Remove tube and provide perianal care as needed.

SAFETY ALERT

Take client's pulse. **RATIONALE:** Alterations in pulse can indicate vagal stimulation; rectal tube may need to be removed. This occurs mostly in clients with cardiac conditions.

CLINICAL NOTE

Instruct client that chewing gum, sucking on candy, drinking liquids through a straw, drinking carbonated beverages, and smoking tend to promote swallowing of air and increased abdominal distention.

CHARTING

- Time rectal tube inserted and removed
- Size of tube
- Presence, absence, or change in abdominal distention

- Pulse rate before and following procedure
- Unexpected outcomes and interventions needed

ENEMA ADMINISTRATION

An enema is a solution that is introduced into the rectum and reaches the large intestine. The purpose of all enemas is to increase peristalsis and promote the expulsion of feces and flatus. There are four basic types of enemas: cleansing, carminative, retention, and return-flow. The enema type prescribed for the client is based on the individual client need.

RATIONALE

- To relieve constipation
- To reduce amount of flatus
- To relieve fecal impaction
- To cleanse bowel before and/or following surgery or diagnostic examination
- To stimulate peristalsis
- To obtain fecal specimen

ASSESSMENT

- Evaluate client's diet for amount of high-bulk foods and amount of daily fluid intake.
- Assess current medical regimen.
- Assess use of drugs that can lead to constipation.
- Assess client's present status and past elimination patterns.
- Assess the following related to elimination:
  - —Time and consistency of last bowel movement
  - —Degree of abdominal distention
  - —Perianal area for tears, ulcerations, or excoriation
  - —History of constipation and/or fecal impaction
  - —Degree of sphincter control
  - —Need for enema
  - —Amount of enema solution client can tolerate

CLINICAL NOTE

TYPES OF ENEMAS

Classification	Type

■ **Cleansing**
Stimulates peristalsis through irritation of colon and rectum by distention.
	1. Soapsuds
	  a. Mild soap solutions stimulate and irritate intestinal mucosa. Dilute 5 mL of castile soap in 1000 mL of water.
	  b. Avoid strong soap solutions, as they can cause severe irritation of mucous membrane of colon.
	2. Tap water
	  a. Give with caution to infants or adults with altered cardiac and renal function as tap water is a hypotonic solution and can be absorbed and alter electrolyte status.
	3. Saline
	  a. Saline solutions are mildly irritating to mucous membrane of colon.

(continued on next page)

CLINICAL NOTE

TYPES OF ENEMAS (CONT'D)

Classification	Type

■ **Retention**
Solution or nutrient is retained for a specified time.
	1. Emollient (oil)
	  a. Lubricates rectum and colon, protecting intestinal mucous membrane.
	  b. Feces absorb oil and become softer and easier to expel.
	  c. Client retains enema for several hours.
	2. Nutrient
	  a. Provides nourishment in temporary or emergency situations.
	  b. Enema solution is retained.

■ **Distention reduction**
Provides relief from flatus causing distention and improves ability to expel flatus.
	1. Carminative
	  a. 1-2-3 enema.
	    ■ 30 g magnesium sulfate.
	    ■ 60 g glycerine.
	    ■ 90 mL warm water.
	  b. Milk and molasses (180–240 mL of equal amounts).
	2. Return-flow (Harris flush)
	  a. Mild colonic irrigation using 100–200 mL enema solution.
	  b. After instillation, enema container is lowered and solution siphoned back into container.

■ **Medicated**
Enemas containing drugs used for reducing bacteria or removing excess potassium.
	1. Kayexalate
	  a. Resin is introduced into large intestine, removing excess potassium by exchanging it for sodium ions.
	2. Neomycin
	  a. Antibiotic solution is used to reduce bacteria prior to bowel surgery.

ADMINISTER AN ENEMA

Equipment

- Fluid container with attached rectal tube size 22 to 30 straight (French) for adults
- Normal saline, tap water, soap solution
- Water-soluble lubricant
- Bath blanket
- IV pole
- Clean bedpan with cover; bed protector
- Skin care items (e.g., soap, water, towels)
- Two pairs of clean gloves
- Toilet tissue

SKILL

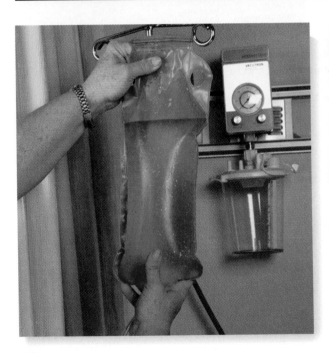

1 Fill container with 750 to 1000 mL of lukewarm solution at 105 to 110°F. **RATIONALE:** Solutions that are too hot or too cold can cause cramping, damage to rectal tissues, and extreme shock.

- Hang container of solution on IV pole next to bed.

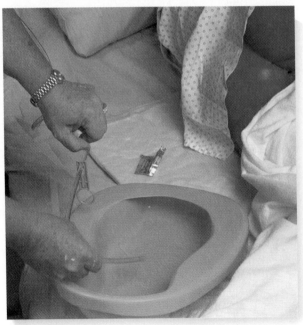

2 Allow solution to run through tubing so that air is removed. Clamp tube. **RATIONALE:** If air is instilled during procedure, client experiences discomfort as a result of distention of colon.

- Place bedpan within easy reach.

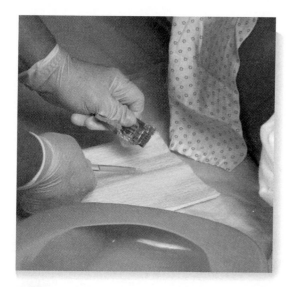

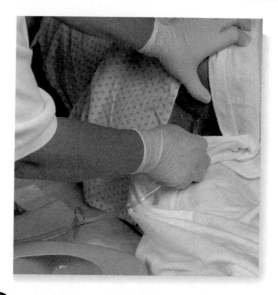

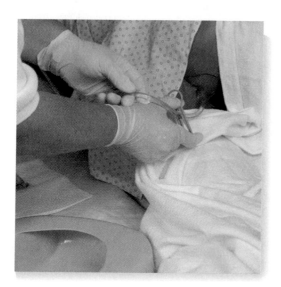

 3 Place client on left side in Sims' position. **RATIONALE:** To facilitate flow of solution using contour of bowel.

- Provide privacy and drape client with bath blanket.
- Lubricate tip of tubing with generous amount of water-soluble lubricant.

4 Gently spread buttocks, instructing client to take slow breath, and insert tubing 3 to 4 in.

- Raise solution container to maximum height of 18 in when giving high enema and 12 to 18 in when giving low enema. **RATIONALE:** The higher the solution container, the higher the solution travels up the colon.

SAFETY ALERT

If client experiences cramping, inability to retain solution, or anxiety during administration of enema solution, lower solution container or momentarily clamp tubing. Resume after a few minutes when symptoms subside.

5 Open regulating clamp and allow solution to flow slowly. **RATIONALE:** Solution that flows too quickly can cause cramping, damage to rectal tissue, and extreme shock. If flow is slow, client experiences fewer cramps and will be able to tolerate and retain greater volume of solution.

- Hold tubing in place in client's rectum at all times. Keep bedpan nearby in case client needs it immediately.

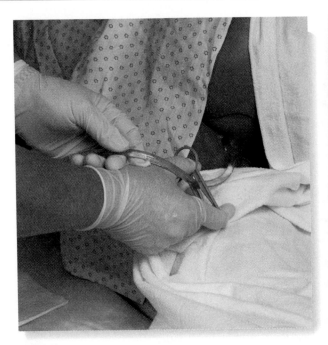

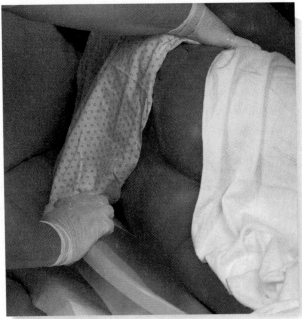

6 After solution is instilled, clamp tubing. **RATIONALE:** To prevent siphoning out enema solution as tube is removed.

- Gently remove tubing.
- Instruct client to hold solution for 10 to 15 min or as long as it can be tolerated. **RATIONALE:** Results are more effective if client holds solution.
- Assist client to bathroom or commode.

7 If client is on bed rest, place on bedpan and elevate head of bed so that client can assume squatting position on bedpan to facilitate evacuation.

- Provide privacy until client has expelled total volume of instilled solution.
- Remove bedpan, assist client with perineal care, resume comfortable positioning.

SAFETY ALERT

If client is on strict I&O, measure the fluid portion of returns of the enema to make certain that the total volume of the enema solution is expelled. If the total volume is not expelled and the difference is less than 100 mL, subtract from the output. If the deficit is greater than 100 mL, notify physician for further orders. If client complains of continued cramping and total volume is not expelled, notify physician immediately.

ADMINISTER A DISPOSABLE ENEMA

Equipment

- Commercially prepared enema
- Water-soluble lubricant
- Bedpan or commode
- Two pairs of clean gloves
- Bed protector
- Skin care items (e.g., soap, water, towels)

SKILL

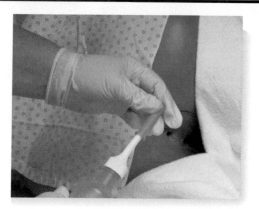

🖐 **1** Read directions on enema container.

- Remove outer cap on tip of container.
- Lubricate tip with water-soluble lubricant if necessary. (Rectal tube is usually prelubricated).
- Expose anal opening to assist in inserting tube without traumatizing tissue.

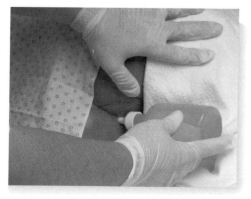

2 Insert rectal tube 3 to 4 in.

- Gently squeeze container and empty entire 120 mL of hypertonic solution into rectum.
- Keep pressure on container while removing from rectum. **RATIONALE:** To prevent solution from being drawn back into container.
- *For Fleet's enema:* Instruct client to hold solution for 5 to 7 min. Continue with step 2, "Administer an Enema."
- *For retention enema:* Instruct client to retain oil solution for 1 to 3 hrs. **RATIONALE:** Purpose of enema is to soften stool.
- A cleansing enema may be given to remove oil and stimulate defecation.

CLINICAL NOTE

HARRIS FLUSH ENEMA

- Fill fluid container with 100 to 200 mL of ordered solution.
- Check temperature to ensure that it is between 105 and 110°F.
- Explain benefits of relaxing and taking periodic deep breaths during procedure.
- Follow with steps 2 to 5 in "Administering an Enema."
- Lower solution container below level of rectum and allow all fluid to flow back into container.
- Raise container 18 in above rectum and allow solution to flow back into rectum.
- Repeat inflow-outflow process five to six times, changing solution when it becomes thick with feces. **RATIONALE:** This assists in stimulating intestinal peristalsis with expulsion of flatus.
- Follow step 7 in "Administer an Enema."

TEST FOR OCCULT BLOOD

Equipment

- Clean bedpan or bedside commode
- Tongue blade
- Guaiac test (Hemoccult) or Gamma Fe-Cult packet

- Guaiac solution
- Glacial acetic acid
- Hydrogen peroxide
- Clean gloves

SKILL

Hemoccult

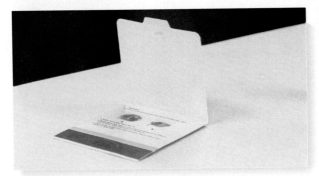

1 Obtain stool specimen.

- Use tongue blade to smear thin layer of stool on panel number 1.
- Obtain second specimen from different part of stool specimen and smear thin layer on panel number 2.
- Wait 3 to 5 min. to process test.

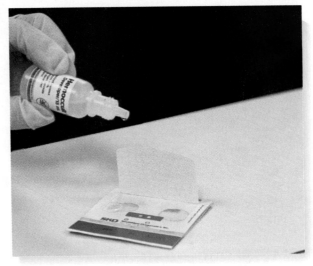

2 Turn packet over, and lift flap.

- Apply two drops of Hemoccult developer over each smear.
- Read and record test results within 60 sec. Blue color indicates guaiac-positive result.

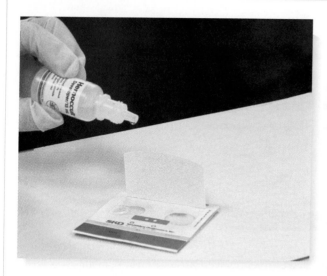

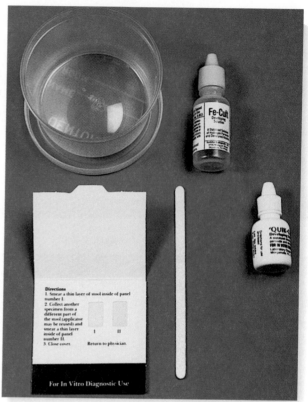

3 Apply one drop of Hemoccult developer between the + and − performance monitor test strip (orange section at bottom of packet).

- Interpret results within 10 sec. If positive side turns blue, test slide is accurate.
- Discard filter paper or packet.

4 Alternate method using Gamma Fe-Cult Plus: Use tongue blade to smear thin layer of stool on panel number 1 and second specimen (from different part of stool specimen) on panel number 2.

- Turn packet over and remove perforated flap (marked *Not To Be Opened By Patient*).
- Add two drops of Fe-Cult developing solution to test area over smear of stool.
- Read and record test results within 30 sec. **RATIONALE:** Color reaction fades within 2 to 3 min. Any trace of blue indicates positive result. No trace of blue indicates negative result.

CLINICAL NOTE

Bleeding from a gastric ulcer or the intestinal tract may be a slow process. If you suspect gastrointestinal bleeding, a guaiac test for occult blood is indicated. Steps for testing for occult blood must be followed in sequence.

CHARTING

- Time and type of enema administered
- Volume of solution used
- Length of time client held solution
- Results obtained: amount expelled, consistency, and color

- Unexpected outcomes and required interventions
- Relief of flatus
- Results of stool guaiac test; if positive, who notified

SECTION THREE

COLOSTOMY IRRIGATION

A colostomy is a surgically created diversionary procedure of the colon in which a small segment of the colon is brought through the abdominal wall to form a stoma. The colostomy can be created using any segment of the large intestine. The character of effluent from the colostomy depends largely upon which section of the large intestine is opened onto the abdominal wall. Colostomy irrigations may be used to reestablish regularity of bowel elimination when necessary; however, most clients are able to reestablish their preoperative bowel routines within a short period of time.

An ileostomy produces a constant liquid effluent due to the portion of the colon resected. An ileostomy is not irrigated. If an obstruction occurs, an enterostomal therapist or physician is notified.

RATIONALE

- To manage regular bowel elimination
- To evacuate stool from colon
- To prepare colon for reanastamosis

ASSESSMENT

- Assess type of colostomy.
- Determine whether colostomy is temporary or permanent.
- Assess for stomal complications: periostomal hernia, stenosed stoma, prolapsed stoma.
- Assess bowel sounds and check abdomen for distention.
- Assess preoperative bowel habits.
- Assess client's ability to sit for a prolonged period of time.
- Assess client's level of alertness and ability to learn.

Equipment

- Solution container with 1000 mL warm water
- Irrigating tubing with cone
- Two pairs of clean gloves
- Irrigating sleeve cut long enough to reach water level in toilet
- Items to clean skin and stoma (e.g., washcloths or gauze sponges)

- Plastic bag for disposal of used pouch
- Clean pouch and closure device
- Skin barriers
- Water-soluble lubricant
- IV pole

SKILL

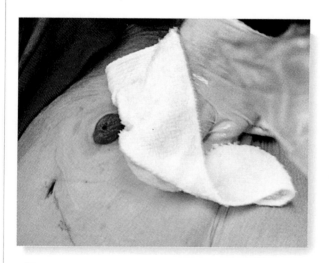

 SAFETY ALERT

A distended colon can cause a vagal response that results in hypotension, bradycardia, and loss of consciousness due to a decrease in cardiac output. Assess pulse and blood pressure in susceptible clients before procedure and monitor closely during procedure for early signs of difficulty.

1 Remove and dispose of used pouch in plastic bag.

- Assess pulse and blood pressure.

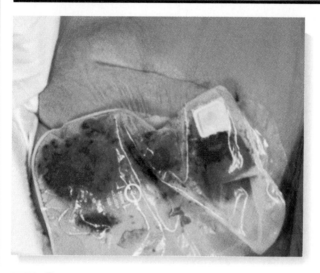

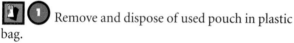

3 Assess for signs of irritation or breakdown.

2 Clean stoma and skin with warm water and soft cloth.

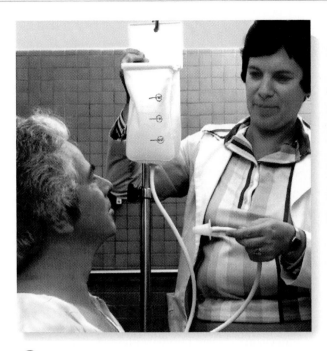

4 Prepare irrigation solution as in steps 1 and 2 in "Administer an Enema" and hang solution on hook or IV pole in bathroom.

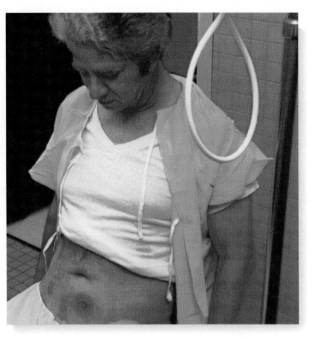

5 Assist client to sit on toilet or on chair in front of toilet.

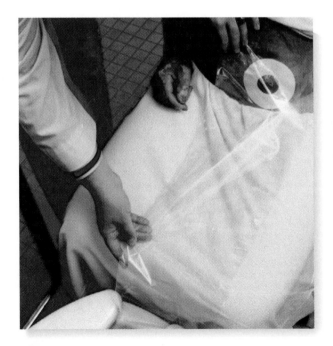

6 Place sleeve between client's thighs and direct end into toilet.

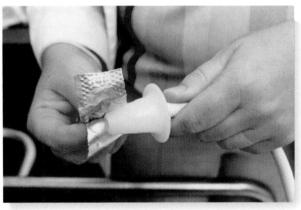

7 Lubricate cone tip with water-soluble lubricant. **RATIONALE:** Danger of perforation of colon is greater when using catheter for irrigation. Use of irrigation cone results in safer administration and better water flow.

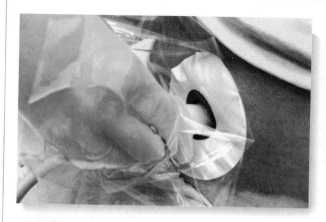

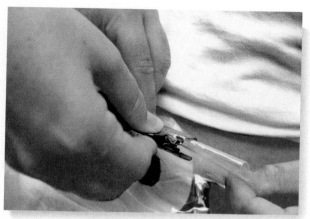

8 Position cone in sleeve by placing top through opening. If cone cannot be inserted easily, do not force it.

- Hold cone snugly against stoma. **RATIONALE:** This prevents backflow of solution.

9 Remove cone and close off or fold over top of sleeve after solution is instilled.

- Allow client to remain seated while majority of stool and solution return, usually 10 to 15 min.
- Clean client's skin and stoma with warm water; dry thoroughly.
- Apply skin barriers and clean pouch.

CHARTING

- Time irrigation administered
- Amount and type of solution used
- Results obtained; amount, color, consistency of returns

- Condition and color of stoma
- Condition of periostoma skin

SECTION FOUR

FECAL OSTOMY POUCH

Proper application and adherence to the skin of the fecal ostomy pouch is critical to prevent leaking of the effluent onto the skin. If leakage occurs, the client is at risk for irritation and excoriation of the periostoma skin. The client also may experience problems accepting the altered body image and route of elimination when "accidental" leakage occurs. Accurate performance of the skill and proper teaching of the client are of paramount importance in the care of a client with a colostomy. The nurse must be accepting of the ostomy if the client is going to accept it.

RATIONALE

- To collect effluent for accurate assessment of output
- To collect effluent for client comfort and body image
- To protect periostoma skin from erythema, excoriation, and infection

ASSESSMENT

- Assess type and location of stoma.
- Observe stoma color (normal is beefy red and moist).
- Inspect client's periostoma skin for signs of erythema, excoriation, ulceration, or fistula formation.
- Evaluate size of stoma and how far stoma protrudes above skin surface.
- Assess output of effluent, including amount, consistency, and odor.
- Assess client's learning abilities, age, manual dexterity, and visual acuity.

Equipment

- Clean drainable pouch with attached skin barrier
- Skin barriers (e.g., Skin Gel or Skin Prep)
- Warm water in basin
- Soft cloths
- Bath blanket
- Plastic bag for disposal of old pouch
- Tail closure for pouch

- Clean gloves
- Measuring guide
- Deodorant (optional)
- Hypoallergenic paper tape (optional)
- Tissues
- Scissors

SKILL

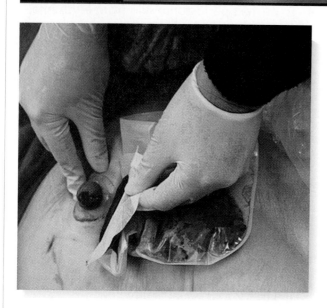

1 Place bath blanket over client, and fanfold top linen to bottom of bed.

- Observe placement of colostomy stoma. **RATIONALE:** To determine expected amount and consistency of output. A transverse colostomy produces stool that is semiliquid to very soft; sigmoid colostomy produces solid, formed stool.
- Empty old pouch. Pouches should be emptied when one-third to one-half full of feces or flatus. **RATIONALE:** This prevents the weight of pouch contents from loosening pouch.
- Remove old pouch by pushing against skin as you pull backing from skin and discard in plastic bag. Save tail closure from pouch.
- Measure output if liquid effluent is returned.

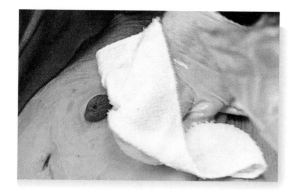

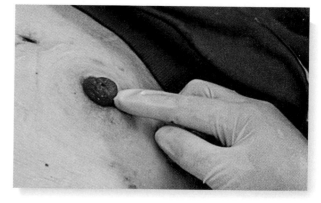

2 Clean client's skin with soft cloth. **RATIONALE:** Soap causes irritation and should be used only if stool is difficult to remove. Oily substances interfere with pouch adhesive.

- Dry client's skin with soft cloth. Keep tissues available in case stoma evacuates stool while pouch is off.

3 Observe skin and stoma for changes in size, protrusion above skin, ulceration, or color (color should be a healthy, beefy red).

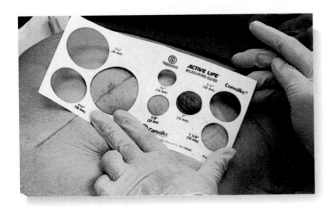

4 Prepare clean pouch:

- Measure stoma with measuring guide.
- Trace measured pattern on wafer.

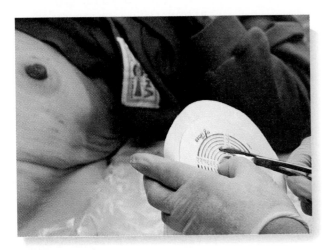

5 Cut pouch size about ⅛ in larger than measurement. **RATIONALE:** Accurate size of opening protects periostoma skin and stoma from trauma or effluent leaks.

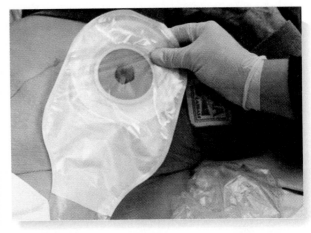

6 Check to ensure opening is large enough to encircle stoma without pushing on edges.

- Remove paper from skin barrier on wafer.

7 Apply skin barrier paste to periostoma area.

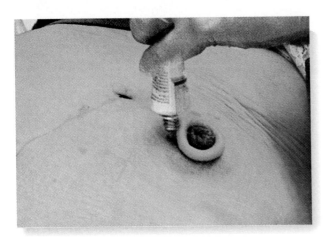

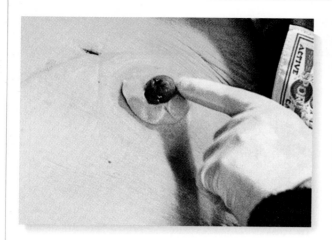

8 Wet fingers and spread paste around stoma.

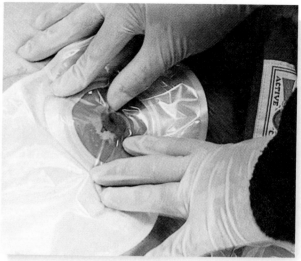

9 Center and apply clean pouch. Pouch may be applied over incision. **RATIONALE:** Incisions are sealed within 24 hrs; therefore contamination from fecal material does not occur.

- Instruct client to "puff out" abdomen. **RATIONALE:** This prevents wrinkles from occurring when pouch is applied.

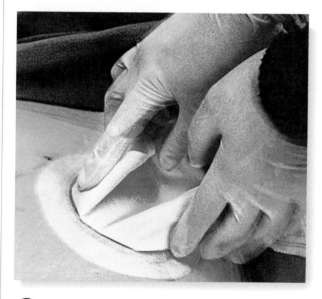

10 Press adhesive around stoma to form seal. Do not allow adhesive to wrinkle. **RATIONALE:** This prevents leakage from pouch.

- Check that adhesive ring is wrinkle free. **RATIONALE:** Prevents seepage of effluent from pouch onto skin.

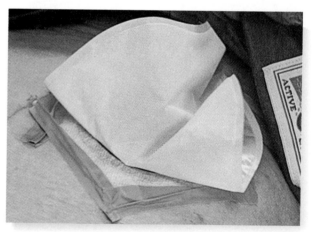

11 Reinforce ring with tape to balance weight of pouch and prevent edges from loosening when client showers.

- Instruct client to lie quietly for 3 to 5 min to allow pouch to seal.

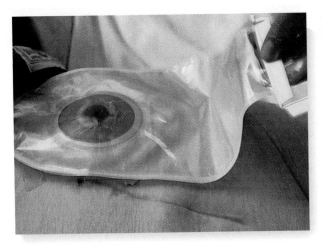

12 Close and secure end of pouch with tail closure.

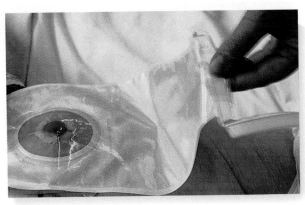

13 Ensure that bowed end of clamp is next to body. **RATIONALE:** This provides better fit to body and prevents outpouching of clamp through clothing.

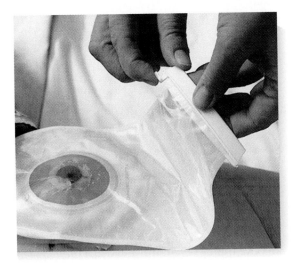

14 Lay hook on top of bag and fold bag 1 in over end of pouch.

- Squeeze clamp together to close.
- Check to see that clamp is positioned correctly; bowed end is toward body, hook is in top left corner.
- Lift up and push clamp in to open clamp.

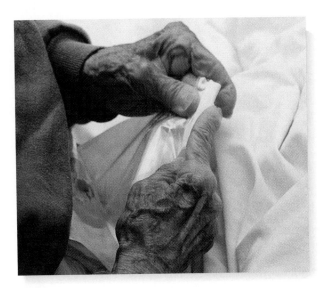

15 Encourage client to practice closing clamp.

- Attach belt to faceplate of pouch (optional).

CHARTING

- Type of pouch and skin barrier used
- Time pouch change completed
- Amount, color, and consistency of stool emptied from pouch
- Presence or absence of flatus through stoma

- Location, condition, and color of stoma
- Condition of periostoma skin
- Condition of incision line
- Condition of abdomen
- Client teaching done

CRITICAL THINKING FOCUS

SECTION ONE ▪ Rectal Tube

Unexpected Outcomes

- Client does not experience relief of abdominal distention.

- Fecal impaction lower in rectum prevents insertion of rectal tube.

Alternative Nursing Actions

- Reposition client at angle that raises lower part of body (e.g., prone position with foot of bed raised).
- Instruct client to circle, raise, and lower legs.
- Reinsert tube 2 to 3 hrs later.
- Remove tube and check for feces that may have clogged outlet. Clean tube and reinsert.

- Perform digital examination with gloved finger and water-soluble lubricant. Break up impaction if present.
- Position client on left side in Fowler's position.
- Reinsert rectal tube.

SECTION TWO ▪ Enema Administration

Unexpected Outcomes

- Client expels solution prematurely.

- Client complains of severe and sudden abdominal pain, nausea, and distention.

- Flow of water is impeded or obstruction is felt.

- Client cannot return enema solution.

Alternative Nursing Actions

- Decrease client's anxiety and distress by reassuring him or her that this is not a problem.
- Place bedpan under client. Place client in semi-Fowler's position with knees flexed.
- Hold rectal tube in client's rectum between thighs. Slow water flow and continue with enema.

- Remove tubing, and notify physician immediately of possible perforation.
- Assess vital signs. If you suspect cardiac dysrhythmias, remove bedpan and notify physician immediately.
- Be prepared to administer emergency drugs, such as atropine.
- If IV is not in place, have IV of 5 percent dextrose in water with a large-bore needle ready for RN to start. This is for emergency use.

- Open clamp on tubing. Allow small amount of solution to flow. Warm solution may help relax internal sphincter.
- Withdraw tube gently and reinsert.
- Gently perform digital examination to check for fecal impaction. Break up impaction if present.
- Obtain order for retention enema, followed by cleansing enema 2 to 3 hrs later.

- Gently massage client's abdomen, if not contraindicated.
- Replace rectal tube. Lower enema bag below level of bed to act as siphon.

SECTION THREE ▪ Colostomy Irrigation

Unexpected Outcomes	Alternative Nursing Actions

Unexpected Outcomes

- Stool leaks out and under irrigation sleeve.

Alternative Nursing Actions

- Secure belt to sleeve.
- Ensure skin is dry before applying sleeve.
- Flatten abdomen before applying sleeve.
- Use self-adhering irrigation pouch.
- Reposition client.

Unexpected Outcomes

- Solution does not flow easily into colostomy.

Alternative Nursing Actions

- Change cone angle or position slightly.
- Check for kinks in tubing from solution container.
- Check height of solution container.
- Remove cone; stool may be expelled.
- Ask client to relax and take deep breaths.
- Reposition client.
- Instill small amounts of water to loosen stool.

Unexpected Outcomes

- Client experiences cramping, nausea, or dizziness during irrigation.

Alternative Nursing Actions

- Stop flow of water, leaving cone or catheter in place.
- Do not resume infusion of water until cramping has passed.
- Check water temperature. Water that is too hot can cause vertigo.
- Check height of water bag. Water that flows too rapidly can cause vertigo.
- Apply drainable pouch.
- Have client increase fluid intake; client may be dehydrated and solution absorbed.
- Repeat irrigation next day.

Unexpected Outcomes

- Client experiences continual spillage of stool between irrigations.

Alternative Nursing Actions

- Reassess type of colostomy—only those in descending or sigmoid colon are to be irrigated.
- Be sure client uses and returns 1000 mL (or amount infused) of solution.
- Assess client's past bowel habits prior to surgery. Clients who have had very irregular bowel habits or frequent stools may not be candidates for irrigation.

Unexpected Outcomes

- Client experiences poor returns due to constipation or fecal impaction.

Alternative Nursing Actions

- Assess client's diet. Dietitian may need to be notified to provide more bulk foods.
- Assess medications client is taking. (Drugs such as codeine, iron, and vincristine can be very constipating.)
- Stool softener or mild laxative may be needed.
- Assess client's fluid intake. Increasing amount of fluids may be necessary.
- Perform digital examination to check for impaction. If impaction or severe constipation persists, colostomy may be irrigated with 30 mL soap, 60 mL oil, and 500 mL water. (Warn client that this can cause severe cramping). This procedure requires physician's order.

- Obtain physician's order to add liquid Colace, milk, molasses, or mineral oil to irrigating solution to soften stool. Soft rubber catheter may be used to put liquid medication nearer to obstruction.
- Administer low volume (100 to 200 mL) of solution; keep cone in place so solution remains in place to assist with stool softening.

SECTION FOUR ▪ Fecal Ostomy Pouch

Unexpected Outcomes	**Alternative Nursing Actions**
▪ Stoma appears dark, dusky-colored, or black.	▪ Notify physician of findings and document in chart. Usually indicates stoma is ischemic.
▪ Stoma becomes ulcerated or cut.	▪ Examine pouching system to see if opening of pouch may be rubbing or cutting into stoma.
	▪ Recut opening ⅛ in larger than stoma to avoid traumatizing stoma.
	▪ Notify physician of findings.
	▪ Assess placement of client's waistband and belt.
▪ Stoma remains a persistent pale pink.	▪ Request physician to order Hgb, Hct, and blood test. This is usually result of low Hgb.
	▪ Instruct client to monitor effluent for constipation if iron preparation is ordered.
▪ Stoma appears taut and shiny after surgery.	▪ Observe and note—caused by postoperative edema, which is expected.
▪ Bleeding occurs under stoma postoperatively.	▪ Observe and note—usual occurrence postoperatively.
▪ Erythematous vesicular rash occurs at site of pouch.	▪ Assess for allergic reaction to product being used.
	▪ Apply corticosteroid skin cream or spray prescribed by physician.
▪ Papular rash appears on periostoma skin.	▪ Assess for possible *Candida albicans* rash from antibiotic use or client immunosuppression.
	▪ Apply antifungal powder prescribed by physician with each pouch change.
▪ Skin is eroded.	▪ Clean skin with tepid water and pat dry.
	▪ Apply hydrocolloid wafer (e.g., DuoDerm, Restore) in addition to usual wafer.
	▪ Change wafer every day.
	▪ Place ostomy paste in ring around stoma or on barrier with each pouch change.
	▪ Use new product, such as Durahesive skin barrier or Flextend barrier, to produce secure fit without paste. These materials swell around stoma.
▪ Pouching system does not provide skin protection.	▪ Reassess abdomen and pouching system for weak points. Modify system to eliminate leakage.
	▪ Change pouch a little more frequently (once per day or every other day) until periostomal skin is healed.

- Client experiences itching, burning, or feeling of irritation under ostomy appliance.

- Assess for allergy to products being used.
- Prepare to change pouch—this is usually a sign of periostomal skin irritation.
- Remove pouch and thoroughly clean skin with warm water and soap. Dry thoroughly.
- Apply new pouch.

- Client is not coping with altered body image.

- Refer to United Ostomy Association, Crohn's and Colitis Foundation of America, American Cancer Society, or Ostomy Rehabilitation Program.

SELF-CHECK EVALUATION

PART 1 ▪ Matching Terms

Match the definition in column B with the correct term in column A.

Column A

_____ a. Perianal
_____ b. Hypermotility
_____ c. Constipation
_____ d. Impaction
_____ e. Defecation
_____ f. Sims' position
_____ g. Harris flush enema
_____ h. Oil retention enema
_____ i. Fleet's enema
_____ j. Soapsuds enema

Column B

1. Small cleansing enema
2. Process of having a bowel movement
3. Left side-lying position
4. 750- to 1000-mL cleansing enema
5. Enema given to soften hard stool
6. Decreased intestinal peristalsis
7. Less than usual number of bowel movements
8. Term designating tissues surrounding the anus
9. Hardened stool that cannot be evacuated by client
10. Distention reduction enema

PART 2 ▪ Multiple Choice Questions

1. Which of the following statements is true regarding rectal tubes?

a. A #22 Foley catheter is used as a rectal tube.
b. The tube is attached to a plastic bag to collect flatus.
c. The tube is inserted 6 to 8 in for best results.
d. The tube is left in for no longer than 60 min.

2. Digital stimulation can result in more effective bowel evacuation if the client performs the procedure:

a. When the urge to defecate is strong.
b. At the same time each day.
c. In conjunction with a daily enema.
d. And maintains fluid intake at 2000 mL/day.

3. Which of the following interventions assists in effective bowel evacuation?

a. Administer bowel training program before meals.
b. Administer bulk-forming medications.
c. Include more complex carbohydrates in the diet.
d. Maintain fluid intake at 2000 mL/day.

4. Which of the following is done when administering an enema?

   a. Insert 100 to 200 mL slowly.
   b. Insert the enema tube 6 to 8 in into the rectum.
   c. Raise the enema container to a height of 18 in.
   d. Warm the enema solution to 99°F.

5. The purpose of administering a Harris flush enema is to:

   a. Cleanse the lower colon to facilitate visualization in x-ray studies.
   b. Decrease bowel motility and flatus formation.
   c. Soften stool for easier evacuation.
   d. Stimulate peristalsis and expel flatus.

6. An inflow-outflow process for the Harris flush enema is usually continued until:

   a. The client is exhausted.
   b. Flatus has subsided.
   c. Return fluid is clear.
   d. Stool is evacuated.

7. When assessing a client's stoma, the nurse notices it appears dark and dusky-colored. The initial intervention is to:

   a. Document findings and continue to assess stoma.
   b. Do nothing, as this is a normal finding.
   c. Notify physician of findings, as the stoma is receiving inadequate blood supply.
   d. Replace pouch using a different type of sealant, as this is an allergic reaction.

8. After a fecal impaction is removed, an elderly client complains of feeling light-headed and has a pulse rate of 44 beats per minute. The appropriate nursing action is to:

   a. Begin CPR.
   b. Call the physician.
   c. Monitor all vital signs.
   d. Place client supine with legs elevated.

9. The most probable cause of the client's bradycardia and light-headedness is:

   a. Anxiety.
   b. Hemorrhage.
   c. Sympathetic nervous system stimulation.
   d. Vagal stimulation.

10. A client is receiving a hypertonic formula continuously through a Keofeed tube. She has not had a bowel movement in 4 days. After checking for and removing a fecal impaction, the most appropriate nursing action is to:

   a. Administer a laxative.
   b. Discontinue tube feeding.
   c. Increase rate of tube feeding.
   d. Review ingredients in formula with dietitian.

11. The most important reason why a cone is preferred over a catheter for colostomy irrigations is that the:

   a. Solution can be instilled at a more rapid rate.
   b. Risk of bowel perforation is less with a cone.
   c. Risk of trauma to the stoma is greater with the cone.
   d. Cone is easier to handle for the client.

12. A nursing intervention to assist a client to adapt emotionally and physically to a new ostomy is to:

   a. Use humor when "accidents" occur.

   b. Insist that client look at stoma and handle it.

   c. Matter-of-factly teach client how to secure pouch to prevent accidents.

   d. Spray room with air freshener before and after procedure.

PART 3 ▪ Critical Thinking Application

You assess Mrs. Jacob, a 65-year-old who had a colostomy performed 6 days ago for cancer of the descending colon. When you tell her you will be instructing her on how to apply a new pouch, she starts to cry and says, "No, I don't want to know how because all it does is leak all over everything."

1. Identify the initial nursing intervention and discuss additional actions you would take to resolve this problem.

2. Describe the assessment database that should be completed before a plan can be implemented.

3. Outline the steps in designing a client teaching plan for a client with an ostomy.

23

RESPIRATORY SKILLS

INTRODUCTION

The role of the respiratory system is to provide for the exchange of gases between the blood and the external environment. The respiratory structures involved in air exchange between the atmosphere and the alveoli include the upper airway (nose, pharynx, larynx), which filters, warms, and humidifies inhaled air, and the lower airway (trachea, bronchi, smaller bronchioli, alveoli). The lower airway is considered a sterile environment, and it is protected by upper airway defense mechanisms.

Oxygen is drawn into the lungs by the inhalation phase of ventilation; it then moves or diffuses across the alveolar membrane into the pulmonary capillaries that circulate past or perfuse the alveoli. The high pressure (PO_2) of diffused oxygen forces it into the red blood cell hemoglobin molecule, thereby arterializing the blood. Oxygen-enriched blood is then delivered to the left side of the heart to be pumped into the systemic circulation and perfused to body tissues. At the tissue capillary level, oxygen is exchanged for carbon dioxide, the acid waste product of cellular metabolism. Carbon dioxide diffuses into the hemoglobin and is carried or perfused back to the lungs to be eliminated by the exhalation phase of ventilation.

(continued on next page)

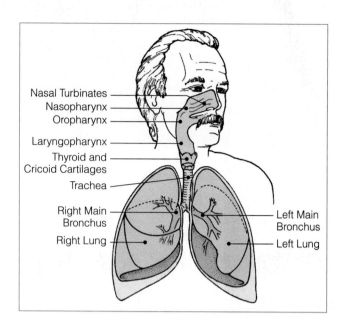

● **FIGURE 23-1** *The anatomy of the respiratory system.*

Inhalation requires active contraction of the diaphragm and external intercostal muscles to expand the thorax. When thoracic expansion occurs, intrapulmonic pressure drops below atmospheric pressure and air flows into the lungs. Surfactant is a phospholipid substance produced by the alveoli to facilitate their inflation. Its production is enhanced by deep breathing, yawning, and sighing—all measures that help prevent atelectasis or alveolar collapse. Exhalation is the passive phase of breathing. It occurs when alveolar pressure increases due to the elastic recoil of lung tissue and the relaxation of the respiratory muscles, causing air to flow out of the lungs and back into the atmosphere.

Inadequate ventilation due to respiratory depression or airway obstruction results in atelectasis with abnormal arterial blood gases, including hypoxemia (low P_{O_2}, low percent saturation of hemoglobin) and eventually an increase in P_{CO_2} (respiratory acidosis). The P_{CO_2} is considered the best measure of ventilation. Hyperventilation due to anxiety or pain results in a low P_{CO_2}, while hypoventilation causes an increased P_{CO_2} (hypercarbia). Excessive levels of carbon dioxide depress the respiratory center and can result in CO_2 narcosis and death.

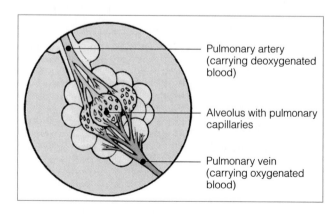

● **FIGURE 23-2** *Air exchange system of the lungs.*

Diffusion is the process of gas exchange between the alveoli and the blood. Gases passively diffuse from an area of high pressure to an area of low pressure. Inhaled air is rich in oxygen and low in carbon dioxide. In contrast, venous blood that perfuses alveolar capillaries is low in oxygen and high in carbon dioxide. These pressure differences between venous blood and the alveoli cause oxygen to diffuse into the blood (PO_2 90 to 100 mm Hg) and bind to red blood cells' hemoglobin (98 percent saturation). Carbon dioxide diffuses out of the hemoglobin and into the alveoli to be eliminated on exhalation. The blood gas value of PO_2 is the best measure of diffusion. If alveoli are inflamed (e.g., pneumonia), thickened (e.g., fibrosis), unable to expand (e.g., atelectasis), or separated from their perfusing capillaries by interstitial fluid (e.g., heart failure), arterial blood oxygenation is decreased, resulting in a low PO_2 (hypoxemia).

Normal perfusion matches circulating blood with ventilated alveoli. If alveoli are inadequately ventilated (e.g., atelectasis), or if blood flow through alveolar capillaries is obstructed (e.g., pulmonary embolism), PO_2 will fall (hypoxemia). Adequate perfusion to peripheral tissues depends on normal blood volume, an adequate amount of hemoglobin that is capable of combining with oxygen, effective cardiac pumping, and competent vasculature. Pathology that interferes with alveolar diffusion, blood cell production, maintenance of blood volume, cardiac pump function, or vascular patency can result in inadequate tissue perfusion and tissue hypoxia. Nursing interventions related to respiratory function focus on maintaining and improving or restoring the critical processes of ventilation, diffusion, and perfusion.

PREPARATION PROTOCOL: FOR RESPIRATORY SKILLS

Complete the following steps before each skill.

1. Validate physician's order for chest physiotherapy, sputum specimen, oxygen therapy, airway suctioning, chest drainage, or other prescribed skills.
2. Wash hands.
3. Validate client's room number, bed number, and identity (check identaband and have client state name).
4. Explain skill and its purpose to client.
5. Assess client's breath sounds to determine areas for focused intervention.
6. Assess client's breath sounds, heart rate, and rhythm before and after suctioning.
7. Place client in appropriate position for skill performance.
8. Don gloves and other protective gear if indicated for skill.

COMPLETION PROTOCOL: FOR RESPIRATORY SKILLS

Make sure the following steps have been completed.

1. Reposition client for comfort.
2. Discard disposable equipment in appropriate receptacle.
3. Clean reusable equipment and return to storage area.
4. Remove and dispose of gloves if used; then wash hands.
5. Ensure that the client with an artificial airway has a means of communication and summoning emergency assistance.
6. Evaluate effectiveness of intervention.
7. Document skill completion as well as pre- and postcare assessment findings and client's tolerance for interventions.

PREVENTIVE MEASURES

The goal of respiratory care interventions is to improve air flow and gas exchange. Standard nursing care for all clients includes independent nursing measures to help prevent pulmonary dysfunction, especially in clients with known pulmonary problems and those at risk for pulmonary complications (e.g., immobilized or surgical clients). Assessing for diminished breath sounds or the development of adventitious sounds (extra sounds superimposed upon usual breath sounds) helps the nurse to individualize care planning and to evaluate the client's response to care measures.

Crackles (fizzing or popping sounds) heard at the end of inspiration indicate hypoventilation of alveoli. These sounds are commonly heard in dependent areas of the lung and signal the need for deep breathing and turning. Wheezes are musical sounds heard on inhalation or exhalation. They indicate secretion retention or airway spasm. Interventions that promote airway clearance and pharmacologic bronchodilator therapy can help to reestablish unobstructed airflow. Clinical manifestations of inadequate ventilation include:

- Crackles at the end of inspiration, usually heard in dependent lung areas
- Dyspnea—difficulty in breathing; the client's sensation of being short of breath
- Restlessness or loss of muscle coordination
- Use of accessory muscles for breathing
- Change in cognition or level of response
- Tachycardia—heart rate over 100 beats per minute
- Tachypnea—breathing rate over 24 breaths per minute
- Increased blood pressure
- Cyanosis—bluish discoloration of mucous membranes ($P_{O_2} < 60$ mm Hg or $Sp_{O_2} < 85$ percent)

Early recognition of these indicators of possible hypoxemia should prompt further investigation and appropriate intervention. One simple measure to support respiratory function is adequate hydration. Fluid intake helps to keep secretions thin and easy to mobilize. Another simple measure is to assist the client to a comfortable Fowler position with pillows supporting the arms to promote optimal ventilation. Turning clients and encouraging deep breathing, especially when clients are receiving respiratory-depressing agents (e.g., opioid analgesics), helps to stimulate surfactant production and ventilate dependent, hypoventilated lung

areas. Studies have shown that deep breathing is the most effective way to prevent postoperative pulmonary complications. The incentive spirometer is a device that encourages clients to monitor and improve their own breathing efforts, but it has not proven to be any more effective than deep breathing alone without such a device.

Encouraging clients to cough while splinting operative sites helps remove retained secretions that increase airflow resistance and lessens the risk of nosocomial infection. Range of motion exercises (passive or active) stimulate both the rate and depth of breathing, while early ambulation promotes greater air exchange (tidal volume) and reduces the risk of other complications of immobility that negatively impact pulmonary function (e.g., pulmonary embolism).

Bronchopulmonary hygiene chest physiotherapy, sometimes called *pulmonary toilet,* includes postural drainage, percussion, and vibration. These medically prescribed therapies are indicated when the client has excessive amounts of thick secretions that become difficult to mobilize. Their beneficial effect on pulmonary function measurements is unclear.

RATIONALE

- To improve pulmonary function
- To prevent hypoventilation and atelectasis
- To prevent pulmonary infection
- To promote client's awareness of breathing capacity
- To loosen secretions and promote airway clearance

ASSESSMENT

- Assess client's ability to perform breathing exercises.
- Evaluate client's operative pain before breathing exercises are encouraged.
- Identify if client is able to independently continue breathing exercises at regular intervals.
- Assess client's breath sounds for improvement following breathing interventions.

DEEP BREATHING AND COUGHING

Equipment

- Chair or hospital bed in upright position
- Pillows for positioning and incisional support
- Tissues for secretions
- Gloves as indicated

SAFETY ALERT

While deep breathing is indicated, coughing is contraindicated for the client following eye, ear, brain, neck, or back surgery.

SKILL

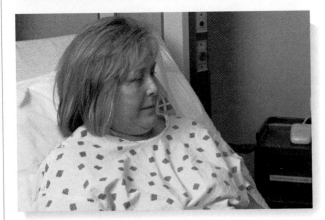

1 With client sitting upright, instruct client to breathe in slowly through nose to expand chest and abdomen, and to hold sustained inspiration for 3 to 5 sec, then exhale slowly through mouth. **RATIONALE:** Inhalation through nose helps to warm, humidify, and filter inspired air. Sustained inhalation stimulates surfactant production and prevents alveolar collapse (atelectasis).

- Provide tissues for client to use while coughing.

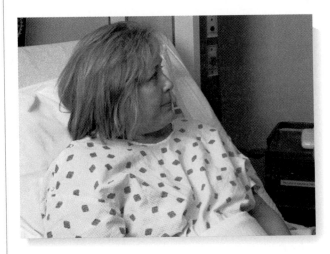

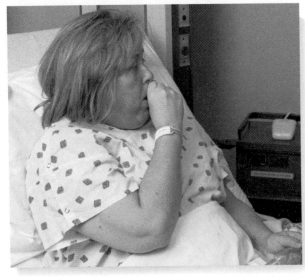

2 After several deep breaths, instruct client to inhale deeply, hold breath for several seconds, lean forward, and cough rapidly through an open mouth, using abdominal, thigh, and buttock muscles. **RATIONALE:** Effectiveness of cough depends on amount of air inhaled and speed with which it is exhaled.

3 Instruct client with pulmonary condition to exhale through pursed lips and to cough throughout exhalation in several short bursts (not at end of deep inhalation). **RATIONALE:** This helps prevent high expiratory pressures that collapse diseased airways and thus facilitates movement of secretions along tracheobronchial tree.

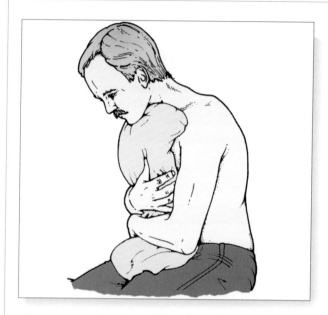

④ Instruct client with abdominal incision to cross arms over pillows as abdominal muscles contract during cough.

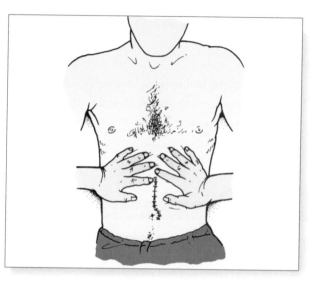

⑤ Instruct client to use manual pressure on wound, or support incision with palms of your hands. **RATIONALE:** This prevents incisional strain and encourages client to cough more effectively.

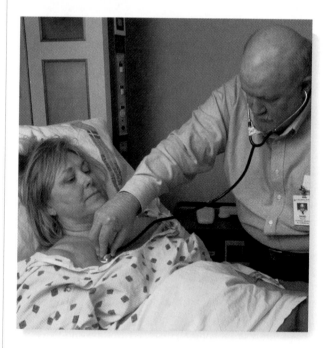

⑥ Assess client regularly and provide positive reinforcement. Encourage client to repeat deep breathing exercises several times hourly. **RATIONALE:** Deep breathing helps to inflate alveoli and mobilize secretions.

■ Repeat cough only if it is productive of secretions. **RATIONALE:** Accumulated secretions promote bacterial growth and interfere with ventilation, but coughing is a Valsalva maneuver and is not indicated unless it is productive of secretions.

INCENTIVE SPIROMETRY

Equipment

- Chair or hospital bed in upright position
- Pillows for positioning (optional)

- Incentive spirometer with flow rate indicator (save bag for storage of device)

SKILL

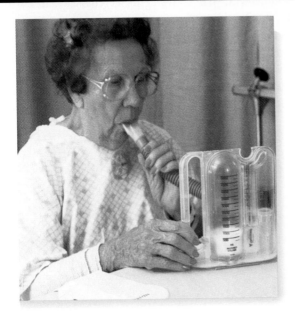

1 Attach open end of tubing to stem on front of exerciser. Instruct client to hold exerciser, place mouth tightly around mouthpiece, and sip in a trial breath. **RATIONALE:** Client can see flow rate indicator on side of unit to visualize appropriate rate for inhalation.

- Explain that a slow deep breath is better than a fast breath. Instruct client to exhale completely, then place mouth tightly around mouthpiece.
- Instruct client to inhale slowly to raise and maintain flow rate indicator at best flow rate range, and continue inhaling to try to raise piston to prescribed (or preoperatively measured) volume level.
- Encourage client to use spirometer hourly, to replace unit in bag when not in use, and to keep unit in an accessible place.

CHEST PHYSIOTHERAPY (CPT)

Equipment

- Gown or towel
- Hospital bed or other method to place client in Trendelenburg position

- Tissues or receptacle for sputum

SKILL

Postural Drainage

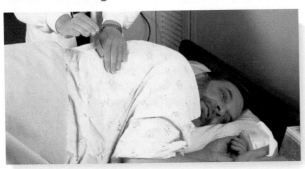

1 Lower head of bed so that client's head is positioned in a 30° downward angle with head lower than chest. If indicated, percuss upper lung areas before placing client in head-down position. Have client remain in each position for 15 min for pulmonary toilet (5 min in position; 5 min for percussion, vibration, and coughing; 5 min for bronchial drainage).

Percussion

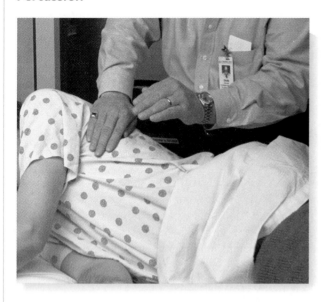

1 Cup your hands with thumbs and fingers closed. Keep wrists loose and relaxed and rhythmically flex and extend wrists to clap over area. **RATIONALE:** This motion produces vibrations that loosen secretions for easier removal with postural drainage and coughing.

- Alternate hands to percuss, and listen for hollow sounds with wrist movements. Percuss each area for 3 to 5 min.
- Do not percuss over bony prominences, such as vertebral column or scapula. **RATIONALE:** Vibrations are not transmitted to the chest wall through bony prominences and percussion there can cause discomfort.

Vibration

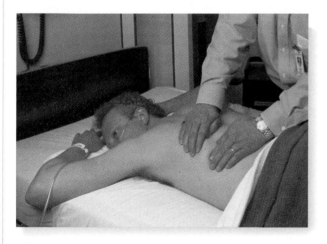

1 Place hands flat over area to be vibrated (may use one hand on top of the other). Keep arms and shoulders straight and wrists stiff.

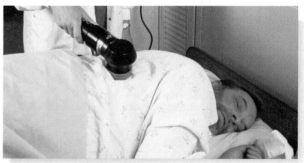

2 Alternate method: Use a vibrating machine in place of manual vibration. Have client take a deep breath in through the nose. As client exhales through pursed lips, vibrate client's chest by quickly contracting and relaxing your arms and shoulders. **RATIONALE:** This increases the turbulence and velocity of exhaled air and loosens and mobilizes secretions from peripheral airways.

- Vibrate area for three to four exhalations. Provide tissues or receptacle for client to expectorate secretions.
- Instruct client to turn to other side, and then supine, repeating sequence of percussion and vibration in each position. **RATIONALE:** This facilitates drainage, percussion, and vibration of all lung areas.
- Discard sputum container in biohazard receptacle, or send sputum specimen to laboratory if ordered.

SPUTUM SPECIMEN COLLECTION

Equipment

- Sputum specimen receptacle with label
- Biohazard bag for specimen transport
- Tissues
- Clean gloves
- Gown, mask, and goggles if needed
- HEPA or N95 respirator for protection against TB

SAFETY ALERT

Sputum testing for TB (acid-fast bacilli) requires specimen collection on three consecutive days. Sputum induction by aerosol therapy may be necessary and, because this procedure places staff at risk for infection, it must be carried out only in AFB isolation rooms or special cubicles. The nurse must wear a HEPA or N95 respirator for protection against TB.

SKILL

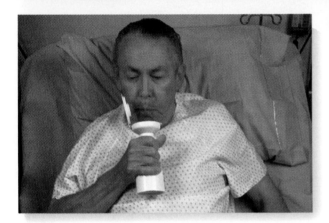

CLINICAL NOTE

Sputum specimens should be collected early in the morning, before the client's teeth are brushed. Have the client rinse the mouth with water before coughing, to help reduce contamination of the sputum sample with oral flora. Do not obtain a specimen immediately after a meal.

1 Place client in sitting position. Instruct client to lift hinged lid of sputum collection system, take several deep breaths, cough, and expectorate sputum (not saliva) directly into sterile container. **RATIONALE:** Deep coughs produce sputum rather than saliva.

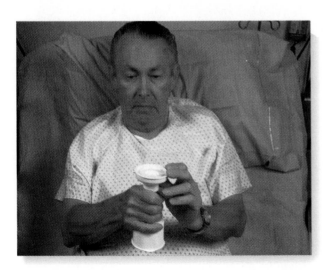

2 Instruct client to obtain 1 to 2 tablespoons of sputum in container; close and seal lid.

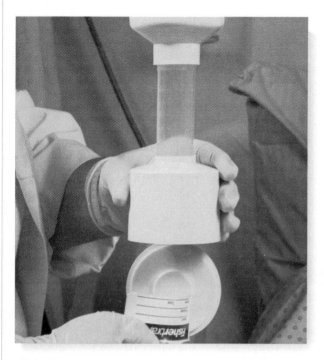

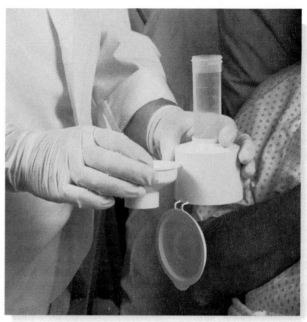

3 Without tipping tube, open hinged bottom and remove client label inside.

4 Remove top housing from collection tube, then remove tube with sputum specimen.

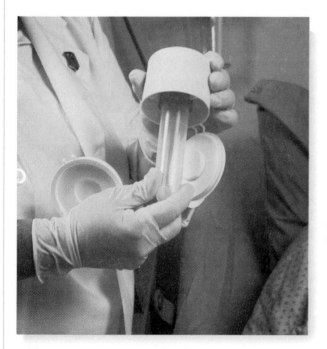

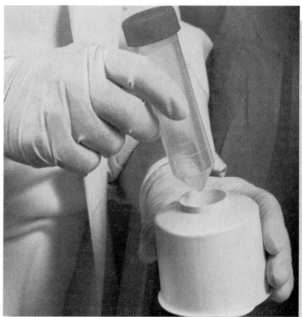

5 Screw specimen tube into cap in bottom of base unit, then remove capped tube.

6 Place specimen tube in unit housing. Label specimen tube directly. **RATIONALE:** If label is placed on tube housing, rather than specimen tube itself, specimen identification may be lost when the two are separated.

- Place housing in biohazard specimen transport bag and deliver to laboratory for analysis.

PEAK FLOW MEASUREMENT

Equipment

- Peak flow meter with instructions for client

SKILL

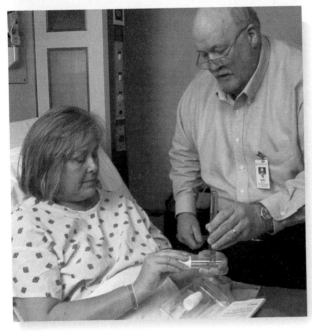

1 Attach mouthpiece to peak flow meter, if desired. **RATIONALE:** Most meters can be used with or without mouthpiece.

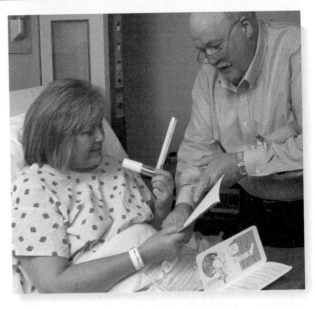

2 Follow product instructions to assemble meter.

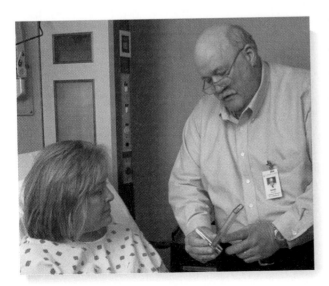

3 Slide indicator to bottom of meter scale. **RATIONALE:** To bring indicator to zero position.

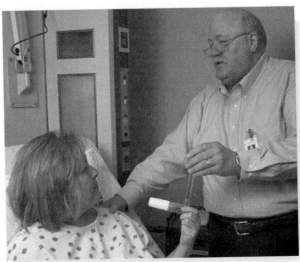

4 Instruct client to inhale as deeply as possible, then place mouth around mouthpiece, forming a tight seal. If possible, client should be standing. **RATIONALE:** Tight seal is necessary for accurate reading.

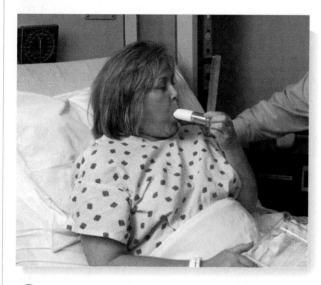

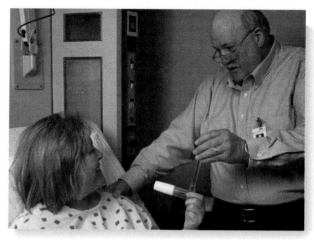

5 Have client blow out through mouth as hard and fast as possible. **RATIONALE:** As client forcefully exhales, indicator moves up scale to record client's peak expiratory flow (liters per minute).

6 Repeat peak flow measurement three times and record highest value. **RATIONALE:** Client may keep daily record of peak flow values and report significant changes.

- Clean unit weekly, following manufacturer's instructions.

CLINICAL NOTE

The peak flow meter is a device used to evaluate lung function by measuring maximum expiratory flow rates. Many asthma clients are able to perceive when their condition is worsening, but some, especially those with severe asthma, are less sensitive to increasing airway obstruction. The peak flow meter can be used on a daily basis for self-assessment to note changes in readings that may indicate a worsening condition (e.g., sudden decline in flow rate by 20 percent). Serial measurements help the physician make decisions about altering the client's medical regimen (e.g., bronchodilator or steroid therapy).

CHARTING

- Rate and character of breath sounds before and after skill
- Quantity and character of sputum produced
- Client's subjective tolerance of therapy

- Dispensation and description of obtained sputum specimen and rationale (laboratory tests to be performed)

OXYGEN THERAPY

Oxygen and carbon dioxide are gases transported or perfused by blood under pressure. These pressures are measured and recorded in mm Hg of Po_2 or Pco_2 by arterial blood gas analysis (ABGs). High or low values of Po_2 or Pco_2 may be indicative of respiratory dysfunction. Hemoglobin saturation with oxygen is dependent upon adequate Po_2 driving pressure. The percentage loading of hemoglobin is called the oxygen saturation. When the Po_2 is 90 mm Hg or greater, there is sufficient hemoglobin saturation to meet tissue needs. Measuring oxygen saturation by noninvasive, readily available and inexpensive pulse oximetry (Spo_2) has become a popular means of determining oxygenation status. Spo_2 values < 90 to 92 percent reflect less than optimal saturation of the hemoglobin and may indicate the need for supplemental oxygen therapy.

Carbon dioxide is a volatile acid that is eliminated by the lungs to help maintain an alkaline blood pH. Hypoventilation due to restrictive or obstructive lung disease results in an increased Pco_2 (respiratory acidosis) and an abnormal acid state of the blood (low pH). Conversely, hyperventilation causes a decreased Pco_2 (respiratory alkalosis) and may result in an abnormally high blood pH.

Although CO_2 is the major stimulus for breathing, high sustained CO_2 levels depress the respiratory center and can cause respiratory arrest due to CO_2 narcosis. Individuals who have chronically elevated Pco_2 levels due to chronic obstructive pulmonary disease (COPD) may become insensitive to Pco_2 as a stimulus for breathing. Instead, their central nervous system respiratory centers respond to a lower than normal Po_2 (<60 mm Hg) to stimulate breathing. Administration of high flows of oxygen to such hypoxic-dependent breathers can eliminate their breathing stimulus. These individuals are at high risk for CO_2 narcosis.

CLINICAL NOTE

PULMONARY ASSESSMENT

- Pulmonary function tests (spirometry) measure lung volume and capacity; they help differentiate restrictive and obstructive defects of ventilation or reveal a combination of both

  VC (vital capacity): maximum amount of air that can be exhaled after normal inhalation; should be 75 to 80 percent of that predicted by age, sex and height; decreased in restrictive disease.

  FVC (forced vital capacity): vital capacity with forced inhalation and exhalation.

  FEV (forced expiratory volume): 65 to 85 percent of VC in 1 sec and 95 percent in 3 sec; decreased in obstructive disease.

  FEV$_1$ (forced expiratory volume in 1 sec): normal is 75 percent of client's VC; decreased in obstructive disease.

  FEV$_{25-75}$ (midportion of FVC): measures expiratory flow capacity of small airways; reduced in obstructive disease.

- Normal pulmonary ventilation and perfusion are reflected by normal arterial blood gas (ABG) values.

  pH (normal 7.35 to 7.45): reflects the normal alkaline state of the blood. Hypoventilation can cause the blood to be abnormally acid, whereas hyperventilation can cause the blood to be abnormally alkaline.

  Pco_2 (normal 35 to 45 mm Hg): reflects adequacy of ventilation. Increased levels indicate hypoventilation; decreased levels indicate hyperventilation.

  HCO_3 (normal 22 to 26 mEq/L): reflects the body's ability to buffer fixed or volatile acids.

  Po_2 (normal 80 to 100 mm Hg): reflects the diffusing capacity of the alveoli. Decreased levels reflect hypoventilation or alveolar diffusion or perfusion problems.

  Sao_2 (normal 96 to 100 percent): reflects how well hemoglobin is saturated with oxygen; reduced saturation occurs with reduced Po_2.

Oxygen is considered a drug that requires a physician's prescription for administration. The nurse must know the indication, dosage, route of administration, and potential complications of its use. While oxygen is not flammable, it is combustible and will support fire.

SAFETY ALERT

Precautions for Oxygen Administration

- Set up "No Smoking" and "Oxygen in Use" signs at the site of administration and at the door, according to agency policy.
- Provide cotton gown—synthetics and wool may generate sparks of static electricity.
- Remove matches, lighters, and ashtrays from the bedside (these items should only be present with physician's orders, since hospitals are smoke-free facilities).
- Disconnect ungrounded electrical equipment.
- Remove all volatile or flammable materials (alcohol, oils, petroleum products).
- Make sure all electrical monitoring equipment is properly grounded.
- Locate fire extinguishers and oxygen meter turn-off lever.

A variety of devices are available for the delivery of oxygen; they vary in the degree to which they enclose the client. High-flow devices separate inhaled and exhaled gases with one-way valves to prevent dilution of inspired gas with exhaled CO_2. These devices have a reservoir capacity to ensure delivery of variable minute volumes, and the delivered oxygen concentration (FIO_2) does not vary with changes in the client's breathing pattern. Examples include the Venturi mask and the nonrebreathing mask. Low-flow devices allow air from the atmosphere to supply part of the inspired volume as well as some reinspiration of exhaled CO_2. These devices are more comfortable, but the oxygen concentration will vary with the client's breathing pattern. Examples include the partial rebreathing mask, the simple mask, and nasal cannulae (prongs).

RATIONALE

- To return arterial PO_2 and SpO_2 to normal or acceptable range
- To monitor client's oxygen saturation noninvasively
- To evaluate client's SpO_2 response to therapies
- To return respiratory rate to within normal limits
- To decrease respiratory distress
- To improve client's activity tolerance

ASSESSMENT

- Review ABGs or pulse oximetry values for baseline measurement.
- Assess client's vital signs, H&H, and medical status.
- Note client's subjective statement and objective signs of breathing effort.
- Monitor client's SpO_2 response shortly after oxygen flow rate is altered.
- Determine if client has had recent tests using IV dyes, since some of these dyes may make oximetry readings inaccurate.

OXYGEN THERAPY

Equipment

- Oxygen supply source
- Oxygen delivery device
- Oxygen flowmeter
- Humidifier, if indicated

OXYGEN DELIVERY DEVICES

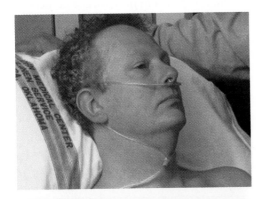

Nasal Cannulae

This equipment is easily tolerated by most clients and is simpler than a mask. The fraction of inhaled oxygen (FIO_2) varies depending on the oxygen liter flow and the rate and depth of client breathing (examples: FIO_2 24 to 38 percent, flow 1 to 2 LPM; FIO_2 30 to 35 percent, flow 3 to 4 LPM; FIO_2 38 to 44 percent, flow 5 to 6 LPM).

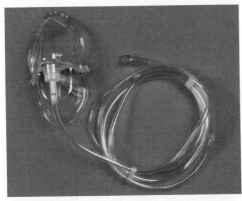

Simple Face Mask

This equipment requires fairly high oxygen flow to prevent rebreathing of carbon dioxide. About 75 percent of the inspired volume is room air drawn in through side holes in the mask. Accurate FIO_2 is difficult to estimate (example: FIO_2 35 to 65 percent, flow 8 to 12 LPM).

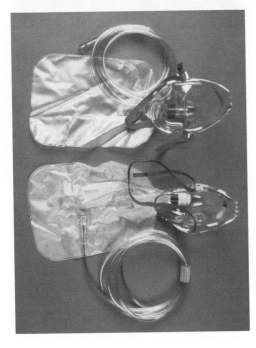

Mask with Reservoir Bag

This equipment provides a reservoir that allows higher FIO_2 to be delivered. At flows of less than 6 LPM, the risk of rebreathing carbon dioxide increases. Two types of these masks are available:

Partial Rebreathing Mask

No inspiratory valve, so that the beginning portion of exhaled air returns to the bag and mixes with the inhaled air. Ports are present so that most exhaled air escapes. The reservoir bag remains partially inflated (example: FIO_2 40 to 60 percent, flow 6 to 10 LPM).

Nonrebreathing Mask

Valve closes during exhalation so that exhaled air does not enter the reservoir and is not rebreathed. Valves on the mask side ports allow exhalation, but close on inhalation to prevent inhalation of room air (example: FIO_2 60 to 100 percent, flow 6 to 15 LPM).

(continued on next page)

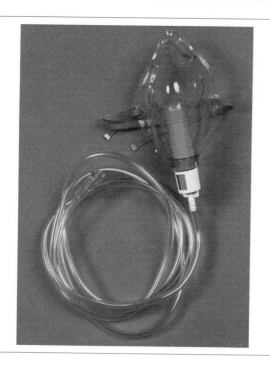

Venturi Mask

This system utilizes different-sized adapters (frequently color coded) to deliver a fixed or predicted rate of FIO_2. The FIO_2 is dependent upon oxygen liter flow and entrainment port size. This mask is used effectively on clients with COPD when precise FIO_2 is necessary (example: FIO_2 24 to 50 percent). Carbon dioxide buildup is kept at a minimum; humidifiers usually are not used.

SKILL

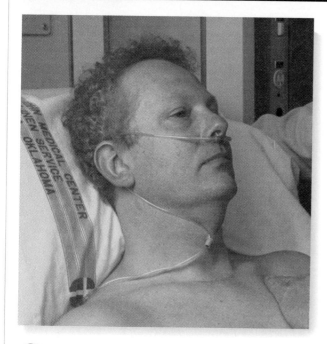

1 Insert oxygen flowmeter into wall outlet. Connect oxygen delivery device tubing to oxygen flowmeter. Place client in Fowler or semi-Fowler position. Apply prescribed oxygen delivery device to client.

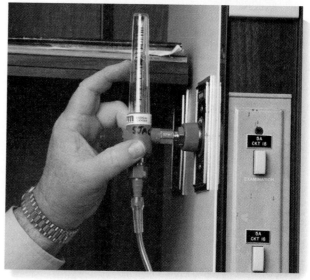

2 Set oxygen flow to prescribed liters per minute (LPM).

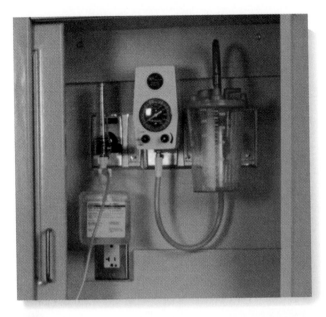

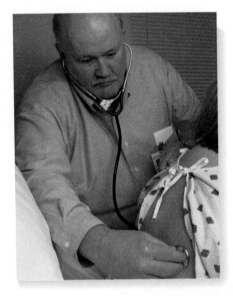

3 If ordered, humidify oxygen when flow rate is greater than 4 LPM. **RATIONALE:** This prevents excessive drying of mucosa.

4 Monitor client's vital signs, breath sounds, level of consciousness, breathing effort, and SpO_2. **RATIONALE:** These measures are used to evaluate effectiveness of therapy.

BAG-VALVE-MASK VENTILATION

Equipment

- Self-inflating resuscitation bag with nonrebreathing valve

- Oxygen source and tubing
- Airway adapter or face mask

Preparation

1 Summon an assistant if client is not intubated. **RATIONALE:** If client does not have an artificial airway, two responders are essential. Assistant holds mask while nurse compresses resuscitator bag.

- Connect mask or airway adapter to resuscitation bag.
- Connect oxygen tubing to bag inlet.

SKILL

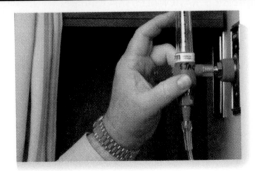

1 Turn oxygen flowmeter wide open to "flush." **RATIONALE:** This provides maximum enrichment of air delivered to client.

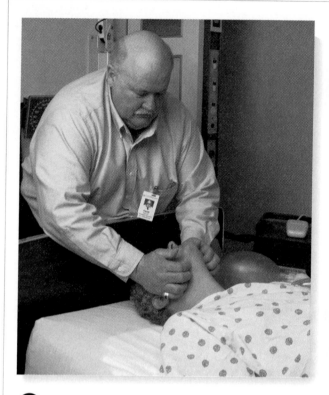

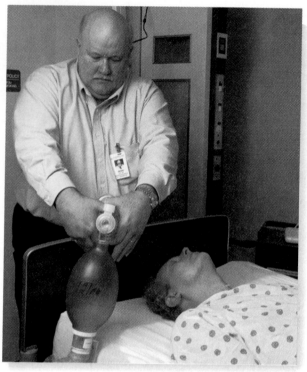

2 When using mask, stand at client's head and use both hands (one on each side of jaw) to lift mandible upward and outward. **RATIONALE:** This maneuver will lift client's tongue off airway.

3 Place apex of mask over client's nose; place base of mask between lower lip and chin. **RATIONALE:** This ensures that mask conforms to client's face for tight seal.

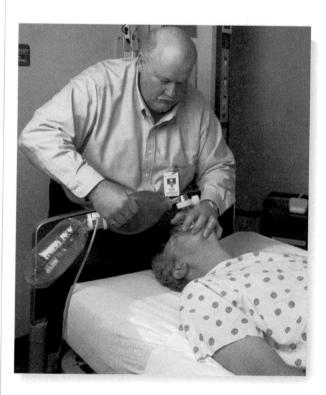

4 Holding client's head in extension, seal mask tightly by pressing it down with thumb and index finger and lifting up client's mandible (jaw lift) with remaining fingers. Compress resuscitator bag over 2 sec every 5 sec. **RATIONALE:** Sustained compression optimizes tidal volume delivered.

- If client is able to breathe spontaneously, give compressions in synchrony with client's breathing.
- Observe that client's chest rises and falls with each compression. **RATIONALE:** This validates ventilation.

PULSE OXIMETRY

Equipment

- Oximeter (battery or line power operated)
- Clip-on sensor probe

SAFETY ALERT

If the client's hemoglobin is greatly reduced, a normal Spo₂ may be present in spite of inadequate tissue oxygenation.

SKILL

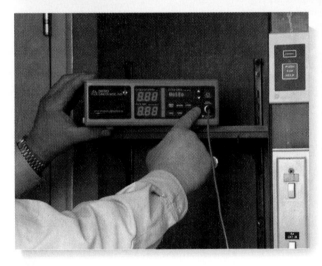

1 Turn oximetry unit power to ON.

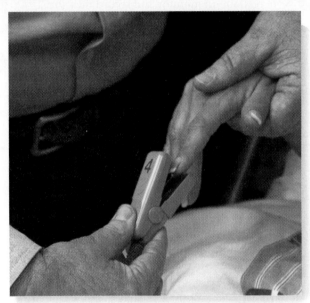

2 Apply sensor probe securely, flush with skin, making sure that both sensor probes are aligned directly opposite each other. **RATIONALE:** Oximeter sensors contain both red and infrared light-emitting diodes (LEDs) and a photodetector. The photodetector measures light absorption by oxygenated and deoxygenated Hgb in arterial blood.

- *Note:* Only very dark nail polish interferes with pulse oximetry measurements.
- If using continuous monitoring, set alarms to predetermined saturation levels and pulse rate limits.

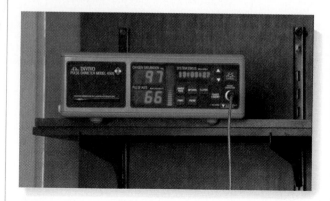

3 Note readout on monitor and record measure.

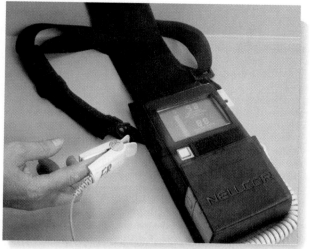

4 Read oxygen saturation level on portable digital unit and record.

- Compare finding with previous saturation levels and change in oxygen therapy (FIO_2).
- Change location of clip-on probe every 4 hrs if continuous readings are monitored.

CHARTING

- Type of device used for oxygen administration
- Oxygen liter flow rate (LPM)
- Measurements obtained with SpO_2 monitoring device (pulse oximetry)

- Client's vital signs and SpO_2 before therapy and 30 min after initiating therapy or any change in oxygen flow rate (LPM or FIO_2)
- Client's subjective response to therapy

SECTION THREE

RESTORATIVE MEASURES

ntubation with an artificial airway helps to provide patency for air exchange and the removal of obstructive secretions. Clients requiring airway maintenance include those with airway obstruction due to upper airway relaxation (e.g., nonresponsive client with relaxed oropharynx) and those who require assistance in ventilation (e.g., on mechanical ventilation) or airway clearance. Endotracheal intubation through the nose or mouth provides immediate ventilatory support, but cannot be prolonged because it insults laryngeal tissue and becomes uncomfortable for the client. Direct access to the lower airway via the trachea, below the larynx, provides a route for continuous airway support for such clients.

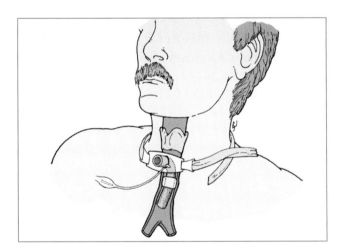

● FIGURE 23-3 *Tracheal intubation below the larynx.*

When the client breathes through an artificial apparatus—either an endotracheal or tracheostomy tube—atmospheric air is drawn directly into the lower airway, bypassing the defense mechanisms of the upper airway. There is no humidification or warming of inspired air, and inhaled foreign particles are not filtered. The client becomes susceptible to drying of secretions within the tube, making them difficult to mobilize and possibly providing a culture medium for infection. And, since the opening to inspired air is below the glottis, the client is unable to perform a Valsalva maneuver, making efforts to cough ineffective. The tube's presence in the airway activates production of secretions that cannot voluntarily be removed. In addition, since the client with an artificial airway exhales air below the larynx through an endotracheal or tracheostomy

tube, normal vocal cord vibration cannot occur to produce oral communication. The client is dependent upon artificial means for communicating with and summoning the emergency assistance of others.

Clients with artificial airways have critical needs that require nursing measures to assure and promote ventilation and to protect the invaded environment. Airway clearance and tracheostomy wound care are standard concerns. Suctioning to remove secretions is necessary, but must be performed only as needed, using sterile technique and careful instrumentation since the lower airway is considered a sterile environment that is vulnerable to trauma. In addition, the tracheostomy inner cannula must be cleaned or changed to prevent obstruction and decrease the risk of infection. Providing oral hygiene reduces pharyngeal bacteria, which also helps prevent pulmonary infection in clients with artificial airways.

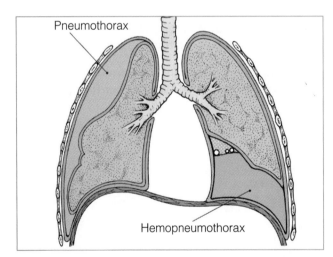

Pneumothorax

Hemopneumothorax

● FIGURE 23-4 *Pneumothorax and hemopneumothorax.*

If air or fluid collects in the pleural space (pneumothorax/hemothorax) due to disease, trauma, or thoracic surgery, the lung cannot expand. Excessive accumulation of air or fluid can increase intrathoracic pressure, impede venous return to the heart, and compromise cardiac output. Clients with pneumothorax or hemothorax may require the insertion of intrapleural chest tubes to drain fluid or air to reestablish the negative pressure normally present in the intrapleural space. Clients undergoing cardiac surgery often have mediastinal chest tubes placed to drain pericardial wound exudate and blood. Just as in the client with pneumothorax, if there is no outlet for postoperative mediastinal fluid, its accumulation can lead to excessive pressure that impairs cardiac function.

The traditional method of chest drainage used a three-bottle system. The first bottle collected chest fluid drainage. The second bottle established a water seal to allow air to exit the system and also to prevent atmospheric air from entering the client's chest. If necessary, a third bottle was used to apply negative pressure to the system to facilitate chest drainage. Today's sterile, disposable three-chamber chest drainage units (e.g., Pleur-Evac) utilize the same principles as the older three-bottle system to eliminate air and fluid from the chest. The functional principles of bottle systems include:

- **One bottle**—Here the bottle functions as a drainage collection bottle as well as a water seal and is used mainly to reestablish negative intrapleural pressure to reinflate the lung after pneumothorax.

- **Two bottles**—Here the water seal and drainage collection bottles are separate and the system is usually not connected to a suction source. These systems are used following thoracic or cardiac surgery.

- **Three bottles**—The third bottle is connected to an external suction source that adds negative pressure to the two-bottle system. These systems are used following thoracic or cardiac surgery.

Careful monitoring and maintenance of chest drainage systems are essential to prevent tension pneumothorax or cardiac tamponade, potentially lethal conditions of increased pressure within the thoracic cavity that impede venous return to the heart and compromise cardiac output.

RATIONALE

- To maintain airway patency for ventilation
- To provide a means for removal of secretions
- To compensate for bypassed airway protective mechanisms
- To provide a technique that minimizes airway contamination and trauma to the respiratory tract
- To provide a means for client communication
- To promote drainage of intrapleural or mediastinal fluid
- To reestablish negative intrapleural pressure for lung expansion

ASSESSMENT

- Assess client for unresponsiveness and need for oral airway maintenance.
- Assess client for double-cannula tracheostomy tube.
- Assess client's need for suctioning to clear airway secretions.
- Check client's pre- and posttherapy vital signs, objective breath sounds, and subjective response.

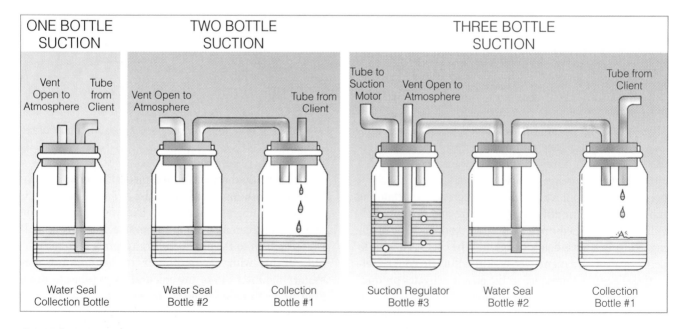

● **FIGURE 23-5** *Methods of chest drainage.*

- Assess that client obtains adequate hydration to help mobilize respiratory secretions.
- Check tracheal tube cuff pressure to assure adequate tissue perfusion.
- Make sure client with artificial airway has a means of communication and summoning immediate help (call bell, paper and pencil, magic slate).

- Make sure physician's written order for amount of negative pressure in the drainage system is followed.
- Check chest drainage system for proper function.
- Assess quantity and character of chest tube drainage.

OROPHARYNGEAL AIRWAY TUBE INSERTION

Equipment

- Oropharyngeal airway
- Tongue depressor
- Clean gloves

- Suction catheter
- Suction source
- Tape

SKILL

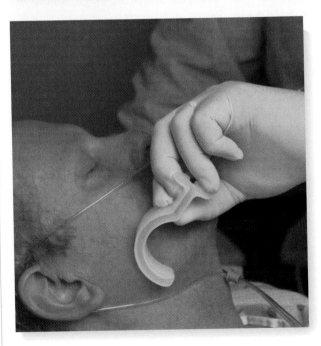

1 Ensure client is unresponsive and has no gag reflex. **RATIONALE:** Conscious client may vomit and aspirate or develop laryngospasm during tube insertion.

- Select appropriate size artificial airway. (Length should be from teeth to end of jawline.)
- Gently open client's mouth with crossed-finger technique; you may need to use modified jaw thrust to insert airway.
- Perform oral suctioning to clear pharyngeal secretions.
- Hold tongue down with tongue depressor and advance airway tube to back of tongue.

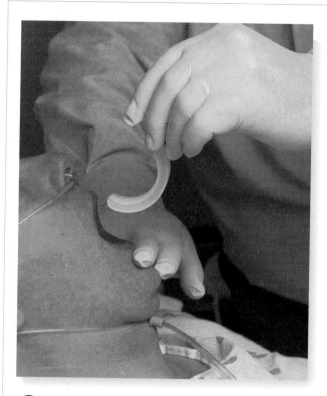

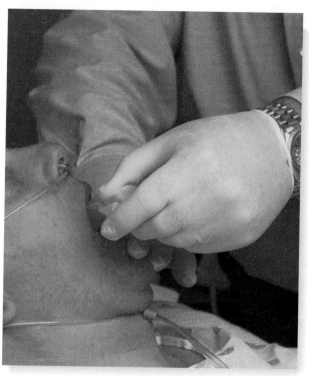

2 Alternate method: Advance airway tube upside down (curve upward).

3 As airway passes uvula, rotate airway 180°.

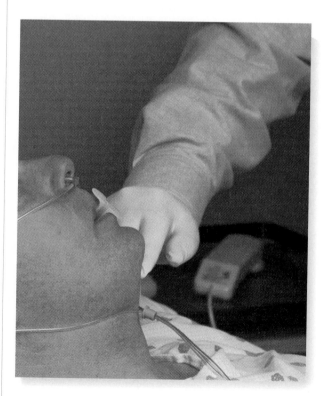

4 Check that curve fits over tongue. Airway should extend from lips to pharynx, displacing tongue anteriorly. **RATIONALE:** Proper positioning helps prevent injury to lips, teeth, tongue, and posterior pharynx.

- Tape top and bottom of airway tube in position. **RATIONALE:** Stabilization of tube prevents injury.
- Position client on side. **RATIONALE:** To facilitate drainage of airway secretions.

TRACHEOSTOMY SUCTIONING

Equipment

- Manual resuscitator bag with tracheostomy tube adapter for hyperoxygenation
- Oxygen source
- Suction source (e.g., wall suction or portable suction machine) with tubing
- Clean gloves (for catheter in sleeve)
- Gown, goggles, and mask as needed if splash is anticipated
- Suctioning kit with suction catheter (no greater in diameter than half the inner diameter of the tracheostomy tube), small container for normal saline solution, sterile gloves, or suction catheter with sleeve
- Bottle of sterile normal saline solution
- Stethoscope

CLINICAL NOTE

To determine suction catheter size, multiply the artificial airway's diameter times 2 (e.g., for an 8-mm tube, use a 16 French suction catheter).

SAFETY ALERT

Clients with artificial airways must have a means of communicating and summoning emergency assistance. Make sure a call bell or other summoning device is within the client's reach and an alternative form of verbal communication is provided (e.g., paper and pencil or magic slate).

Preparation

1 Instruct an assistant to manage resuscitator bag to hyperoxygenate client's airway before and after suctioning. **RATIONALE:** Skill is more safely performed with an assistant.

2 Attach resuscitator bag to oxygen tubing and open oxygen flowmeter to maximum (to flush).

SAFETY ALERT

Instillation of saline into airways for suctioning purposes leads to greater hypoxemia than suctioning without saline instillation. In addition, bacteria are dispersed through airways with saline instillation.

SKILL

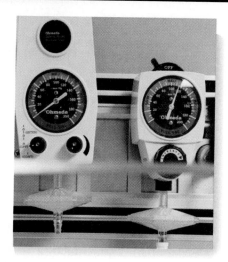

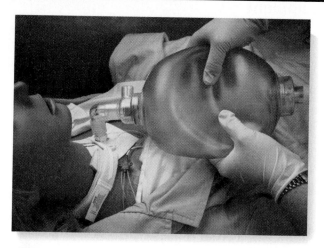

① Turn suction on at 80 to 120 mm Hg pressure. **RATIONALE:** Higher suction pressure increases risk of mucosal injury.

- Don goggles, mask, and gown as needed.
- Open trach kit to display sterile items.
- Open normal saline flush container (box) and fill with sterile saline solution.
- Don sterile gloves. (Dominant hand will be sterile and other hand will be clean.)
- Have client take several deep breaths to hyperoxygenate.

② Alternative method: Have assistant (if present) disconnect client's oxygen source and connect resuscitator bag to tracheostomy tube, then compress for 2 sec to hyperoxygenate lungs with 100 percent oxygen for five breaths, then disconnect bag and place nearby. **RATIONALE:** Suctioning causes tachycardia, then hypoxemia and vagal responses with bradycardia and other cardiac arrhythmias. Pre- and postsuctioning hyperoxygenation helps to prevent these potentially lethal complications.

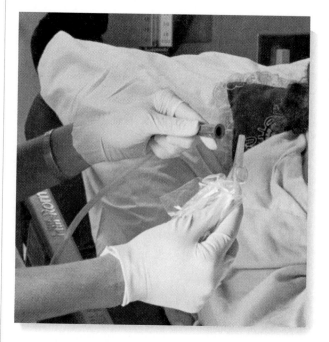

③ Using *sterile gloved dominant hand,* pick up sterile suction catheter and connect to wall (or machine) suction tubing held with *nondominant hand* that now becomes nonsterile.

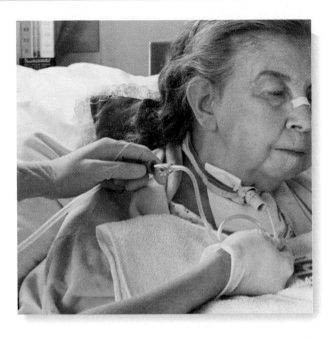

4 Holding suction catheter with sterile gloved dominant hand, dip catheter into box of sterile saline to lubricate and, without applying suction, advance catheter into client's tracheostomy tube. **RATIONALE:** Suction application during tube insertion inhibits tube advancement.

- Using nondominant hand (gloved, but no longer sterile), apply intermittent occlusion to suction tube opening, while using sterile gloved dominant hand to rotate and withdraw the catheter from the tracheostomy tube. **RATIONALE:** Intermittent suctioning and catheter rotation reduce damage to mucosal lining during suctioning.
- Apply suction for no more than 10 sec. **RATIONALE:** This helps prevent hypoxemia and resultant cardiac arrhythmias.

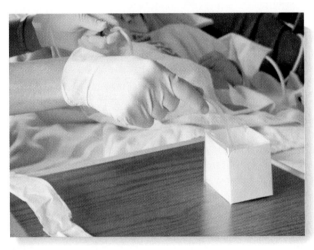

 SAFETY ALERT

Hyperoxygenate the client before and after each time the airway is entered for suctioning, and wait 2 to 3 min before suctioning again to prevent severe hypoxemia.

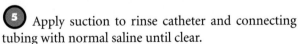

5 Apply suction to rinse catheter and connecting tubing with normal saline until clear.

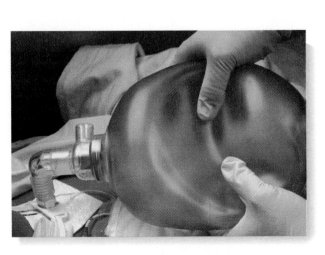

6 Hyperoxygenate client's lungs with resuscitator bag as in step 2, or reattach oxygen source and have client take several deep breaths for postsuctioning hyperoxygenation.

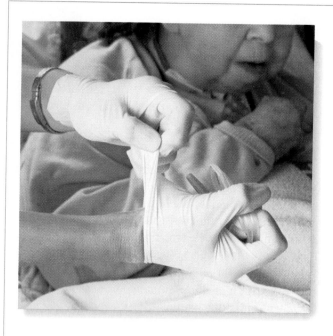

7 Dispose of suction catheter by disconnecting it from suction tubing, coiling catheter around fingers, and removing glove back over catheter. Discard gloves with gloved catheter into appropriate receptacle.

- Auscultate client's lung sounds and assess heart rate and rhythm to compare with baseline assessment.
- Turn off suction source.

CLINICAL NOTE

SUCTIONING WITH CATHETER IN SLEEVE
Sterile suction catheters are available in protective external sleeves. These devices are commonly used in short-term care settings for intubated clients (e.g., in postanesthesia care unit). The sleeve allows suctioning without requiring the nurse to don sterile gloves.

Wearing clean gloves, the nurse advances the catheter through the protective sleeve into the client's airway. While intermittent suction is applied, the catheter is withdrawn back into the sleeve. The sleeve protects the catheter for immediate reuse, if necessary, and at the same time protects the nurse from exposure to the client's secretions.

SAFETY ALERT

Any time the tracheostomy cuff is to be deflated, it is important to first suction the oropharynx (clean technique using catheter or Yankauer device) so that upper airway secretions do not fall into the lower airway upon cuff deflation.

TRACHEOSTOMY CARE

Equipment

- Tracheal cleaning tray (sterile basin, pipe cleaners, 4 × 4 gauze squares)
- Sterile applicators
- Clean gloves
- Sterile gloves
- Sterile hydrogen peroxide (H_2O_2)
- Sterile normal saline
- Sterile 4 × 4 presplit gauze dressing or 4 × 4 gauze squares
- Tracheal ties (twill or foam)
- Scissors
- Forceps

Preparation

1 Open trach tray, remove lids of liquid containers, and pour H_2O_2 into sterile basin.

2 Open sterile packet of 4 × 4s, leaving them inside package (sterile) cover. Open pipe cleaner packet for availability.

3 Fold end of twill ties over 1½ inches and cut a slit across the folded edge.

SKILL

Tracheostomy Tube Inner Cannula Care

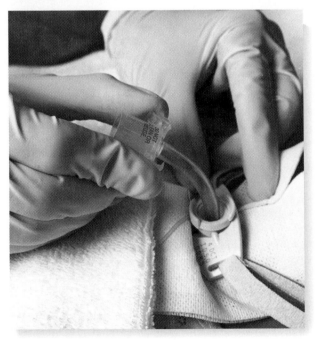

1 Using nondominant hand, secure client's tracheostomy tube outer cannula neck plate with index finger and thumb and use dominant hand to unlock inner cannula by turning counterclockwise 90°. Then gently pull inner cannula upward and outward toward you to remove. Place nondisposable inner cannula in sterile basin filled with H_2O_2 to soak and remove dried secretions.

- Don sterile gloves. Cleanse lumen and outer surface of inner cannula with pipe cleaners moistened in H_2O_2, rinse with sterile water or saline, place on sterile 4 × 4 gauze, and dry thoroughly.

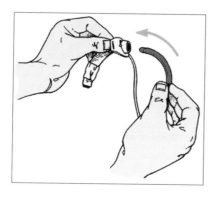

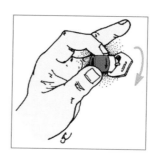

3 Lock by rotating clockwise.

2 Stabilize outer flange of tracheostomy tube and replace inner cannula.

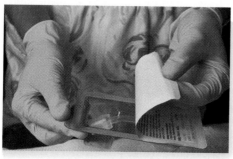

CLINICAL NOTE

The use and changing of disposable inner cannulas has eliminated the necessity for inner cannula cleaning in many care settings. Increased cost, combined with inconclusive benefit of this practice, indicate a need for further research.

4 Alternately, discard and replace disposable inner cannula with new sterile one.

Tracheostomy Tube Ties

CLINICAL NOTE

TRACHEOSTOMY TUBE TIES

- Have another nurse secure tracheostomy tube outer cannula. Cut, remove, and discard old trach ties. Securing the tube helps prevent accidental extubation if the client coughs.
- Leave the old trach tie in place if you are changing the ties without assistance. This prevents accidental dislodging of the trach tube during care.

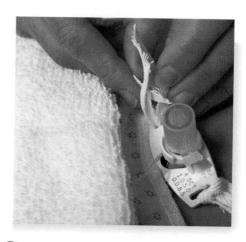

SAFETY ALERT

An obturator is kept at the bedside for emergency use. If the tracheostomy tube is inadvertently dislodged, it can be reinserted immediately using the obturator.

1 Pass slit end of ties through flange loop of trach tube about 2 to 3 in.

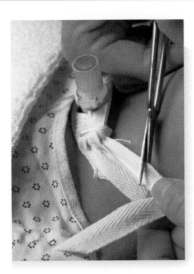

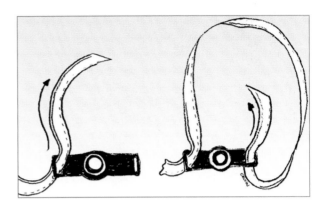

2 Thread other end of tie all the way through slit. Pull tie firmly into place. Repeat actions for other side of tracheostomy tube.

- Bring the two ties around client's neck and tie in square knot to one side of neck, leaving one fingerbreadth of slack under tie. **RATIONALE:** This is more comfortable and prevents pressure on neck and jugular vein.

3 Alternate method: Use Velcro ties or a long piece of twill. Pull end through flange slit and bring tape around back of client's neck, thread end through flange on other side of trach tube, double back around client's neck to other end, and tie in square knot.

Tracheostomy Dressing

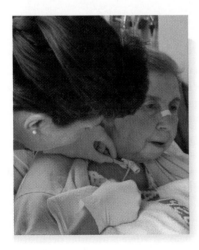

1 Don sterile gloves. Using separate sterile applicators soaked in normal saline or dilute H_2O_2, cleanse outer cannula and tracheostomy site.

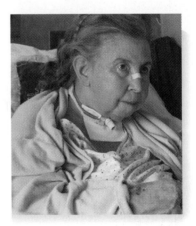

2 Apply presplit (nonraveling) sterile trach dressing up and around insertion site.

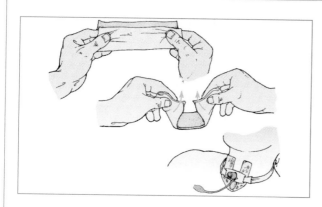

③ Alternate method: Fold sterile 4 × 4 gauze square in half and chevron ends up under tracheostomy flanges.

TRACHEAL TUBE CUFF INFLATION

Equipment

- 10-mL syringe
- Suction equipment
- Stethoscope

SKILL

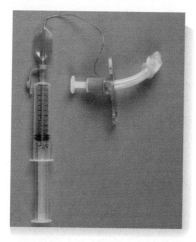

① Attach 10-mL syringe to distal end of inflatable cuff.

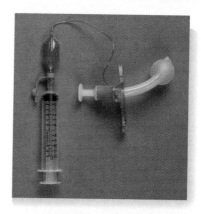

② Inflate cuff for minimal leak using minimal occlusive pressure. **RATIONALE:** To prevent undue pressure on tracheal tissue.

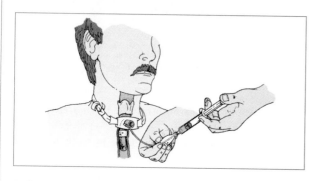

③ To measure appropriate tracheal tube cuff pressure, use stethoscope to auscultate at client's suprasternal notch. Noting hissing sound at end of inspiration indicates desired minimal occlusive pressure in cuff. Ask client to speak: If voice is audible, occlusion is inadequate.

TRACHEOSTOMY TUBE CAP INSERTION

Equipment

- Passey-Muir speaking valve or cap
- Suction source
- Suction catheter or oral suction device (e.g., Yankauer)
- Clean gloves
- Sterile gloves
- Empty 10-mL syringe

CLINICAL NOTE

If the client is considered to be ready for weaning from an artificial airway, obtain a physician's order to change to a fenestrated uncuffed tracheostomy tube.

SKILL

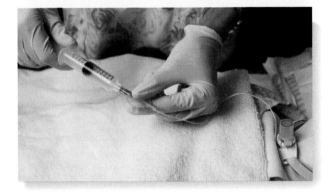

 1 Suction nasopharynx if cuffed tube is in place. **RATIONALE:** This removes secretions that have pooled above cuff, preventing their mobilization into lower airways upon cuff deflation.

- Attach syringe and deflate tracheal cuff if present. **RATIONALE:** If tracheostomy tube is capped and cuff is not deflated, client has no airway.

SAFETY ALERT

If the tracheostomy tube is capped to allow exhaled air to flow over the larynx so that the client can speak, the cuff must be deflated to allow an outlet for exhalation of air and an inlet for inhalation of air through the client's natural airway. If the tracheostomy tube is capped and the cuff remains inflated, the client has no access to air for ventilation, and will suffocate.

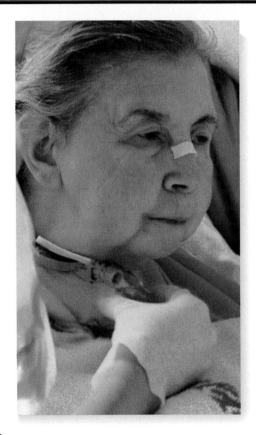

2 Don sterile gloves. Place speaking valve or cap over opening of tracheostomy tube. Observe client for respiratory distress. **RATIONALE:** Tube's presence increases resistance to airflow dramatically, thus increasing the work of breathing.

- Stay at bedside until client is comfortable and exhibits no difficulty breathing. Cut pilot balloon tube so that cuff cannot be inflated, or post notices on pilot balloon, over bed, and on client's chart: "Do not inflate cuff with cap in place."

CHEST TUBE DRAINAGE SYSTEM

Equipment

- Disposable water seal suction unit with stand
- 60-mL sterile syringe with irrigating/catheter tip
- Bottle of sterile water
- Tape
- Suction source
- Padded hemostats

SKILL

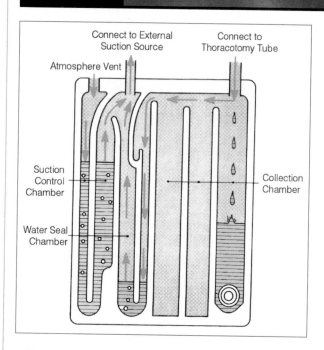

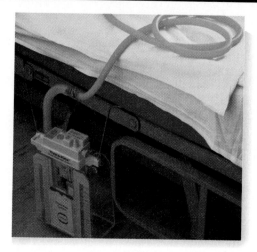

1 Insert syringe (as a funnel) and fill water seal chamber with sterile water to 2-cm level. **RATIONALE:** This level provides sufficient fluid to create a one-way valve to prevent room air from entering but to allow air to exit client's intrapleural space.

- Remove plastic plug of suction control chamber, fill suction control chamber with sterile water to prescribed (e.g., 20-cm) level, and replace plug. **RATIONALE:** This level dictates amount of negative pressure applied to intrapleural space.

- Maintaining asepsis, connect tube on fluid collection side of unit to long flexible tubing of client's chest tube, taping connection sites securely. **RATIONALE:** Taping helps prevent air entry from atmosphere into system.

2 Coil excess flexible tubing on bed, but provide straight line of tubing from bed to collection system. **RATIONALE:** Straight line of tubing prevents pooling of fluid in dependent loops, which creates excess pressure in tubing and prevents evacuation of air and fluid.

- Attach tubing on water seal chamber to suction source. **RATIONALE:** This establishes negative pressure equivalent to water level (e.g., 20 cm).

- *Or,* if no suction source is used, keep water seal chamber tubing open to air to provide vent. **RATIONALE:** This maintains underwater seal and allows evacuation of air from intrapleural space.

- To establish suction, turn on suction source slowly, just until bubbling occurs in unit's suction control chamber.

- Encourage client to deep-breathe, turn, and cough, supporting surgical incision. **RATIONALE:** When client coughs, increased intrapleural pressure helps to force air from client's chest.

- Monitor water levels daily in both water seal chamber and suction control chamber. Refill to prescribed level with sterile water as needed. **RATIONALE:** Bubbling will cause water to evaporate over time, altering level of negative pressure applied.

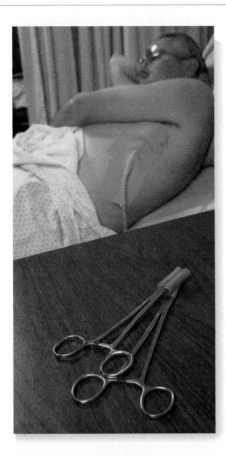

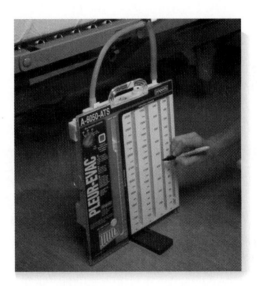

3 For emergency purposes only, keep rubber-tipped hemostat at client's bedside. **RATIONALE:** In case of emergency, tube can be clamped close to client's chest insertion site to prevent atmospheric air from entering client's pleural space and causing pneumothorax.

■ Always keep drainage collection system level and below client's chest. **RATIONALE:** This promotes drainage and prevents siphoning of fluid contents back into client's intrapleural space.

4 Mark quantity of drainage on receptacle regularly, and report drainage exceeding 100 mL/hr. **RATIONALE:** Excessive or unusual increase in drainage must be reported to physician.

CLINICAL NOTE

"Stripping" and "milking" chest tubes may help eliminate clots, but may also create sudden extreme sub-atmospheric pressures in the intrapleural space, resulting in potential injury to lung tissue.

■ If there is a physician's order to strip, use your nondominant hand to support the drainage tube; use your dominant thumb and forefinger over an alcohol sponge to compress and slide down the tube, stripping any obstruction (e.g., clot) toward the drainage receptacle.

■ To milk the chest drainage tubing, fold, squeeze to compress, then release the tubing, repeating sequence and moving out from client to drainage receptacle. This measure also creates excessive intrapleural negative pressure.

CHARTING

- Clinical manifestations indicating need for oral airway
- Preoxygenation and postoxygenation provision with suctioning
- Frequency of suctioning
- Character and quantity of secretions obtained by suctioning
- Pre- and postskill vital signs and breath sounds
- Client's subjective response to interventions (e.g., "less dyspnea")

- Type and frequency of tracheostomy tube care and site dressing change
- Description of tracheostomy site
- Measures employed to ensure client communication
- Time and type of tracheostomy tube cap inserted and client's response
- Amount of negative pressure in chest tube drainage system
- Quantity and description of chest tube drainage

CRITICAL THINKING FOCUS

SECTION ONE ▪ Preventive Measures

Unexpected Outcomes

- Client is unwilling to deep breathe because of pain or fear of wound dehiscence.

- Client is unable to master use of incentive spirometer.

- Client forgets to use incentive spirometer.

- Slapping sounds are produced with chest percussion.

- Client becomes nauseated while coughing up secretions following chest PT exercises.

- Adventitious lung sounds continue.

- Client's breathing becomes more rapid and labored.

Alternative Nursing Actions

- Review importance of maintenance measures.
- Assist in supporting incision, using your gloved hands.

- Optimize ventilatory capacity by placing client in Fowler position.
- Assure that client does regular deep breathing if device interferes with adherence.

- Suggest that client use spirometer or perform deep sustained inspiration, coordinating with TV commercials as a reminder.

- Cup hands more and assure that clapping is with wrist flexion and extension only.

- Perform treatments between or before but not after meals.

- Identify area of lung that requires focused chest PT and administer to specific area.

- Evaluate need for additional treatments or potential need for intubation and assisted mechanical ventilation.

SECTION TWO ▪ Oxygen Therapy

Unexpected Outcomes	Alternative Nursing Actions
▪ Client develops atelectasis.	▪ Encourage deep breathing and turning, range of motion, and ambulation if possible. ▪ Discuss need for chest PT with physician. ▪ Use sedatives or other respiratory depressants carefully.
▪ Oxygen saturation findings vary considerably.	▪ Check that sensor probes are aligned to prevent photodetector picking up light from sources other than sensor.
▪ Oximeter artifact or alarms sound.	▪ Encourage client to keep sensor site still. Movement scrambles signals from photodetector, interfering with readings. ▪ Place sensor on different site. ▪ Avoid placing sensor on hand of arm used for continuous blood pressure monitoring.
▪ Oximeter pulsations are inadequate.	▪ Carefully assess client for possible reason for change in peripheral perfusion. ▪ Evaluate need for different type of sensor if site is vasoconstricted or edematous.
▪ Single nurse cannot manage adequate compression of manual bag resuscitator.	▪ Assure optimum mask fit and use your body to compress bag to obtain larger tidal volume.

SECTION THREE ▪ Restorative Measures

Unexpected Outcomes	Alternative Nursing Actions
▪ Secretions and coughing are excessive while inner cannula is cleansed.	▪ Perform oral suctioning before trach tube is deflated. ▪ Provide new inner cannula as alternate while cleansing old inner cannula.
▪ Arrhythmias occur during tracheal suctioning.	▪ Limit suctioning time to less than 10 sec. ▪ Oxygenate lungs with 100 percent oxygen before and after suctioning. ▪ Ensure that suction catheter is not larger than 50 percent of the size of the tube being suctioned.
▪ Tracheostomy tube is obstructed.	▪ Deflate cuff immediately to allow airflow. ▪ Remove obstructed tracheostomy tube and insert obturator or forceps to establish and maintain airway if necessary. ▪ Seal client's stoma (by pinching) and provide bag–valve–face mask ventilation for resuscitation if signs of respiratory distress are present. ▪ Insert new tracheostomy tube as soon as possible.
▪ There is continuous bubbling in the water seal chamber of chest drainage unit.	▪ Check connections for tight seal. ▪ Reinforce client's tube site dressing.

■ There is no fluctuation of fluid in the seal chamber.

■ Chest drainage tube is accidentally disconnected from drainage collection system.

■ Use padded hemostat to clamp tubing, briefly, starting at client and moving toward collection unit. When bubbling ceases, you have passed site of air leak.

■ Check to be sure client is not lying on chest tube.

■ If lung reexpansion has occurred, lung will press against tube; check for return of breath sounds.

■ Milking or stripping to dislodge clots may be indicated if tube is obstructed. Obtain physician's order to perform this skill.

■ Submerge distal tip of drainage tube under 1 inch of sterile water to reestablish water seal. Have client cough to help evacuate intrapleural space.

SELF-CHECK EVALUATION

PART 1 ■ Matching Items

Match the definition in column B with the correct term in column A.

Column A

_____ a. Hypoxemia
_____ b. Perfusion
_____ c. Diffusion
_____ d. Ventilation
_____ e. Adventitious sounds
_____ f. Dyspnea
_____ g. Atelectasis
_____ h. Acidosis
_____ i. Acidemia
_____ j. Surfactant

Column B

1. Alveolar collapse, frequently due to inadequate ventilation or surfactant activity
2. Phospholipid produced by alveoli that reduces alveolar surface tension and prevents alveolar collapse
3. Acid state in which the blood pH is less than 7.35
4. State of inadequate saturation of hemoglobin with oxygen (less than 90 percent), resulting in inadequate tissue oxygenation
5. Circulation of blood to peripheral tissues
6. Condition of inadequate acid buffering by the kidneys (low HCO_3) or inadequate acid elimination by the lungs (high P_{CO_2}) resulting in an acid state of the blood (low pH)
7. Subjective feeling of difficulty breathing
8. Passive movement of a gas from an area of higher to an area of lower pressure
9. Abnormal sounds in addition to breath sounds normally auscultated during inhalation and exhalation
10. Active process of airflow from the atmosphere into the airways due to the creation of negative pressure on inspiration

PART 2 ▪ Multiple Choice Questions

1. The most effective way to prevent postoperative pulmonary complications is:

a. Sustained deep breathing.
b. Airway suctioning.
c. Coughing.
d. Chest physical therapy.

2. The Sp_{O2} is directly related to the:

a. P_{CO_2}.
b. P_{O_2}.
c. HCO_3.
d. Serum pH.

3. The major stimulus for breathing is:

a. Hypoxia.
b. Decrease in carbon dioxide.
c. Rise in carbon dioxide.
d. High serum pH.

4. Percussion and vibration are effective measures to:

a. Strengthen pulmonary muscles.
b. Liquify thick secretions.
c. Loosen retained secretions.
d. Enhance oxygen diffusion.

5. The peak flow meter is used to determine:

a. Need for oxygen therapy.
b. Inspiratory flow rate.
c. Increased airway secretions.
d. Expiratory flow rate.

6. The goal of oxygen therapy for the client with COPD is to obtain a(n):

a. Sp_{O_2} of 90 percent.
b. P_{O_2} of 100 mm Hg.
c. Normal P_{CO_2}.
d. Normal respiratory rate.

7. The oxygen delivery system that provides the highest concentration of oxygen is:

a. Nasal prongs.
b. Partial rebreathing mask.
c. Nonrebreathing mask with reservoir bag.
d. Venturi mask.

8. The rationale for humidifying high flows of oxygen is to:

a. Provide moisture to mucous membranes.
b. Prevent infection of upper airways.
c. Promote patency of the airways.
d. Increase oxygen delivery.

9. To obtain a reliable pulse oximetry measure, the client must have:

a. Normal capillary refill.
b. Normal respiratory rate.
c. Nails free of polish.
d. Normal hemoglobin level.

10. Pulse oximetry is a noninvasive method of measuring:

a. P_{O_2}.
b. P_{CO_2}.
c. Sa_{O_2}.
d. Capillary refill.

11. Suctioning places the client at risk for:

a. Cardiac depression.
b. Respiratory arrest.
c. Neurologic insult.
d. Tracheal perforation.

12. The best method to prevent hypoxia when suctioning is to:

a. Suction routinely.
b. Hyperoxygenate for 1 to 2 min before suctioning.
c. Suction for no more than 15 sec.
d. Use only a large catheter.

13. The priority concern for the client with a capped tracheostomy tube is:

a. Continuous tube cuff deflation.
b. Providing a means of communication.
c. Aspiration precautions.
d. Continuous pulse oximetry monitoring.

14. Which of the following is an important intervention before deflating the cuff of a tracheostomy tube?

a. Instilling 10 mL normal saline.
b. Preoxygenating with 100 percent oxygen.
c. Providing oral hygiene.
d. Suctioning the oropharynx.

PART 3 ▪ Critical Thinking Application

Mrs. Harvey, age 72, has a history of chronic obstructive pulmonary disease (COPD) with components of emphysema and chronic bronchitis. She has frequent recurrence of respiratory infection requiring hospitalization. With her most recent hospitalization, she has developed pulmonary hypertension and right-sided heart failure with weight gain and systemic edema. After treatment with IV antibiotics, she is ready for discharge, but will be sent home with continuous low-flow (1.5 LPM) oxygen therapy. Her ABGs at the time of discharge show elevated P_{CO_2} (respiratory acidosis), elevated bicarbonate level (metabolic alkalosis), P_{O_2} of 60 mm Hg, and O_2 saturation of 90 percent. Her blood pH is low normal due to the compensated respiratory acidosis.

1. What is the rationale for home oxygen therapy for Mrs. Harvey?

2. What are the hazards that accompany home oxygen therapy?

3. What should the client know about home oxygen therapy?

4. What are the objective expected outcomes of home oxygen therapy (ABGs)?

24

CARDIOVASCULAR SKILLS

INTRODUCTION

The heart and vessels comprise a closed unit that circulates oxygen- and nutrient-enriched blood to the tissues by way of arteries. This system then picks up the waste products of cellular metabolism and, by way of veins, returns them to the heart to be delivered to appropriate organs of excretion (lungs and kidneys). It is within the capillaries, between the arteries and veins, that this exchange takes place.

The blood that carries waste products flows through veins to the right side of the heart. Veins are low-pressure, thin-walled structures that lack the elastic propelling force found in arteries. The muscle pump of the lower extremities and the negative intrathoracic pressure created by breathing help veins return blood to the heart against the force of gravity. In contrast, arteries are strong, elastic structures that perpetuate the rhythmic pumping of the heart to propel blood under pressure to the body tissues.

The role of the heart is to receive blood from the veins (preload) and to pump arterial blood into arteries (afterload) to meet the needs of the body. When metabolic demand increases (e.g., through exercise or illness), the heart must handle an increased

(continued on next page)

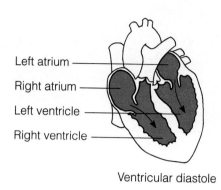
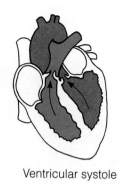

Left atrium

Right atrium

Left ventricle

Right ventricle

Ventricular diastole

Ventricular systole

● **FIGURE 24-1** *Functioning of the heart.* (SOURCE: *Lemone and Burke,* Medical Surgical Nursing, *2nd ed., Prentice Hall Health, 2000.)*

venous return and augment its cardiac output. In sickness and in health, efficient heart function requires that the heart fill adequately and empty by contracting effectively.

The heart is a two-phase pump. *Ventricular diastole* is the relaxed, filling phase during which the mitral and tricuspid valves are open so that the atria and ventricles function as one. This allows the right ventricle to fill with venous blood coming from the systemic circulation, while the left ventricle receives arterialized blood from the pulmonic circulation. During filling, the ventricular walls are stretched, and pressure rises to enhance contraction. Also during this diastolic filling phase, the coronary arteries perfuse the heart. If diastole is shortened due to premature ectopic contractions or rapid ventricular rates, ventricular filling and coronary perfusion are both compromised, potentially resulting in decreased cardiac output.

During the second phase, *systole,* the ventricles contract to close the mitral and tricuspid valves and eject approximately 50 percent of the blood received. Right ventricular contraction forces the pulmonic valve open as blood is ejected into the pulmonic circulation via the pulmonary artery. At the same time, left ventricular contraction forces the aortic valve open as blood is ejected into the systemic circulation via the aorta.

Effective pumping of the heart requires synchronized muscle stimulation, a contractile response for ejection, and then relaxation for filling. Specialized myocardial cells within the heart are responsible for the electrical stimulation of this pumping action. These cells initiate and conduct electrical impulses with regularity and consistency. In response, myocardial working cells of first the atria and then the ventricles depolarize (become positively charged due to ion influx), their cells shorten, and contraction occurs. Following depolarization, atrial and then ventricular cells return to their resting negative charge (as ions leave the cells) and the chambers relax to fill with blood for the next contraction. This sequence of atrial followed by ventricular activity along with the resulting closure and opening of valves propels the blood through the heart in a one-way forward direction. The heart normally pumps the entire circulating blood volume each minute, but can increase this work manyfold in times of metabolic need (e.g., during exercise or stress). Irregularities of electrical impulse formation or transmission can adversely affect this important synchronized pumping of the heart.

Insults to the left ventricle (e.g., myocardial infarction, sustained hypertension, arrhythmias) alter its ability to fill in diastole and eject during systole. As less blood is ejected, ventricular filling pressure rises (increased preload). When left heart pressure rises, blood pools in the pulmonary veins, constricting alveolar expansion. Dyspnea due to backward congestion, and fatigue due to decreased ejection, are the major symptoms of pump dysfunction. As pulmonary vascular pressure rises, the right heart is strained and becomes overly full and less able to receive systemic venous return. This results in an increase in central venous pressure (CVP) and congestion (edema) in gravity-dependent areas of the body.

Serious pump dysfunction can lead to cardiogenic shock, a state of reduced cardiac output that results in inadequate tissue perfusion. This state is characterized by elevated filling pressures within the heart and an abnormally high CVP. In contrast, significant internal or external fluid loss results in hypovolemia (reduced preload). Low-volume states are characterized by an abnormally low central venous pressure. Hypovolemic shock may be due to hemorrhage or fluid loss from another cause (e.g., dehydration), or may be the result of massive expansion of the vascular bed (relative hypovolemia), as occurs in septic shock.

One of the most common peripheral vascular disorders is deep vein thrombosis (DVT) in the lower extremities and pelvis. Illness, immobility, and surgery are frequently accompanied by circulatory stasis, vessel damage, and hypercoagulability. These factors predispose to development of venous thrombosis, which usually begins silently in the deep veins of the calf. Platelets adhere to the vessel wall; then fibrin and white blood cells aggregate and propagate along the vein to create a free-floating clot. Since it takes several days for the inflammatory response to bind the clot to the vein wall, 50 percent of clients have no early indications of thrombophlebitis. When the clot attaches, the client may notice subjective aching tightness in the affected calf, especially when walking. Objective signs include calf swelling, distended superficial veins, low-grade fever, and tachycardia. While these signs indicate clot attachment, the free-floating tail of the clot continues as a threat for detachment and potentially lethal pulmonary embolism.

PREPARATION PROTOCOL: FOR CARDIOVASCULAR SKILLS

Complete the following steps before each skill.

1. Review physician's orders to validate skill intended.
2. Review manufacturer instructions for application of devices and care directions.
3. Evaluate client's medical status.
4. Wash hands.
5. Verify client's identity (check identaband and have client state name).
6. Provide privacy; explain procedure and purpose of skill to client.

COMPLETION PROTOCOL: FOR CARDIOVASCULAR SKILLS

Make sure the following steps have been completed.

1. Monitor equipment regularly for appropriate application, fit, and function.
2. Assess neurovascular status and provide skin care to lower extremities regularly.
3. Encourage thrombus-deterrent activities (ankle exercises, hydration, deep breathing).
4. Document assessment findings and interventions.
5. Save compression (T.E.D.) hosiery package instructions for client's future use.

(continued on next page)

PREPARATION PROTOCOL: FOR CARDIOVASCULAR SKILLS (CONT'D)

7. Ensure client's skin is clean and dry for electrode placement.
8. Check that client's lower extremities are free of lesions, ischemic vascular disease, or phlebitis.
9. Ensure client has peripheral pulses before application of compression elastic stockings (T.E.D. hose).
10. Assess sensory and motor status of client's extremities for baseline.
11. Place client in supine position and elevate bed to a level of working comfort.

COMPLETION PROTOCOL: FOR CARDIOVASCULAR SKILLS (CONT'D)

6. Remove T.E.D. hosiery two or three times daily for 30 min and launder regularly.
7. Discard disposable equipment when therapy is discontinued.
8. Return nondisposable units to central area for cleaning and storage.

SECTION ONE

CARDIAC MONITORING

The electrical impulses that stimulate the heart to pump blood can be amplified and recorded from the surface of the body; the electrocardiogram (ECG) is a graphic recording of these events. As such, it provides a highly specialized tool for client assessment that may enhance, but does not take the place of, physical assessment of the client's heart rate through auscultation. Additionally, evaluation of the heart's mechanical pumping function requires physical assessment of the client's peripheral pulses, mentation, blood pressure, urinary output, and other reflective determinants of vital organ perfusion.

Adhesive discs (electrodes) placed on standard designated areas of the client's skin transmit the electrical signals of atrial and ventricular depolarization and repolarization. These electrodes connect to lead wires that are then connected to corresponding terminals of a cable (or battery-operated radio transmitter), which amplifies and transmits the heart signals to a monitor.

The monitor screen (oscilloscope) displays the client's ECG and can be brightened or darkened, centered, or otherwise adjusted for optimal monitoring. Monitor screen alarms can be set to notify personnel of heart rates that exceed or fall below predesignated limits (e.g., 50 [low] to 140 [high]) depending on anticipated need. Setting very wide ranges obviously defeats the purpose of the alarm system.

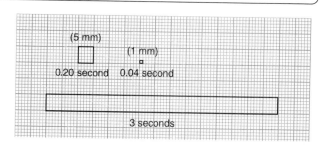

● **FIGURE 24-2** *ECG grid paper.*

Special grid paper is used to record a client's ECG. This paper moves at a speed of 1 inch (25 mm) per second as the ECG is being displayed and recorded. The horizontal and vertical lines provide a tool for measuring the client's waveform, rate, and rhythm. It is important to understand that the larger outlined squares are 5 mm apart (representing 0.20 sec); within these outlined squares, the five smaller squares are 1 mm apart (representing 0.04 sec).

The client's transmitted cardiac impulses are recorded on ECG paper, which displays features of atrial (P wave) and ventricular (QRS complex) depolarization. Ventricular repolarization is represented by a T wave following the QRS complex. In the normal cardiac cycle, the P, QRS, and T waves recur sequentially and rhythmically at a rate of 60

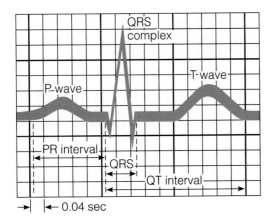

● **FIGURE 24-3** *Measurement of electrical impulses on ECG paper.*

to 100 per minute. Cardiac ventricular pumping correlates with the QRS complex on the ECG, and these responses are heard on cardiac auscultation as heart rate or beats per minute. However, if pumping is ineffective (e.g., premature), radial pulse rate may be less than auscultated heart rate (pulse deficit).

Electrode placement determines the lead or particular view of cardiac electrical activity that is recorded on the ECG. Good-quality wave depiction is not always the major criterion for selecting a particular monitoring lead. The care setting, along with individual client factors and risk for critical changes in cardiac function, helps determine which lead (electrode placement) is most appropriate for the client. Once selected, electrode placement should remain consistent so that personnel become familiar with the client's cardiac complex in the chosen lead. If lead selection is changed, documentation and oral communication with all involved personnel are essential. Commonly, MCL$_1$ is used for single-lead monitoring. For double-lead monitoring, leads MCL$_1$ and MCL$_6$ (positive electrode at 5th intercostal space [ICS], midaxillary line) are favored.

Environmental interference can distort the client's ECG, making waveform distinction difficult. Loose electrodes, muscle tremors, client movement, and 60-cycle (alternating current) interference from ungrounded equipment are sources of such artifact.

The central venous pressure (CVP) approximates right ventricular filling pressure and is used to estimate cardiac pump function and fluid status. The normal CVP is between 2 and 6 mm Hg or between 4 and 11 cm H$_2$O. If the CVP is low, hypovolemia is suspected. If the CVP is high, fluid overload or right ventricular dysfunction is assumed. The client's need for fluid resuscitation or pharmacologic management is often based on CVP determinations.

RATIONALE

- To select most appropriate lead for monitoring client's ECG
- To monitor cardiac rate and rhythm
- To evaluate cardiac response to activity or medical therapy
- To detect significant changes in cardiac rate or rhythm
- To immediately recognize potentially life-threatening alterations of cardiac electrical activity
- To determine central venous pressure (right ventricular filling pressure)
- To assess fluid volume status

ASSESSMENT

- Verify physician's order for CVP or cardiac monitoring.
- Make sure client understands rationale for noninvasive cardiac monitoring.
- Ensure that electrode gel is moist and that expiration date has not passed.
- Check that monitoring electrodes are adherent and that a clear, readable signal is displayed.
- Check that established lead is appropriate for monitoring purpose.
- Make sure monitor alarms are programmed and functioning.
- Make sure client has an established central venous catheter.
- Assess that CVP catheter site is without signs of inflammation.

CONTINUOUS ECG MONITORING

Equipment

- Adhesive electrodes
- Alcohol swabs
- Color-coded lead wires
- Telemetry transmitter or cardiac monitor and cable

Preparation

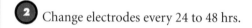

1 Prepare selected site with alcohol and rub briskly with gauze to enhance electrode adherence and impulse transmission.

2 Change electrodes every 24 to 48 hrs.

CLINICAL NOTE

As with any electrically operated piece of machinery, you cannot assume that the heart's electrical integrity (normal ECG) means that the heart pump is functioning properly. The ECG is merely a record of electrical stimulation of the myocardial pumping cells, not a guarantee of the pump's contractile response. A normal ECG can accompany a nonfunctioning heart. Conversely, some hearts, despite chaotic electrical stimulation, pump sufficiently to meet the needs of the body. Evaluation of cardiac mechanical function requires physical assessment of the client's heart rate through auscultation, as well as assessment of peripheral pulses, mentation, blood pressure, urinary output, and other reflective determinants of vital organ perfusion.

SKILL

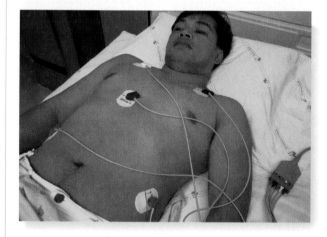

1 Peel off paper backing and apply five clamp- (or snap)-type electrodes to client's chest:

- **White** to right shoulder (negative electrode)
- **Black** to left shoulder (Lead I positive electrode or MCL_1 negative electrode)
- **Red** to left midclavicular upper abdominal area (Lead II positive electrode)
- **Brown** to 4th intercostal space, right sternal border (MCL_1 positive chest electrode), or left sternal border, or alternatively at 5th intercostal space, midaxillary line (V_6 position)
- **Green** to right abdomen or other convenient area (ground electrode)

Note: Limb leads and any one chest lead can be monitored using these electrode positions.

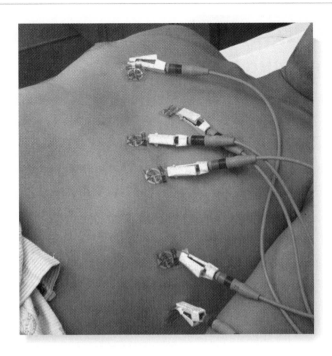

2 Additionally, brown electrode (chest lead) can be placed in any one of the following locations:

- V_1—at 4th right intercostal space, next to sternum
- V_2—at 4th left intercostal space, next to sternum
- V_3—between V_2 and V_4
- V_4—at 5th left intercostal space, midclavicular
- V_5—at 5th left intercostal space, anterior axillary
- V_6—at 5th left intercostal space, midaxillary
- Attach color-coded lead wires to corresponding electrode positions. *Note:* If using snap-type electrodes, attach lead wires before applying electrodes to client's chest. **RATIONALE:** Eliminates need to push on client to attach lead wires.

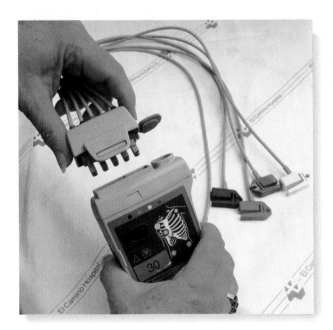

3 Connect lead wire terminals to corresponding-color recipient on client's monitor or telemetry transmitter case cable. Observe pattern on oscilloscope to ensure clarity of discrete waveforms.

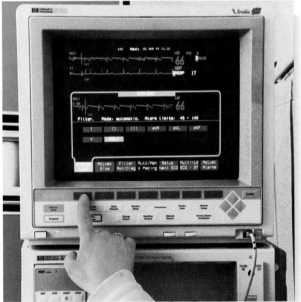

4 Select appropriate lead(s) for monitoring client (see Beyond the Skill box). Record sample rhythm strip for baseline and place in client's record. Set high and low wave rate alarm limits appropriate for client (e.g., 50 [low], 140 [high]).

BEYOND THE SKILL

CONTINUOUS CARDIAC MONITORING LEAD SELECTION

Select the lead that reveals the most helpful features of the ECG tracing for your client.

Lead I

This lead records electrical activity between a positive electrode placed below the left clavicle and a negative electrode placed below the right clavicle.

- Atrial arrhythmic activity is poorly identified.

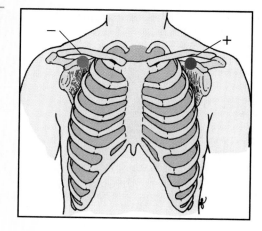

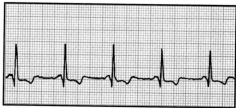

ECG Pattern–Lead I

Lead II

This lead records electrical activity between a positive electrode placed at the midclavicular line on the left flank and a negative electrode placed below the right clavicle.

- Lead position is parallel to the force and direction of normal cardiac depolarization.
- Deflections are upright.
- Provides good identifiable P waves for atrial activity.
- Shows deceptively narrow QRS complexes, so does not identify bundle branch block or differentiate aberrant atrial conduction from ectopic ventricular impulses (PVCs).
- Poor choice for most major arrhythmias.

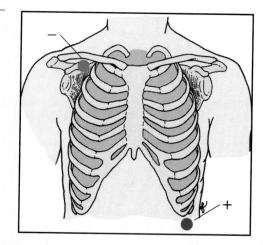

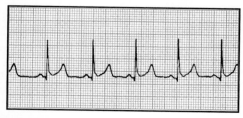

ECG Pattern–Lead II

(continued on next page)

Lead III

This lead records electrical activity between a negative electrode placed below the left clavicle and a positive electrode placed at the midclavicular line on the left flank.

- Lead position is perpendicular to the normal force and direction of cardiac depolarization, so waves are not strong.
- Wave forms may be too similar in height for continuous monitoring.
- Computer may erroneously double client's heart rate.

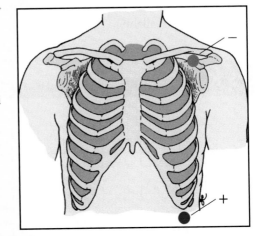

MCL_1

This lead records electrical activity between a positive electrode placed at the right of the sternum, 4th intercostal space, and a negative electrode placed under the left clavicle. It is similar to the V_1 chest lead of the 12-lead electrocardiogram.

- This is the lead preferred in critical settings for continuous monitoring; differentiates wide QRS due to atrial aberrancy from that due to ventricular ectopy.
- Used along with MCL_6 (chest lead V_6) to differentiate left and right bundle branch block.

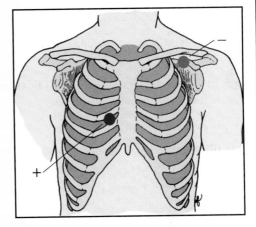

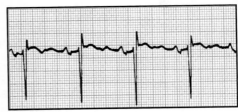

ECG Pattern–MCL

MCL_6

This lead records electrical activity between a positive electrode placed at the left 5th intercostal space, midaxillary line, and a negative electrode placed under the left clavicle.

- Used along with MCL_1 (chest lead V_1) to differentiate left and right bundle branch block.

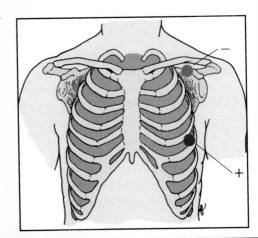

ECG RHYTHM STRIP ANALYSIS

Equipment

- Calipers (if available)
- Strip of client's ECG tracing

SKILL

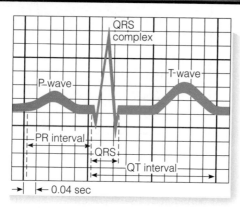

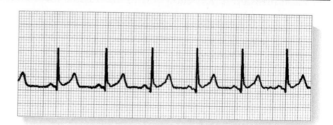

Normal Sinus Rhythm

1 To analyze strip, compare client's ECG features to criteria for normal sinus rhythm:

- QRS width: 0.05 to 0.10 sec
- QRS (ventricular) rate: 60 to 100 per minute
- QRS (ventricular) rhythm: regular
- P (atrial) wave rate: 60 to 100 per minute
- P (atrial) rhythm: regular
- PR interval: 0.12 to 0.20 sec

2 Generally inspect strip to identify specific waves. Analyze ventricular activity (QRS complexes). Measure width of QRS complexes (from beginning of Q wave to end of S wave if all are present). **RATIONALE:** Normal duration is 0.04 to 0.10 sec (less than three small squares). If QRS is wider, abnormal intraventicular conduction is occurring. *Note:* Impulse may be of ventricular origin, indicating potential lethal arrhythmia.

- Estimate ventricular (QRS) rate by counting number of QRS complexes in 6 in (6 sec) and multiplying by 10 to get rate per minute. **RATIONALE:** Normal QRS rate is 60 to 100 per minute. Faster QRS rate is tachycardia; slower QRS rate is bradycardia.

Alternatively, count number of large squares between QRS complexes and divide into 300. **RATIONALE:** This method is convenient to use for regular rhythms.

Or, count number of small squares between QRS complexes and divide into 1500. **RATIONALE:** This method is convenient for calculating very fast rates.

- Determine ventricular (QRS) rhythm. Are QRS complexes equally spaced? Use calipers or other measuring device to determine regularity. **RATIONALE:** QRS complexes should recur with regularity.

- Analyze atrial activity (P waves). Determine atrial (P wave) rate per minute (number of P waves in 6 sec × 10) **RATIONALE:** Normally there is one P wave for every QRS complex (rate same as QRS rate); if more than one P wave exists per QRS complex, then atrial arrhythmia or atrioventricular (AV) block is present.

- Determine atrial (P wave) rhythm. **RATIONALE:** Premature P waves indicate atrial ectopy.

- Analyze atrioventricular relationship (PR interval). Measure PR interval to determine conduction time through atria, AV node, and His-Purkinje system (from beginning of P wave to beginning of QRS complex). **RATIONALE:** Normal measure is 0.12 to 0.20 sec (three to five small squares); longer interval indicates conduction block between atria and ventricles.

- Analyze ventricular repolarization time (if indicated). Measure QT interval (from beginning of QRS complex to end of T wave) to determine duration of ventricular repolarization. **RATIONALE:** Normal is 0.39 ± 0.04 sec at any heart rate.

BEYOND THE SKILL

RECOGNITION OF POTENTIALLY LETHAL ARRHYTHMIAS

Multiform (polymorphic) Premature Ventricular Contractions (PVCs)

PVCs are usually due to irritability of ventricular muscle cells. Frequent (over 6 per minute) and consecutive PVCs can develop into ventricular tachycardia (three or more consecutive PVCs). Multiform PVCs are considered more serious than uniform PVCs.

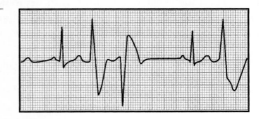

Multiform Premature Ventricular Contractions (PVCs)

Characteristics

- QRS width is greater than 0.12 sec for premature beats (distorted morphology varies within strip).
- QRS wave rate varies.
- QRS rhythm is irregular due to prematurities (e.g., PVCs occurring after every normal beat result in a regularly irregular bigeminal rhythm).
- T wave is opposite in polarity to the final part of the PVC.
- P waves are regular, but none occur with premature beats because the impulse originates in the ventricle.
- Atrial rate is less than ventricular rate due to PVCs.
- PR interval is absent with premature beat.

Etiology

- Sympathetic nervous system stimuli (caffeine, drugs, hypoxia, anxiety)
- Myocardial ischemia
- Electrolyte imbalance
- Drug toxicity (especially digitalis)

Treatment

- Correct underlying cause (e.g., KCl or Mg supplementation).
- Ensure pain management (e.g., in MI).
- Withdraw drug or give antidote for toxicity.
- Give medication (procainamide, sotalol, amiodarone, lidocaine).

Ventricular Tachycardia

A nonsustained (less than 30 sec) episode of stable ventricular tachycardia (client has pulse) may lead to unstable ventricular tachycardia with hemodynamic instability (loss of pulse and measurable blood pressure). VT is usually associated with coronary artery disease or cardiomyopathy.

Ventricular Tachycardia

Characteristics

- QRS width is greater than 0.12 sec (uniform morphology).
- QRS rate is usually 130 to 170 per minute.
- QRS rhythm is regular.
- P waves are usually unidentifiable or may be dissociated.
- PR interval is unidentifiable.

Etiology

- Cardiac disease
- Digitalis toxicity

(continued on next page)

Treatment

- For a stable client, give any one of the following medications: procainamide, sotalol, amiodarone, lidocaine.
- For a client with poor ejection fraction (systolic heart failure), give Amiodarone (150 mg IV bolus over 10 min) or lidocaine (0.5 to 0.75 mg/kg IV push) followed by synchronized cardioversion.

- For a client with serious signs and symptoms related to the tachycardia, if ventricular wave rate is over 150 per minute, perform immediate synchronized cardioverision (100 J, 200 J, 300 J, 360 J); premedicate if possible.

Ventricular Fibrillation

Chaotic electrical activity causes ineffective quivering of the ventricles. The client is unresponsive with no detectable signs of life.

Characteristics

- QRS width shows fibrillating waves only.
- QRS rate cannot be determined.
- QRS rhythm is irregular.
- P waves are unidentifiable.
- Client is unresponsive.

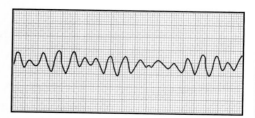

Ventricular Fibrillation

Etiology

- Coronary artery disease
- Cardiomyopathy

Treatment

- Perform immediate defibrillation.
- Start CPR.
- Initiate advanced cardiac life support.

Third-Degree Heart Block

Electrical impulses originate in the SA node, but all impulses are blocked from conduction through the atrioventricular pathways. A slow ventricular escape rhythm develops, with wide QRS complexes that have no association with the P waves (two pacemakers exist). The client may have hemodynamic deterioration due to severe bradycardia and symptoms such as chest pain, dyspnea, or decreased level of consciousness.

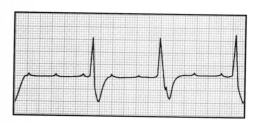

Third-Degree Heart Block

Characteristics

- QRS width is normal if the pacemaker is in the AV junction, greater than 0.12 sec if the pacemaker is in the ventricle.
- QRS rate is 40 to 60 per minute if the escape focus is in the AV junction, 20 to 40 per minute if the escape focus is in the ventricle.
- QRS rhythm is regular.
- P wave rate is greater than QRS rate.
- P wave rhythm is regular.
- PR interval varies; there is no association between P waves and QRS complexes.

(continued on next page)

Etiology

- Anterior MI (most common cause)
- Drug intoxication

Treatment

- For a symptomatic client, give atropine 0.5 to 1.0 mg IV.
- Institute transcutaneous pacing (do not delay if atropine is unavailable).
- Give dopamine 5 to 20 µg/kg/min.
- Give epinephrine 2 to 10 µg/min.
- Begin preparation for transvenous pacemaker placement.

CENTRAL VENOUS PRESSURE MEASUREMENT

Equipment

- D$_5$W IV solution
- IV administration set
- Disposable CVP manometer with stopcock
- Extension tubing with needleless cannula (for central catheter access)
- Povidone iodine prep swabs
- Syringe with 5 mL normal saline (NS) to flush central line
- Marker (to identify manometer leveling point on client's skin)
- Carpenter's level

SAFETY ALERT

The disposable manometer and administration set comprise a closed system and should be changed using aseptic technique every 96 hrs or if contamination is suspected.

Preparation

1. Connect CVP manometer to IV pole.

2. Aseptically spike solution bag with administration tubing and prime (see Chap. 17).

3. Aseptically connect administration tubing to CVP manometer and open stopcock to fill manometer to 18 to 20 cm.

4. Aseptically connect extension tubing to manometer and prime extension tubing by turning stopcock's flat side perpendicular (OFF) to manometer.

5. Prep with povidone iodine swabs and flush client's central access lumen (5 mL NS), then affix extension tubing needleless cannula to client's central line (see Chap. 17).

SKILL

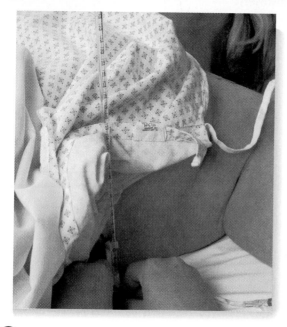

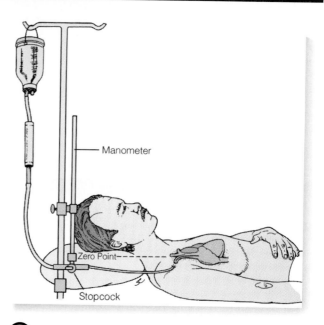

① Locate client's right atrium (midaxillary line at 4th intercostal space), and mark location on client's skin. **RATIONALE:** Marking promotes consistent placement for ongoing CVP measurements.

② Using carpenter's level, adjust manometer so zero is level with client's phlebostatic level mark. **RATIONALE:** Leveling manometer with this point is essential for accurate CVP measurement.

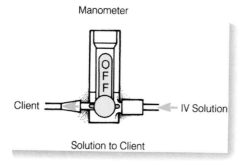

③ Turn flat side of stopcock perpendicular (OFF) to manometer to initiate infusion to client at slow rate (e.g., 10 mL/hr).

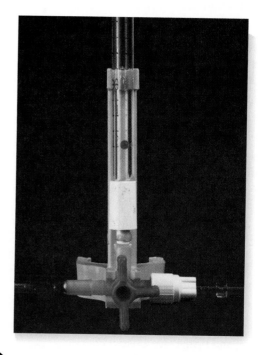

④ Turn stopcock so that solution flows into manometer (flat side to client). Fill manometer to 18 to 20 cm, then stop infusion. **RATIONALE:** Overfilling manometer may expose client to contamination.

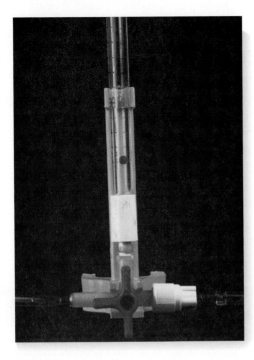

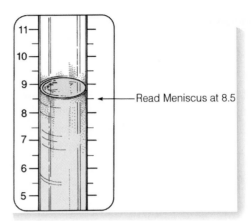

Read Meniscus at 8.5

6 Observe meniscus at eye level and note that fluid level rises with client's exhalation and falls with inhalation. **RATIONALE:** Fluid fluctuations reflect normal changes in intrathoracic pressure with breathing.

■ Take reading at end of exhalation (rise of fluid in manometer). **RATIONALE:** End exhalation provides closest comparison to atmospheric level pressure.

5 Turn stopcock OFF (flat side) to infusion bag and OPEN to manometer so manometer solution infuses into client. Note manometer level at which solution ceases to infuse. **RATIONALE:** This level reflects central venous (right atrial) pressure, normally 4 to 11 cm H_2O.

7 Turn stopcock to resume infusion of solution from bag to client (flat side to manometer).

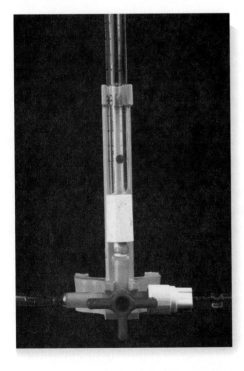

CHARTING

- Client's monitored heart rate and rhythm (recorded hourly)
- Sample of client's ECG strip every 8 hrs, or more often if events occur
- Type and frequency of any arrhythmias
- Client activity at time arrhythmia emerged
- Client assessment associated with arrhythmia (vital signs, subjective findings)

- Interventions in response to symptomatic arrhythmia
- Date and time of CVP reading (may use flow sheet for frequent readings because trends are more relevant than isolated values)
- Any unusual assessment findings and actions taken

SECTION TWO

PREVENTION OF VENOUS THROMBOSIS

Clients at risk for venous thrombosis include those over age 40, those with a history of vein problems, and those who are obese or immobilized, have heart failure, or are undergoing lengthy surgery or surgery below the umbilicus (especially orthopedic surgery).

Standard measures to support venous return from the lower extremities to prevent deep vein thrombosis (DVT) include passive or active leg and foot exercises, leg elevation (by raising the foot of the bed 15 to 20° rather than using pillows), adequate hydration, prevention of leg crossing or placement of any other obstructive device under the knees, and early ambulation.

In addition to standard measures and anticoagulant prophylaxis, many high-risk clients benefit from the use of graduated compression elastic stockings (e.g., T.E.D. hosiery) or intermittent pneumatic compression devices. Similarly to the normal physiologic pumping mechanisms of the muscles, these devices enhance venous return by applying continuous or intermittent external compression to the tissues and veins.

Graduated compression hose are available in a variety of sizes and colors. They are expensive, but last for months with proper care. They should be applied before getting out of bed, and preferably with the legs elevated. They can be removed at bedtime.

Pneumatic compression devices consist of an air pump connected to tubes that inflate and deflate lower extremity sleeves or wraps. Single-chamber devices inflate intermittently, then deflate while the sleeve on the oppo-

site extremity inflates. Devices with three chambers provide sequential compression with cycles that move incrementally up the leg. All pneumatic devices have safety valves that prevent overinflation.

RATIONALE

- To promote venous return
- To prevent venous thrombus formation
- To promote comfort

ASSESSMENT

- Assess that client is a candidate for venous support therapy (hose, wraps).
- Assess that client's skin is free of lesions.
- Assess that client's extremities are without excessive edema or signs of circulatory insufficiency.
- Make sure stockings are clean, have no wrinkles, and fit appropriately.
- Ensure device fits and functions appropriately, and is removed regularly to allow for assessment and skin care.
- Make sure client's peripheral neurovascular status is not adversely affected by thrombotic deterrent therapy.

GRADUATED COMPRESSION ELASTIC HOSE (T.E.D. HOSE)

Equipment

- Tape measure
- Below-the-knee or above-the-knee hosiery (e.g., T.E.D. hose)
- Talcum powder or cornstarch (optional)

SKILL

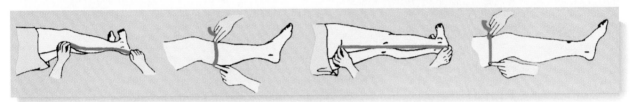

Length
Measure leg from bottom of heel to popliteal fold

Circumference
Measure calf at largest circumference

Length
Measure leg from bottom of heel to fold of buttocks

Circumference
Measure thigh at largest circumference

1 To order correct hosiery size, place client in supine position for measurements:

- Measure distance from bottom of heel to popliteal fold.
- Measure midcalf circumference.
- Measure distance from gluteal fold to bottom of heel.
- Measure largest thigh circumference.
- Refer to manufacturer's chart to obtain correctly sized hosiery; two pairs are usually needed.

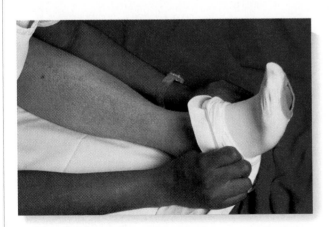

2 With client in supine position, gather stocking to foot area, pull foot of stocking over client's foot, then pull hose up over client's leg. Legs may be powdered for easier application if desired. *Note:* Stockings should be applied before client gets out of bed. **RATIONALE:** Venous hydrostatic pressure is minimal before ambulation.

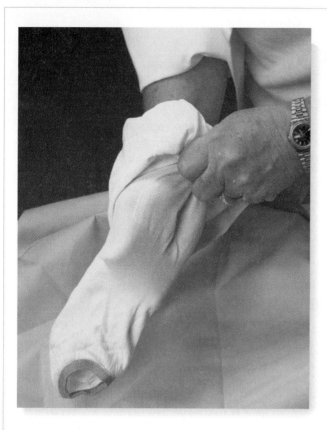

3 Alternatively, turn stocking inside out down to heel (foot of stocking is now inverted inside of stocking). Place thumbs inside foot of stocking and slip stocking onto client's foot until heel is properly aligned; then pull remainder of stocking up over client's leg.

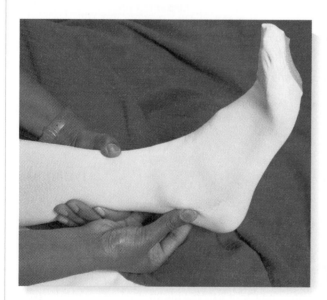

4 Ensure stocking fits properly and smoothly over toe and heel.

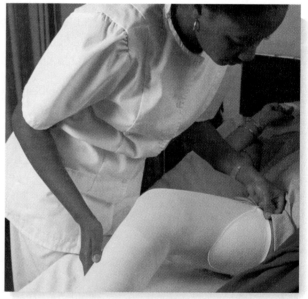

5 Pull stocking up over client's leg, positioning support section on inner thigh. **RATIONALE:** If pad is on outer thigh, stocking is on wrong leg.

- Remove stockings at bedtime, if ordered. **RATIONALE:** Stockings are not necessary at bedtime because venous hydrostatic pressure is minimized by recumbency.

PNEUMATIC EXTERNAL COMPRESSION DEVICE (SEQUENTIAL SLEEVES)

Equipment

- Disposable leg wraps or sleeves (knee length or thigh length) of appropriate size
- Tubing assembly
- Compression controller (motor)

SAFETY ALERT

Always read manufacturers' instructions for operating compression devices. Pressure should be set between 45 and 60 mm Hg. Clients with severe peripheral arterial disease, phlebitis, skin lesions, recent skin graft, or absent pedal pulses are not candidates for these devices.

SKILL

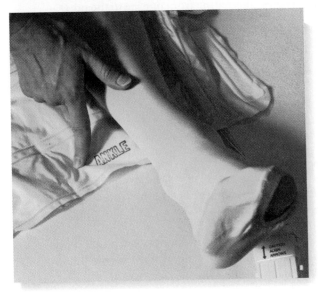

1 Place client's leg on white side (lining) of wrap and note markings on lining for ankle and popliteal areas.

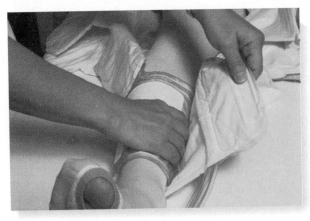

2 Starting at side opposite clear plastic tubing, wrap device securely around client's leg, distally to proximally. **RATIONALE:** To promote venous return, device applies more external compression at ankle and less compression more proximally.

- Secure hook (or Velcro) edge to wrap.

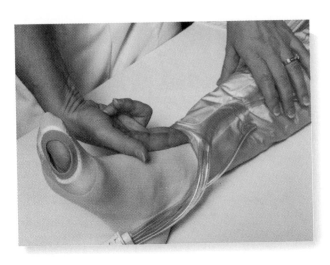

3 Place two fingers between client's leg and compression wrap to determine if wrap fits properly. **RATIONALE:** Two fingers of slack indicates wrap is not constricting circulation.

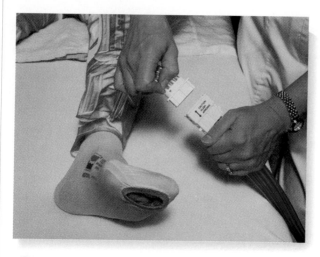

4 Connect tubing assembly to plugs of compression wrap, then connect tubing assembly plug to controller at tubing assembly connector site. Ensure tubing is free of kinks or twists. **RATIONALE:** To prevent restriction of air flow through tubing.

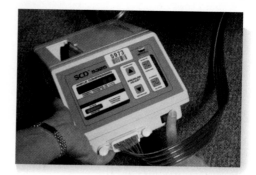

5 Plug controller power cable into grounded electrical outlet and turn controller power switch to ON.

- For intermittent device, sleeve inflates, then deflates, alternating from one leg to the other. Check that pressure indicator lights and cooling light are functioning properly.
- For sequential compression sleeve, light is ON when pressure is applied to each specific segment. Distal to proximal sections inflate in sequence, then deflate. When cooling light is ON, compression lights go OFF.

6 Assess skin and neurovascular status every 2 hrs; immediately discontinue device if client complains of numbness.

- To remove sleeve, turn power switch OFF and disconnect tubing assembly from sleeve at connection site. Unwrap sleeve from leg.

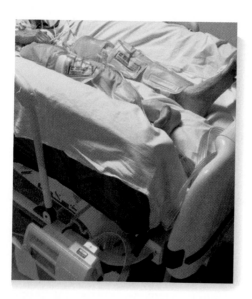

CHARTING

- Date and time skill was performed
- Neurovascular assessment of extremities for baseline
- Condition of client's skin
- Size and type of elastic hose or compression device applied

- Pneumatic compression sleeve pressure
- Frequency of hose/compression device release
- Presence of peripheral pulses and neurovascular status
- Additional measures to promote venous return

CRITICAL THINKING FOCUS

SECTION ONE ▪ Cardiac Monitoring

Unexpected Outcomes	Alternative Nursing Actions
▪ Telemetry signal is lost at base monitor station.	▪ Check that client is not out of range for telemetry monitoring.
▪ Artifact interferes with identification of waveforms.	▪ Check that equipment in environment is properly grounded (can cause 60-cycle interference, creating wide, dark baseline).
	▪ Turn off all equipment in environment (IV pump, etc.), then turn on items one at a time, noting when interference reappears. Notify biomedical engineer of defective equipment.
	▪ Replace electrodes if loose (causes wandering baseline).
	▪ Assess client for interfering activity (e.g., brushing teeth or bathing causes irregular baseline).
▪ Electrodes fail to stick due to client's hairy chest.	▪ Clip hair, but do not shave skin. Cleanse skin well to remove oil.
	▪ Abrade for better electrode contact only if necessary.
	▪ Notify monitor technician of change in electrode position.
▪ ECG monitor shows troubling arrhythmia.	▪ Immediately assess client to determine if intervention is indicated.
	▪ If client is asymptomatic, arrhythmia does not require treatment.
▪ CVP system does not infuse.	▪ Check line for kinks; change client's position.
	▪ Validate that manometer stopcock is in the IV-to-client position.
▪ CVP readings vary greatly.	▪ Verify that manometer zero is level with client's right atrium (4th ICS, midaxillary). Adjust when head of bed or entire bed is elevated or lowered.
	▪ Mark zero leveling point on client's chest for consistent positioning of manometer.

SECTION TWO ▪ Prevention of Venous Thrombosis

Unexpected Outcomes	Alternative Nursing Actions
▪ Elastic hosiery is unavailable.	▪ Elastic wraps can be substituted: Anchor bandages on top of foot and in front of leg using tape or safety pin. Overlap one-third of bandage width with each turn with distal-to-proximal application.
	▪ Check peripheral pulse to ensure that elastic bandages are tight enough for support but do not obstruct arterial flow.

- Elastic hosiery becomes loose.

- Elastic stockings are difficult to apply.

- Client complains of numbness or tingling.

- Initiate other measures to promote venous return: adequate hydration, ankle exercises, early ambulation, and deep breathing.
- Remeasure legs and compare to chart to determine correct size.
- Preserve elasticity by line-drying after laundering. Do not use a clothes drier. (Client should have two pairs of stockings.)
- Sprinkle legs with powder or cornstarch before application. Wear rubber gloves to strengthen grip on hose.
- Ensure that you can slip two fingers between compression device sleeve and leg. Wrap may be too tight.
- Turn device off immediately, remove sleeve, and complete neurovascular assessment. Recheck and reprogram device pressure limits.

SELF-CHECK EVALUATION

PART 1 ▪ Matching Items

Match the definition in column B with the correct term in column A.

Column A	Column B
_____ a. Arrhythmia	1. Muscular pumping chamber of the heart
_____ b. Telemetry	2. Pressure of blood that distends the ventricle at the end of diastole
_____ c. Electrode	3. Phase during which the cell becomes positively charged
_____ d. CVP	4. Positioning placement of two electrodes of opposite polarity to obtain a view of cardiac electrical activity
_____ e. Depolarization	5. Abnormal heart rate or irregular rhythm
_____ f. Afterload	6. Relaxation phase of ventricular filling
_____ g. Ventricle	7. Remote radiofrequency-transmitted monitoring
_____ h. Lead	8. Impedance against which the cardiac chamber must eject volume
_____ i. Preload	9. Measure of blood volume and right ventricular filling pressure
_____ j. Diastole	10. Device that adheres to the skin to detect and relay electrical information from the heart to monitoring equipment

PART 2 ▪ Multiple Choice Questions

1. When measuring to fit knee-high elastic hose, you should measure:
   a. From heel to buttocks while client is standing.
   b. From heel to knee with client lying prone.

    c. Ankle and calf circumference with client supine.

    d. Calf circumference and length from heel to knee bend.

2. Clients who are candidates for venous compression devices/hose include those with:

    a. Total hip replacement surgery.

    b. Peripheral arterial disease.

    c. Existing deep vein thrombosis.

    d. Pulmonary edema.

3. The P wave of the ECG represents:

    a. Ventricular depolarization.

    b. Ventricular repolarization.

    c. Atrial depolarization.

    d. Atrial repolarization.

4. The QRS complex of the ECG represents:

    a. Ventricular repolarization.

    b. Ventricular depolarization.

    c. Conduction through the bundle branches.

    d. Conduction through the Purkinje fibers.

5. Select the statement that correctly identifies a normal ECG strip:

    a. The PR interval precedes the QRS complex.

    b. The T wave follows the QRS and is inverted.

    c. The QRS is no longer than 0.20 sec.

    d. The PR interval is less than 0.12 sec.

6. Events that occur during the PR interval include:

    a. Atrial depolarization and delay in the AV node.

    b. Depolarization of bundle branches and ventricules.

    c. Transmission of impulse from the sinoatrial (SA) node to Purkinje fibers.

    d. Depolarization of atria and ventricles.

7. The central venous pressure is a measurement of:

    a. Left ventricular filling pressure.

    b. Right ventricular filling pressure.

    c. Blood pressure.

    d. Extent of peripheral edema.

8. Maximum duration of a normal QRS complex is less than:

    a. 0.04 sec.

    b. 0.06 sec.

    c. 0.12 sec.

    d. 0.20 sec.

9. Normal pneumatic compression pressure range is:

    a. 10 to 40 mm Hg.

    b. 20 to 40 mm Hg.

    c. 35 to 55 mm Hg.

    d. 40 to 60 mm Hg.

10. The major role of the heart is to:

    a. Oxygenate blood.

    b. Pump blood.

    c. Perfuse peripheral tissues.

    d. Provide nutrients to tissues.

11. Which of the following events occur during ventricular diastole?
    a. Ventricular filling and coronary perfusion.
    b. Ventricular ejection and opening of the aortic valve.
    c. Atrial contraction and closing of the mitral and tricuspid valves.
    d. Atrial contraction and opening of the aortic and pulmonic valves.

12. Which of the following is the most accurate way to count a client's heart rate?
    a. Count QRS complexes in a 6-in strip and multiply by 10.
    b. Count QRS complexes in a 10-in strip and multiply by 3.
    c. Auscultate the heartbeat for 1 min.
    d. Count the radial pulse for 1 min.

13. To correctly measure the CVP, the manometer zero should be level with the:
    a. Client's bed.
    b. Bag of infusing fluid.
    c. Client's clavicle.
    d. Client's right atrium.

14. A seriously low central venous pressure (e.g., 2 cm H_2O) indicates that the client needs:
    a. Volume replacement.
    b. Diuretic therapy.
    c. Blood transfusion.
    d. Vasoconstrictor therapy.

PART 3 ▪ Critical Thinking Application

Mr. Nelson has recently undergone surgical repair of an abdominal aortic aneurysm. He has a history of myocardial infarction and arrhythmias, and has been admitted to a monitored surgical unit for his postoperative recovery. He has been having frequent premature ventricular contractions, but has remained asymptomatic with these. Just as you pass the monitoring station, a high rate alarm sounds. The technician recognizes that Mr. Nelson has gone into ventricular tachycardia (VT). Quickly glancing at the oscilloscope, you validate the technician's interpretation.

1. What should the nurse's first action be?
2. What are the electocardiographic characteristics of VT?
3. Describe the hemodynamic consequences of ventricular tachycardia.

25

CARDIOVASCULAR AND PULMONARY EMERGENCIES

INTRODUCTION

Cardiac arrest continues to be the number one cause of death in the United States. Each year, 15 percent of deaths in the United States (360,000) are due to cardiac arrest or sudden death caused by ventricular fibrillation, a lethal arrhythmia. While sudden death can accompany a number of noncardiac conditions, it is usually associated with coronary artery disease. Fifty percent of those with symptoms of acute coronary syndrome die before reaching the hospital. Most victims, however, are healthy and socially active, have a mean age of 65 years, and experience sudden death without warning, most in their own homes. Cardiac arrest is their first and last symptom of this silent disease.

Since biblical times, humans have used a variety of techniques to attempt to resuscitate the dead or near-dead. This historical development is reflected in the **ABCD** sequence of actions used today when responding to a cardiopulmonary emergency. The earliest efforts focused on providing an **A**irway by inserting a tube into the trachea. Later, a bellows was added for mechanical **B**reathing. Chest compression to pump the heart for **C**irculation was introduced in the early 1800s. Late in the nineteenth century,

(continued on next page)

it was hypothesized that sudden death was due to ventricular fibrillation, but the role for electrical **D**efibrillation emerged only in the twentieth century.

In the early 1960s the combination of ventilation, chest compression, and the use of electrical countershock to convert ventricular fibrillation was described as lifesaving. Since 1966, it has been recommended and widely accepted that all health care personnel, as well as the general public, should be trained in cardiopulmonary resuscitation (CPR) according to standards outlined by the American Heart Association. Important progress continues to be made and guidelines have evolved to include new concepts and technological advances. As a result, there is widespread acceptance of CPR training as a guide for standardized management of cardiopulmonary emergencies.

Today, basic life support (BLS) and total community-wide emergency cardiovascular care (ECC), which includes advanced cardiovascular life support (ACLS) and a comprehensive system of emergency medical services (EMS), form the "Chain of Survival," response for effective cardiopulmonary resuscitation. Emergency cardiac care requires effective teamwork in which all citizens and trained rescuers participate in a coordinated and standardized attempt to optimize the victim's outcome. Since these services are medical in nature, but must be initiated without the presence of a prescribing physician, all states have enacted "Good Samaritan laws" that authorize health care personnel (and trained citizens) to administer needed emergency medical procedures without fear of liability. These laws are based on the assumption that individuals consent to emergency treatment, encourage health care providers to assist strangers in need of assistance, and recognize providers as a protected class.

In spite of more than 35 years of sustained efforts to improve life support skills through education and research, however, there has been little increase in cardiac arrest survival rates. What was once considered to be a successful public health initiative has proven to be ineffective. The chance of surviving cardiac arrest remains at approximately 5 percent, and even if spontaneous circulation is restored after 8 to 10 min, the frequency of serious, permanent neurological damage is unacceptably high. The primary obstacle to successful resuscitation is time. Knowing what to do for victims of cardiac arrest is simple compared with having the ability to provide the necessary intervention within 5 min. Since the vast majority of cardiac arrests occur outside of the hospital, and since early defibrillation is the highest-priority intervention for victims of out-of-hospital sudden death, availability of widespread public access defibrillation (PAD) has become an important health care initiative. Automated external defibrillators (AEDs) are being placed throughout communities for use by trained laypersons in airports, at large gatherings, on aircraft, in gated communities and shopping malls, and especially at remote sites. Statistically, communities with such programs have strengthened their Chain of Survival with successful resuscitation rates as high as 49 percent.

Skills based on standards of care that follow concepts and principles of basic life support consistent with the new International Guidelines 2000 published by the American Heart Association can improve the outcome for victims of cardiovascular and pulmonary emergencies (*International Guidelines 2000 for CPR and ECC: A Consensus on Science, 2000*).

PREPARATION PROTOCOL: FOR CARDIOVASCULAR AND PULMONARY EMERGENCY SKILLS

Complete the following steps before each skill.

1. Determine that client does not have an order for DNAR (DNR or no CPR).
2. Determine that client is unresponsive. Summon help if client is unresponsive.
3. Determine that client is not breathing.
4. Determine that client has no pulse.
5. Determine that client is choking.
6. Determine that resuscitation is indicated.

COMPLETION PROTOCOL: FOR CARDIOVASCULAR AND PULMONARY EMERGENCY SKILLS

Make sure the following steps have been completed.

1. Continue client assessment.
2. Report specifics of event to rescue support team and client's physician.
3. Ensure that client is stabilized and transported or transferred for advanced care if indicated.
4. Discard disposable resuscitation equipment in appropriate receptacle.
5. Document events and interventions on appropriate forms.
6. Send equipment suspected to be contaminated with blood or other body fluids to be disinfected.
7. Replace emergency equipment used.

SECTION ONE

BASIC LIFE SUPPORT

Basic life support (BLS) stands for a sequence of actions designed to recognize cardiovascular and pulmonary emergencies and rapidly respond with appropriate on-site care. These steps include:

- Prompt recognition of myocardial infarction and stroke and actions to prevent respiratory and cardiac arrest
- Early access to EMS personnel (calling a code if in the hospital)
- Rescue breathing for victims of respiratory arrest
- Chest compression and rescue breathing for victims of cardiopulmonary arrest
- Attempted defibrillation of clients with ventricular fibrillation (VF) or ventricular tachycardia (VT) with an automated external defibrillator (AED)
- Recognition and relief of foreign body airway obstruction (FBAO)

When the heart stops pumping effectively, timely and appropriate resuscitation must restore cardiac activity before permanent brain damage has occurred. While cerebral resuscitation is the major goal, rapid restoration of a beating heart and establishment of effective perfusion is the first step toward this goal. Early recognition and prompt response are crucial to these efforts. Since effective treatment is time dependent, decisions must be made quickly. CPR protocol provides a well-formulated and widely accepted plan of action (standard of care) by instilling a systematic way of thinking and responding to an individual experiencing a cardiovascular or pulmonary emergency.

While early CPR is of significant value, it is only temporizing and loses value if the next life support links—early defibrillation and ACLS—are delayed. Most adult sudden death is due to ventricular fibrillation, but basic CPR cannot convert this chaotic arrhythmia to a sustained perfusing cardiac rhythm; it only prolongs it. Reducing the time lapse to defibrillation is the greatest challenge. If defibrillation is attempted within 2 min after the onset of ventricular fibrillation, over 80 percent of victims will convert to a perfusing rhythm. In contrast, delayed defibrillation (over 5 min) usually results in an irreversible pulseless rhythm or ventricular asystole.

Early defibrillation is now included in the standard of care. It is recognized as an important link in the Chain of Survival and facilitated by availability of the automated external defibrillator (AED). As more portable AED units are placed in agencies and on every hospital unit, the time parameter to begin defibrillation (less than 3 min) will be more easily met. Until AED units are accessible, the protocol is still to call a code and begin CPR.

The AED is a portable, laboratory- and clinically tested unit that has proven to be safe and effective. Before its advent, the decision to defibrillate required training in interpreting a cardiac monitor or rhythm strip to recognize ventricular fibrillation. The AED eliminates the need for training in rhythm interpretation, allowing minimally trained or even untrained lay rescuers to institute this life-saving link in care. It analyzes the victim's cardiac rhythm, confirms the presence of a lethal arrhythmia, then charges and defibrillates the victim automatically, or instructs an operator to do so. The use of adhesive defibrillation pads reduces impedance, thereby eliminating the need to press paddles on the victim's chest, allowing safe, hands-off defibrillation and promoting consistent shock placement and delivery. This new technology allows widespread public access so that automated defibrillation is more readily available at the site of the emergency; it is therefore regarded as a major care breakthrough.

We must note that in contrast with older victims (i.e., 90 percent of victims), in whom sudden death is primarily a cardiac mechanism triggered by ventricular fibrillation, cardiac arrest in younger victims is predominantly due to impaired ventilation. Ventilatory failure may be due to obstruction of the large or small airways, drowning, or impaired breathing due to drugs, nervous system injury or disease, or anaphylaxis. Cardiac arrest in these cases is usually preceded by signs of respiratory distress and bradyarrhythmias. The use of AEDs in infants and children under the age of 8 years is not recommended.

RATIONALE

- To save a life
- To recognize serious cardiac and respiratory compromise
- To summon emergency medical service (EMS) for advanced life support
- To provide early defibrillation (within 2 min)
- To institute emergency life support CPR (ventilation and circulation) within 3 min
- To reduce death and disability
- To decrease risk of disease transmission during exposure to body fluids

ASSESSMENT

- Check that hospitalized client does not have a written order for *do not attempt to resuscitate* (DNAR), no CPR, or DNR; CPR is an intervention that is automatic unless there is a written order not to resuscitate.
- Determine if partial code is ordered.
- Assess that **A**ctivation of emergency medical service (EMS) is indicated.
- Make sure that an **A**irway is established.
- Make sure that **B**reathing is provided if victim is not exchanging air.
- Make sure that chest compressions to establish **C**irculation are provided if victim has no pulse.
- Assess that **D**efibrillation is indicated due to presence of lethal arrhythmia.
- Assess that Heimlich maneuver is indicated (i.e., victim's airway is obstructed).

CLINICAL NOTE

State Living Will laws provide guidelines that support our rights to register preferences about medical care (including the right to refuse resuscitative measures) in the event that our decision-making capacity is lost or interrupted. While these documents are legally enforceable, some states require that a physician determine whether the client is terminally ill or in a persistent vegetative state before living wills are honored. Because this determination has not been made in most emergency cases, resuscitation efforts should be initiated on all persons found in a pulseless and/or nonbreathing state in settings outside of the hospital. Currently, only 26 states allow recognition of a client's DNAR orders in the out-of-hospital setting.

CARDIOPULMONARY RESUSCITATION (CPR)

Equipment

- Cardiac board or firm surface
- Mask with one-way valve (if available)
- Automated external defibrillator (if available)
- Assistive personnel (if available)

CLINICAL NOTE

Good Samaritan laws vary significantly from state to state. Some states extend protection solely to licensed health care providers (some states to RNs but not LPNs). Some states require that assistance be rendered to those in need; in other states there is no legal duty to do so. All agree, however, that once assistance is initiated, the legal duty is one of reasonable emergency care that is provided without compensation (money or gifts). You must familiarize yourself with local Good Samaritan laws so you know which persons and what activities are protected under the laws in your state, as well as in other states, before rendering assistance. Fortunately, beneficent values usually guide us to respond in an emergency situation with our best possible efforts, and we do so in good faith rather than in fear of legal liability.

SAFETY ALERT

Early defibrillation and advanced cardiovascular life support (ACLS) increase the probability of survival and cerebral resuscitation. If a single rescuer has immediate access to an AED, early defibrillation takes precedence over other resuscitative measures:

- Verify unresponsiveness
- Give two ventilations
- Check for pulse
- If no pulse, attach AED

The EMS system is not activated until there is a NO SHOCK INDICATED readout command on the AED or someone else arrives to call for help.

If there are two rescuers, one establishes the defibrillator while the other begins CPR. Other activities are deferred (e.g., oxygen setup, IV line establishment) unless other rescuers are available.

SKILL

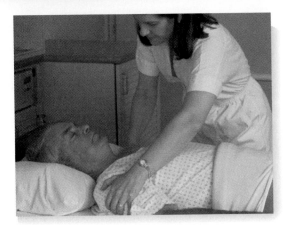

1 **Determine unresponsiveness:** Shake victim's shoulders and shout, "Are you OK?" **RATIONALE:** To ensure that client is unresponsive and to recognize need for immediate action.

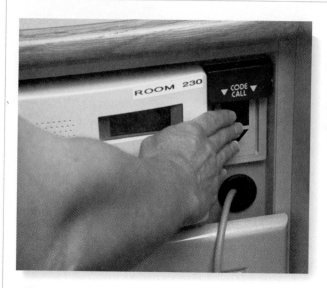

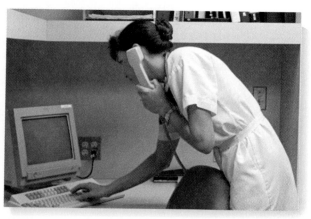

3 Alternatively, call or have someone else phone for help (e.g., 911 or other local emergency number). *Do not hang up until you are told to do so!* **RATIONALE:** To ensure that EMS personnel have all necessary information.

2 **Call for help:** Activate emergency medical service (EMS) System. If in an agency, such as a hospital, press STAT button or call a code (per policy). **RATIONALE:** Emergency assistance and supplies for ACLS should be available in minutes.

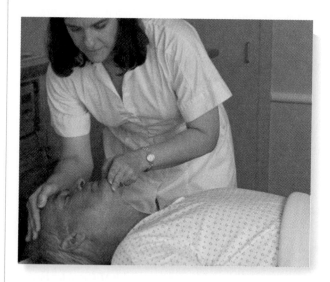

4 Place victim flat on firm surface, and kneel down next to victim. **RATIONALE:** A flat position improves blood flow to the brain and makes CPR easier.

- **Establish airway:** Tilt victim's head back by placing your palm on victim's forehead and pressing backward. **RATIONALE:** This position opens airway.

- Place fingers of your other hand under victim's chin, but do not use thumb. Lift victim's chin up and forward. **RATIONALE:** This helps tilt head back to establish airway.

SAFETY ALERT

If you suspect neck injury, do not tilt or turn the victim's head. Keep the cervical spine immobilized and open the airway by a jaw thrust, using both hands (one on each side of the jaw) to lift the mandible upward and outward. This maneuver will lift the tongue off of the victim's airway (see Chap. 23).

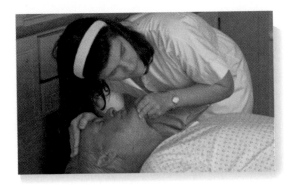

Gasping (agonal) respirations often occur early in cardiac arrest and should not be confused with effective breathing. If respirations appear inadequate, proceed with rescue breathing.

5 **Determine breathlessness:** Place your ear down near victim's mouth: Do you feel air movement? Is there chest movement? **RATIONALE:** If chest rises and falls, but air movement is neither heard nor felt, airway is obstructed.

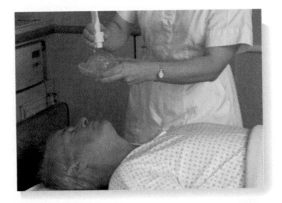

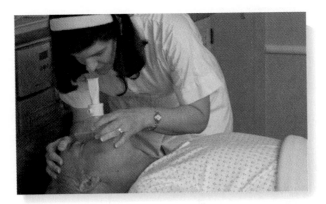

6 If victim is not breathing, place mask over victim's mouth and nose (use bridge of nose as a guide). Place index finger and thumb of hand closest to victim's forehead on top border of mask and place thumb of other hand on lower margin of mask. **RATIONALE:** To ensure a good airtight seal.

- If mask is not available, pinch victim's nostrils closed with your hand that is pressing on victim's forehead. **RATIONALE:** Pinching nose closed prevents air from escaping.
- Take deep breath and seal lips around victim's mouth.

7 **Begin mouth-to-mask or mouth-to-mouth breathing:** Exhale your breath into victim's airway with long (2 sec) ventilations. **RATIONALE:** Slow ventilation reduces risk of gastric inflation. Mask's one-way valve diverts victim's exhaled air away from rescuer.

- Note that victim's chest rises with rescue breathing. **RATIONALE:** Victim's head should be repositioned if chest is not rising with ventilations.
- Keep victim's airway patent; listen and feel for exhalation. **RATIONALE:** Maintaining airway promotes air exchange and minimizes gastric distention.
- Take a fresh breath, then repeat ventilation. Provide 700 to 1000 mL tidal volume over 2 sec per breath. **RATIONALE:** Rescuer's exhaled air provides enough oxygen for victim.
- If available, ventilate with bag-valve-mask resuscitation unit with supplemental delivery of oxygen at maximum flow rate (see Chap. 23). **RATIONALE:** Lower tidal volumes can be delivered with resuscitator unit, reducing risk of gastric inflation.

SAFETY ALERT

There has been no documentation of transmission of hepatitis B or C virus or HIV during mouth-to-mouth resuscitation. Hepatitis B virus (HBV)-positive saliva has not been shown to be infectious to oral mucous membranes and saliva has not been implicated in the transmission of HIV (CDC National Prevention Information Network, 1999).

   If there is exchange of blood as in trauma situations, or if the victim or rescuer has breaks in the skin or mucosa, there is theoretical risk of HBV and HIV transmission during mouth-to-mouth resuscitation. Transmission of other pathogens such as herpes simplex virus or *Neisseria meningitidis* and enteric pathogens has been linked to mouth-to-mouth ventilation.

Rescuers with a duty to provide CPR should follow precautions and guidelines established by the Centers for Disease Control (CDC) and the Occupational Safety and Health Administration (OSHA) that include use of latex gloves and manual ventilation equipment such as a bag mask and other masks with valves that divert the victim's exhaled air away from the rescuer. While face masks with one-way valves prevent transmission of bacteria from victim to rescuer, face shields have not proven to be as reliable a barrier.

SAFETY ALERT

While mouth-to-mouth breathing is effective and safe, many would-be rescuers are reluctant to provide it to strangers. If you are unwilling or unable to perform mouth-to-mouth rescue breathing, provide chest compressions only. This is better than no CPR at all in adult arrest cases. Studies show that positive-pressure ventilation is not essential during the first 6 to 12 min of adult CPR, especially if the victim has gasping respirations.

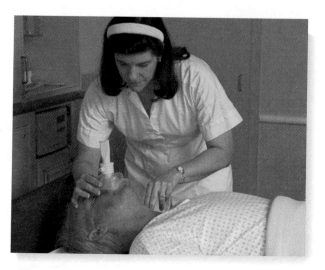

8 **Determine pulselessness:** Briefly (5 sec) check for carotid pulse (on side closest to rescuer) or other signs of circulation (e.g., movement, swallowing). If pulse is present, but victim is not breathing, continue rescue breathing at 10 to 12 breaths per minute. If there are no signs of circulation, or if pulse is absent, prepare for chest compressions.

SAFETY ALERT

Ventricular fibrillation is the most common rhythm accompanying cardiac arrest, and it tends to convert to asystole in just a few minutes. If pulse is absent, retrieve an AED for immediate rhythm analysis. The earlier defibrillation occurs, the better the prognosis. The goal of early defibrillation by first responders is a collapse-to-shock interval of 5 min in the community or less than 3 min in a health care facility.

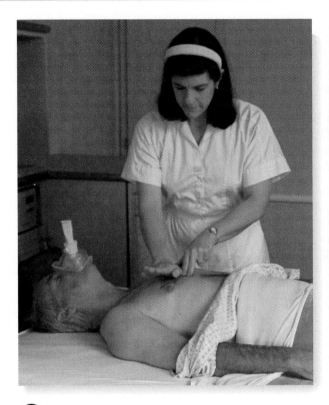

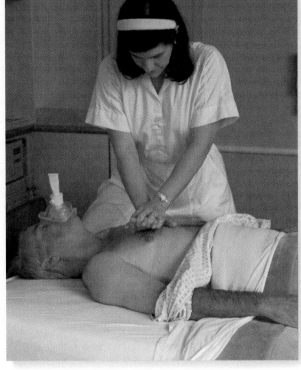

9 Locate xiphoid notch (where lower ribs meet bottom of sternum). Position heel of one hand on lower half of sternum (long axis of heel on long axis of sternum), two fingers above xiphoid process. Superimpose other hand on top of first hand, keeping hands parallel. **RATIONALE:** Compressions at this site decrease risk of damage to victim's liver.

10 Interlace and extend fingers, keeping them off victim's chest so that only supported heel of hand has contact. **RATIONALE:** This helps prevent rocking motion and damage to victim's ribs.

- Position your shoulders over your hands, keeping arms straight and elbows locked. **RATIONALE:** Your body weight helps to depress victim's sternum, which increases intrathoracic and intracardiac pressures.

- **Begin chest compressions:** Compress sternum 1.5 to 2 in at a rate of 100 compressions per minute. **RATIONALE:** This rate improves coronary blood flow.

- Establish an equal timing for compression/release (50 percent for each) to a "one-and, two-and, three-and" rhythm. **RATIONALE:** Rhythmic release reduces intrathoracic pressure and allows time for venous blood to return to heart.

- Do not lift hands from sternum while releasing pressure. **RATIONALE:** This prevents loss of proper hand positioning between compressions.

SAFETY ALERT

If administering CPR to a pregnant victim, place pillows or other object under the woman's right buttock to move the uterus off the vena cava and increase venous return.

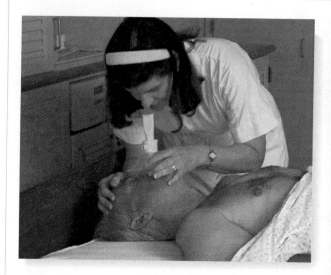

11 Pause after 15 compressions to give another two breaths. A 15:2 compression-to-ventilation ratio is used for either one or two rescuers.

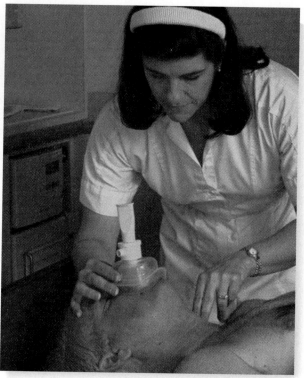

12 **Reassess victim:** After the fourth cycle's ventilations (1 min), check briefly (3 to 5 sec) for return of carotid pulse. Reassess every few minutes.

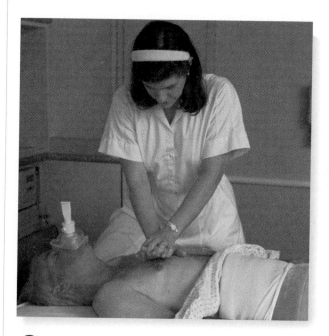

13 If pulse is still absent, resume CPR, beginning with sternal compressions. **RATIONALE:** Ventilation has just been delivered.

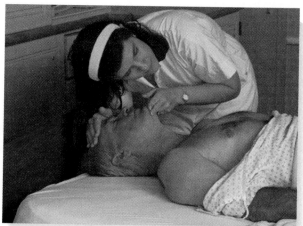

14 If pulse is now present, check breathing. If breathing is present, place victim in recovery position (rolled to side), unless trauma is suspected, and continue to monitor. **RATIONALE:** Recovery position helps maintain open airway.

■ If breathing is absent, continue rescue breathing 10 to 12 times per minute.

CPR BY TWO RESCUERS

Rescuer A
- Initiates CPR

Rescuer B
- Retrieves AED and summons EMS (if not already done)
- Returns for brief reassessment and early defibrillation if indicated
- Positions self behind victim's head, or on opposite side of rescuer A at victim's head
- Maintains victim's airway by holding barrier mask and performing chin lift with both hands
- Delivers rescue breathing, monitors carotid pulse periodically, and reports to rescuer A (compression-to-ventilation ratio is the same as for a single rescuer—15:2)

Rescuer A
- Compresses at 100 times per minute, stops briefly after 15th compression for rescuer B to ventilate victim two times; several compressions are required to resume adequate blood flow each time compressions are interrupted to deliver a breath.

(*Note:* When rescuer A becomes fatigued, positions and roles are exchanged after ventilations and resumed with compressions.)

CALLING A CODE

Preparation

1 Identify hospitalized clients at risk for cardiovascular or pulmonary arrest.

2 Check at-risk client's code status (partial code or do not attempt resuscitation [DNAR, DNR, or no CPR]).

3 Assess if client has patent IV for administration of fluids and medications in event of code.

4 Note any client allergies.

5 Review agency code policy.

6 Determine accessibility and location of crash cart.

Resuscitation efforts should be provided for all clients unless the client has refused these measures or there is clear evidence of futility. Do not attempt resuscitation (DNAR) orders are initiated upon the hospitalized client's request and are recorded on the client's record by the physician per agency policy. The nurse must become familiar with the agency's policy regarding these directives. The DNAR is appropriate if:

- The client has a valid consent (living will).
- The client has a terminal condition.
- The client is permanently unconscious.
- Resuscitation would be medically futile (the client's chance of survival versus the decision maker's goal may be defined by state statute).

DNAR orders do not preclude the administration of IV fluids, nutrition, oxygen, analgesia, sedation, or cardiovascular agents. Some clients may accept defibrillation and chest compression but not intubation and mechanical ventilation. The DNAR order can be individualized and must be reviewed regularly.

Equipment

- Method of summoning emergency response system (e.g., STAT button)
- Crash cart

SAFETY ALERT

The nurse must be familiar with the location and contents of the unit's crash cart and equipment use. Contents vary among agencies and among units within agencies. Contents generally include ECG monitoring supplies, defibrillator, respiratory equipment, emergency medications, IV equipment, stopcocks, needles, syringes, tape, swabs, tourniquets, cutdown supplies, checklist, and code flowsheets. Drawers are kept locked when the cart is not in use.

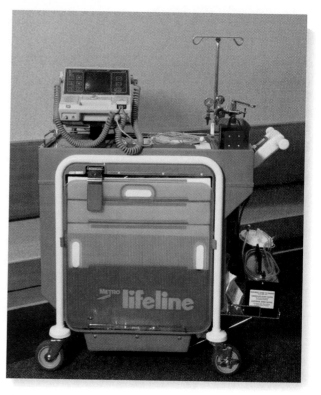

● **FIGURE 25-1** *Crash cart.*

SKILL

1 Determine that client's condition has changed significantly or is rapidly deteriorating. **RATIONALE:** It is not necessary that client's heart and breathing stop before code is called.

2 Initiate code if client is unresponsive, has stopped breathing, or is pulseless.

3 Press bedside STAT button and call out for help: "Code in room 1223! Bring the crash cart!" **RATIONALE:** Unit secretary usually summons code team.

4 Place client in supine position and initiate CPR, continuing measures until code team arrives.

5 Ask assistant to close curtain for privacy and clear area to make room for code cart and team.

6 Quickly communicate details of situation when code team arrives. **RATIONALE:** This aids team leader's decision making.

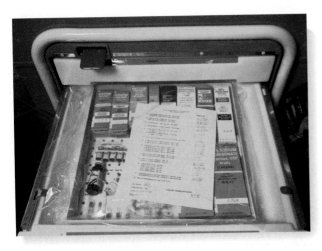

● **FIGURE 25-2** *Crash cart drawer.*

7 Assist code team as necessary with the following (per agency):

- Positioning cardiac board (or head board) to facilitate chest compressions
- Establishing IV with 0.9 percent sodium chloride or lactated Ringer's infusion
- Providing bag-valve-mask ventilation with 100 percent oxygen delivery (see Chapter 23)
- Cardiac monitoring
- Airway intubation and suctioning
- Advanced cardiac life support protocol
- Documentation of interventions and client responses

CLINICAL NOTE

Code team member roles include:

Staff nurse from unit
- Maintains crowd control
- Communicates with family members as time allows
- Places phone calls for additional assistance (lab, ECG, physician, x-ray, clergy) or client arrangements (e.g., transfer to critical care unit)

Crash cart nurse
- Sets up equipment
- Prepares medications and/or hands medications to code team member
- Replaces used equipment and medications following code

Critical care nurse (code team RN)
- Administers medications
- Defibrillates client
- Prepares for external pacing if needed
- Assists with intubation if needed

Documentation nurse
- Communicates with person in charge (physician or nurse)
- Reports when last dose of medication was given, number of doses of each medication, ABG (or other lab) results, ECG findings
- Records on code flowsheet: client's condition and time of code initiation, ongoing client responses (e.g., vital signs), time of each event and treatment, and time of code discontinuation (uses one clock or watch consistently)

Team leader (physician or specially prepared nurse)
- Documents resuscitation process
- Writes summary narrative of code proceedings
- Signs completed code sheet

AUTOMATED EXTERNAL DEFIBRILLATION (AED)

Equipment

- Adhesive defibrillatory electrode pads with connecting cables
- Battery-operated automated external defibrillator (AED) unit.

SAFETY ALERT

AEDs should be used only on victims who are unconscious, who are not breathing, and who have no detectable pulse. Do not place pads over a nitroglycerin patch, or over implanted devices such as pacemakers (avoid both by 5 inches).

SKILL

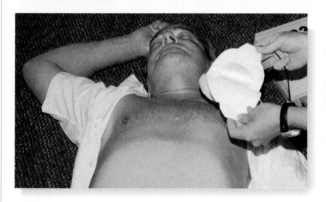

1 Place AED close to victim's left ear, if possible. **RATIONALE:** This gives better access to defibrillator controls and allows easier placement of pads.

- Connect defibrillator pad cable to AED unit, and turn unit power ON.
- If using semiautomated unit, follow AED commands (AEDs provide digitized readout or voice-synthesized instructions).
- Open package, and remove backing from adhesive chest defibrillation pads.

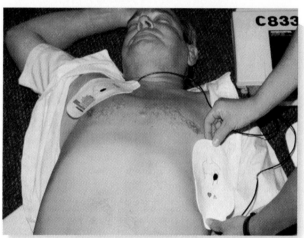

2 Apply adhesive pads to victim's bare chest in modified Lead II: one pad to the upper right subclavicular area, and pad marked with ♥ to lower left ribs over cardiac apex. Cease any motion of victim (including CPR). **RATIONALE:** Unit will not function reliably if there is any movement.

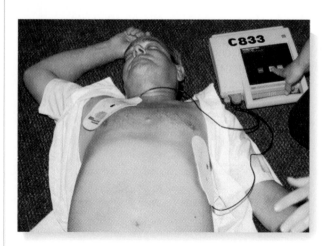

3 Keep victim **clear** and initiate rhythm ANALYZE, allowing 5 to 15 sec to process. **RATIONALE:** Charging of capacitors is initiated; handling client interferes with analysis. Fully automated units are usually found in lay settings and will charge and deliver shock to victim if initiated.

- Command loudly for all nearby to "STAND CLEAR." **RATIONALE:** Rescuer is accountable for preventing injury to others; shock must be confined to victim.

SAFETY ALERT

Under no circumstance should anyone handle the victim (or the bed) while the AED is analyzing, charging, or delivering sequential shocks.

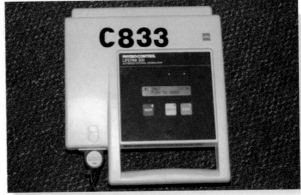

4 Deliver shock if PUSH TO SHOCK is indicated and it is safe to do so. Victim's muscles will suddenly contract.

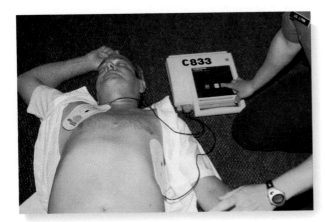

5 Following each shock, quickly press ANALYZE for follow-up rhythm report; do not resume CPR at this time.

- If ventricular fibrillation persists, AED will command repeat for second and third (stacked) shocks; do not delay process by checking for pulse between shocks. **RATIONALE:** If ventricular fibrillation persists, shocks should be delivered in sets of three; many AEDs increase energy level with subsequent shocks (e.g., 200 J to 360 J). Sequential stacked shocks reduce impedance to energy transmission across chest and internal organs.

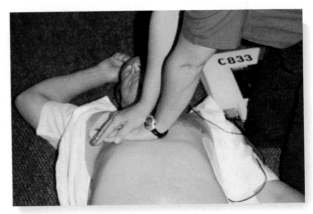

6 If ventricular fibrillation persists after three shocks, perform chest compressions for 1 min. Again analyze rhythm and follow AED commands for three more shocks if indicated.

7 Continue process (analyze, three shocks, CPR for 1 min) until NO SHOCK INDICATED appears.

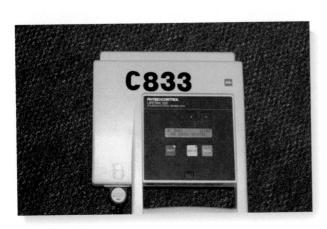

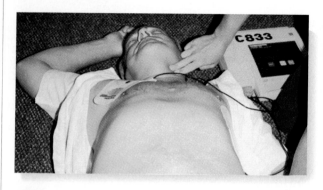

8 Check for pulse; if no pulse obtained, resume CPR.

CLINICAL NOTE

DISCONTINUATION OF BLS

Most efforts at resuscitation of people in cardiac arrest will fail. The majority of resuscitation attempts end in death; or, in some cases, the brain suffers seriously during the resuscitation attempt. Resuscitation is inappropriate and unjustifiable in futile cases and was never intended to be used in cases of terminal, irreversible illness when death is not unexpected.

Discontinue efforts if the victim's ventilation and circulation are restored, or care is transferred to other trained individuals who can continue life support. No matter how long you persist, appropriate efforts beyond 30 min are futile if there is no "flicker of life" response. With few exceptions (e.g., drug overdose), in-hospital interventions will not resuscitate victims who fail out-of-hospital efforts.

ABDOMINAL THRUST (HEIMLICH) MANEUVER

Equipment

- Rescuer's hands, arms, and understanding of skill

SKILL

Conscious Victim (Standing or Sitting)

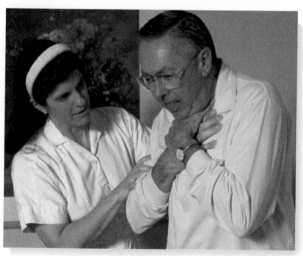

1 Note signs of airway obstruction: poor air exchange; weak, ineffective cough; high-pitched noise with inhalation; cyanosis. **RATIONALE:** Obstructed airway impedes airflow and leads to oxygen desaturation.

- Ask victim to hold hand on neck if choking. **RATIONALE:** This is universal distress signal for foreign body airway obstruction.
- Ask if victim can speak. **RATIONALE:** Victim is unable to speak with complete airway obstruction.

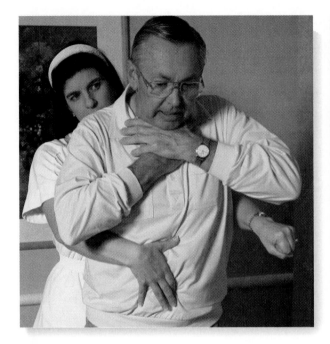

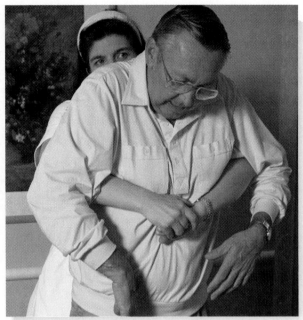

2 If choking and inability to speak are confirmed, position hands for subdiaphragmatic abdominal thrusts. Stand behind victim and wrap your arms around victim's waist. Locate landmarks of xiphoid process and umbilicus.

3 Make a fist with one hand and press thumb side of fist into victim's abdomen slightly above umbilicus, but well below xiphoid process. **RATIONALE:** Fist position near xiphoid or lower ribs can result in serious injury to abdominal or thoracic organs.

- Place your other hand over your fist and, with a rotating upward motion, forcefully thrust your hands into victim's abdomen.
- Repeat thrusts five times until foreign body is expelled or victim becomes unconscious.

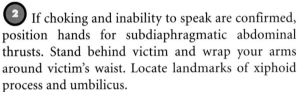

Unconscious Victim

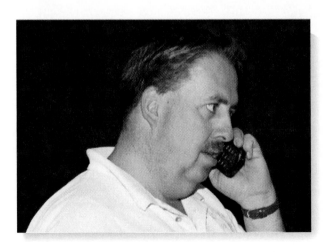

1 If unresponsiveness is known to be caused by foreign body airway obstruction, activate the emergency response system, or have someone else do so.

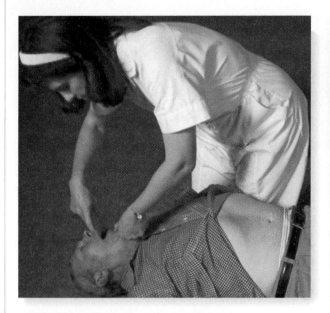

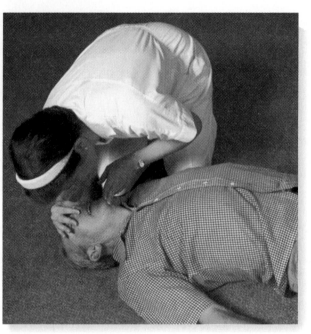

2 Tilt victim's head back, grasp tongue and lower jaw between your thumb and fingers, and lift mandible. **RATIONALE:** This lifts tongue away from back of the throat and possibly away from foreign body lodged there.

3 Open airway and try to ventilate; if unsuccessful, reposition head and try again.

- Perform finger sweep: Use index finger to hook and press object to one side of throat and work it toward mouth for removal.

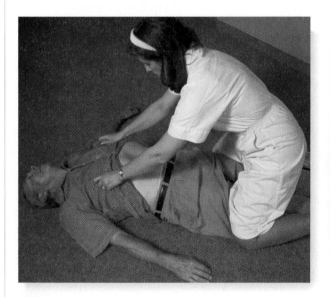

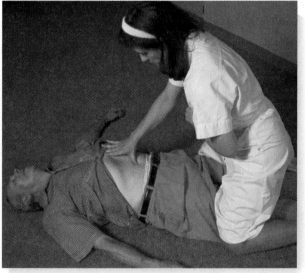

4 If unable to ventilate, kneel to straddle victim's thighs and prepare for Heimlich maneuver. **RATIONALE:** Inability to ventilate even with repositioning of victim's head increases probability of foreign object obstructing airway.

5 Locate landmarks (umbilicus and xiphoid process). **RATIONALE:** This identifies subdiaphragmatic area.

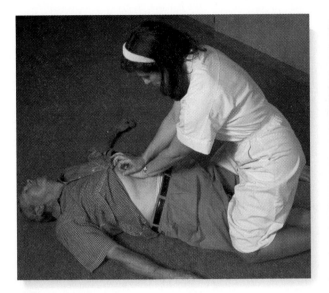

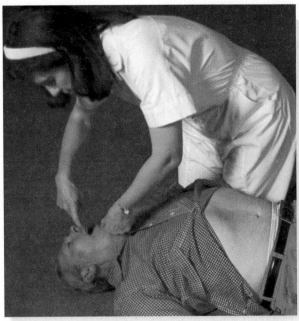

6 Position heel of one hand on victim's midabdomen, slightly above umbilicus and well below xiphoid. **RATIONALE:** Avoiding subxiphoid area helps reduce risk of internal injuries.

■ Place other hand on top, press into victim's abdomen, and quickly thrust upward up to five times until foreign object dislodges. **RATIONALE:** Maneuver forces diaphragm upward, raises intrathoracic pressure, and creates artificial cough.

7 Move to victim's head, perform tongue-jaw lift to open mouth, and use index finger to perform finger sweep. **RATIONALE:** This helps secure and retrieve object.

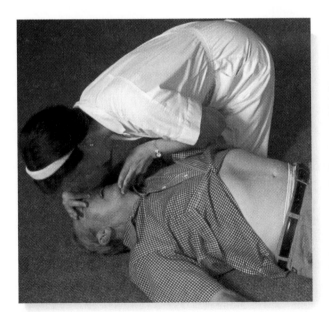

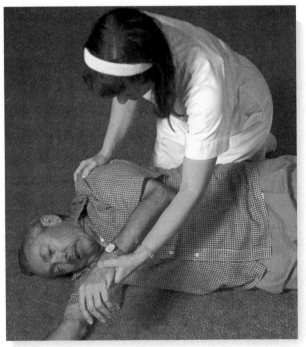

8 Attempt to ventilate victim. Continue repeating sequence of efforts to dislodge and remove foreign object: tongue-jaw lift, finger sweep, attempt ventilation, reposition and try again, then perform Heimlich maneuver up to five times.

9 When victim resumes effective breathing, turn to side-lying recovery position, and continue to observe.

CHARTING

- Time and description of circumstances around victim's becoming unresponsive or requiring immediate action
- Time of calling code or summoning EMS and time of arrival
- Initial resuscitation efforts
- Name(s) of responders and their actions: respiratory measures, IV fluids, medications and dosages, etc. (use flow sheet if available at the time)

- Number of attempts at defibrillation
- Duration of resuscitative efforts
- Summary ECG strips from AED (if available)
- Victim's responses to efforts

CRITICAL THINKING FOCUS

SECTION ONE ▪ Basic Life Support

Unexpected Outcomes

- Victim requiring resuscitation is in a burning building.

- Rescuer of cardiac arrest victim is alone, but must summon help.

- Gastric distension develops during CPR.

- Attempts at ventilation for rescue breathing are ineffective; chest does not rise, no air is felt.

- Rescuer just cannot continue efforts at unsuccessful resuscitation.

- AED fails to analyze rhythm after 15 sec.

- No pulse returns after three AED shocks.

- Victim of airway obstruction is obese and rescuer cannot reach around victim's abdomen.

Alternative Nursing Actions

- Move victim to safety before initiating CPR.

- It is more important to activate EMS; delay CPR momentarily.

- Decrease ventilation volume and slow ventilation flow rate—take 1.5 to 2 sec to ventilate.

- Perform Heimlich maneuver several times, open victim's mouth for finger sweep (only in unconscious victim), then resume attempts to ventilate. Abdominal thrust (Heimlich) maneuver may be indicated.

- The benefit of CPR beyond 30 min is questionable. Discontinue efforts if unable to continue due to exhaustion or endangerment.

- Cease CPR or any movement of victim as soon you activate the ANALYZE function.

- Resume CPR for 1 min, reanalyze rhythm, check for pulse, and deliver three more rounds of stacked shocks if ventricular fibrillation persists.

- Stand behind victim and place your arms around victim's chest up under armpits. Make a fist and press thumb side against victim's *midsternum*. Support fist with other hand and thrust backward toward yourself to dislodge object.
- Place victim supine and deliver abdominal thrusts as you would for unconscious victim.

SELF-CHECK EVALUATION

PART 1 ▪ Matching Terms

Match the definition in column B with the correct term in column A.

Column A

_____ a. CPR
_____ b. EMS
_____ c. BLS
_____ d. Ventricular
            fibrillation
_____ e. AED
_____ f. ECG
_____ g. Defibrillate
_____ h. Xiphoid
_____ i. ACLS
_____ j. Abdominal thrust
            Heimlich maneuver

Column B

1. Personnel who dispatch emergency responders to scene of emergency
2. Lethal arrhythmia with no cardiac output
3. Pointed cartilage connected to lower sternum
4. Automatic or semiautomatic defibrillating unit
5. Life support including CPR, airway intubation, defibrillation, and IV medications
6. Application of an electrical impulse to the heart to correct lethal arrhythmia
7. Subdiaphragmatic thrust to create artificial exhalation
8. Emergency cardiac care, referring to CPR, EMS activation, ACLS, and professional and community training programs
9. Recognition of cardiac arrest, access to EMS system, and basic CPR
10. Maneuvers of rescue breathing and chest compression

PART 2 ▪ Multiple Choice Questions

1. During CPR, the compression-to-ventilation ratio for two rescuers is:

   a. 5:1.
   b. 12:3.
   c. 15:1.
   d. 15:2.

2. Slow ventilation is recommended for rescue breathing because it:

   a. Reduces rescuer anxiety.
   b. Prevents gastric distention.
   c. Improves oxygen diffusion.
   d. Allows cardiac filling.

3. The best way to improve a cardiac arrest victim's chance of survival is to immediately:

   a. Deliver a sternal blow.
   b. Defibrillate.
   c. Perform the abdominal thrust (Heimlich) maneuver.
   d. Start cardiac compressions.

4. In order to establish an airway, the rescuer:

   a. Tilts the head back and lifts the chin.
   b. Holds the tongue against the upper palate.
   c. Tilts the head back and holds the mouth closed.
   d. Presses the victim's chin to the chest.

5. The most common arrhythmia that occurs with cardiac arrest is:
   a. Complete heart block.
   b. Ventricular tachycardia.
   c. Ventricular fibrillation.
   d. Asystole.

6. The use of a mask or shield device for ventilation during CPR:
   a. Promotes better ventilation.
   b. Protects against exposure to body fluids.
   c. Maintains the victim's head positioning.
   d. Delays the rescue process.

7. To establish pulselessness, the rescuer:
   a. Palpates the carotid artery.
   b. Palpates the femoral artery.
   c. Listens for a heartbeat.
   d. Notes pupil dilation.

8. The use of automated external defibrillators:
   a. Expands the availability of defibrillation.
   b. Is reserved for emergency medical technicians (EMTs).
   c. Requires special training.
   d. Needs further research.

9. The most common cause of cardiac arrest is:
   a. Drowning.
   b. Stroke.
   c. Electrocution.
   d. Heart disease.

10. The AED should be placed at the:
   a. Victim's left side.
   b. Victim's right side.
   c. Foot of the bed.
   d. Head of the bed.

11. The first step when responding to cardiopulmonary emergency is:
   a. Summoning help.
   b. Assessing the victim.
   c. Initiating ventilation.
   d. Initiating circulation.

12. If the victim's chest is rising and falling but no air movement can be felt or heard, the likely cause is:
   a. Cardiac arrest.
   b. Agonal breathing.
   c. Brainstem stroke.
   d. Airway obstruction.

13. For recovery positioning following CPR, the victim is placed:
   a. Supine (on the back).
   b. Prone (face down).
   c. Turned to the side.
   d. On the back, head elevated.

14. Positioning of the fist to deliver the Heimlich maneuver is:

    a. At the umbilicus.
    b. At the xiphoid process.
    c. Just above the umbilicus.
    d. Just below the xiphoid process.

PART 3 ▪ Critical Thinking Application

While you are dining with friends at a restaurant, it becomes apparent that a pregnant woman at the table next to you is in distress—violently coughing and wheezing, still conscious but in serious trouble, holding her throat. You notice chunks of chopped brisket on her plate.

1. What should your intervention be at this time?

2. The woman fails to clear her airway, her cough becomes weak, and she develops an audible inspiratory stridor and signs of increasing distress. What is your analysis of these signs?

3. You decide that an abdominal thrust (Heimlich) maneuver is essential. How will you adapt this technique for a victim in advanced pregnancy?

4. What are the major causes of airway obstruction?

5. How can airway obstruction be prevented?

APPENDIX A: CONVERTING DOSAGE SYSTEMS AND CALCULATING DOSAGES

 ## CONVERTING DOSAGE SYSTEMS

Procedure

1. To make conversions from the metric to apothecaries' or household systems, it is necessary to memorize or refer to equivalency tables.

2. To convert milligrams to grains, use the following formula:

$$\frac{1 \text{ gr}}{\text{milligrams per grain}} = \frac{\text{Dose desired}}{\text{Dose on hand}}$$

$$\frac{1}{60} = \frac{x}{180}$$

$$60x = 180$$
$$x = 3 \text{ gr}$$

3. You may also make this conversion as a ratio:

1 gr:60 mg: :x gr:180 mg

$$60x = 180$$
$$x = 3 \text{ gr}$$

4. To convert milligrams to milliliters, you can set up a direct proportion and, following the algebraic principle, cross-multiply.

5. Check conversion tables in Appendix C.

 ## CALCULATING DOSAGES

Equipment

Orders for dosage of medication needed
Dosage of medication on hand

Procedure

1. To calculate oral dosages, use the following formula. (*D* and *H* must be in same unit of measure.)

$$\frac{D}{H} = X$$

where D = dose desired; H = dose on hand; and X = dose to be administered.

EXAMPLE: Give 500 mg of ampicillin sodium when the dose on hand is in capsules containing 250 mg.

$$\frac{500 \text{ mg}}{250 \text{ mg}} = 2 \text{ capsules}$$

2. To calculate dose when in liquid form, use the following formula:

$$\frac{D}{H} \times Q = X$$

where D = dose desired; H = dose on hand; Q = quantity; and X = amount to be administered.

EXAMPLE: Give 375 mg of ampicillin when it is supplied as 250 mg/5 mL.

$$\frac{375 \text{ mg}}{250 \text{ mg}} \times 5$$

$$1.5 \times 5 = 7.5 \text{ mL}$$

3. To calculate parenteral dosages, use the following formula:

$$\frac{D}{H} \times Q = X$$

EXAMPLE: Give client 40 mg gentamicin C complex sulfate. On hand is a multidose vial with a strength of 80 mg/2 mL.

$$\frac{40}{80} \times 2 = 1 \text{ mL}$$

4. Check your calculations before drawing up the medications.

5. See calculations of solutions in Appendix B.

APPENDIX B: CALCULATIONS OF SOLUTIONS

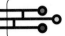 ## CALCULATIONS OF SOLUTIONS

Types of Solutions

1. Volume to volume (vol/vol): a given volume of solute is added to a given volume of solvent.
2. Weight to weight (wt/wt): a stated weight of solute is dissolved in a stated weight of solvent.
3. Weight to volume (wt/vol): a given weight of solute is dissolved in a given volume of solvent, which results in the proper amount of solution.

Preparing Solutions

■ **Solutions of Varying Strengths**

Determine the strength of the solution, the strength of the drug on hand, and the quantity of solution required.

Use this formula for preparing solutions:

$$\frac{D}{H} \times Q = X$$

where D = desired strength; H = strength on hand; Q = quantity of solution desired; and X = amount of solute.

EXAMPLE: You have a 100% solution of hydrogen peroxide on hand. You need a liter of 50% solution.

$$\frac{50}{100} \times 1000 \text{ mL} = 500 \text{ mL (solute)}$$

If the strength desired and strength on hand are not in like terms, you need to change one of the terms.

EXAMPLE: You have 1 L of 50% solution on hand. You need a liter of 1:10 solution. 1:10 solution is the same as 10%.

$$\frac{10\%}{50\%} \times 1000 \text{ mL} = 200 \text{ mL (solute)}$$

Add 200 mL of the drug to 800 mL of the solvent to make a liter of 10% solution.

■ **Volume to Volume Solutions**

Use the formula:

$$\frac{D}{H} \times Q = X$$

EXAMPLE: Prepare a liter of 5% solution from a stock solution of 50%.

$$\frac{5\%}{50\%} \times 1000 \text{ mL} = 100 \text{ mL}$$

Add 100 mL to 900 mL of diluent to make 1 L of 5% solution.

■ **Solutions from Tablets**

Use the formula:

$$\frac{D}{H} \times Q = X$$

where X = amount per number of tablets used.

EXAMPLE: Prepare 1 L of a 1:1000 solution, using 10-gr tablets.

$$\frac{1/1000}{10 \text{ gr}} \times 1000 \text{ mL} = X$$

First convert 10 gr to grams so the numerator and denominator are in the same unit of measure. 1 g = 15 gr; therefore 10 gr = ⅔ g. Now substitute the new numbers in the formula and solve for X.

$$\frac{1/1000}{2/3} \times \frac{1000}{1} \text{ mL} = X$$

$$\frac{3}{2000} \times \frac{1000}{1} = X$$

X = ¾ or 1½ tablets

Place 1½ tablets into the liter of solution and dissolve.

APPENDIX C: ABBREVIATIONS AND SYMBOLS AND CONVERSION TABLES

ABBREVIATIONS AND SYMBOLS

aa	of each	p.c.	after meals
a.c.	before meals	per	by, through
ad lib.	freely, as desired	prn *or* PRN	whenever necessary
b.i.d.	twice each day	q.d.	every day
c̄	with	q.h.	every hour
C	carbon	q.i.d.	four times each day
Ca	calcium	q.s.	as much as required, quantity sufficient
Cl	chlorine		
dr *or* ℨ	dram	q2h	every 2 hours
et	and	q3h	every 3 hours
GI	gastrointestinal	q4h	every 4 hours
gt *or* gtt	drop(s)	R_x	treatment, "take thou"
H_2O	water	s̄	without
H_2O_2	hydrogen peroxide	s̄s̄	one-half
IM	intramuscular	STAT	immediately
in.	inch	t.i.d.	three times each day
K	potassium	tsp	teaspoon
lb *or* #	pound	WBC	white blood count
m	minimum (a minimum)	°	degree
Mg	magnesium	−	minus, negative, alkaline reaction
N	nitrogen, normal	+	plus, positive, acid reaction
Na	sodium	%	percent
n.p.o.	nothing by mouth	v	Roman numeral 5
oob	out of bed	vii	Roman numeral 7
os	mouth	ix	Roman numeral 9
oz *or* ℨ	ounce	xiii	Roman numeral 13

CONVERSION TABLES

Household Equivalents (Volume)

Metric	Apothecary	Household
0.06 mL	1 minim	1 drop
5(4) mL	1 fluid dram	1 teaspoonful
15 mL	4 fluid drams	1 tablespoonful
30 mL	1 fluid ounce	2 tablespoonfuls
180 mL	6 fluid ounces	1 teacupful
240 mL	8 fluid ounces	1 glassful

Apothecary Equivalents (Volume)

Metric		Apothecary
1 mL	=	15 minims
1 cc	=	15 minims
0.06 mL	=	1 minim
4 mL	=	1 fluid dram
30 mL	=	1 fluid ounce
500 mL	=	1 pint
1000 mL (1 L)	=	1 quart

Apothecary Equivalents (Weight)

Metric				Apothecary
1.0 g	*or*	1000 mg	=	gr xv
0.6 g	*or*	600 mg	=	gr x
0.5 g	*or*	500 mg	=	gr viiss
0.3 g	*or*	300 mg	=	gr v
0.2 g	*or*	200 mg	=	gr iii
0.1 g	*or*	100 mg	=	gr 1½
0.06 g	*or*	60 mg	=	gr 1
0.05 g	*or*	50 mg	=	gr ¾
0.03 g	*or*	30 mg	=	gr ½
0.015 g	*or*	15 mg	=	gr ¼
0.010 g	*or*	10 mg	=	gr ⅙
0.008 g	*or*	8 mg	=	gr ⅛
4 g			=	1 dr
30 g			=	1 oz
1 kg			=	2.2 lbs

GLOSSARY

 A

ABDUCTION: movement of a bone away from the midline of the body or body part, as in raising the arm or spreading the fingers.

ABRASION: the scraping away of a portion of skin or of a mucous membrane as a result of injury.

ABSCESS: a localized collection of pus in any part of the body.

ABSORPTION: the passage of a substance from an administration site into the bloodstream.

ACIDOSIS: accumulation of acids (metabolic or respiratory), potentially disturbing the acid-base balance and causing acidemia (low pH).

ACLS: advanced cardiac life support—resuscitative measures that include CPR, defibrillation, airway intubation, and administration of IV medications.

ACUPRESSURE: Chinese method of treatment that involves compression of certain areas of the body by following a system of meridians or energy flow.

ADDUCTION: movement of a bone toward the midline of the body or part.

ADHESIONS: formation of fibrous scar tissue around an incision as a result of surgical intervention. Adhesions can cause obstruction or malfunction by distorting an organ.

ADJUNCTIVE: accessory to or assisting with.

ADMISSION: the process of signing a client into the hospital.

ADVENTITIOUS: abnormal extra sounds (crackles, wheezes) superimposed on breath sounds.

AED: automated or semiautomatic defibrillating unit.

AEROBE: a microorganism that lives and grows in the presence of free oxygen.

AEROSOL: liquid particles suspended in a gas, especially a suspension of a drug or other substance to be dispensed in a fine spray or mist.

AFTERLOAD: impedance to ventricular ejection (e.g., systemic vascular resistance).

AIDS: acquired immune deficiency syndrome—a serious condition characterized by a defect in natural immunity against disease. When the immune system is suppressed, the individual is vulnerable to a host of opportunistic infections.

ALIGNMENT: arrangement in a straight line. Also, referring to posture, the relationship of body parts to one another.

ALKALOSIS: condition in which the alkalinity of the body tends to increase beyond normal, potentially resulting in alkalemia (high pH).

ALLERGY: an altered reaction of body tissues to a specific substance, essentially an antibody-antigen reaction; may be due to the release of histamine.

AMBIENT AIR TEMPERATURE: the temperature of the air surrounding a person.

AMBULATE: to walk.

ANABOLISM: constructive phase of metabolism.

ANAEROBE: an organism that lives and grows in the absence of molecular oxygen.

ANAL FISSURE: a small linear ulcerated area in the anal area.

ANALGESIA: absence of the normal sense of pain.

ANAPHYLAXIS: a hypersensitive shock state due to a foreign substance, protein, or drug.

ANEMIA: a condition in which the number of circulating red blood cells, or hemoglobin, is reduced.

ANESTHESIA: partial or complete loss of sensation induced by administration of a drug or gas.

ANESTHESIA (SURGICAL, RECOVERY) BED: a bed made in a specific manner for the client returning to the unit after anesthesia or surgery.

ANGINA: a sense of suffocation or pain and feeling of pressure in region of the arms, jaw, or heart resulting from lack of oxygen.

ANOREXIA: loss of appetite for food.

ANTIBACTERIAL: any substance that fights against or suppresses bacteria.

ANTIBIOTIC: a substance that has the power to inhibit or destroy other organisms, especially bacteria.

ANTIBODY: protein substance developed by the body to fight disease organisms. Not effective against a virus that is inside the cells.

ANTICOAGULANT: any substance that suppresses or counteracts coagulation of blood.

ANTIEMBOLIC: measure used to help prevent formation of an embolism, such as elastic hosiery.

ANTIEMETIC: an agent that prevents or relieves nausea and vomiting.

ANTIMICROBIAL: an agent that prevents the development or pathogenic action of microbes.

ANTIPYRETIC: an agent that reduces febrile temperatures.

ANTISEPTICS: agents that are applied to body tissues, such as skin or mucous membrane, to destroy or retard the growth of microorganisms.

ANURIA: a total suppression or lack of production of urine.

ANXIETY: a troubled or apprehensive feeling; a sense of dread or fear.

APEX: the pointed end of a cone-shaped part or organ (e.g., lower heart, upper lung).

APNEA: cessation of breathing; usually of a temporary nature.

ARC: AIDS-related complex—characterized by a prolonged history of fever, unexplained weight loss, swollen lymph nodes, or fungus infection of the mouth and throat. A certain but unknown percentage of persons with ARC will develop AIDS.

ARRHYTHMIA: deviation from normal cardiac rate, rhythm, or time intervals.

ARTERIOSCLEROSIS: an arterial disease characterized by inelasticity and thickening of the vessel walls resulting in altered blood flow to tissues and organs.

ARTHRITIS: inflammation of a joint, usually accompanied by pain and sometimes by change in structure.

ARTIFACT: abnormal waves or spikes showing erratic electrocardiographic activity on an ECG as a result of man-made sources, such as electrical interference, loose electrodes, or client movement.

ASEPSIS: sterile condition; a condition free from germs; the absence of disease-producing microorganisms; prevention of contact with microorganisms.

ASEPTIC: sterile; free from bacteria and infection.

ASEPTIC TECHNIQUE: a method to eliminate contamination, germs, or infection.

ASPIRATION: the removal of fluids or gases from a cavity by the application of suction.

ASSESSMENT: critical evaluation of information; the first step in the nursing process.

ATHEROSCLEROSIS: accumulation of lipid-containing material localized within the internal walls of the blood vessels.

ATRIAL: pertaining to the upper cardiac chambers that receive blood from the lungs and systemic circulation.

ATRIAL FIBRILLATION: a chaotically irregular pulse rhythm with a pulse deficit.

ATROPHY: a wasting of any organ or body part due to lack of nutrients or oxygen.

AUSCULTATION: the act of listening to sounds produced by the body using a stethoscope.

AUTOIMMUNITY: immunity produced by an attack of disease or by processes occurring within the body.

AUTOINFECTIONS: infections that arise from an individual's own body flora.

AUTONOMIC NERVOUS SYSTEM: the part of the nervous system that regulates the functioning of internal organs and glands, such as digestion, respiration, and cardiovascular activity.

AUTOREGULATION: the intrinsic ability of an organ or tissue to maintain blood flow despite changes in arterial pressure.

AXILLA: armpit.

B

BACTERIA: unicellular plantlike microorganisms lacking chlorophyll.

BACTERICIDAL: able to destroy bacteria.

BACTERIOSTATIC: a substance that prevents the growth or multiplication of bacteria.

BARRIER NURSING: any technique that reduces the risk of cross-contamination.

BASE OF SUPPORT: surface area on which an object rests (e.g., for a client lying in prone position, the base of support is the entire undersurface of the body).

BEDSORE: a synonym for decubitus or pressure ulcer—area of cellular necrosis due to decreased circulation.

BEHAVIOR: a person's total activity; actions or reactions, especially conduct that can be observed.

B.I.D.: two times daily.

BIGEMINAL PULSE: a regularly irregular pulse occurring with premature beats that is a disturbance in rhythm.

BIOFEEDBACK: a training technique that uses monitoring instruments to assist people to control stress-related disorders through self-regulation of internal functions.

BIOT RESPIRATIONS: abrupt interruptions between a faster, deeper respiratory rate.

BLANCHING: a whitish hue to an area of the skin.

BLS: basic life support—resuscitative measures that include recognition of cardiac arrest, access to EMS system, basic CPR, and defibrillation.

BODY MECHANICS: movement of the body in a coordinated and efficient way so that proper balance, alignment, and conservation of energy are maintained.

BOLUS: rapid administration of a volume of fluid or a drug intravenously.

BOWEL: the intestine.

BOWEL MOVEMENT: the emptying of the intestinal tract.

BRACHIAL PLEXUS: network of spinal nerves supplying the arm, forearm, and hand.

BRADY-: prefix indicating slow.

BRADYCARDIA: slow heart rate (below 60 BPM).

BRADYPNEA: slow, regular respirations. Rate is below 10 per minute.

BRONCHIAL BREATH SOUNDS: loud, harsh, high-pitched sounds; heard over the trachea, bronchi, and main bronchus.

BRONCHODILATATION: dilatation of the airways.

BRONCHOVESICULAR BREATH SOUNDS: blowing sounds of moderate intensity and pitch; heard over large airways.

BUCK'S TRACTION: a type of skin traction used in the client with a hip fracture prior to surgery.

C

CALLUS: localized hyperplasia of the horny layer of the epidermis, usually due to pressure or friction.

CALORIE: the amount of heat necessary to raise the temperature of 1 kilogram of water by 1°C. The dietary (large) Calorie represents 1000 of these calories, or 1 kilocalorie.

CANNULA: a tube inserted into the body using a trocar or wire. Removal of the trocar or wire allows body fluid to pass through the cannula.

CANTHUS: the angle at either end of the slit between the eyelids.

CAPILLARY: minute blood vessels forming a network connecting the venous and arterial systems.

CARBOHYDRATES: a group of chemical substances, including sugars, glycogen, starches, dextrin, and cellulose, that contain only carbon, oxygen, and hydrogen.

CARDIAC ARREST: cessation of cardiac mechanical activity confirmed by absence of detectable pulse, unresponsiveness, and apnea or anginal gasping respiration.

CARDIAC TAMPONADE: external compression inhibiting diastolic filling of the heart (e.g., pericardial fluid, pneumothorax).

CARDIO-: prefix that pertains to the heart.

CARDIOVASCULAR: term that pertains to the heart and blood vessels; e.g., cardiovascular system.

CARMINATIVE: an agent that removes gases from the gastrointestinal tract.

CARRIER: a person or animal that does not show signs of illness but carries pathogens on or within the body that can be transferred to others.

CARTILAGE: bonelike tissue of the very young that is replaced by bone tissue through the process of ossification. In adults cartilage is found in such areas as the nose, ears, and joints.

CATABOLISM: Destructive phase of metabolism.

CATHARTIC: a drug to induce emptying of the intestinal tract; a laxative.

CATHETERIZATION: a sterile tube inserted for the injection of or removal of fluids from a vessel or body cavity.

CENTER OF GRAVITY: midpoint or center of the body weight. In an adult it is the midpelvic cavity between the symphysis pubis and umbilicus.

CHAIN OF SURVIVAL: concept of cardiac arrest treatment that includes early access, early CPR, early defibrillation, and early ACLS. One weak link results in poor community survival rates.

CHARTING: process of recording information about a client concerning the progress of his or her disease and treatment.

CHARTING BY EXCEPTION: documenting only exceptions to predetermined nursing standards in a narrative format.

CHEMORECEPTOR: a sense organ or sensory nerve ending that is stimulated by and reacts to chemical stimuli.

CHEYNE-STOKES RESPIRATIONS: respirations that become deeper and faster than normal, followed by a slower rate and progressing to periods of apnea lasting from 15 to 60 sec.

CIRCULATION: movement of blood in a circular course, exiting through the aorta and coming back into the heart via the vena cava.

CLIENT CARE PLAN: a plan for care of a specific client or one designed especially for one client.

CLIENT EDUCATION: the process of influencing behavior and teaching the client self-care techniques so that he or she can resume responsibility for certain aspects of health care following discharge from the health facility.

CLINICAL PATHWAYS: interdisciplinary client care plans using specific assessments, interventions, and outcomes for specified health-related conditions.

CLOSED BED: a bed not being used by a client. The linens are left to cover the bed.

COLITIS: inflammation of the colon.

COLLAGEN FORMATION: formation of the protein substance of the white fibers of skin, bone, and cartilage.

COLON: the large intestine, which extends from the cecum to the anus.

COLOSTOMY: an artificially created opening from the colon to the abdominal surface for the elimination of waste.

COMFORT: to ease physically; to relieve, as of pain.

COMMUNICATION: conveying or transmitting knowledge, information, or messages to another person.

COMPLETE BATH: all areas of the body are bathed. This bath can be done completely by the nurse or by the client.

COMPLETE CARE: the client requires total assistance from the nurse because he or she is able to do little or nothing for him- or herself.

COMPRESS: a pad of cloth applied firmly to a part of the body; may be dry or wet, cold or warm.

COMPUTED TOMOGRAPHY: CT—a scanning technique that provides a series of detailed visualizations.

COMPUTER-ASSISTED CHARTING: client information is entered into the computer for storage and retrieval at a later time.

CONDUCTION: transfer of heat by direct contact through fluids, solids, or any suitable substance.

CONGENITAL: present at birth.

CONSENT: to agree; to be of the same mind.

CONSTIPATION: difficult defecation; the passage of dry, hard fecal material.

CONSTRICTION: a narrowing or closing in.

CONTAGIOUS DISEASE: a disease conveyed easily to others.

CONTAMINATION: introduction of disease, germs, or infectious materials into or on normally sterile objects.

CONTOUR SHEETS: sheets that have elastic at each corner; fitted sheets.

CONTRACTILITY: the ability to contract or shorten muscle tissue or cells.

CONTRACTURE: abnormal shortening of muscle tissue, making the muscle resistant to stretching.

CONVECTION: transfer of heat by air.

COUNSELING: giving support or providing guidance.

CPR: cardiopulmonary resuscitation—maneuvers of rescue breathing and chest compression.

CRACKLES: discontinuous popping, crackling, bubbling, moist breath sounds; heard on inspiration.

CRISIS: sudden drop in fever to a normal value. Also, a crucial point or situation in the course of anything; turning point.

CRITERION: a standard, rule or test on which a judgment or decision can be based.

CULTURE: to grow microorganisms or living tissue cells in a special medium.

CYANOSIS: bluish discoloration of the skin and the mucous membrane resulting from reduced oxygenation of red blood cells.

D

DANGLE: to have a client sit on the edge of the bed with feet in a dependent position.

DECUBITUS ULCER: see pressure ulcer.

DEFECATION: emptying of the intestinal tract; bowel movement.

DEFIBRILLATE: to apply an electrical impulse to the heart to correct lethal arrhythmia.

DEHISCENCE: a bursting open, as of a graafian follicle or wound, especially abdominal wounds.

DEHYDRATION: the process of losing water, as in depriving the body tissues of water.

DEPOLARIZATION: development of positive intracellular electrical charge due to rapid entry of sodium into a cell.

DERMATITIS: inflammation of skin evidenced by itching, redness, and skin lesions.

DERMIS: synonym for corium; the skin layer beneath the epidermis; contains vascular connective tissues.

DIAGNOSIS: method or art of identifying the disease or condition a person has or is believed to have.

DIAGNOSTIC TEST: a test used to determine a diagnosis or to determine the cause and nature of a pathological condition.

DIAPHORESIS: an excessive amount of perspiration, as when a person's skin is moist and perspiring.

DIARRHEA: frequent passage of unformed liquid stool.

DIASTOLE: the period in which the heart relaxes and fills with blood.

DIGESTION: the process by which food is broken down, mechanically and chemically, in the gastrointestinal tract.

DILATATION: expansion of an organ or vessel.

DIPLOPIA: double vision.

DISABILITY: a disabled state or condition; incapacity; a handicap.

DISINFECTANTS: chemical agents that are used to destroy or reduce microorganisms on inanimate surfaces and objects.

DISINFECTION: a process that employs physical and chemical means to remove, control, or destroy most of the organisms that may be present on equipment or materials.

DISTAL: area farthest away from point of reference (fingers are the most distal part of upper extremity).

DISTENTION: stretching out or inflating of an organ such as the bladder.

DIURESIS: the excessive production and elimination of urine.

DIURETIC: a chemical agent that increases the production of urine.

DORSAL: pertaining to the back.

DORSIFLEXION: flexion of the foot at the ankle joint; the act of turning the foot and toes upward, as in standing on the heel.

DRAWSHEETS: sheets made of fabric, plastic, or rubber that are placed across the shoulder-to-knee area of the bed and tucked in on the sides.

DYSPNEA: a subjective feeling of difficulty in breathing.

DYSRHYTHMIA: abnormality of heart rate or rhythm.

DYSURIA: difficult or painful urination.

E

EARLY MORNING CARE: may include bathing the hands and face, use of the bedpan or urinal, oral care, and other preparations before breakfast.

ECC: emergency cardiac care—refers to CPR, EMS activation, early defibrillation, ACLS, and professional and community training programs.

ECCHYMOSIS: large irregularly formed hemorrhagic area of the skin that is initially blue-black, changing to greenish-brown or yellow in color; a bruise.

ECG: electrocardiogram—graphic representation of the variations in electrical potential caused by depolarization of the heart muscles.

ECG LEAD: two electrodes of opposite polarity.

EDEMA: a local or generalized condition in which there is excess fluid in the tissues. Also, an excessive amount of extracellular fluid.

EDEMATOUS: the presence of abnormally large amounts of fluid in the intercellular tissue spaces of the body.

EFFLEURAGE: long stroking motions of the hands up and down the back. Hands do not leave the skin surface. Pressure is light.

ELECTRODE: a device that adheres to the skin to detect and transmit electrical information from the heart to monitoring equipment.

ELECTROLYTE: a chemical composed of acids, bases, and salts; a compound that dissociates into ions when placed into solution and becomes a conductor of electricity.

EMBOLISM: obstruction of a blood vessel by a foreign substance or a blood clot.

EMBOLUS: a mass of undissolved matter present in a blood or lymphatic vessel carried by the blood or lymph current.

EMESIS: vomiting.

EMS: emergency medical service—personnel who dispatch emergency responders or respond at the scene of an emergency.

ENDOCARDIUM: endothelial membrane lining the inner surface and cavities of the heart.

ENDOGENOUS: organisms natural to an individual's own body.

ENDORPHINS: naturally occurring body chemicals similar to morphine but many times stronger.

ENEMA: the introduction of fluid through a tube into the lower intestinal tract.

ENTERIC PRECAUTIONS: isolation practices designed to prevent transmission of pathogens through contact with fecal matter and vomitus.

EPIDERMIS: superficial, top, or outer layer of skin.

EPITHELIUM: outer covering of the body; top layer of skin.

ERYTHEMA: a redness of the skin due to congestion or vasodilatation of capillaries or associated with rashes, infections, or allergic responses.

EVALUATE: to examine and judge; to appraise.

EVAPORATION: to convert from a liquid or solid state to a gaseous state.

EVENING CARE: H.S. care, hour of sleep care—includes oral care, partial bathing, skin care and a soothing back massage, straightening or changing the bed linen, and offering the bedpan or urinal. The client should also be assessed for the need for food, drink, or medication before sleep.

EVERSION: turning outward; movement of the foot at the ankle joint so that the sole faces outward.

EVISCERATION: protrusion of the viscera; removal of the viscera.

EXCORIATION: a breakdown or abrasion of the epidermis.

EXCRETION: elimination of products from the body.

EXOGENOUS: organisms external to an individual's own body.

EXPECTORATION: expulsion of mucus or phlegm from the throat or lungs.

EXTENSION: a movement that increases the angle between two bones, straightening a joint.

EXTERNAL FIXATION DEVICE: a metal frame with attached metal percutaneous pins that are held in place by the frame. The pins are inserted into or through a bone to maintain alignment.

EXTRAVASATION: inadvertent administration of a vesicant medication into surrounding tissue.

EXUDATE: accumulation of fluid in a cavity. Also, material obtained from a wound as the result of the inflammatory process.

F

FALSE NEGATIVE: a negative test in someone who in fact has been infected by a microorganism but for some reason has not developed antibodies.

FEBRILE: feverish, increased body temperature.

FECES: intestinal waste products consisting of bacteria and secretions of the liver, in addition to a small amount of food residue and water.

FIBRILLATION: quivering, involuntary contraction of individual muscle fibers.

FIBROTIC: pertinent to fibrosis, the formation of fibrous material.

FISSURE: a groove, slit, or natural division; an ulcer or cracklike sore.

FISTULA: an abnormal tubelike passage from a normal cavity or tube to a free surface or another cavity.

FLATULENCE: excessive gas in the stomach and intestines.

FLEXION: a movement that decreases the angle between two bones; the act of bending a joint. Also, the act or condition of being bent.

FLOSS: a waxed or unwaxed tape or thread used to clean between teeth.

FLOWSHEETS: forms on which client data is recorded or graphed to show patterns or alterations in findings.

FOCUS CHARTING: charting on one "focus" area or one problem. Uses data, action, response (DAR) format.

FOLEY CATHETER: a type of indwelling tube that is inserted through the urethra into the bladder to provide continuous urinary drainage.

FOOTDROP: a falling or dragging of the foot from paralysis of the flexors of the ankle or peroneal nerve injury.

FOWLER'S POSITION: head of bed is at a 45° angle; client's knees may or may not be flexed.

FRACTURE: any break or crack in a bone.

FULL SHEETS: regular full-length flat sheets that can be used as top or bottom sheets.

FUNGUS: a vegetable cellular organism that subsists on organic matter.

G

GASTRO-: prefix that denotes the stomach.

GASTROINTESTINAL: having to do with the stomach and intestines.

GAVAGE: introduction of nourishment into the stomach by mechanical means.

GENERIC: common or general name for a drug as opposed to a brand name.

GENITOURINARY: pertaining to the genital and urinary systems.

GRANULATION: formation of granules; fleshy projections formed on the surface of a gaping wound that is not healing by the normal joining together of skin edges.

GRAVITY: the force that pulls objects toward the earth's surface.

GUAIAC: test for blood in stool.

H

HEMATURIA: the presence of blood in the urine.

HEMO-: prefix meaning blood.

HEMORRHAGE: abnormal internal or external escape of blood from the vessels.

HEMOTHORAX: accumulation of blood within the pleural sac, creating positive pressure in the intrapleural space.

HERNIA: the protrusion or projection of an organ or part of an organ through the wall of the cavity that normally contains it.

HIGH FOWLER'S POSITION: head of bed is at a 60° angle; often used to achieve maximum chest expansion.

HOLISTIC: the philosophy that an individual must be cared for as a whole rather than a sum of parts.

HOMEOSTASIS: an internal state of equilibrium or balance.

HOST: an animal or person on which or within which microorganisms live.

HOYER LIFT: a mechanical device that enables one person to safely transfer a client from bed to chair.

HUMORAL IMMUNITY: acquired immunity in which the circulating antibody is predominant.

HYDRATION: the chemical combination of a substance with water.

HYDROMETER: instrument used to determine the specific gravity of urine.

HYGIENE: study of health and observance of rules pertinent to health.

HYPEREMIA: influx of blood into an area causing redness to the skin.

HYPEREXTENSION: continuation of extension beyond the anatomic position, as in bending the head backward.

HYPERGLYCEMIA: condition characterized by an increase in blood sugar levels.

HYPERPNEA: abnormal, increased respiratory rate with deeper breathing.

HYPERTHERMIA: a body temperature much higher than the normal range.

HYPERTONIC: a solution having a higher osmotic pressure or tonicity than a solution to which it is compared.

HYPERVENTILATION: abnormally deep breathing that results in a decrease in P_{CO_2} (respiratory alkalosis).

HYPERVOLEMIA: abnormal increase in the volume of circulating body fluid.

HYPOALLERGENIC: deemed to cause very little, if any, allergic response.

HYPOGLYCEMIA: condition characterized by a deficiency of sugar or glucose in the blood.

HYPOTENSION: decrease of systolic blood pressure below normal.

HYPOTHALAMUS: the part of the brain that lies below the thalamus; it maintains or regulates body temperature, certain metabolic processes, and other autonomic activities.

HYPOTHERMIA: a body temperature below the average normal range.

HYPOVENTILATION: reduced rate and depth of breathing resulting in retention of carbon dioxide (respiratory acidosis).

HYPOVOLEMIA: diminished circulating blood volume.

HYPOXEMIA: insufficient oxygenation of the blood (decreased P_{O_2}).

I

IDENTABAND: a band, usually worn on a client's wrist, with the client's name and medical record number.

ILEOSTOMY: an artificially created opening from the ileum to the abdominal surface for the elimination of wastes.

IMMOBILIZE: to render a part or limb immovable.

IMMUNOSUPPRESSIVE: acting to suppress the body's natural immune response to an antigen.

IMPACTION: condition of being tightly wedged into a place, as of feces in the bowel.

INCIDENT REPORT: recording of an unusual happening or event that could affect client or staff safety; also commonly referred to as unusual occurrences.

INCISION: a cut made with a knife.

INCONTINENT: unable to retain urine or feces through loss of sphincter control.

INCONTINENT PADS: large, disposable pads that can be placed under the buttocks area, head, drains, or any place where excess moisture or fluid may collect on the bed.

INCURVATE: curved, especially inward.

INFECTION: establishment of a disease process that involves invasion of the body tissue by a pathogenic agent (microorganism or virus) that may multiply and produce effects that are injurious, and the reaction of the tissues to the agent's presence or the toxins generated by it.

INFILTRATION: inadvertent administration of a nonvesicant medication into surrounding tissue.

INFLAMMATION: swelling, pain, heat, and redness of tissue.

INFLAMMATORY PROCESS: localized response when injury or destruction of tissue has occurred; destroys, wards off, or dilutes the causative agent or the injured tissue.

INFUSION: a liquid substance introduced into the body via a vein for therapeutic purposes.

INSPECTION: the process of examining the surface of the body and its movements utilizing the visual, auditory, and olfactory senses to gather information.

INTERVENTION: one or more actions taken in order to modify an effect.

INTRAMUSCULAR: within the muscle area rich in blood vessels and nerves.

INTUBATION: inserting a tube into a body opening, as into the trachea.

INVASIVE: involving puncturing or incising the skin for insertion of a tube or instrument into the body.

INVERSION: turning inward; movement of the foot at the ankle joint so that the sole faces inward.

IRRIGATE: to rinse or wash out with a fluid.

IRRIGATION: the flushing of a tube, canal, or area with solution.

ISCHEMIA: decreased, insufficient blood supply to body area. Also, local and temporary tissue hypoxia due to obstruction of the circulation.

ISOLATION: limitation of movement and social contacts of a client; used especially with clients who have communicable diseases to prevent the spread of an infectious agent.

ISOLATION TECHNIQUE: practices designed to prevent the transmission of communicable diseases.

J

JAUNDICE: yellowish appearance caused by deposition of bile pigment in the skin.

JEJUNOSTOMY: surgical creation of an opening into the jejunum.

JOINT: the portion of the body where two or more bones join together.

K

KARDEX: a system of cards that contain pertinent medical information about clients.

KOROTKOFF SOUNDS: low-frequency sounds that are regarded by the American Heart Association as the best index of blood pressure in an adult.

KUSSMAUL RESPIRATIONS: deep, gasping breathing. An attempt to blow off carbon dioxide as respiratory compensation for metabolic acidosis (e.g., diabetic ketoacidosis).

L

LABIA: the lips of the vulva.

LARGE, BOUNDING PULSE: felt as a slapping against the fingers because of the rapid upstroke and quick downstroke.

LAVAGE: to wash out.

LAXATIVE: a mild-acting drug to induce emptying of the intestinal tract.

LEAD: record of electrical activity of the heart sensed by electrodes of opposite polarity placed on the skin.

LESION: an injury, wound, or area of broken skin; a single infected patch in a skin disease.

LIPIDS: emulsion containing fats used to correct fatty acid deficiencies via parenteral nutrition.

M

MAGNETIC RESONANCE IMAGING: MRI—a noninvasive test that uses a magnetic field with radio frequency waves to produce cross-sectional images of the body.

MALNUTRITION: a condition characterized by a lack of necessary food substances or improper absorption and distribution of food substances in the body.

MARROW: soft tissue that is contained in the compact bone hollow.

METABOLISM: the sum of all physical and chemical changes that take place within an organism; all energy and material transformations that occur within living cells.

MICROORGANISM: a minute living body such as a bacterium or protozoon not perceptible to the naked eye.

MINERALS: inorganic elements or compounds.

MOBILITY: state or quality of being mobile; facility of movement.

MUCOSA: mucous membrane lining passages and cavities communicating with the air.

MUSCULO-: prefix pertaining to muscles.

MYCOTIC: fungal infection on nails.

MYOCARDIUM: the middle muscle layer of the walls of the heart.

N

NARCOTIC: a controlled substance that depresses the central nervous system, thus relieving pain and producing sedation.

NARES: the nostrils.

NAUSEA: a feeling of sickness accompanied by the urge to vomit.

NECROSIS: cellular death. Also, death of areas of tissue or bone caused by enzymatic action or lack of circulation.

NECROTIC: affected by death of a portion of tissue.

NEURO-: prefix pertaining to nerves.

NOCTURIA: excessive urination during the night.

NONCOMPLIANCE: failure or refusal to comply or go along with something.

NOSOCOMIAL INFECTION: an infection acquired while in the hospital that was not present or incubating at the time of admission.

NPO: nothing by mouth.

NURSING PROCESS: a set of actions that includes assessment, planning, intervention, and evaluation.

NUTRIENT: nourishing item that supplies the body with necessary elements.

O

OBSTIPATION: the act or condition of obstructing; extreme constipation due to obstruction.

OCCULT BLOOD: blood in minute quantities, can be recognized only by microscopic examination or by chemical means.

OCCUPIED BED: the client remains in the bed while it is being made.

OLIGURIA: the diminished production of urine by the kidneys.

OPPORTUNISTIC INFECTIONS: illness or diseases that would not be a threat to anyone whose immune system is functioning normally, but may be responsible for death.

ORAL: concerning the mouth.

ORTHOSTATIC: concerning an erect or standing position.

ORTHOSTATIC HYPOTENSION: blood pressure that falls upon standing.

OSTEOBLASTS: immature cells that on maturation play a role in bone production.

OSTOMY: a surgically formed artificial opening that serves as an exit site for the bowel or intestine.

P

PAIN: a sensation in which a person experiences discomfort, distress, or suffering.

PALLOR: paleness; absence of skin coloration; loss of reddish hue due to superficial vasoconstriction produced by sympathetic stimulation.

PALPATE: to examine by touch; to feel.

PALPATION: Using touch to gather information about temperature, turgor, texture, moisture, vibration, and shape.

PALPITATION: rapid, violent, or throbbing pulsation, as an abnormally rapid, throbbing, or fluttering heart.

PARALYSIS: temporary or permanent loss of function, especially loss of sensation or voluntary motion.

PARESTHESIA: pertains to an abnormal sensation.

PARTIAL CARE: the client performs as much of his or her own care as possible. The nurse completes the remaining care.

PATENCY: the state of being freely open.

PATHOGEN: disease-producing organism.

PEDICULOSIS: infestation of lice.

PEG: percutaneous endoscopic gastrostomy.

PEJ: percutaneous endoscopic jejunostomy.

PERCUSSION: the art of striking one object with another to create sound so the location, size, and density of underlying tissues can be assessed.

PERFUSION: passing of fluid through spaces.

PERI-: prefix meaning around or about.

PERINEUM: the external region between the vulva and anus in a female or between the scrotum and anus in a male.

PERIPHERAL: pertinent to the periphery, away from the central structure.

PERIPHERAL VASCULAR DISEASE: indicates diseases of the arteries and veins of the extremities, especially those conditions that interfere with adequate flow of blood.

PERIPHERY: outer part or surface of a body.

PERISTALSIS: a progressive wavelike movement that occurs involuntarily in hollow tubes in the body, especially the alimentary tract.

PETRISSAGE: pinching of the skin, subcutaneous tissue, and muscle as you move up and down the client's back.

PHLEBITIS: inflammation of a vein.

PHLEBOTOMY: obtaining a blood specimen from a peripheral vein.

PILOERECTION: hair standing on end when heat production is stimulated through vasoconstriction.

PLANTARFLEXION: extension of the foot at the ankle joint; the foot and toes are turned downward toward the sole of the foot, as in standing on tiptoe.

PLAQUE: a patch on the skin, a mucous surface, or vascular endothelium.

PLEURA: two-layer sac that surrounds the lungs and maintains negative pressure (compared to atmospheric pressure) to support lung inflation.

PLEURAL FRICTION RUB: dry, grating breath sounds heard on both inspiration and expiration.

PNEUMOTHORAX: accumulation of air within the pleural sac, creating positive pressure in the intrapleural space resulting in the lung collapsing.

POLYURIA: the excessive production and elimination of urine.

POMR: problem-oriented medical record—a client record that is organized according to the person's specific health problems.

POSTURE: attitude or position of body.

PRELOAD: ventricular filling pressure.

PREMATURE BEATS: a pacemaker outside the sinus node fires earlier than the sinus node, the normal pacemaker of the heart. The stroke volume may be less because the ventricles do not have time to fill. This condition causes a pause in rhythm, which may result in a pulse deficit.

PRESSURE POINT: area for exerting pressure to control bleeding; an area of skin that can become irritated with pressure, especially over bony prominences.

PRESSURE ULCER: skin changes that generally occur over bony prominences of the heels, sacrum, hip, and shoulder. Also, a synonym for bedsore or pressure sore area of cellular necrosis due to decreased circulation.

PRONATION: rotation of the forearm so that the palm faces backward or downward; movement of the whole body so that the face and abdomen are downward.

PRONE: lying horizontal with face downward.

PROSTHESIS: replacement of a part by an artificial substitute.

PROTECTIVE ISOLATION: practices designed to protect a highly susceptible person from contagious diseases; reverse isolation.

PROTEIN: substance that contains amino acids essential for growth and repair of tissues.

PROTOCOL: description of steps taken in exact order.

PROXIMAL: nearest the point of attachment or reference point.

PULL SHEETS: sheets placed across the shoulder-to-knee area of the bed. The sides are not tucked under the mattress. The sheet is kept wrinkle-free and folded under the client. Pull sheets are used to lift the client in the bed.

PULSE: the rhythmic dilation of an artery caused by contraction of the heart.

PULSE DEFICIT: occurs when the heart rate counted at the apex by auscultation is greater than the heart rate counted by palpation of the radial pulse. The pulse wave is not transmitted to the periphery to produce a palpable radial pulse.

PULSUS ALTERNANS: rhythm is regular but amplitude alternates from beat to beat.

PULSUS PARADOXUS: detected by blood pressure measurement. The disappearance of Korotkoff sounds during the inspiration phase of breathing with sounds appearing throughout the respiratory cycle (during inspiration and exhalation) at a pressure 10 mm Hg lower than heard during exhalation alone.

PURPURA: hemorrhage into the skin, mucous membranes, internal organs, and other tissues that causes a reddish-purple area.

PURULENT: containing pus, or caused by pus.

PUS: an inflammation product containing leukocytes and exudate.

PYROGEN: any substance that produces fever.

PYURIA: the presence of pus in the urine.

R

RADIATION: transfer of energy (heat) in the form of waves.

REFERRED PAIN: pain felt in a part removed from its point of origin.

REFLUX: a return of or backward flow.

REPOLARIZATION: development of negative intracellular electrical charge caused by the release of potassium from the cell.

REPORT: to give an account of something that has been seen, heard, done, or considered.

RESTORATIVE: promoting a return to health.

REVERSE TRENDELENBURG'S POSITION: mattress remains unbent, but head of bed is raised and foot is lowered.

RHONCHI: rumbling breath sounds heard on expiration.

ROTATION: movement of a bone around its own axis, as in moving the head to indicate "no" or turning the palm of the hand up and then down.

RUSSELL'S TRACTION: type of skeletal traction used to treat fractures of the shaft of the femur.

S

SCLEROSIS: hardening or induration of an organ or tissue due to excessive growth of fibrous tissue.

SECOND-INTENTION HEALING: second stage in wound healing in which granulation occurs.

SEDIMENT: a substance settling at the bottom of a liquid.

SEMI-FOWLER'S POSITION: head of bed is at a 30° angle; often used for clients with cardiac and respiratory problems.

SEPSIS: condition resulting from the presence of pathogenic bacteria and its poisonous products in the bloodstream. Also, a pathologic state, usually febrile.

SEPTIC: pertinent to pathologic organisms or their toxins.

SEPTICEMIA: presence of pathologic bacteria in the blood.

SHEARING FORCE: layers of skin moving on each other.

SHIVERING: trembling of the body, usually in response to coolness. It is the result of reflex action coordinated by the hypothalamus.

SHIVERING THERMOGENESIS: production of body heat by shivering or muscle contraction (tremors).

SHOCK: state of inadequate tissue perfusion resulting from circulatory failure, precipitated by many factors and identified by various signs and symptoms. Also, a term used to designate a clinical syndrome with varying degrees of disturbances of oxygen supply to the tissues and return to the heart.

SINUS ARRHYTHMIA: the heart rate accelerates with inspiration and slows with expiration. Common in children and young adults.

SITZ BATH: bath to sit in with water above the hips.

SMALL, WEAK PULSE: pulse pressure is diminished. It is smooth and rounded but is felt as a gradual upstroke and prolonged downstroke. It is commonly seen in conditions resulting in decreased cardiac output, such as heart failure and shock, and with obstruction to left ventricular ejection, such as aortic stenosis.

SOAPIE: nursing notes similar to SOAP with additional data—Implementation and Evaluation.

SOAP NOTES: nursing notes organized consistently by what the client feels Subjectively; what the nurse observes Objectively; how the nurse Assesses the situation; and what the nurse Plans.

SONOROUS: loud breathing.

SOURCE-ORIENTED CHARTING: information in the chart is organized according to its source, for example, physician's progress notes, nurses' notes.

SPECIFIC GRAVITY: weight of a substance compared with an equal volume of water. The specific gravity of water is 1.000.

SPHYGMOMANOMETER: instrument for indirectly determining arterial blood pressure.

SPRAIN: injury caused by wrenching or twisting of a joint that results in tearing or stretching of the associated ligaments.

STAMINA: constitutional energy; strength; endurance.

STERILE: free from any living microorganisms.

STERTOROUS: loud, noisy breathing.

STOMA: an artificially created opening between two passages or between a passage and the body surface.

STOOL: waste matter discharged from the bowels.

STRAIN: injury caused by excessive force or stretching of muscles or tendons around the joint.

SUBCUTANEOUS: third layer of tissue that contains fat, few blood vessels, and nerves.

SUBLINGUAL: under the tongue.

SUPINATION: rotation of forearm so that the palm faces forward or upward; movement of the whole body so that the face and abdomen are oriented upward.

SUPPOSITORY: cone-shaped mass of solid medicated substance for introduction into the rectum or vagina, where it dissolves and is absorbed.

SURGICAL ASEPSIS: practice to keep area free from microorganisms, as by a surgical scrub.

SYNCOPE: fainting; transient loss of consciousness due to inadequate blood flow to the brain.

SYSTEMIC: pertinent to the whole body rather than to one of its parts.

SYSTEMS CHARTING: charting or documentation relative to the assessment data obtained during the physical assessment of the client.

T

TACHY-: prefix meaning fast.

TACHYCARDIA: abnormal rapidity of heart action; above 100 BPM.

TACHYPNEA: respiratory rate increased above 24 breaths per minute.

TAPOTEMENT: alternate striking of fleshy part of hands on client's back as you move up and down the back.

TERTIARY HEALING: using open method of wound healing; allows granulation to occur.

THERAPEUTIC: having medicinal or healing properties; a healing agent.

THERMOGENESIS: heat production by the body.

THERMOREGULATION: the body's physiological function of heat regulation to maintain a constant internal body temperature.

THOMAS SPLINT: skeletal traction used for long-term immobilization of fractures.

TINNITUS: subjective ringing in the ear.

TONICITY: the state of tissue tone or tension; the effective osmotic pressure equivalent.

TOPICAL: pertinent to a particular area; local.

TRACHEOSTOMY: an opening through the neck to establish a route for passage of air (airway) into the lungs.

TRACTION: process of drawing or pulling, often by weights, to keep the body or parts in proper alignment.

TRANSFUSION: injection of blood or a blood component into the blood vessels of a person.

TRAUMA: a physical injury or wound caused by external force or violence; an emotional or psychologic shock that may produce disordered feelings or behavior.

TRENDELENBURG'S POSITION: mattress remains unbent but the head of the bed is lowered and the foot is raised. "Shock blocks" may be used under the feet of the bed to achieve this position.

TROCHANTER: either of the two bony prominences below the neck of the femur.

TUMOR: uncontrolled new growth or tissue forming an abnormal mass that performs no physiologic function.

U

ULCER: an open sore or lesion of the skin or mucous membrane of the body.

UNOCCUPIED BED: the client is out of the bed while it is being made.

UREMIA: toxic condition associated with end-stage renal disease and the retention of nitrogenous substances in the blood.

URETHRA: canal for the discharge of urine extending from the bladder to outside the body.

URINARY DIVERSION: an interruption in normal flow of urine through the urinary system by surgical intervention.

UTI: urinary tract infection—an infection of the urinary tract, including all or part of the organs and ducts participating in the secretion and elimination of urine.

V

VALIDATE: to substantiate or verify.

VASCULAR: pertinent to or composed of blood vessels.

VASO-: prefix meaning vessel, as a blood vessel.

VASOCONSTRICTION: a narrowing or constriction of the blood vessels and stimulation of heat production.

VASODILATION: dilation of blood vessels and the inhibition of heat production.

VASODILATOR: an agent that causes blood vessels to dilate.

VASOMOTOR: pertaining to nerves having muscular control of the blood vessel walls.

VASOPRESSOR: causes contraction of the muscular tissue of the arteries and veins.

VASOSPASM: constriction of a vessel due to spasm.

VENOUS: pertaining to the veins; unoxygenated blood.

VENTRICULAR FIBRILLATION: lethal arrhythmia with no cardiac output.

VERTIGO: sensation of moving or having objects around you move when they are actually still, due to a disturbance of balance.

VESICANT: medication that causes blisters and tissue injury when it escapes into surrounding tissue.

VESICULAR BREATH SOUNDS: soft, breezy sounds; heard over the peripheral lung areas.

VIRUS: minute, parasitic organism that depends on nutrients inside cells for its metabolic and reproductive needs. These organisms cause a variety of infectious diseases and stimulate host antibodies. Unlike a bacteria, viruses are unable to survive for long periods on their own and are not affected by antibodies.

VITAMINS: a group of organic substances essential for life.

VOID: to urinate.

W

WHEEZES: high-pitched musical breath sounds; heard during both inspiration and expiration. Caused by airway spasm, retained secretions, or other obstruction.

WOUND DEHISCENCE: the separation of layers of a surgical wound.

WOUND EVISCERATION: protrusion of the internal viscera or organs through an opened incisional site.

X

XIPHOID: pointed cartilage connected to the lower sternum.

BIBLIOGRAPHY

Abrams, A. C., (1991). *Clinical Drug Therapy: Rationales for Nursing Practice* (3rd ed.). Philadelphia: Lippincott.

Abrutyn, E., Goldmann, D. A., Scheckler, W. E. (1998). *Saunders Infection Control Reference Service.* Philadelphia: Saunders.

AHCPR. (1992). *AHCPR Clinical Practice Guideline: Acute Pain Management.* Washington, DC: U.S. Department of Health and Human Services.

Alfaro-LeFevre, R. (1998). *Critical Thinking in Nursing: A Practical Approach* (2nd ed.). Philadelphia: Saunders.

Alpers, D., Stenson, W., Bier, D. (1995). *Manual of Nutritional Therapeutics* (3rd ed.). Boston: Little, Brown.

American Heart Association. (1997). *Advanced Cardiac Life Support, 1997–1999.* Emergency Cardiovascular Care Programs.

American Heart Association. (1997). *Basic Life Support for Healthcare Providers, 1997–1999.* Emergency Cardiovascular Care Programs.

American Nurses Association. (1973). *Standards of Nursing Practice.* Washington, DC: American Nurses Association.

American Nurses Association. (1985). *Code for Nurses with Interpretive Statements.* Washington, DC: American Nurses Association.

American Nurses Association. (1998). *Standards of Clinical Nursing Practice* (2nd ed.). Washington, DC: American Nurses Publishing, American Nurses Foundation/American Nurses Association.

American Nurses Association Press Release. http://www.needlestick.org/pressrel/2000/pr0915a.html.

Anderson, F., Maloney, J. (1994). Taking blood pressure correctly: It's no off-the-cuff matter. *Nursing94,* 24(11):34–38.

Anderson, K., Anderson, L., Glanze, W. (1997). *Mosby's Medicine, Nursing, and Allied Health Dictionary* (5th ed.). St. Louis: Mosby.

Bandman, E., Bandman, B. (1995). *Critical Thinking in Nursing* (2nd ed.). Norwalk, CT: Appleton & Lange.

Barnes, H. (1993). Alternating transparent and hydrocolloid dressings. *Nursing93,* 23(3):59–61.

Bates, B. (1999). *A Guide to Physical Examination* (7th ed.). Philadelphia: Lippincott Williams & Wilkins.

Beare, P., Myers, J. (1998). *Adult Health Nursing* (3rd ed.). St. Louis: Mosby.

Beck, V. (1998). On the lookout for impaired wound healing. *Nursing98,* 28(1) 32H:1–4.

Beyea, S., (1996). *Critical Pathways for Collaborative Nursing Care.* Menlo Park: Addison-Wesley.

Black, J., Matassarin-Jacobs, E. (1997). *Medical-Surgical Nursing: Clinical Management for Continuity of Care* (5th ed.). Philadelphia: Saunders.

Blank-Reid, C. A., Reid, P. C. (1999). Taking the tension out of traumatic pneumothoraxes. *Nursing* 29(4):41–47.

Bliss, D., Lehmann, S. (1999). Tube feeding: Administration tips. *RN* 62(8):29–31.

Bockus, S. (1993). When your patient needs tube feedings. *Nursing* 23(7):34–43.

Booker, M., Ignatavicius, D. (1996). *Infusion Therapy Techniques & Medications.* Philadelphia: W.B. Saunders.

Bowers, S. (1996). Tubes: A nurse's guide to enteral feeding devices. *MEDSURG Nursing* 5(5):313–325.

Boyce, John, M. D. It is time for action: Improving hand hygiene in hospitals. *Annals of Internal Medicine.* January 19, 1999. 130:153–155.

Boyer, M. J. (1994). *Math for Nurses: A Pocket Guide to Dosage Calculations and Drug Preparations* (3rd ed.). Philadelphia: Lippincott.

Braun, A. (1991). Defibrillation or cardioversion. *Nursing91,* 21(7):50–54.

Bright, L., Georgi, S. (1994). How to protect your patient from DVT. *American Journal of Nursing* 94(12):28–32.

Brody, H. (2000). The placebo response. *Journal of Family Practice* 49(7):649–654.

Brooks-Brunn, A. (1998). Validation of a predictive model for postoperative pulmonary complications. *Heart & Lung* 27(3):151–158.

Brungardt, G. (1994). Patient restraints: New guidelines for a less restrictive approach. *Geriatrics,* 49(6):43–50.

Burns, S., et al. (1998). Are frequent inner cannula changes necessary? A pilot study. *Heart & Lung* 27(1):58–62.

Business & Legal Reports, Inc. (1998). OSHA's bloodborne pathogens standard: Protecting yourself from AIDS & hepatitis B. Madison, CT.

Buttaro, M. (1994). Staying on top of transdermal drug patches. *Nursing94,* 24(11):41–44.

Calianno, C. (1996). Actionstat. Aspiration pneumonia. *Nursing* 26(10):47.

Calianno, C., Clifford, D. W., Titano, K. (1995). Oxygen therapy: Giving your patient breathing room. *Nursing* 25(12):33–39.

Camp, D., Otten, N. (1990). How to insert and remove nasogastric tubes. *Nursing* 20(9):59–64.

Campolo, S. (1997). Spontaneous pneumothorax. *American Journal of Nursing* 97(2):30.

Carroll, P. (1994). Safe suctioning. *RN Magazine,* 57(5):32–36.

Carroll, P. (1995). Chest tubes made easy. *RN* 58(12):46–55.

Carroll, P. (1998). Preventing nosocomial pneumonia. *RN* 61(6):44–47.

Catalano, J. (1993). *Guide to ECG Analysis.* Philadelphia: Lippincott Williams & Wilkins.

CDC National Prevention Information Network. (1999). HIV and its transmission (White Paper, pp. 1–4). available at www.cdcnpin.org.

Chambers, C., et al. (2000). Asthma: Getting the priorities straight. *Patient Care* April 30:56–81.

Christianson, D. (1994). Caring for a patient who has an implanted venous port. *American Journal of Nursing,* 94(11):40–44.

Chulay, M., Guzzetta, C., Dossey, B. (1997). *AACN Handbook of Critical Care Nursing.* Stamford, CT: Appleton & Lange.

Church, V. (2000). Staying on guard for DVT and PE. *Nursing* 30(2):34–43.

Colizza, D. (1995). Actionstat: Dislodged chest tube. *Nursing* 25(5):41–47.

Conover, M. (1998). *Electrocardiography* (4th ed.). St. Louis: Mosby.

Corbett, J. (1996). *Laboratory Tests and Diagnostic Procedures with Nursing Diagnoses* (4th ed.). Norwalk, CT: Appleton & Lange.

Cuzzell, J. (1994). Back to basics: Test your wound assessment skills. *American Journal of Nursing,* 94(6):34–35.

Dennison, R. (1994). Making sense of hemodynamic monitoring. *American Journal of Nursing,* 94(8):24–31.

Department of Health and Human Services: CDC. Draft Guidelines for Isolation Precautions in Hospitals. Available: *Federal Register,* 59 (214) November 7, 1994.

deWit, S. (1998). *Essentials of Medical-Surgical Nursing* (4th ed.). Philadelphia: Saunders.

Doenges, M., Moorhouse, M. (1998). *Nurse's Pocket Guide: Diagnosis, Interventions, and Rationales* (6th ed.). Philadelphia: Davis.

Dracup, K. (1995). *Meltzer's Intensive Coronary Care: A Manual for Nurses* (5th ed.). Norwalk, CT: Appleton & Lange.

Ehrhardt, B. S., Graham, M. (1990). Pulse oximetry: An easy way to check oxygen saturation. *Nursing90,* 20(3):50–54.

Eisenberg, P. (1994). Gastrostomy and jejunostomy tubes. *RN Magazine,* 57(11):54–59.

Elder, A. N. (1991). Setting up and using a cardiac monitor. *Nursing 91,* 21(3):58–63.

Ellenberger, A. (1999). Starting an IV line. *Nursing* 29(3):56–59.

Ellstrom, K., DellaBella, L. (1990). Understanding your role during a code. *Nursing90,* 20(5):37–43.

Epps, C. (1996, November). The delicate business of ostomy care. *RN Magazine,* 59(11):32–36.

Epstein, C., Henning, R. (1993). Oxygen transport variables in the identification and treatment of tissue hypoxia. *Heart & Lung* 22(4):328–445.

Erickson, R. (1994). Accuracy of infrared ear thermometry and traditional temperature methods in young children. *Heart Lung,* 23(3):181–195.

Ernst, D. (1995). Flawless phlebotomy: Becoming a great collector. *Nursing95,* 25(10):54–57.

Ernst, D. (1999). Reduce your risk when you draw blood. *RN* 62(12):65–68.

Erwin-Toth, P. (1995). Wound care: Selecting the right dressing. *American Journal of Nursing,* 95(2):46–51.

Faller, N., Lawrence, K. (1993). Comparing low-profile gastrostomy tubes. *Nursing* 23(12):46–48.

Fater, K. (1995). Determining nasoenteral feeding tube placement. *MEDSURG Nursing* 4(1):27–32.

Fenstermacher, K. (1998). *Dysrhythmia Recognition and Management.* Philadelphia: Saunders.

Finkelstein, L. (1996). Sputum testing for TB. *American Journal of Nursing* 96(2):14.

Fischbach, F. (1996). *A Manual of Laboratory and Diagnostic Tests* (5th ed.). Philadelphia: Lippincott Williams & Wilkins.

Fredrickson, L. (1997). *MiniMed Certified Pump Trainer Manual.* Sylmar, CA: MiniMed, Inc.

Gahart, B. (1995). *Intravenous Medications: A Handbook for Nurses and Allied Health Professionals* (11th ed.). St. Louis: Mosby.

Gazarian, P. (1997). Teaching your patient to use a metered-dose inhaler. *Nursing97,* 27(1).

George, R., et al. (1996). *Current pulmonary and critical care medicine.* St. Louis: Mosby.

Gever, M. P. (1998). Transdermal patches. *Nursing98,* 28(5):58–59.

Green, L., Gerlach, C. J. (1994). Central lines have moved out. *RN Magazine,* 57(5):26–30.

Gritter, M. (1998). The latex threat. *American Journal of Nursing,* 98(9):26–32.

(1998). Guidelines for infection control in health care personnel. *American Journal of Infection Control* 26(3): 294–297.

(1999–2000). Guidelines for the use of parenteral and enteral nutrition in adult and pediatric patients. *American Society of Parenteral and External Nutrition.*

Hadaway, L. (1999). IV infiltration. *Nursing* 29(9):41–47.

Hambleton, N. (1994). Dealing with complications of epidural analgesia. *Nursing94,* 24(10):55–57.

Harovas, J., Anthony, H. (1993). Your guide to trouble-free transfusions. *RN Magazine,* 56(11):27–34.

Higgins, D., et al. (1997). Dysphagia in the patient with a tracheostomy. *Heart & Lung* 26(3):215–220.

Hoare, K., et al. (2000). Comparing three patient-controlled analgesia methods. *MEDSURG Nursing* 9(1):33–39.

Howland, W. (1995). Defending your patient against nosocomial pneumonia. *Nursing* 25(8):62–63.

Ignatavicius, D., Workman, M., Mishler, M. (1999). *Medical-Surgical Nursing Across the Health Care Continuum* (3rd ed.). Philadelphia: Saunders.

(2000). International Guidelines 2000 for CPR and ECC: A Consensus on Science. *Circulation* 102 (Suppl. I):I 1–370. Hagerstown, MD: Lippincott Williams & Wilkins.

(1998). Intravenous nursing. Standards of practice. Intravenous Nurses Society (practice guidelines). *Journal of Intravenous Nursing* 21(1 Suppl.):S1–91.

Jagger, J., Perry, J. (1999). Exposure prevention, point by point. *Nursing* 29(6):32–42.

Jarvis, C. (1995). *Physical Examination and Health Assessment* (2nd ed.). Philadelphia: Saunders.

Jarvis, W. R. (1996). Selected aspects of the socioeconomic impact of nosocomial infections: Morbidity, mortality, cost, and prevention. *Infection Control and Hospital Epidemiology* 17(8):552–557.

Jensen, L., et al. (1998). Meta-analysis of arterial oxygen saturation monitoring by pulse oximetry in adults. *Nursing98* 28(6):387–408.

Jones, A., Rowe, B. (2000). Bronchopulmonary hygiene physical therapy in bronchiectasis and chronic obstructive pulmonary disease: A systematic review. *Heart & Lung* 29(2):125–135.

Jones, L., Brooks, J. (1990). The ABCs of PCA. *RN Magazine,* 53(5):54–60.

Keddington, R. (1994). Emergency cardiac care: New pediatric guidelines. *RN Magazine,* 57(5):44–51.

Keen, M. F. (1990). Get on the right track with Z-track injections. *Nursing90,* 20(8):59.

Kinney, M., Packa, D. (1996). *Andreoli's Comprehensive Cardiac Care* (8th ed.). St. Louis: Mosby.

Kinsey, G. (1995). Combating infection: Preventing contamination during enteral feedings. *Nursing* 25(3):20.

Kohn-Keeth, C. (2000). How to keep feeding tubes flowing freely. *Nursing* 30(3):58–59.

Konstantinides, N. (1993). The impact of nutrition on wound healing. *Critical Care Nursing,* 13(5):25–33.

Kozier, B., Erb, G., Olivieri, R. (1998). *Fundamentals of Nursing: Concepts, Process and Practice* (5th ed.). Redwood City, CA: Addison-Wesley.

Krasner, D. (1990). *Chronic Wound Care.* King of Prussia, PA: Health Management Publications.

Krasner, D. (1992). The 12 commandments of wound care. *Nursing92,* 22(12):34–41.

Krasner, D. (1995). Wound care: How to use the red-yellow-black system. *American Journal of Nursing,* 95(5):44–47.

Kuhn, M. (1998). *Pharmacotherapeutics: A nursing process approach* (4th ed.). Philadelphia: F. A. Davis.

Larson, E., Kretzer, E. K. (1995). Compliance with handwashing and barrier precautions. *Journal of Hospital Infection* 30(Suppl.):88–106.

Lavin, J., Enright, B. (1996). Charting with managed care in mind. *RN Magazine* 59(8):47–48.

Lazzara, D. (1999). Shocking facts about semiautomatic defibrillation. *Nursing* 29(4):55–57.

Leahy, J., Kizilay, P. (1998). *Foundations of Nursing Practice: A Nursing Process Approach.* Philadelphia: Saunders.

Lehman, C. (1998). Preventing pressure ulcers with something old and SUMPINU. *Nursing98,* 28(6) 32H:14–16.

LeMone, P., Burke, K. (2000). *Medical-Surgical Nursing: Critical Thinking in Client Care* (2nd ed.). Saddle River, NJ: Prentice Hall Health.

Lewis, S., Collier, I., Heitkemper, M. (1996). *Medical-Surgical Nursing* (4th ed.). St. Louis: Mosby.

Lewis, S. M., Collier, I. C., Heitkemper, M. (1996). *Medical-Surgical Nursing: Assessment and Management of Clinical Problems* (4th ed.). St. Louis: Mosby.

Little, C. (2000). Manual ventilation. *Nursing* 30(3):50–51.

Loan, T., Magnuson, B., Williams, S. (1998). Debunking six myths about enteral feeding. *Nursing98,* 28(8):43–48.

Lord, L. (1997). Enteral access devices. *Nursing Clinics of North America,* 32(4):685–703.

Lorenz, B. L. (1990). Are you using the right IV pump? *RN Magazine,* 53(5):31–36.

Maloney, J., et al. (2000). Systemic absorption of food dye in patient with sepsis. *The New England Journal of Medicine.* 343(14):1047–1048.

Malseed, R., Goldstein, F., Baldon, N. (1995). *Pharmacology: Drug Therapy and Nursing Considerations* (4th ed.). Philadelphia: Lippincott.

Mancini, M. (1997). Saving lives with automated external defibrillators. *Nursing97,* 27(10):42–43.

Mancini, M., Kaye, W. (1999). AEDs: Changing the way you respond to cardiac arrest. *American Journal of Nursing,* 99(5):26–30.

Markus, K. (1999). Latex and the law. *NurseWeek* 12(14):19.

Marriott, H., Conover, M. (1998). *Advanced Concepts in Arrhythmias.* St. Louis: Mosby.

Marriott, H., Conover, M. (1999). *Mastering Documentation* (2nd ed.). Springhouse, PA: Springhouse.

Masoorli, S. (1998). Managing complications of central venous access devices. *Nursing98,* 27(8):59–63.

Mathews, J. (1991). How to use an automated vital signs monitor. *Nursing91,* 21(2).

McCaffery, M., Ferrell, B. (1994). How to use the new AHCPR cancer pain guidelines. *American Journal of Nursing* 94(7):42–46.

McCaffery, M., Ferrell, B. (1994). Understanding opioids and addiction. *Nursing* 24(8):56–59.

McCance, K., Huether, S. (1998). *Pathophysiology* (3rd ed.). St. Louis: Mosby-Yearbook.

McConnell, E. (1995). Clinical do's and dont's: Putting on sterile gloves. *Nursing95,* 25(10):30.

McConnell, E. (1996). Ensuring electrical safety. *Nursing96,* 26(10):20.

McConnell, E. A. (1997). Inserting a nasogastric tube. *Nursing* 27(1):72.

McConnell, E. A. (2000). Infusing packed RBCs. *Nursing* 30(2):17.

McGaffigan, P. A. (1996). Hazards of hypoxemia: How to protect your patient from low oxygen levels. *Nursing* 26(5):41–47.

Meares, C. (1992). PICC and MLC lines: Options worth exploring. *Nursing92*, 22(10):52–55.

Mehler, E. (1994). Preparing your patient to use a fecal occult blood test. *Nursing94*, 24(5).

Mergaert, S. (1994). STOP and assess chest tubes the easy way. *Nursing* 24(2):52–53.

Metheny, N. (1998). pH, color and feeding tubes. *RN* 61(1):25–27.

Metheny, N. (2000). *Fluid and Electrolyte Balance* (4th ed.). Philadelphia: Lippincott Williams & Wilkins.

Metheny, N., et al. (1990). Effectiveness of the auscultatory method in predicting feeding tube location. *Nursing Research* 39(5):262–267.

Metheny, N., et al. (1999). pH and concentration of bilirubin in feeding tube aspirates as predictors of tube placement. *Nursing Research* 48(4):189–197.

Murphy, J., Burke, L. J. (1990). Charting by exception: a more efficient way to document. *Nursing90*, 20(5):65–69.

Newton, M., Newton, D., Fudin, J. (1992). Reviewing the "Big Three" injection routes. *Nursing92*, 22(2):34–41.

Noah, V. (1990). Preop teaching is the key to PCA success. *RN Magazine*, 53(5):60–63.

O'Brien, B., et al. (1999). G-tube site care: A practical guide. *RN* 62(2):52–56.

O'Hanlon-Nichols, T. (1996). Commonly asked questions about chest tubes. *American Journal of Nursing* 96(5):60–64.

OSHA http:/www.osha.gov/ Enforcement procedures for the occupational exposure to bloodborne pathogens standards.

OSHA http:/www.osha.gov/ Part II Recommendations for isolation precautions in hospitals.

Parkman, C., Calfee, B. (1997). Advance directives: Honoring your patient's end-of-life-wishes. *Nursing97*, 98(4):48–53.

Pasero, C., McCaffery, M. (1996). Managing postoperative pain in the elderly. *American Journal of Nursing* 96(10):39–45.

Patel, C., Koperski-Moen, K. (2000). Vacuum-assisted wound closure. *American Journal of Nursing* 100(12):45–48.

Phillips, L. (1997). *Manual of IV Therapeutics* (2nd ed.). Philadelphia: F. A. Davis.

Phipps, W., Sands, J., Marek, J. (1999). *Medical Surgical Nursing: Concepts & Clinical Practice* (6th ed.). St. Louis: Mosby.

Physicians' Desk Reference to Pharmaceutical Specialties and Biologicals (53rd ed.). (1999). Montvale: Medical Economics.

Pinderman, M. (1994). Indwelling urinary catheters: Reducing infection risks. *Nursing94*, 24(9):66–68.

Pittet, D., Mourouga, P., Perneger, T. V. (1999). Compliance with handwashing in a teaching hospital. Infection control program. *Annals of Internal Medicine* 130(2):126–130.

Pettinicchi, T. A. (1998). Troubleshooting chest tubes. *Nursing* 28(3):58–59.

Polaski, A., Tatro, P. (1996). *Luckmann's Core Principles of Medical-Surgical Nursing.* Philadelphia: Saunders.

Porth, C. (1998). *Pathophysiology Concepts of Altered Health States* (5th ed.). Philadelphia: Lippincott.

Possanza, C. (1997). Special delivery: Using a syringe pump to administer IV drugs. *Nursing97*, 27(9):43–45.

Quinn, C. A. (1994). The four A's of restraint reduction: attitude, assessment, anticipation, avoidance. *Orthopaedic Nursing*, 13(2):11–18.

Quraishi, Z. A., McGuckin, M., Blais, F. X. (1984). Duration of handwashing in intensive care units: A descriptive study. *American Journal of Infection Control* 12(2):83–87.

Riley, M. (1997). Elective cardioversion. *RN Magazine*, 60(5):27–29.

Rubenfeld, M. G., Scheffer, B. K. (1999). *Critical Thinking in Nursing: An Interactive Approach* (2nd ed.). Philadelphia: Lippincott.

Rutter, K. (1995). Actionstat! Tension pneumothorax. *Nursing* 28(12):42–46.

Sarver-Steffensen, J. (1999). When MRSA reaches into long-term care. *RN Magazine* 62(3):39–41.

Saul, L. (1991). Arrhythmia mimics. *American Journal of Nursing* 91(3):40–43.

Shelton, B. (1998). Mounting an offense against lobar pneumonia. *Nursing* 28(12):42–46.

Sieggreen, M., Maklebust, J. (1996). Managing leg ulcers. *Nursing96*, 26(12):41–46.

Sims, L., et al. (1995). *Health Assessment in Nursing.* Menlo Park: Addison-Wesley.

Smeltzer, S., Bare, B. (1996). *Brunner & Suddarth's Textbook of Medical-Surgical Nursing* (8th ed.). Philadelphia: Lippincott.

Smith, R. (1995). Underwater chest drainage: Bringing the facts to the surface. *Nursing* 25(2):60–63.

Smith, S. (2000). *Sandra Smith's Review for NCLEX-RN* (10th ed.). Upper Saddle River, NJ: Prentice Hall Health.

Smith, S., Duell, D., Martin, B. (2000). *Clinical Nursing Skills* (5th ed.). Upper Saddle River, NJ: Prentice Hall Health.

Snowberger, P. (1994). Premature ventricular contractions. *RN Magazine*, 57(10):59–61.

Springhouse Corporation. (1990). *Normal & Abnormal Heart Sounds.* Springhouse, PA: Springhouse.

Springhouse Corporation. (1994). *Illustrated Manual of Nursing Practice* (2nd ed.). Springhouse, PA: Springhouse.

Stewart, K., Murray, H. (1997). How to use crutches correctly. *Nursing97*, 27(5).

Stotts, N. (1990). Seeing red and yellow and black: The three color concepts of wound care. *Nursing90*, 20(2):59–61.

Strevy, S. (1998). Myths and facts about pain. *RN* 61(2):42–47.

Sullivan, G. (2000). Keep your charting on course. *RN Magazine* 63(5):75–59.

Swearingen, P. L. (ed.). (1996). *Photo-Atlas of Nursing Procedures* (3rd ed.). Menlo Park: Addison-Wesley.

Tasota, F., Wesmiller, S. (1994). Assessing ABGs: Maintaining the delicate balance. *Nursing94,* 24(5):34–45.

The Blue Book: Guidelines for the Control of Infectious Disease. http://hna.ffh.vic.gov.au(phb/hprot/inf_dis/bluebook/app4.htm.

Thomas-Masoorli, S. (1996). Intravenous therapy handbook. *Nursing* 26(10):48–51.

Thompson, J. et al. (1995). *Mosby's Manual of Clinical Nursing* (3rd ed.). St. Louis: Mosby.

Thompson, J. (2000). A practical guide to wound care. *RN Magazine* 63(1):48–52.

Tierney, L., et al. (eds.). (1999). *Current Medical Diagnosis and Treatment* (38th ed.). Stamford, CT: Appleton & Lange.

Trombley, J. (1996). Listen up: Don't trust tympanic thermometers. *Nursing96,* 26(2):58–59.

Turner, J., McDonald, G., Larter, N. (1994). *Handbook of Adult and Pediatric Respiratory Home Care.* St. Louis: Mosby.

US Department of Agriculture and US Department of Health and Human Services. (1992). *Food Guide Pyramid—A Guide to Daily Food Choices.* Washington, DC: USDA/HNIS.

Urdang, L., (ed.). (1995). *Mosby's Medical and Nursing and Allied Health Dictionary and Data Base.* St. Louis: Mosby.

Veenstra, D. L., et al. (1999). Efficacy of antiseptic impregnated central venous catheters in preventing catheter related bloodstream infection. *JAMA,* 281(3):261.

Viall, C. (1995). Taking the mystery out of TPN, Part I. *Nursing95,* 25(4):34–41.

Viall, C. (1995). Taking the mystery out of TPN, Part II. *Nursing95,* 25(5):57–59.

Weber, J. (1997). *Nurses' Handbook of Health Assessment* (3rd ed.). Philadelphia: Lippincott Williams & Wilkins.

Weil, M., Tang, W. (2000). *CPR: Resuscitation of the Arrested Heart.* Philadelphia: W.B. Saunders.

Weinstein, S. (1997). *Plumer's Principles and Practice of Intravenous Therapy.* Philadelphia: Lippincott Williams & Wilkins.

Whitman, M. (1995). The push is on: Delivering medications safely by IV bolus. *Nursing* 25(8):52–54.

Whitney, E., Cataldo, C., Rolfes, S. (1998). *Understanding Normal and Clinical Nutrition* (5th ed.). St. Paul, MN: West-Publishing.

Wilkinson, J. (1996). *Nursing Process: A Critical Thinking Approach* (2nd ed.). Redwood City, CA: Addison-Wesley.

Winslow, E. (1996). ECG lead selection shouldn't be automatic. *American Journal of Nursing* 96(1):53.

ANSWERS TO SELF-CHECK EVALUATIONS

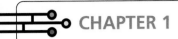 CHAPTER 1

Part 1 ■ Matching Terms

a. 2
b. 4
c. 5
d. 1
e. 3
f. 6

Part 2 ■ Multiple Choice Questions

1. b
2. a
3. d
4. c
5. c
6. c
7. d

Part 3 ■ Critical Thinking Application

1. Advance directives: living will, durable power of attorney for health care, consent to receive health service.

2. Advance directives allow clients to participate in choosing their health care providers, decide who has access to their medical records, the type of medical treatment they desire, consent or refusal of treatments, and choosing the agent who will make health care decisions if they are unable to do so. These documents should be written and signed before the client needs health care.

   - Living will: This is a statement indicating the client's wishes regarding prolonging life using life support measures, refusing or stopping medical interventions, or making decisions about his or her medical care when the client is diagnosed as having a terminal or permanent unconscious condition.

   - Durable power of attorney: This document gives the power to make health care decisions to a designated individual in the event the client is unable to make competent decisions for him- or herself.

   - Consent to receive health services: Signing this statement, the client approves to have his or her body touched by specific individuals, such as doctors, nurses, and laboratory technicians.

3. The nurse is only responsible for the consent to receive health services document. This is usually completed in the admission office of the facility; however, the nurse admitting the client should check to be sure it has been signed. The other documents are signed before they enter the hospital. If they haven't been signed, the client should be informed that hospital personnel cannot witness these documents, and therefore the client will need to have his or her relatives arrange for these documents to be signed.

CHAPTER 2

Part 1 ■ Matching Terms

a. 2, 4
b. 4, 6, 7
c. 1, 3, 4, 5
d. 3, 4, 5, 8

Part 2 ■ Multiple Choice Questions

1. a
2. b
3. b
4. a
5. d
6. a
7. a

Part 3 ■ Critical Thinking Application

Nurses' Notes

TIME	MEDICATIONS/TREATMENT	OBSERVATIONS	SIGNATURE
11:30 p	Demerol 50 mg & Phenergan IM LUOQ	c/o inc. pain	DD, SN
1:00 a		sleeping	DD, SN
3:00 a		awake. drsg. dry & intact. turns independently TCDB. unproductive cough.	DD, SN

CHAPTER 3

Part 1 ■ Matching Terms

a. 2
b. 1
c. 4
d. 5

Part 2 ■ Multiple Choice Questions

1. b
2. c
3. c
4. b
5. d
6. d

Part 3 ■ Critical Thinking Application

1. Use of medical asepsis: Handwashing is carried out whenever client care is completed. This includes providing assistance with ambulation, taking vital signs, and administering medications.

2. Gloves (do not use latex gloves if either the client or nurse has a latex allergy):

   Client 1. When checking dressings or emptying bedpan or urinal. When moving or turning only if drainage is present; otherwise it is not necessary. Clean gloves would be indicated unless a dressing change is required; then sterile gloves would be used.

   Client 2. Checking dressings, restarting the IV. Clean gloves are used to check the dressings and to start the IV.

   Client 3. None indicated, unless an IV is started before surgery. Clean gloves would be used to start the IV.

3. Both clients 1 and 2 may require the use of surgical asepsis if a dressing change needs to be completed. Surgical asepsis is necessary to prevent the spread of microorganisms to the surgical site. This requires the use of both sterile gloves and sterile supplies for the dressing change.

CHAPTER 4

Part 1 ■ Matching Terms

a. 3
b. 4
c. 1
d. 5
e. 6
f. 2

Part 2 ■ Multiple Choice Questions

1. b
2. a
3. d
4. b
5. d
6. c

Part 3 ■ Critical Thinking Application

1. Yes. Tuberculosis is spread by airborne droplets. With proper handwashing and barrier nursing protocol, the client with the abdominal resection will not be in jeopardy.

2. Client with abdominal resection: Medical asepsis will be carried out. Surgical asepsis will be used when changing the dressing. Handwashing will be before and after caring for the client. You must adhere to barrier nursing principles. It would be best to provide care for the client with the abdominal surgery first. Use of appropriate isolation equipment when caring for the TBC client is imperative.

3. Clients with TBC are to be placed in private rooms. If a private room is not available, they may be placed with another TBC client. Isolation precautions will be adhered to. Gown, respirator mask, and gloves will be used when providing care for the client. If possible, the client will be placed in a room with a directional air-flow, negative-pressure ventilation system.

4. It is best to take the vital signs on the client with TBC and complete a quick visual assessment to determine if there are any emergent problems. This requires only the use of the respirator mask. It should take no more than 10 to 15 min. Next, the abdominal surgical client should be cared for. Completing the vital signs, focus assessment, IV monitoring, and hygienic care should take about 30 to 45 min. Since the abdominal surgery client is a fresh postop client, he or she will need a pain assessment and perhaps pain medication administration. The dressing change can be done at this time or perhaps later in the shift. Much of this decision is based on the client's strength.

5. Remove gloves and gown; wash hands. After leaving the room, wash hands, remove respirator mask and place it in plastic bag, and wash hands again.

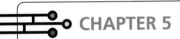

CHAPTER 5

Part 1 ■ Matching Terms

a. 2
b. 6
c. 3
d. 9
e. 8
f. 1

Part 2 ■ Multiple Choice Questions

1. d
2. a
3. d
4. b
5. c
6. d
7. a
8. b
9. d
10. c
11. a
12. a
13. a
14. c
15. d

Part 3 ■ Critical Thinking Application

1. Assessment should include overall mental status, physiologic status (current health problems), sensory status (vision, hearing), and medications. Is there a history of falls? What environmental obstacles exist that would increase risk for falls?

2. Initial action should be to measure and reorient the client to reality, then to provide a safe environment, reminding the client to call for assistance when she wants to get up. Place ¾ side rails on bed. Put bedside commode near bed and toilet every 2 hr. Place on bed-check program. All alternative actions must be tried before any form of physical restraint can be implemented.

3. Determine if all other alternatives to protect the client have been exhausted before restraints are applied. Determine if the client is a risk to self or others. Determine if the client is a risk for falling or for removing devices such as IVs or endotracheal tubes.

4. Documentation includes type of restraint applied, time applied, level of consciousness, response, resolution, and effect. The restraints are monitored every 15 min and documentation is completed after each assessment. Restraints are removed every 2 hr. Skin and circulation are assessed, range-of-motion exercises are done, and fluids and nourishment and toileting are provided.

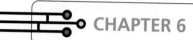 **CHAPTER 6**

Part 1 ▪ Matching Terms

a. 4
b. 5
c. 1
d. 6
e. 7
f. 3
g. 2

Part 2 ▪ Multiple Choice Questions

1. b
2. c
3. d
4. c
5. c

6. c
7. b
8. d

Part 3 ▪ Critical Thinking Application

1. First establish a nurse-client relationship with Mr. Chavez. When you feel the time is right, you could say something like, "Mr. Chavez, I notice you have not had a bath for the past 3 days. Could you tell me why you have been refusing the bath?" Depending on the answer, indicate that bathing is essential to help prevent infection at the surgical site. It may be that culturally, the client does not want a female nurse caring for him. Ask him if he would prefer a male nurse or attendant to help bathe him. Usually by day 3 patients can shower. Suggest a shower, if orders allow.

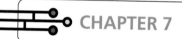 **CHAPTER 7**

Part 1 ▪ Matching Terms

a. 5
b. 4
c. 7
d. 3
e. 1
f. 6
g. 2

Part 2 ▪ Multiple Choice Questions

1. c
2. d
3. b
4. c
5. c
6. d
7. d
8. b

Part 3 ▪ Critical Thinking Application

1. It is very important that all aspects of personal care be provided for this client. He is a high-risk client for infection. Client teaching would be most important for him. It would be essential that he understand the reason for good personal hygiene. It should be determined if he is depressed or has other psychological disturbances that interfere with his ability to care for himself. It may be necessary to refer him to other agencies once he is discharged from the hospital.

2. Establish a nurse-client relationship with the client. Discuss need for hygienic care. Explain the benefits of personal hygiene care. You may need to discuss how privacy will be maintained. Discuss issue of male or female nurse providing care. The client may not want a female nurse bathing him. If necessary, only some personal hygiene tasks may need to be done at one time.

3. Perineal and oral care. Perineal care will help prevent urinary tract infections and yeast infections. The condition of the oral cavity has a direct influence on an individual's overall state of health. Dental disease leads to loss of teeth and perhaps infection of the oral cavity.

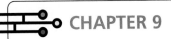

CHAPTER 8

Part 1 ■ Matching Terms

a. 3
b. 5
c. 6
d. 1
e. 2
f. 4

Part 2 ■ Multiple Choice Questions

1. c
2. c
3. c
4. d
5. b
6. a
7. d
8. c
9. d
10. c
11. a
12. d
13. c

Part 3 ■ Critical Thinking Application

1. Neurological data: possible depressed responsiveness (decreased LOC); eyes deviated to the left (possible perceptual loss on right side); flaccid extremities, right side, edematous; no reflexes on right side (no DTRs, no plantar response); inability to express self (expressive aphasia); difficulty swallowing (diminished gag reflex); flaccid right side of face, drooling; possible incontinence.

2. Nursing diagnoses are related to physical losses and the effect of immobility on all body systems. Alteration in perfusion and venous stasis; risk for aspiration; body image disturbance; bowel incontinence, constipation; self-care deficit; grieving; nutritional deficiency; physical mobility impairment; self-esteem disturbance; urinary elimination, alteration; verbal communication impairment; high risk for injury (falls, skin integrity); sensory or perceptual alteration.

3. Immediate priority concerns and planning:
   - Airway patency (potential for aspiration).
   - Circulation (control hypertension, monitor heparin drip response); venous thrombosis due to stasis and flaccidity—TEDS and PTT.
   - Decreased mobility (turn, do not leave on paralyzed side for more than 30 min), ROM.
   - Integument support—elevate edematous extremities, inspect skin, turn every 90 min, massage bony areas if not reddened.
   - Plan for airway, elevate HOB, check gag reflex, check ability to swallow with semisoft liquid food.
   - For drooling, turn to side; keep suction equipment available; perform careful oral hygiene; may be NPO and will need enteral nutrition.

CHAPTER 9

Part 1 ■ Matching Terms

a. 4
b. 3
c. 7
d. 9
e. 6
f. 10
g. 5
h. 8
i. 2
j. 1

Part 2 ■ Multiple Choice Questions

1. c
2. b
3. c
4. d
5. c
6. d
7. c
8. b
9. a
10. c

11. b

12. c

13. c

14. d

Part 3 ▪ Critical Thinking Resolution

1. Diagnosis is fluid volume deficit; hyperthermia.

2. Fever triggers baroreceptors to increase heart rate and respiration, and vasodilation to radiate heat (also triggers baroreceptors). BP initially increases, but may decrease with volume deficit due to fever.

3. Other findings in this case may include reduced urine output (more intake, less output) with increased specific gravity, decreased skin turgor (remains pinched, although difficult to assess in elderly), dry mouth and thirst, or weight loss.

4. The elderly have a diminished sense of thirst, so they may not respond to decreased volume! The elderly also have a decreased ability to sweat to reduce body temperature; volume deficit compounds this problem. The elderly may be medicated with diuretics, beta-blocking agents, or medications that decrease cardiac output or blood pressure—all of which affect the parameters evaluated and hemodynamic responses to volume changes. The restricted income of many elderly people often makes the purchase of an air conditioner prohibitive.

5. Plan of care includes monitoring hydration (I&O, daily weight, skin turgor, mucous membranes and tongue, vital signs); providing fluids (isotonic and hypotonic, PO if able, or IV); removing excess clothing and blankets (exposing skin, knees, and elbows); using evaporative cooling techniques and cool PO fluids; keeping room cool (spray with water and evaporate to cool); and dampening clothing. Teaching: Keep fluid intake regular in spite of lack of thirst; report diarrhea; control temperature over 101°F; increase fluid with electrolytes (cola, diluted broth); avoid salt tablets (these increase need for water intake); do not add extra heat (e.g., blankets) to "break fever."

6. Evaluative outcomes: more dilute urine, input equals output, decreased temperature, decreased pulse, decreased respirations, decreased BP, decreased thirst, increased skin turgor, increased weight, decreased diarrhea with treatment, increased client understanding of risk for volume deficit and preventive measures.

CHAPTER 10

Part 1 ▪ Matching Terms

a. 6

b. 5

c. 4

d. 3

e. 2

f. 1

Part 2 ▪ Multiple Choice Questions

1. b

2. a

3. b

4. b

5. a

6. c

7. d

8. c

9. d

Part 3 ▪ Critical Thinking Application

1. Assess client for clinical manifestations of a respiratory complication, urinary tract infection, or wound infection. Administer an acetaminophen agent to decrease temperature. Take vital signs in 30 min. The acetaminophen should decrease the temperature.

2. If an inflammatory process is present, manifestations may include soft tissue injury, muscle pain, or joint injury. Heat produces vasodilation, decreases pain by its relaxation effect on muscles, and increases capillary permeability and cellular metabolism.

3. Do not apply a heat treatment in excess of 110°F; burning of the skin can occur. Check the skin 5 min after the heat treatment is applied to check for skin effects. Apply petroleum jelly to sensitive skin before placing heat treatment on skin surface, to prevent burning of the skin. Remove pack after 20 to 25 min; otherwise the opposite effect of the treatment can occur.

4. Call physician for order for DuoDerm dressing. If there are no blisters, Tegaderm can be used.

CHAPTER 11

Part 1 ▪ Matching Terms

a. 1
b. 2
c. 3
d. 4
e. 5
f. 6
g. 7
h. 8
i. 9

Part 2 ▪ Multiple Choice Questions

1. b
2. d
3. b
4. c
5. d
6. c
7. d
8. a
9. b
10. b
11. b
12. d
13. a
14. c

Part 3 ▪ Critical Thinking Application

1. Full-thickness skin loss involving damage or necrosis of subcutaneous tissue that may extend down to but not through underlying facia. The ulcer presents clinically as a deep crater with or without undermining of adjacent tissue.

2. Hydrocolloid can remain in place for up to 7 days. It absorbs exudate. These dressings contain hydroactive particles that absorb exudate to form a hydrated gel over the wound. When the dressing is removed, the gel separates from the dressing, thereby protecting newly formed tissue. The dressing is impermeable to oxygen and maintains a moist environment that promotes autolysis.

3. Follow the skills outlined in the textbook for applying the hydrocolloid dressing.

4. The description matches the definition of a stage III pressure ulcer.

CHAPTER 12

Part 1 ▪ Matching Terms

a. 5
b. 7
c. 4
d. 3
e. 8
f. 2
g. 1
h. 12
i. 11
j. 6
k. 10
l. 9

Part 2 ▪ Multiple Choice Questions

1. b
2. c
3. c
4. d
5. b
6. a
7. b
8. a
9. d
10. b

Part 3 ▪ Critical Thinking Application

1. The options for solving this problem are limited. Do not try to move the client yourself. Wait until there is a male staff member available to help, or find two female staff members to assist you in moving the client. Another option is to use the Hoyer lift for moving the client. A safety belt can also be used. A physical therapist may also be able to assist you. In many facilities, a physical therapist is assigned to nursing units. The role of the physical therapist in this instance is to ambulate and move clients. You might even suggest that the hospital provide a pool of two strong male staff members to move clients in and out of bed, especially at mealtimes.

2. This client may experience difficulty positioning him- or herself in bed; potential pressure ulcer formation; and possibly respiratory problems.

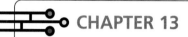

CHAPTER 13

Part 1 ▪ Matching Terms

a. 2
b. 6
c. 5
d. 1
e. 8
f. 3
g. 7
h. 4

Part 2 ▪ Multiple Choice Questions

1. c
2. b
3. d
4. b
5. b
6. d
7. a
8. d
9. a
10. c
11. c

Part 3 ▪ Critical Thinking Application

1. The general health and the projected health of the client is not good for the following reasons. Early ambulation decreases hospitalization time and prevents complications such as paralytic ileus and thrombophlebitis. This client may not recover quickly and may potentially develop complications. The sooner the client begins to ambulate after being on bedrest, the more easily she will regain her strength.
   - Exercise improves physical and mental well-being.
   - Ambulation increases muscle strength and joint mobility; without movement, the client will lose muscle strength and may become immobile.
   - Exercise also increases respiratory exchange, gastrointestinal muscle tone, and circulation; refusal to ambulate will cause all of these systems to not function to their optimum level.

2. Explain the danger of a sedentary existence, especially following surgery, so the client understands the consequences of this behavior.

3. Formulate a plan of care involving the client. Determine how exercises will be increased throughout the hospital stay. Plan how this exercise regimen can be maintained at home. Examples could include walking around the yard several times a day, walking the dog around the block, swimming daily if a pool is accessible, and doing stretching exercises.

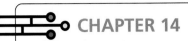

CHAPTER 14

Part 1 ▪ Matching Terms

a. 4
b. 7
c. 6
d. 3
e. 2
f. 1
g. 5

Part 2 ▪ Multiple Choice Questions

1. d
2. b
3. a
4. c
5. a
6. b
7. b
8. d
9. d
10. a

Part 3 ▪ Critical Thinking Applications

1. Instruct the client in postoperative routine to prevent complications of infection and joint dislocation. This includes use of abductor pillows, positioning and turning in bed, ambulation, and exercises. To prevent infection, discuss the antibiotics and keeping the dressings dry.

2. Client care plan goals:
   - Short-term goal: to ambulate by day two with aid of walker
   - Long-term goal: to maintain hip in abduction and external rotation to prevent postoperative complications

   Nursing diagnosis:
   - Injury, high risk for
   - Infection, high risk for
   - Role performance, alteration

   Nursing interventions:
   - Injury, high risk for: Use abductor pillow to maintain right hip in abduction and external rotation; do not flex hip, do not bend over.
   - Infection, high risk for: Keep hip dressings dry and intact; place absorbent pads over hip dressing when using bedpan.
   - Role performance, alteration: Provide opportunities for client to make decisions and encourage client to maintain personal responsibilities as able.

3. Safety issues in this case would be maintaining the hip in alignment and preventing infection. To achieve these goals, use abductor splint and walker and maintain sterility with dressing changes.

4. Instruct client to notify physician if abnormal signs and symptoms appear, such as fever, pain, or increased drainage. Provide instruction on medications, dressing changes, and ambulation. Ensure that client has the necessary services for home care. This includes referral to home health agency, equipment rental, and physician follow-up appointment.

CHAPTER 15

Part 1 ▪ Matching Terms

a. 5
b. 7
c. 6
d. 1
e. 4
f. 8
g. 3
h. 10
i. 2
j. 9

Part 2 ▪ Multiple Choice Questions

1. d
2. b
3. c
4. d
5. d

6. b
7. a
8. c
9. b
10. d
11. b
12. a
13. b
14. a

Part 3 ■ Critical Thinking Application

1. The problem-solving team would include the nurse, speech therapist, physical therapist, occupational therapist, physician, and pharmacist. Collaborate with the physician to order a swallow evaluation. The speech therapist can evaluate the client by performing a modified barium swallow evaluation to determine the best approaches to management of dysphagia.

2. Thickened pureed liquids or very soft foods are easier for the stroke client to swallow than liquids. The client should be placed in an upright sitting position, leaning toward the strong side, with head flexed forward to help lower the risk of aspiration. These instructions should be entered into the plan of care and posted at the client's bedside.

3. Since the Inderal LA 80-mg capsule cannot be opened and its contents mixed with soft food, the dosage could be changed to 20-mg tablets, which can be crushed and mixed with pudding or jelly. In addition, this is more cost effective.

4. To achieve the intended 24-hr coverage of the 80-mg LA dose, the 20-mg tablets should be administered every 6 hr around the clock (e.g., 0600, 1200, 1800, 2400) rather than q.i.d. (within a 12-hr period). After collaborating with the pharmacist, the nurse alters the MAR to indicate the medication, dosage change, and altered hours for administration, also noting to crush the tablets and administer with soft food.

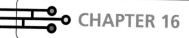

CHAPTER 16

Part 1 ■ Matching Terms

a. 7
b. 10
c. 3
d. 6
e. 8
f. 5
g. 4
h. 1
i. 2
j. 9

Part 2 ■ Multiple Choice Questions

1. b
2. c
3. b
4. c
5. d
6. a
7. d
8. c
9. d
10. c

11. a
12. d
13. b
14. c

Part 3 ■ Critical Thinking Application

1. Valid diagnoses for this situation include: ineffective individual coping, adjustment impairment, health-seeking behaviors, ineffective management of therapeutic regimen, and alteration in role performance.

2. Nancy is in the stage of adolescence where peer group acceptance is very important. Anything that makes her different can be threatening, so denial of her condition and ineffective coping may be present. These may be dealt with by suggesting that Nancy join a support group for teen diabetics or see a private counselor. In addition, Nancy needs specific feedback and information about the consequences of uncontrolled diabetes, both now and for her future.

3. Insulin absorption is quickest in the abdomen, then the arm, then the thigh. Random alteration of injection sites leads to random onset and peak action of the drug. Exercise of the injected extremity enhances absorption and hastens drug action.

4. Because Nancy "hates shots and they hurt" and she is afraid of unpredictable effects when administering into extremities (due to cheerleading activity), an excellent alternative for her is the "button infuser," or Insuflon. This is an 18-mm over-the-needle catheter that is inserted into the abdomen (similar to a Heparin lock) that is dressed and remains in place for 1 wk. Insulin injections are delivered through the transparent film in the center. The catheter site is changed weekly (only one stick per week), moving to another area on the abdomen. Extremity injections are not necessary, and insulin absorption is more constant. Nancy may experience better control (with less hassle and fear) with this alternative method of insulin administration.

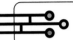 **CHAPTER 17**

Part 1 ■ Matching Terms

a. 8
b. 9
c. 7
d. 4
e. 2
f. 3
g. 5
h. 10
i. 6
j. 1

Part 2 ■ Multiple Choice Questions

1. d
2. c
3. b
4. b
5. a
6. d
7. a
8. d
9. c
10. b
11. c
12. a
13. d
14. c

Part 3 ■ Critical Thinking Application

1. If an IV is infusing properly, the site should not appear swollen or feel cool, and the client should have no subjective complaints.

2. This client displays signs of infiltration by a swollen extremity and coolness to the touch (the best indicator). Other signs might include leaking at the site and subjective tenderness.

   ■ Infiltration is the most common complication of intravenous infusion therapy. It is much more common than phlebitis.

   ■ Infiltration (infusion into tissue rather than into the vein) can occur if the cannula penetrates the vein wall, or if the catheter is in the vein wall but the penetration site does not seal, allowing fluid to escape or leak into tissue. Unfortunately, an IV delivered by pump will continue to infuse even if the fluid is infiltrating (the pump automatically increases pressure to overcome tissue resistance to infiltration). Gravity pumps may be better alarms for infiltration problems.

3. To check for infiltration, first slow the drip rate and remove infusion tubing from the pump. Lower the IV bag (if there is blood return, absolute infiltration is not likely) or place a tourniquet just above the IV insertion site to see if the infusion stops. If it does, the catheter is in the vein. If it continues to drip, the IV is going into the tissue.

   ■ Always select IV insertion sites more proximally on an extremity. There is a possibility that moving distally from an ineffective site may result in leakage into tissues from the previous site.

CHAPTER 18

Part 1 ■ Matching Terms

a. 3
b. 10
c. 2
d. 7
e. 8
f. 1
g. 4
h. 9
i. 6
j. 5

Part 2 ■ Multiple Choice Questions

1. d
2. a
3. a
4. d
5. c
6. b
7. c
8. a
9. b
10. b
11. d
12. a
13. c
14. c

Part 3 ■ Critical Thinking Application

1. Following are methods of assessing pain.
   - Assess type of pain.
     -Acute pain, of short duration, transient, lasting less than 6 mo
     -Chronic pain, lasting longer than 6 mo
     -Intractable pain, severe and constant and resistant to relief measures
   - Choose a pain intensity scale and identify the level or degree of pain the client is experiencing.
   - Assess nonverbal indicators of pain.
   - Assess client's behavioral responses to pain: depressed, angry, withdrawn, stoic or expressive.
   - Assess location, quality, intensity, onset, aggravating factors, associated factors, and alleviating factors.
2. This client would most likely use nonverbal, behavioral responses and possibly verbal responses.
3. Due to this client's medical condition, the nurse cannot depend on clear reporting of the level of pain the client is experiencing. Cognitive impairment interferes greatly with the assessment of pain.
4. This client will require frequent monitoring. Pain assessment may depend on nonverbal behaviors such as restlessness, groaning, moaning, agitation, and/or resistance. The elderly are at risk for adverse responses to pain medication and should be monitored closely.

CHAPTER 19

Part 1 ■ Matching Terms

a. 6
b. 4
c. 5
d. 2
e. 3
f. 10
g. 8
h. 7
i. 1
j. 9

Part 2 ■ Multiple Choice Questions

1. c
2. c
3. a
4. b
5. a
6. b
7. d
8. a
9. c
10. a

11. d

12. a

13. b

14. a

Part 3 ■ Critical Thinking Application

1. Small bowel obstruction causes reduced intestinal motility with resultant accumulation of gas and fluid in the small intestine. Distention of the bowel wall causes large quantities of fluid and electrolytes to move into the gut from surrounding capillaries. Fluid continues to accumulate even though the client is vomiting. Hypovolemia may result due to this extracellular fluid volume shift ("third-spacing").

2. Initial vomiting is an isotonic fluid loss, but as the client becomes hypovolemic and thirsty, water intake and continued vomiting lead to a hypotonic state (reduced serum Na). In addition, vomiting is associated with the loss of electrolytes (K, HCl, Mg). Vomiting can cause hypovolemia (low BP, fast HR) and metabolic alkalosis (high pH, high bicarb).

3. Since gastric secretions are acid (low pH), their loss results in an "oversupply" of bicarbonate buffer, a state called metabolic alkalosis (high serum bicarb). In addition, the loss of potassium causes the kidneys to excrete more hydrogen (acid), while loss of chloride causes the kidneys to produce and reabsorb more bicarbonate (base). These renal responses contribute to the state of metabolic alkalosis. In contrast to gastric fluid, intestinal fluid is alkaline. The loss of intestinal (alkaline) fluid through diarrhea or surgically induced drainage can result in metabolic acidosis (low pH, low bicarb).

4. In a state of *metabolic acidosis* (low pH and low bicarb), the respiratory center is stimulated to increase the rate and depth of breathing. Hyperventilation of volatile acid (CO_2) compensates for the relative increase in metabolic acid (actual loss of bicarb) that causes pH imbalance.

   In a state of *metabolic alkalosis* (high pH, low bicarb, low K), the kidneys must reabsorb more chloride and excrete more hydrogen ion. While the lungs should be stimulated to hypoventilate to retain volatile acid (increase the CO_2) to compensate for metabolic alkalosis, the respiratory center responds to a rise in CO_2 by stimulating breathing. Therefore, respiratory compensation of metabolic alkalosis is never effective.

5. Since *metabolic acidosis* can accompany many pathologic conditions, it is most important to identify its cause, and treatment should address that particular pathology: alkaline fluid loss (intestinal), alkaline ingestion (bicarb), or fixed metabolic acid accumulation (due to renal failure, shock, or diabetes). The administration of bicarbonate is rarely indicated, but isotonic fluid resuscitation is essential for the hypovolemic client.

   In order to correct *metabolic alkalosis* and fluid volume deficit associated with decompression of gastric secretions, the client must receive intravenous fluids that contain KCl. Supplementation of potassium chloride reduces obligatory reabsorption of bicarbonate by the kidney, thus helping to correct the alkalosis problem.

CHAPTER 20

Part 1 ■ Matching Terms

a. 4

b. 5

c. 6

d. 3

e. 2

f. 9

g. 8

h. 10

i. 1

j. 7

Part 2 ■ Multiple Choice Questions

1. b

2. a

3. b

4. c

5. d

6. c

7. d

8. c

9. a

10. c

11. b

12. c

13. d
14. b

Part 3 ▪ Critical Thinking Application

1. If the GI tract is functioning, and feeding can be delivered safely with little risk of aspiration, the oral route is preferred. Supplemental formulas may be taken by mouth. If the oral route is unsafe (e.g., dysphagia), enteral modes into the stomach or intestine are used. If the enteral route is unavailable, or the GI tract is not functioning, parenteral feeding is recommended.

2. Decisions about starting and stopping nutritional support should by made by the client, if he or she is capable. Only the client has the right to consent to or refuse medical care. If the client is unable to make decisions, an advance directive (under the Patient Self-Determination Act) or proxy (if identified) can provide decisions on the client's behalf. In the absence of this, the family usually is empowered to make decisions.

3. No treatment is intrinsically ordinary or extraordinary, and this artificial distinction should never be a basis for decision making. The focus of decision making must be on the client and the balancing of risks and benefits of treatment must be made from the client's perspective.

4. Some health care providers believe there is an ethical distinction between withholding and withdrawing a treatment; in fact, none truly exists. Certainly it is more difficult to discontinue any treatment, especially if doing so allows the client to die, but there is no legal requirement to continue any treatment once it is started.

5. Many believe that ongoing provision of nutritional support is an expression of compassion. Medical therapy, however, is not based on the many social, religious, or symbolic meanings typically associated with food, eating, and nuturing. The decision to withdraw treatment is legal and ethical, even if the client's death is associated with this, because the client's death is truly due to the underlying disease that is allowed to run its course. Food and fluid should be offered to the client when artificial feeding is discontinued, and other acts of care and comfort are continued.

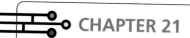

CHAPTER 21

Part 1 ▪ Matching Terms

a. 10
b. 3
c. 6
d. 7
e. 2
f. 4
g. 1
h. 9
i. 8
j. 5

Part 2 ▪ Multiple Choice Questions

1. a
2. a
3. b
4. a
5. b
6. b
7. c
8. a
9. c
10. d
11. c
12. b
13. d
14. b
15. c

Part 3 ▪ Critical Thinking Application

1. Determine if the client can empty her bladder after removal of the Foley catheter. Two hours is not a sufficient time to necessitate recatheterization.

2. Immediately catheterize the client to check for residual urine.

3. A Foley catheter may need to be reinserted. In situations such as this, it is often hospital policy to use a Foley catheter to check for residual urine. If there is a large volume of residual urine, the Foley catheter can be left in place. This prevents the need for an additional catheter insertion.

CHAPTER 22

Part 1 ■ Matching Terms

a. 8
b. 6
c. 7
d. 9
e. 2
f. 3
g. 10
h. 5
i. 1
j. 4

Part 2 ■ Multiple Choice Questions

1. b
2. b
3. b
4. c
5. d
6. b
7. c
8. d
9. d
10. b
11. b
12. c

Part 3 ■ Critical Thinking Application

1. Sit down with the patient, allow her to express her concerns, and discuss her fears and anxieties about the ostomy. Remember that this is probably the anger stage of grieving. You may need to postpone the teaching until the client is ready to listen and participate in the pouch change.
2. Assess the client's readiness to learn, including:
   ■ Environment, to determine appropriateness.
   ■ Client's emotional status and ability to listen to instructions.
   ■ Client's physical state, to determine if she has pain or other situations that could interfere with her ability to listen to instructions.
   ■ Client's knowledge base, if any, about the procedure.
3. Use the principles of client teaching that begin with assessment of the client's motivation and ability to learn.
   ■ Determine readiness to learn.
   ■ Assess client's developmental level and interact on that level.
   ■ Understand the client's expectations for the learning situation; correct misconceptions.
   ■ Identify learning needs and styles.
   ■ Determine appropriate teaching strategy.
   ■ Determine goals with client and discuss steps to meet the goals.
   ■ Determine outcome criteria.
   ■ Implement teaching strategies.
   ■ Evaluate outcome of teaching plan.

CHAPTER 23

Part 1 ■ Matching Terms

a. 4
b. 5
c. 8
d. 10
e. 9
f. 7
g. 1
h. 6
i. 3
j. 2

Part 2 ■ Multiple Choice Questions

1. a
2. b
3. c
4. c
5. d

6. a

7. c

8. a

9. a

10. c

11. a

12. b

13. a

14. d

Part 3 ▪ Critical Thinking Application

1. Low-flow oxygen therapy (2 L/min per nasal cannula) to maintain Po_2 near 60 mm Hg (Spo_2 at 90 percent) prevents pulmonary hypertension and corrects right-sided heart failure (cor pulmonale), polycythemia, weight gain, and systemic edema. It relieves client dyspnea and improves activity tolerance.

2. Oxygen is a drug and must be used according to prescription. The chronic pulmonary client who has chronically elevated Pco_2 has an elevated bicarbonate level (renal compensation, metabolic alkalosis) to help maintain a normal blood pH. This renal compensation blunts the ability of the elevated Pco_2 to stimulate the brain to maintain breathing. Instead, this client depends on a chronically low Po_2 level (around 60 mm Hg) as a breathing stimulus to the brain. Administration of higher flow of oxygen than ordered could eliminate the hypoxic stimulus to breathe and lead to CO_2 narcosis and death. While oxygen is not explosive, it supports combustion, so no spark or flame should occur near the oxygen source.

3. The client (and family) should be taught to monitor for signs of hypoxemia and respiratory failure (change in mentation, lethargy, headache), and report or seek medical evaluation. Changes in sputum production (volume, color, or character), increased cough, and other signs of respiratory infection should also be reported.

4. Expected blood gas values for this client would be Po_2 at 60 mm Hg with saturation near 90 percent and not less than 85 percent. The Pco_2 will remain elevated, as will the bicarbonate level, and the pH should remain in the low normal range.

CHAPTER 24

Part 1 ▪ Matching Terms

a. 5

b. 7

c. 10

d. 9

e. 3

f. 8

g. 1

h. 4

i. 2

j. 6

8. c

9. c

10. b

11. c

12. c

13. d

14. a

Part 2 ▪ Multiple Choice Questions

1. d

2. a

3. c

4. b

5. a

6. c

7. b

Part 3 ▪ Critical Thinking Application

1. When high alarms signal rapid ventricular activity, the nurse quickly assesses the QRS complex width. Wide complex tachycardia can be of atrial or ventricular origin. The client must be assessed physically; the nurse must immediately go directly to the client to determine cardiac function (responsiveness, pulse, respirations, blood pressure).

    If the client is responsive and experiencing no distress, and the burst of VT is brief, no treatment is indicated. Short bursts of VT are common—these episodes usually have a rate less than 150. Correction of hypoxia, pain management, or other possible causative factors should be addressed. Continued close monitoring is indicated. Any persistence or indication of client deterioration must be treated with pharmacologic or immediate electrical intervention. The physician should be notified.

For the stable client, VT may be terminated with administration of antiarrhythmic agents. If conversion to normal sinus rhythm is unsuccessful with medication and the client deteriorates, ventricular fibrillation may develop. Summon emergency medical assistance (e.g., "Code Blue") and prepare for immediate electrical cardioversion. Emergency defibrillation is indicated for pulseless VT or VF.

2. Electrocardiographic characteristics of ventricular tachycardia include wide, distorted QRS complexes with regular to slightly irregular rhythm. The rate is usually between 130 and 170 to 200 BPM. There are no identifiable P waves; therefore, a PR interval is not evident.

3. Ventricular tachycardia can emerge as a brief episode (less than 30 sec) without causing hemodynamic compromise. The client may be asymptomatic. This type of VT usually has a rate of 130 BPM. Faster VT that is sustained over 30 sec is seriously detrimental to the pumping effectiveness of the heart, resulting in hemodynamic deterioration.

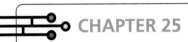

CHAPTER 25

Part 1 ■ Matching Terms

a. 10
b. 1
c. 9
d. 2
e. 4
f. 8
g. 6
h. 3
i. 5
j. 7

Part 2 ■ Multiple Choice Questions

1. d
2. b
3. b
4. c
5. c
6. b
7. a
8. a
9. d
10. a
11. b
12. d
13. c
14. c

Part 3 ■ Critical Thinking Application

1. If air exchange is adequate (i.e., the victim remains conscious, coughs forcefully, and may have wheezing) you need only to monitor at this time. If distress continues, initiate EMS support.

2. These are signs of ineffective air exchange and call for the same assistance you would render to a victim with a complete obstruction. If the airway is completely obstructed, the victim cannot speak. Ask her to clutch her neck if she is choking (universal distress signal).

3. Stand behind the victim with your arms around her chest, high up under her arms. Press the thumb side of your fist onto the middle of her sternum, grasp your fist with your other hand, and perform backward thrusts to help dislodge the object. Or lay the victim supine and kneel close to her side. Place the heel of one hand on the lower half of her sternum as you would for CPR chest compressions (avoid the xiphoid process). Thrust firmly to help dislodge the object (chest thrust maneuver).

4. The airway of any unconscious or sedated client can become obstructed as the tongue relaxes back in the pharynx. Dentures can also obstruct the airway.

   ■ In adults, obstruction due to a foreign body is most often caused by large, insufficiently chewed pieces of meat; excessive consumption of alcohol is also a risk factor for airway obstruction.

   ■ Small children develop airway obstruction with any variety of small objects, including food, especially if running or playing with objects in their mouths.

5. Airway obstruction can be prevented by sufficient cutting and chewing of food, avoiding talking while chewing or swallowing, and temperance in the use of alcohol. Children should not be allowed to run or play while eating and should not be given small, discrete foods such as peanuts, popcorn, or hard candy. Small objects or toys with small parts should be kept away from infants and toddlers. The sedated or unconscious client should be positioned on his or her side for airway maintenance.

INDEX